The Lithium Handbook

Meyer and Stahl's *Lithium Handbook* accomplishes a rare feat - a book for clinicians that is comprehensive, scientifically sophisticated, data-based and clinically wise - all at once! It can be read as an overall review or used as a reference book to explore specific questions. The sections reviewing the renal effects of lithium are particularly detailed and thoughtful. The book covers the use of lithium in all clinical areas imaginable, from bipolar disorder to depression to dementia; provides concrete recommendations in pediatric populations, geriatric populations and pregnant women. Overall, a tour de force!

Michael Gitlin, M.D.
Distinguished Professor of Clinical Psychiatry; Director, Adult Division of Psychiatry; Director, Mood Disorders Clinic, Geffen School of Medicine at UCLA

Dr. Meyer has provided a masterpiece for the field by synthesizing and translating the literature as it relates to Lithium for psychiatric and medical disorders that integrates basic and translational research with accessible clinical application; a must-have for clinicians, academics, researchers, and all persons interested in the best of care of persons living with bipolar disorder.

Roger S. McIntyre, M.D., FRCPC
Professor of Psychiatry and Pharmacology, University of Toronto, Canada

What a timely appearance of this excellent publication! This year, we observe the 60th anniversary of Geoffrey Hartigan's article, which first discovered the prophylactic activity of lithium in mood disorders. In the following years, lithium became a gold standard for preventing affective episodes in bipolar illness. Furthermore, many beneficial psychiatric properties of lithium have been established, such as the augmentation of antidepressant drugs and the great benefits of long-term treatment, including antisuicidal, neuroprotective, and antiviral effects. Yet in recent years, the art of lithium treatment has deteriorated, and the use of this valuable drug decreased, probably due to the introduction of other mood-stabilizing medications and a reluctance to employ lithium by psychiatrists, simply uninformed in this respect. And here comes Stahl's book, with its rectifying and educational message for psychiatrists. The book is bringing hope that, after its careful reading, more patients will become the beneficiaries of lithium therapy.

Janusz Rybakowski
Professor Emeritus and previous Head, Department of Adult Psychiatry, Poznan University of Medical Sciences; Corresponding member of the Polish Academy of Sciences

This is the most authoritative and comprehensive exposition of lithium to date. Lithium is the only medication in psychiatric practice that could be reasonably considered as disease-modifying, and so is worthy of a dedicated exposition of its chemistry, physiological impact, clinical efficacy and safety. Drs Meyer and Stahl deftly explain putative mechanisms of lithium action with both accessibility and nuance. This is a must have for any practitioner prescribing in the mental health space.

Manpreet Kaur Singh, MD MS
Associate Professor of Psychiatry and Behavioral Sciences; Stanford University, Stanford

The Lithium Handbook

Stahl's Handbooks

Jonathan M. Meyer

Voluntary Clinical Professor of Psychiatry,
University of California, San Diego

Stephen M. Stahl

Clinical Professor of Psychiatry and Neuroscience,
University of California, Riverside, and Adjunct Professor
of Psychiatry, University of California, San Diego

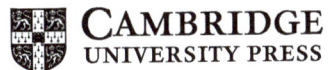
CAMBRIDGE
UNIVERSITY PRESS

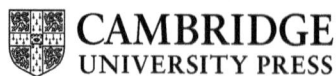

Shaftesbury Road, Cambridge CB2 8EA, United Kingdom

One Liberty Plaza, 20th Floor, New York, NY 10006, USA

477 Williamstown Road, Port Melbourne, VIC 3207, Australia

314–321, 3rd Floor, Plot 3, Splendor Forum, Jasola District Centre, New Delhi – 110025, India

103 Penang Road, #05–06/07, Visioncrest Commercial, Singapore 238467

Cambridge University Press is part of Cambridge University Press & Assessment, a department of the University of Cambridge.

We share the University's mission to contribute to society through the pursuit of education, learning and research at the highest international levels of excellence.

www.cambridge.org
Information on this title: www.cambridge.org/9781009225052

DOI: 10.1017/9781009225069

First published 2023

A catalogue record for this publication is available from the British Library

ISBN   978-1-009-22505-2   Paperback

Contents

Foreword

There is no single medication for mood disorder treatment such as lithium, which has an abundance of clinical and scientific evidence supporting its unique features but which is grossly underutilized [1]. The conclusions of recent reviews reiterate that lithium is the gold standard for long-term treatment of bipolar I disorder (BD-1) [2–4], that it is no less effective than other agents when used in rapid cycling or mixed episode BD patients [1], and that it possesses unparalleled effects on the risk for completed suicide [5, 6] and the incidence of dementia [7, 8]. Sadly, many clinicians are dissuaded from prescribing lithium due to overestimation of its risks and underestimation of its efficacy, misperceptions that are often reinforced by their peers [9]. Stoking these anxieties have been years of counterdetailing by manufacturers of anticonvulsant mood stabilizers and second generation antipsychotics (SGAs) that caused both a decline in lithium use and the loss of a shared cultural memory within the psychiatric profession about lithium's efficacy across the BD spectrum, and its generally favorable risk–benefit profile when prescribed and monitored using the latest recommendations [10, 11].

The net result is that patients suffer. As papers on naturalistic outcomes slowly appear in the literature, it has become apparent that in long-term real world usage BD-1 patients have comparatively high rates of treatment failure on SGA monotherapy compared with lithium monotherapy [12]. Certain anticonvulsants touted as potential mood stabilizers (e.g. gabapentin, oxcarbazepine, topiramate) have no maintenance data to support ongoing use in BD, and have failed to demonstrate efficacy in placebo-controlled acute mania trials [13, 14]; moreover, within-subject mirror image studies also note no anti-suicide effect during periods of valproate treatment [15]. Older BD patients suffer in a different manner when unnecessarily deprived of lithium therapy, specifically because long-term lithium use reduces dementia risk nearly 50% while non-lithium therapies exhibit no impact on dementia risk [7, 16]. Women of childbearing age also suffer greatly when decisions to routinely discontinue lithium are made based on outdated estimates of lithium related risks during pregnancy and lactation [17, 18].

Excellent papers and books have been devoted to educating clinicians about lithium [19, 20], yet there have been dramatic and rapid advances in many areas related to lithium in recent years including: revised estimates of lithium related risks during pregnancy and lactation; new data informing how one alters the frequency and type of laboratory monitoring based not on age but on estimated glomerular filtration rate (eGFR) and the presence of medical comorbidities. There are also newer understandings regarding the mechanisms and early signs of lithium's renal effects, the implementation of monitoring tools to track polyuria, and the use of amiloride and acetazolamide to manage this condition. Outside of renally focused topics, there are recent data indicating a general lack of effects on cardiac conduction, papers reporting nonsurgical options to manage hyperparathyroidism, and evidence based actions that minimize the risk of lithium toxicity from kinetically interacting medications.

In the end, the only way to combat the disconnect between lithium's efficacy and its underuse is through education. Knowledge is indeed power, and once clinicians develop a comfort level with anxiety-inducing topics, such as lithium's journey through the kidney, they are ideally situated to offer the advantages of lithium treatment without undue trepidation. The purpose of the present volume is to provide prescribers with a clinically oriented handbook that gives evidence based and rational approaches to situations commonly encountered during lithium treatment, and that dispels misguided notions regarding lithium's safety and efficacy. Meyer and Stahl have established the standard for such handbooks [21, 22], and have employed the same eye for detail in creating this comprehensive book that covers all aspects of lithium treatment, and, most importantly, leads the clinician through the reasoning process that underlies all of the ideas and recommendations. As both a researcher and a clinician, it is my hope that this handbook will serve as the cornerstone of any clinician's library on mood disorder treatment, and thereby help reverse the trend of lithium underprescribing. Lithium is not a medication to be feared but one which should be used frequently in the management of BD spectrum and other mood disorder patients. This handbook is one of many efforts to facilitate increased lithium use, and arrives at an opportune moment to support those clinicians who want to practice based on knowledge, not on fear, and thus offer their patients the most optimal care by confidently employing the gold standard for BD treatment: lithium.

Paul E. Keck, Jr., MD

Craig and Frances Lindner Professor of Psychiatry and Behavioral Neuroscience – University of Cincinnati College of Medicine

Psychiatrist in Chief, Founding President and CEO Emeritus – The Lindner Center of HOPE, Mason, Ohio

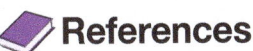 # References

1. Fountoulakis, K. N., Tohen, M. and Zarate, C. A. (2022). Lithium treatment of bipolar disorder in adults: A systematic review of randomized trials and meta-analyses. *Eur Neuropsychopharmacol*, 54, 100–115.

2. Baldessarini, R. J., Tondo, L. and Vazquez, G. H. (2019). Pharmacological treatment of adult bipolar disorder. *Mol Psychiatry*, 24, 198–217.

3. McIntyre, R. S., Berk, M., Brietzke, E., et al. (2020). Bipolar disorders. *Lancet*, 396, 1841–1856.

4. Verdolini, N., Hidalgo-Mazzei, D., Del Matto, L., et al. (2021). Long-term treatment of bipolar disorder type I: A systematic and critical review of clinical guidelines with derived practice algorithms. *Bipolar Disord*, 23, 324–340.

5. Baldessarini, R. J., Tondo, L., Davis, P., et al. (2006). Decreased risk of suicides and attempts during long-term lithium treatment: A meta-analytic review. *Bipolar Disord*, 8, 625–639.

6. Benard, V., Vaiva, G., Masson, M., et al. (2016). Lithium and suicide prevention in bipolar disorder. *Encephale*, 42, 234–241.

7. Velosa, J., Delgado, A., Finger, E., et al. (2020). Risk of dementia in bipolar disorder and the interplay of lithium: A systematic review and meta-analyses. *Acta Psychiatr Scand*, 141, 510–521.

8. Ochoa, E. L. M. (2022). Lithium as a neuroprotective agent for bipolar disorder: An overview. *Cell Mol Neurobiol*, 42, 85–97.

9. Zivanovic, O. (2017). Lithium: A classic drug frequently discussed but, sadly, seldom prescribed! *Aust N Z J Psychiatry*, 51, 886–896.

10. Lin, Y., Mojtabai, R., Goes, F. S., et al. (2020). Trends in prescriptions of lithium and other medications for patients with bipolar disorder in office-based practices in the United States: 1996–2015. *J Affect Disord*, 276, 883–889.

11. Poranen, J., Koistinaho, A., Tanskanen, A., et al. (2022). 20-year medication use trends in first-episode bipolar disorder. *Acta Psychiatr Scand*, 146, 583–593.

12. Wingård, L., Brandt, L., Bodén, R., et al. (2019). Monotherapy vs. combination therapy for post mania maintenance treatment: A population based cohort study. *Eur Neuropsychopharmacol*, 29, 691–700.

13. Rosa, A. R., Fountoulakis, K., Siamouli, M., et al. (2011). Is anticonvulsant treatment of mania a class effect? Data from randomized clinical trials. *CNS Neuroscience & Therapeutics*, 17, 167–177.

14. Kishi, T., Ikuta, T., Matsuda, Y., et al. (2022). Pharmacological treatment for bipolar mania: A systematic review and network meta-analysis of double-blind randomized controlled trials. *Mol Psychiatry*, 27, 1136–1144.

15. Song, J., Sjolander, A., Joas, E., et al. (2017). Suicidal behavior during lithium and valproate treatment: A within-individual 8-year prospective study of 50,000 patients with bipolar disorder. *Am J Psychiatry*, 174, 795–802.

16. Gerhard, T., Devanand, D. P., Huang, C., et al. (2015). Lithium treatment and risk for dementia in adults with bipolar disorder: population-based cohort study. *Br J Psychiatry*, 207, 46–51.

17. Fornaro, M., Maritan, E., Ferranti, R., et al. (2020). Lithium exposure during pregnancy and the postpartum period: A systematic review and meta-analysis of safety and efficacy outcomes. *Am J Psychiatry*, 177, 76–92.

18. Heinonen, E., Totterman, K., Back, K., et al. (2022). Lithium use during breastfeeding was safe in healthy full-term infants under strict monitoring. *Acta Paediatr*, 111, 1891–1898.

19. Bauer, M. and Gitlin, M. (2016). *The Essential Guide to Lithium Treatment*. Basle, Switzerland: Springer International Publishing AG.

20. Malhi, G. S., Masson, M. and Bellivier, F., eds. (2017). *The Science and Practice of Lithium Therapy*. Basle, Switzerland: Springer International Publishing AG.
21. Meyer, J. M. and Stahl, S. M. (2019). *The Clozapine Handbook* (Stahl's Handbooks). Cambridge: Cambridge University Press.
22. Meyer, J. M. and Stahl, S. M. (2021). *The Clinical Use of Antipsychotic Plasma Levels* (Stahl's Handbooks). New York: Cambridge University Press.

Preface: How to Use This Handbook

Most clinicians are aware of lithium's unparalleled efficacy data in bipolar disorder (BD), and evidence pointing to its anti-suicide and neuroprotective properties [1, 2]; however, some may be less familiar with recent long-term observational studies indicating that lithium's renal impact is more modest than previously thought [3–6]. There are many hypotheses surrounding the disconnect between the data supporting lithium as the gold standard mood stabilizer and its low utilization, but the leading contender very much parallels the lack of widespread clozapine use for treatment resistant schizophrenia: clinician fear [7, 8]. Lithium shares a laboratory monitoring burden with anticonvulsant mood stabilizers, but it is those short-term adverse effects unique to lithium (e.g. hypothyroidism, hyperparathyroidism, polyuria) combined with concerns about lithium toxicity and lithium's long-term renal impact which dissuade clinicians from lithium prescribing despite knowledge that it is the superior mood stabilizing option for many BD spectrum patients. (Chapter 4 also documents that this may be compounded by patient fear of lithium derived from a variety of sources and rumors [9].)

   With those thoughts in mind, the core element of this text is Chapter 2, devoted to a detailed explanation of lithium's renal clearance. To understand lithium is to understand how lithium moves through the kidney (Figure P1) [6, 10]. The short- and long-term renal adverse effects, potential for drug interactions, monitoring scheme, and treatment approaches derive from the physiology of lithium's clearance, and an understanding of how lithium enters collecting duct principal cells via the epithelial sodium channel (ENaC) and interferes with urine concentrating ability. That polyuria represents the earliest sign of lithium's renal effects, and that it can be easily tracked with a simple test of urine osmolality and treated with the ENaC inhibitor amiloride is welcome news for many clinicians. This knowledge transforms the inchoate mass of kidney related fears into discrete actionable monitoring and treatment related tasks, with Chapter 2 also reinforcing that use of appropriate maintenance lithium levels, once daily dosing, and management of chronic kidney disease (CKD) risks (e.g. hypertension, diabetes mellitus [DM]) are all central to preserving renal health. The subsequent chapters on kinetic and drug interactions (Chapter 3), laboratory monitoring (Chapter 4), lithium toxicity (Chapter 5) and lithium's use in a variety of patient populations (e.g. older individuals, pregnant women) (Chapter 7) relate to this newfound appreciation of lithium's renal journey. Once this information is assimilated, it becomes clear how to use the estimated glomerular filtration rate (eGFR) to track renal function, why one adjusts the monitoring frequency based on eGFR and not age, why one should add the urine albumin-to-creatinine ratio to the laboratory monitoring scheme to track CKD pathology from non-lithium-related comorbidities (e.g. hypertension, DM), and how to employ urine osmolality and the 24h fluid intake record (FIR) to manage polyuria complaints.

Figure P1 Detailed view of collecting duct principal cells illustrating how lithium enters via the epithelial sodium channel (ENaC) [11]

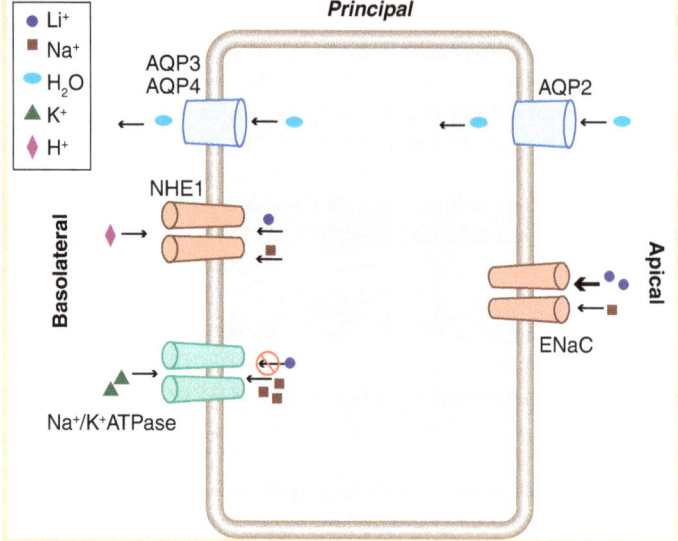

Legend AQP: aquaporin channel; ENaC: epithelial sodium channel; NHE1: sodium-hydrogen exchanger type 1 (Adapted from: J. P. Grünfeld and B. C. Rossier [2009]. Lithium nephrotoxicity revisited. *Nat Rev Nephrol*, 5, 270–276.)

Despite 70 years of literature comprising contributions from numerous scientists and clinical investigators around the world, the sources of renal related consternation among clinicians are readily apparent. Certain important questions are often indirectly addressed in reviews or treatment guidelines, but represent significant clinical decision points. For example:

1. Is there a minimum eGFR to initiate lithium?
2. What is the lowest eGFR to continue lithium and what clinical factors play a role in this decision?
3. What laboratory measures other than eGFR can be used to track changes in renal function from systemic illnesses associated with CKD?
4. Can the prophylactic use of amiloride mitigate lithium's renal related risks by blocking lithium entry into collecting duct principal cells via ENaC?

Although there is a lack of consensus on these topics, by building a foundation of knowledge on lithium's renal profile and how to mitigate risks related to low eGFR, drug interactions and the presence of CKD comorbidities, one can approach the first three decisions with the necessary monitoring tools to manage more challenging situations. The latter question about prophylactic amiloride use is an important research topic. While prophylactic use is not endorsed by any study or guideline presently, amiloride is a strongly evidence based method for treating polyuria, and should be employed as early as possible when this complaint arises during lithium treatment [12].

The purpose of this handbook is to provide a level of detail about lithium prescribing that builds on modern understanding of dosing, lithium kinetics and safety data covering renal and other adverse effects. While the primary use of lithium is for BD spectrum patients, this is not a volume dedicated to covering the natural history and diagnostic dilemmas clinicians encounter with BD patients, nor a compendium of the wide-ranging and extensive preclinical and human research about lithium, or the history of its discovery for mood disorder treatment. Those topics are eloquently covered by other volumes that psychiatric professionals should include in their library [13–16], with the first two chapters of the 2016 book entitled *The Essential Guide to Lithium Treatment* by longstanding mood researchers Professor Michael Bauer (Technische Universität, Dresden, German) and Professor Michael Gitlin (Geffen School of Medicine, University of California, Los Angeles) providing a clear description of mood disorder classification, the natural history of bipolar disorder and implications for treatment [17]. The 2020 Royal Australian and New Zealand College of Psychiatrists clinical practice guidelines for mood disorders is a thoughtful and beautifully illustrated document that covers the course and subtypes of BD, and how to utilize this information in managing the spectrum of BD patients with the evidence-based biological and non-biological therapies [18]. While the pressing clinical question at times can be "Does this patient have a BD spectrum disorder?", the more angst-riddled consideration for many prescribers is not the diagnostic dilemma, but: "Is it safe to use lithium?" Reading Chapter 2 before digesting the later chapters of this handbook will help the reader master the latest information about lithium, and hopefully bolster the confidence of those who want to give their patients the benefits of lithium therapy but did not feel comfortable about their knowledge of its renal issues to use lithium to the fullest extent possible.

References

1. Fountoulakis, K. N., Tohen, M. and Zarate, C. A. (2022). Lithium treatment of bipolar disorder in adults: A systematic review of randomized trials and meta-analyses. *Eur Neuropsychopharmacol*, 54, 100–115.

2. Nestsiarovich, A., Gaudiot, C. E. S., Baldessarini, R. J., et al. (2022). Preventing new episodes of bipolar disorder in adults: Systematic review and meta-analysis of randomized controlled trials. *Eur Neuropsychopharmacol*, 54, 75–89.

3. Werneke, U., Ott, M., Renberg, E. S., et al. (2012). A decision analysis of long-term lithium treatment and the risk of renal failure. *Acta Psychiatr Scand*, 126, 186–197.

4. Clos, S., Rauchhaus, P., Severn, A., et al. (2015). Long-term effect of lithium maintenance therapy on estimated glomerular filtration rate in patients with affective disorders: A population-based cohort study. *Lancet Psychiatry*, 2, 1075–1083.

5. Kessing, L. V., Gerds, T. A., Feldt-Rasmussen, B., et al. (2015). Use of lithium and anticonvulsants and the rate of chronic kidney disease: A nationwide population-based study. *JAMA Psychiatry*, 72, 1182–1191.

6. Davis, J., Desmond, M. and Berk, M. (2018). Lithium and nephrotoxicity: A literature review of approaches to clinical management and risk stratification. *BMC Nephrol*, 19, 305.

7. Rej, S., Elie, D., Mucsi, I., et al. (2015). Chronic kidney disease in lithium-treated older adults: A review of epidemiology, mechanisms, and implications for the treatment of late-life mood disorders. *Drugs Aging*, 32, 31–42.

8. Ott, M., Stegmayr, B., Salander Renberg, E., et al. (2016). Lithium intoxication: incidence, clinical course and renal function – a population-based retrospective cohort study. *J Psychopharmacol*, 30, 1008–1019.

9. Kerner, B., Crisanti, A. S., DeShaw, J. L., et al. (2019). Preferences of information dissemination on treatment for bipolar disorder: Patient-centered focus group study. *JMIR Ment Health*, 6, e12848.

10. Davis, J., Desmond, M. and Berk, M. (2018). Lithium and nephrotoxicity: Unravelling the complex pathophysiological threads of the lightest metal. *Nephrology (Carlton)*, 23, 897–903.

11. Grünfeld, J.-P. and Rossier, B. C. (2009). Lithium nephrotoxicity revisited. *Nat Rev Nephrol*, 5, 270–276.

12. Schoot, T. S., Molmans, T. H. J., Grootens, K. P., et al. (2020). Systematic review and practical guideline for the prevention and management of the renal side effects of lithium therapy. *Eur Neuropsychopharmacol*, 31, 16–32.

13. Bauer, M., Grof, P. and Muller-Oerlinghausen, B., eds. (2006). *Lithium in Neuropsychiatry – The Comprehensive Guide*. Oxford: CRC Press.

14. Soares, J. C. and Young, A. H. (2016). *Bipolar Disorders: Basic Mechanisms and Therapeutic Implications* (3rd edn.). Cambridge: Cambridge University Press.

15. Malhi, G. S., Masson, M. and Bellivier, F., eds. (2017). *The Science and Practice of Lithium Therapy*. Basle, Switzerland: Springer International Publishing AG.

16. Parker, G. (2019). *Bipolar II Disorder: Modelling, Measuring and Managing* (3rd edn.). Cambridge: Cambridge University Press.

17. Bauer, M. and Gitlin, M. (2016). *The Essential Guide to Lithium Treatment*. Basle, Switzerland: Springer International Publishing AG.

18. Malhi, G. S., Bell, E., Bassett, D., et al. (2021). The 2020 Royal Australian and New Zealand College of Psychiatrists clinical practice guidelines for mood disorders. *Aust N Z J Psychiatry*, 55, 7–117.

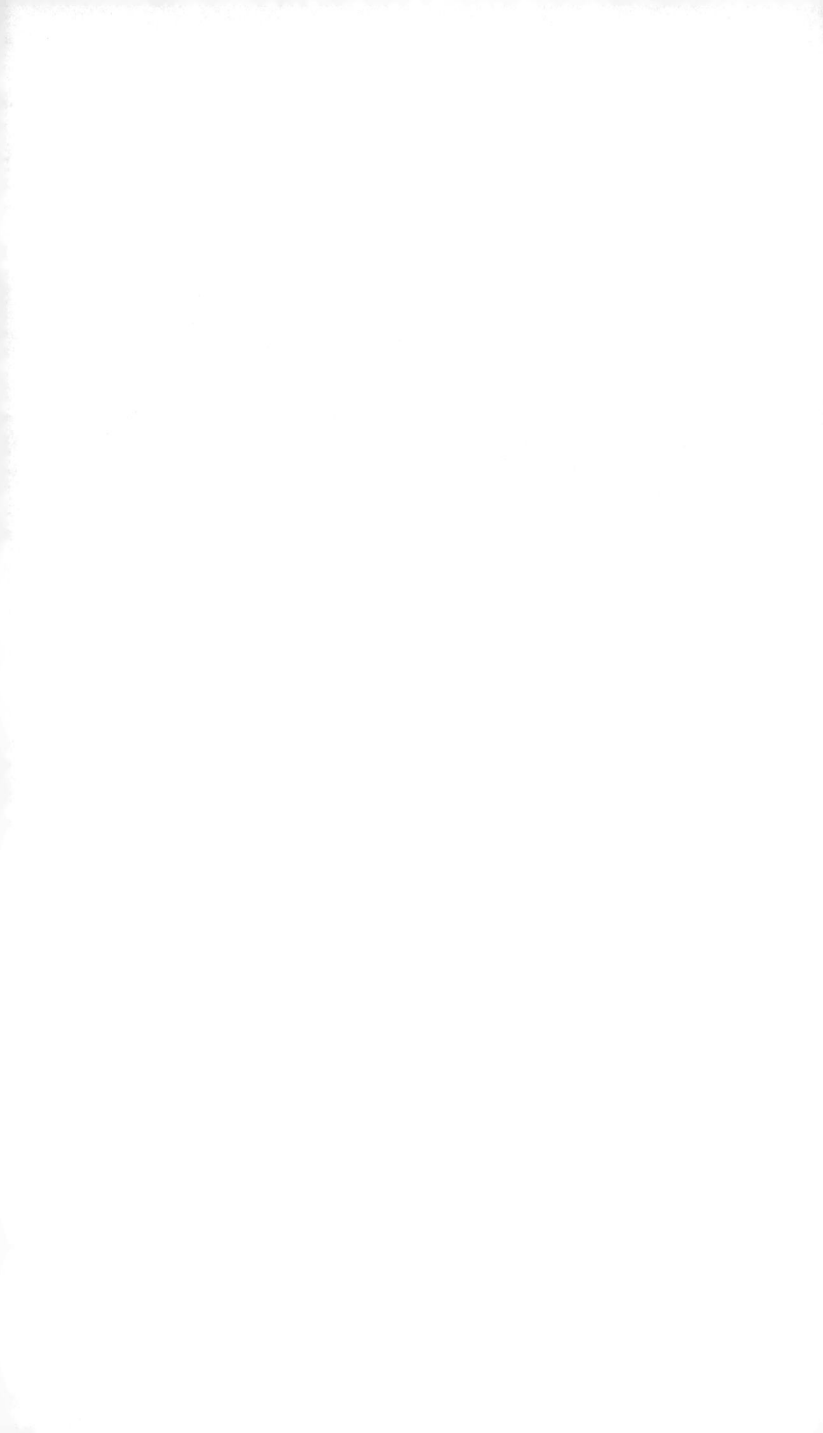

Introduction

As reflected in the number of citations per year, the initial golden age of lithium discovery was indeed 1965–1990. Yet interest in lithium has not waned, and a renaissance in lithium related publications has occurred over the past 20 years (Figure 0.1). This literature is fueled by ongoing exploration of lithium's unique mood stabilizing, anti-suicide and neuroprotective properties, a constellation of activities not seen in any single molecule [1–10]. Delving into how a simple ion conveys such benefits has opened important avenues of research into the neurobiology of both mood and degenerative brain disorders, and the molecular neuropharmacology of intracellular G-protein dependent and G-protein independent 2nd messenger systems [11, 12].

Unfortunately, this recent explosion of scientific interest occurs in the context of low lithium utilization despite the abundant evidence of lithium's advantages [13, 14]. However, rumors of lithium's demise are greatly exaggerated – as seen in Figure 0.2, the declining trend in US lithium use stabilized in 2009, a finding reflected in data sets from European sites [13, 15]. Factors underlying this reversal include: (1) the realization that certain non-lithium therapies have significant efficacy limitations (e.g. lamotrigine, second generation antipsychotics [SGAs]) or may be largely ineffective as mood stabilizers (e.g. gabapentin, oxcarbazepine, topiramate) [16–20]; (2) a greater appreciation for the risk of treatment failure when SGAs are used as maintenance monotherapy for bipolar I disorder (BD-1) [21]; (3) a renewed focus on the cognitive effects of mood disorders and emerging data supporting lithium's neuroprotective effects in older bipolar patients [22–26]; (4) the realization that the negative perception of lithium may be based on misconceptions regarding efficacy and safety that have been dispelled by newer data (Table 0.1) [27, 28]; (5) recent bans on prescribing valproate/divalproex (VPA) to women of reproductive age due to the risk for polycystic ovary syndrome (PCOS), congenital malformations and fetal valproate syndrome; and (6) recently revised lower estimates of the lithium related risk for Ebstein's and other cardiovascular anomalies following 1st trimester exposure [29–33].

A 2021 meta-analysis and critical review of clinical guidelines with derived practice algorithms concluded that lithium remained the gold standard for treatment of BD-1 patients based on its clear efficacy in treating mania and in preventing manic episodes [28]. The clinical course of bipolar II disorder (BD-2) is dominated by the time spent in a depressive phase (50.3%), with very little time spent in a hypomanic or mixed phase (3.6%) [34]. While some BD-2 patients may respond to and tolerate antidepressants for extended periods without undue switch rates [35], there is increasing evidence that the number of prior antidepressant treatment trials decreases likelihood of response, increases the odds of depressive relapse, and shortens the time to relapse in those with BD-2 disorder who previously were antidepressant responders, and in whom antidepressants are used as maintenance therapy [36]. Many BD-2 patients need mood stabilization, and lithium has proven efficacy in preventing mood episodes, although the data are not compelling for lithium as a treatment for acute bipolar depression [37]. Schizoaffective disorder, bipolar type (SAD-BT) patients also experience acute mania, but there is a paucity of prospective data in this patient group compared with other bipolar diatheses or mood disorders. Nonetheless, the available data make the compelling argument that SAD-BT patients also benefit from lithium therapy, and that this group has suboptimal stability on antipsychotic monotherapy [38].

Figure 0.1 70-year trend in lithium references on mood disorders and neuroprotection

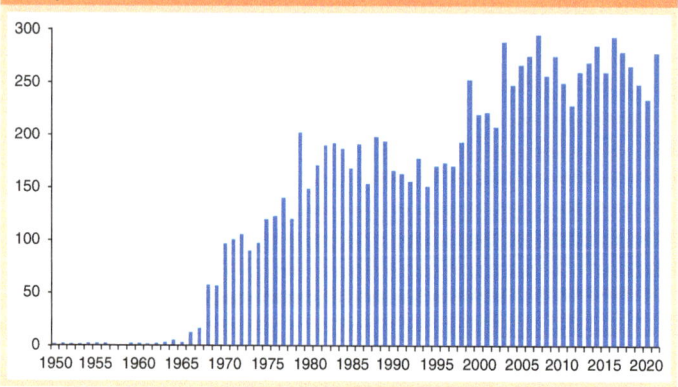

(Data from PubMed search conducted May 1, 2022. Search terms: lithium AND [manic OR mania OR neuroprotection OR major depression OR bipolar disorder].)

Figure 0.2 US trends 1997–2016 in different medication categories prescribed during outpatient visits for bipolar disorder

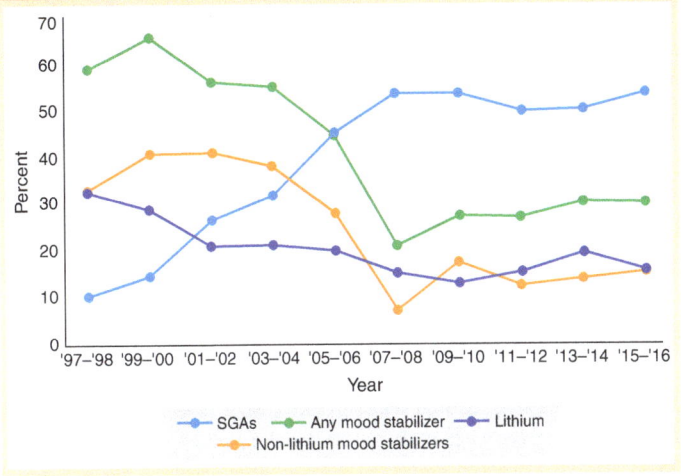

(Adapted from: T. G. Rhee, M. Olfson, A. A. Nierenberg, et al. [2020]. 20-year trends in the pharmacologic treatment of bipolar disorder by psychiatrists in outpatient care settings. *Am J Psychiatry*, 177, 706–715.)

 Dispelling the Misconceptions

This disconnect between the evidence base supporting lithium and its underutilization has not gone unnoticed, with concerted efforts undertaken by leading psychopharmacologists to help clinicians appreciate that current practice is not in line with new insights about lithium's safety and efficacy profile. Among the leading champions is Professor Janusz K. Rybakowski, a Polish researcher from the Department of Adult Psychiatry, Poznań University of Medical Sciences, who has been publishing on lithium for over 50 years [39]. His 2022 mini-review on lithium lamented the dissociation between practice patterns and data, provided a concise summary of lithium's unique features, and called on the mental health profession worldwide to simultaneously promote the long-term use of lithium in mood disorders, and challenge the negative perception that lithium is not suitable as a first-line candidate for BD prophylaxis [40]. Another leading psychopharmacologist and lithium proponent who has been instrumental in shaping BD treatment guidelines is Professor Gin Malhi (Psychiatry Chair at The University of Sydney,

Executive and Clinical Director of the CADE Clinic at the Northern Clinical School, and Head of the Academic Department of Psychiatry at the Royal North Shore Hospital). Crucial to increasing use of lithium is the need to dispel outdated ideas, and Professor Malhi's 2021 editorial "Lithium mythology" provides a list of seven statements frequently elaborated as reasons to avoid prescribing lithium [41]:

1. *Lithium is an old drug; it has nothing new to offer*
2. *Lithium seldom works*
3. *Lithium is not suitable first line*
4. *Lithium is complicated to prescribe and manage*
5. *Lithium is a dirty drug and difficult to tolerate*
6. *Lithium destroys thyroid function*
7. *Lithium ruins kidney function and eventuates in kidney failure*

While Professor Malhi's wording is deliberately provocative, his passion to "make lithium great again" is part of a collective effort to disseminate cutting-edge information, and thereby inspire clinicians to practice psychiatry based on evidence based concepts, and not on anxiety and fear [42]. Underlying these educational efforts is the overarching idea that certain medications such as clozapine and lithium offer distinct efficacy advantages, that the knowledge to prescribe such molecules is easily assimilated, and that depriving patients of such treatments is below the standard of care [42–44]. The tremendous regional variation in Swedish lithium use (Figure 0.3) very much parallels findings related to clozapine prescribing in the United Kingdom and in the United States [45–47], and reflects how local culture either promotes best practices, or sustains a climate where fear, uncertainty and doubt are acceptable reasons for not using pharmacological tools that are inarguably in the patient's best interest [48]. The Swedish data also present a compelling picture of the clinical outcomes associated with variations in lithium use for BD: higher prescription rates were significantly associated with a lower rate of mood recurrence, an association that was even more robust when analyzed separately for the BD-1 cohort [48].

To rectify the underuse of clozapine, governmental entities established resource centers to provide clinicians with data, education and decision support [49, 50]. Education is also the key to rectifying the inequities in lithium use and addressing those areas of greatest concern and misinformation that interfere with evidence based practice. Professor Malhi's use of the term "myth" reflects that certain exaggerated and inexact beliefs *not supported by the latest data* still hold sway in many corners of the mental health profession. While not intended to supplant the

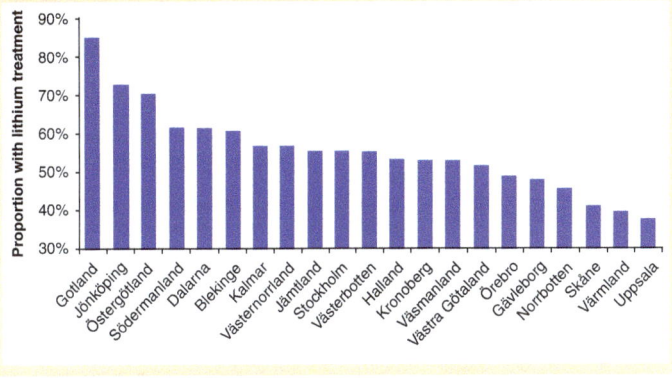

Figure 0.3 Regional variation in proportion of lithium treated bipolar patients by county in Sweden [48]

(Adapted from: M. Sköld, S. Rolstad, E. Joas, et al. [2021]. Regional lithium prescription rates and recurrence in bipolar disorder. *Int J Bipolar Disord*, 9, 18–27.)

list above, in the spirit of cooperativity with all efforts to promote accurate language about lithium, I present a list of misconceptions encountered when discussing lithium with trainees and clinicians throughout the spectrum of care delivery: medical students, physician assistants, pharmacists, nurses, psychiatric nurse practitioners and physicians (Table 0.1). The items largely overlap many of the concerns enumerated in Professor Malhi's list, and the "Modern evidence" column provides the busy reader with some quick rejoinders to erroneous statements made by colleagues or to misperceptions voiced by patients and caregivers.

Table 0.1 A selected list of misconceptions and modern evidence regarding lithium treatment

Efficacy misconceptions	Modern evidence
1. Second generation antipsychotic (SGA) monotherapy is as effective as lithium monotherapy for maintenance treatment of bipolar I disorder	• Naturalistic data indicate that bipolar I patients on SGA monotherapy have higher rates of treatment failure than those on lithium monotherapy [21].

Efficacy misconceptions	Modern evidence
2. Rapid cycling bipolar disorder (RC-BD) patients respond poorly to lithium in general, and lithium is inferior to other options such as divalproex in this patient cohort	• The hallmark of RC-BD (when not iatrogenically induced by use of traditional antidepressant molecules) is frequent, but comparatively shorter, depressive episodes than non-rapid cycling patients [51].
	• The number of prospective controlled studies in general is very sparse for this diagnosis. Clinical decisions must be made based on the few prospective and retrospective studies available [52].
	• RC-BD patients respond comparably to non-RC-BD patients during lithium treatment in terms of time spent ill. RC-BD patients continue to have a greater number of depressive episodes during lithium treatment than non-RC-BD patients but not greater total time spent depressed [53, 54].
	• The prospective studies indicate that lithium is not inferior to divalproex for management of RC-BD [55]. Use of a 2nd agent to treat the depressive phase of the disorder will likely be necessary regardless of mood stabilizer choice [53].
3. Lithium should be avoided in older bipolar disorder patients due to the lack of efficacy data and concerns about safety	• Lithium is as effective as divalproex in acutely manic older bipolar I (BD-1) patients and its tolerability is comparable [56].
	• A 1-year follow-up study of 1388 older BD-1 patients (age ≥ 66 years) found that, after discharge from an acute psychiatric hospitalization for mania, there were no significant differences between lithium- and VPA-treated individuals in the proportion with medical admissions or nonpsychiatric emergency room visits, or in the time to medical admission [57].
	• Older BD patients can be safely maintained on lithium with appropriate eGFR monitoring, and oversight of medications with potential kinetic interactions [58–63].
	• Due to a number of factors (e.g. lifestyle, cardiometabolic comorbidities), BD is associated with a 3-fold increased risk of dementia; treatment with lithium decreases the risk of dementia in BD by almost 50% [22, 26].
Safety misconceptions	**Modern evidence**
4. Use of lithium is associated with high risk for end-stage renal disease or renal failure	• Using modern monitoring principles, and practices that minimize risks for renal insufficiency (e.g. once daily lithium use, keeping maintenance levels < 1.2 mEq/l), no patient should develop severe chronic kidney disease (eGFR 15–29 ml/min) or renal failure (eGFR < 15 ml/min) on lithium therapy [64, 65].

Efficacy misconceptions	Modern evidence
5. There is no easy way to monitor for or manage lithium related polyuria (defined as daily urine output > 3 liters)	• Patients may underreport the inconvenience of polyuria – all patients on lithium should be asked at each visit urinary frequency and volume, and the functional impact [66].
	• The 24h fluid intake recollection (FIR) is an evidence based office screening tool [67].
	• Early morning urine osmolality (EMUO) is an easily obtained laboratory measure to quantify the extent of any concentrating defect [67].
	• Amiloride has emerged as an effective treatment for lithium related nephrogenic diabetes insipidus (NDI), and should be started as soon as any problems are detected [68].
6. Lithium should not be used in women of reproductive age due to an estimated 400-fold increased relative risk for Ebstein's anomaly.	• Using modern statistical methods (e.g. propensity score matching), analysis of the largest data set available revealed three important conclusions regarding risks from 1st trimester lithium exposure [29]:
	a. The adjusted risk ratio (ARR) for non-cardiac defects among infants exposed to lithium was not significantly different than among unexposed infants.
	b. No cases of Ebstein's anomaly were seen among 663 lithium-exposed pregnancies examined.
	c. There was a dose dependent increased risk for any cardiac malformation:
	Dose ≤ 600 mg/d: **RR 1.11** (95% CI 0.46–2.64)
	Dose 601–900 mg/d: **RR 1.60** (95% CI 0.67–3.80)
	Dose > 900 mg/d: **RR 3.22** (95% CI 1.47–7.02)
	d. **Meta-analysis findings:** The number needed to harm (NNH) for any cardiovascular malformation across all lithium doses is 83 when comparing rates between lithium users and non-users with bipolar disorder [69].
7. Other mood stabilizer options (e.g. valproate) are safer and should be routinely used in female bipolar disorder patients of reproductive age in lieu of lithium	• 1st trimester valproate/divalproex (VPA) exposure is associated with unacceptably high rates of congenital malformations and fetal valproate syndrome and should be avoided in women of reproductive age, or only prescribed if a woman understands the risks and uses adequate contraception [70].
	• A meta-analysis of VPA related reproductive adverse effects in bipolar patients revealed statistically significant differences between the VPA treated and non-VPA treated groups in PCOS (odds ratio [OR]: **6.74**), any menstrual disorder (OR **1.81**) and hyperandrogenism (OR **2.02**) [71].

Efficacy misconceptions	Modern evidence
8. Lithium related hypothyroidism is highly prevalent, difficult to screen for and to manage, and often leads to treatment discontinuation	• Prevalence estimates vary, but overt hypothyroidism is only thought to occur in 8%–19% [72], and is easily screened for with TSH added to routine monitoring labs. • In large studies, hypothyroidism is not among the 10 leading somatic causes of lithium discontinuation, with a rate of only 2.0% in a recent surveillance study [73]. • Lithium use is not associated with development of antithyroid antibodies [74, 75]. • Hypothyroidism never justifies lithium discontinuation [72] but, should discontinuation be necessary for other reasons, hypothyroidism is often reversible [76]. • The sensitivity of depressive symptoms to TSH values at the upper limit of the normal range in bipolar patients provides important guidance about when thyroid replacement therapy might be initiated when hypothyroidism is not present by TSH or somatic symptom criteria [77, 78, 79].

B The Efficacy Misconceptions

Broadly speaking, the misconceptions about lithium fall into one of two categories: those which minimize efficacy, or those which exaggerate safety issues. Many of the safety concerns were reinforced by the pharmaceutical industry in promoting VPA and SGAs for BD [40]. As seen in the upward trends toward SGA use and the simultaneous decline in lithium prescriptions, the unopposed message of lithium's harms and management burdens not only led clinicians to eschew lithium, but often to avoid mood stabilization altogether, even in BD-1 patients [13, 21]. Although aripiprazole, olanzapine and long-acting injectable risperidone microspheres have indications for BD-1 maintenance as monotherapy [80], the design of monotherapy maintenance trials is to prove that stable patients who have previously responded to that treatment have lower relapse rates than those on placebo. Importantly, neither aripiprazole, olanzapine or risperidone have demonstrable efficacy for the depressive pole of the disorder. Among the SGAs, only cariprazine and quetiapine have US approvals for acute mania and bipolar depression, but cariprazine has no registrational data for adjunctive use with lithium or VPA, no maintenance indication for BD-1 in the US, and is only approved for schizophrenia by the European Medicines Agency [81].

The results of the naturalistic experiment that unfolded over the past 15 years is becoming apparent, with data indicating that BD-1 patients have higher rates of treatment failure on SGA monotherapy compared with lithium monotherapy [21]. One Swedish group examined treatment failure rates (defined as: treatment discontinuation, switch or rehospitalization) with mood stabilizer and SGA therapies, alone or in combination among 3772 adults discharged from psychiatric inpatient care for mania from July 1, 2006 to December 31, 2014. After excluding those with schizophrenia, SAD-BT, or dementia diagnoses from the analysis, and after adjusting for an extensive list of potential confounding variables related to sociodemographics, severity of the index hospitalization for mania and prior psychiatric history, the investigators found that, compared with lithium monotherapy, VPA monotherapy had a higher rate of medication discontinuation, and that SGA monotherapies (aripiprazole, olanzapine or quetiapine) were associated with the highest rates of all-cause treatment failure and failure due to medication switching (Figure 0.4) [21]. Prospective randomized studies corroborate

Figure 0.4 Time to treatment failure after hospitalization for mania among various treatment options for bipolar I disorder using lithium (dark blue line) as the comparator treatment [21]

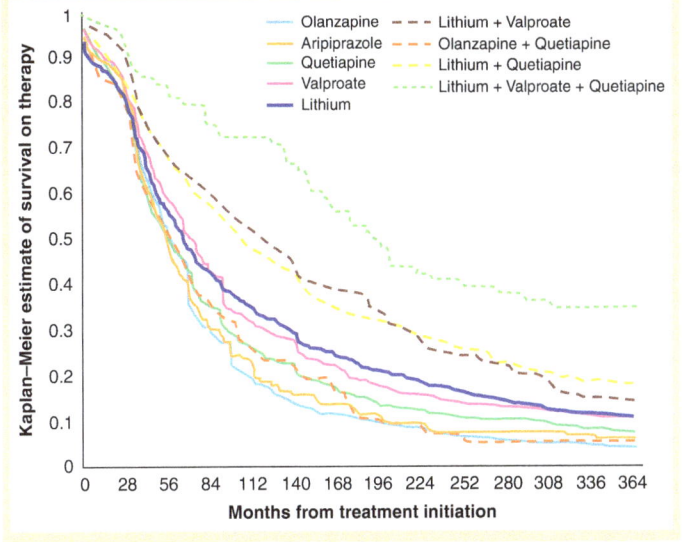

(Adapted from: L. Wingård, L. Brandt, R. Bodén, et al. [2019]. Monotherapy vs. combination therapy for post mania maintenance treatment: A population based cohort study. *Eur Neuropsychopharmacol*, 29, 691–700.)

this naturalistic finding. In a 1-year randomized trial of patients with first episode mania, lithium was more effective than quetiapine during follow-up on every outcome measure, including mood, functioning, cognition, and brain imaging changes, with large differences emerging during the second half of the year [82].

In addition to short-term clinical outcomes when BD patients receive suboptimal treatment (e.g. mood relapse), recent papers have advanced a more nuanced argument that failure to adequately manage this disorder may itself be a disease-modifying event that portends lower long-term treatment response [83]. This argument has been made extensively in the schizophrenia literature as multiple analyses have demonstrated higher response rates when clozapine is initiated earlier for treatment resistant patients [84]. Multiple studies in BD-1 patients substantiate that earlier treatment with lithium is met with higher response rates, and that patients who receive more intensive treatment for just two years following a first manic episode have a longer time to rehospitalization than those randomized to usual care, an effect that persisted and increased during the next six years [85]. The underlying hypothesis for schizophrenia and BD is that failure to minimize symptom severity and recurrence, through treatment delay or suboptimal treatment, may result in epigenetic changes that have long-term impact on neurochemistry and medication response [83]. It is for this reason that treatment guidelines and expert recommendations are substantially in agreement that one must preferentially use lithium as the gold standard core treatment in the maintenance therapy of BD-1 patients and possibly BD-2 individuals, while acknowledging that additional medications may be necessary to manage mood recurrence, especially to the depressive pole [28, 30, 53, 86–88].

Improved characterization of the clinical course of rapid cycling bipolar disorder (RC-BD) has also been helpful in reframing the misguided notion that lithium is either ineffective in this cohort, or less effective than non-lithium options, especially VPA [86]. The hallmark of RC-BD is frequent, brief depressive episodes (by definition ≥ 4 mood episodes in a 12-month period), although total illness duration may not differ from non-RC patients [51]. Papers on lithium response often note that the presence of RC-BD diminishes rates of good clinical outcomes [89, 90]; however, a 2020 meta-analysis on predictors of long-term lithium response came to two important conclusions: (1) there is marked heterogeneity in the quality of outcomes data in this area; (2) among the 4 predictors of poor lithium outcome initially identified in the 31 relevant data sets (alcohol use disorder, personality disorders, higher lifetime number of hospital admissions, rapid cycling), when the analysis was confined to data from the high-quality studies (11 trials, n = 9981), only higher lifetime number of hospitalization admissions remained [91]. Importantly, when studies compare lithium to non-lithium treatments, both retrospective analyses and prospective trials note that RC-BD patients have high substance use comorbidity rates and high rates of mood recurrence, yet lithium treated RC-BD patients respond at rates that are comparable to patients on other therapies, including VPA [54, 55, 92]. The refined message from two decades of research is that the limitations of lithium relate to the neurobiology of RC-BD itself and not a failure of lithium per se, and that no mood stabilizer monotherapy will be sufficient to manage mood recurrence in many of these individuals [53]. Eschewing traditional antidepressants (e.g. selective serotonin reuptake inhibitors, serotonin norepinephrine reuptake inhibitors, etc.), and use of evidence based medications for acute and maintenance treatment of bipolar depression (e.g. lurasidone, cariprazine, quetiapine, lamotrigine), is now understood to be the optimal approach in RC-BD [53].

Another patient cohort in which use of lithium has been unnecessarily avoided is older bipolar patients. While age-related declines in estimated glomerular filtration rate (eGFR) diminish the margin of error for older individuals [93], assumptions that lithium use is inherently poorly tolerated, ineffective or unsafe in this population are largely disproven. Prospective, randomized, double-blind acute mania trials document that lithium is as effective and tolerable as divalproex [56]; moreover, the recent literature documents that long-term lithium use in older BD patients is associated with a close to 50% reduction in dementia risk, a finding not seen with non-lithium therapies [22, 26]. One investigator in particular, Dr. Soham Rej of McGill University Department of Psychiatry, Montréal, Canada, has contributed numerous analyses substantiating that use of lithium is not associated with undue risk for medical complications in comparison to other options such as VPA, and that, with appropriate eGFR monitoring and attention to use of medications with kinetic interactions, lithium is generally well tolerated in patients older than 65 years of age [57–61, 94–96].

 The Safety Misconceptions

The early recognition that use of certain SGAs was associated with inordinate rates of metabolic adverse effects had one important outcome: it focused clinical attention and research on medical comorbidity in patients with serious mental illnesses such as schizophrenia and BD [80, 87]. The high prevalence of cardiometabolic disorders in BD patients is likely a significant contributor to the 3-fold increased dementia risk in this diagnostic group [97, 98]. While lithium is associated with renal adverse effects, some of the long-term risk of renal insufficiency previously ascribed solely to lithium exposure is contributed by chronic kidney disease (CKD) risk factors, such as hypertension, metabolic syndrome, diabetes and smoking, that disproportionately affect BD patients [99]. Echoing the findings for dementia, having a diagnosis of BD is associated with a 3-fold increased risk of CKD *independent of drug treatment* [99]. Not only is the independent effect of lithium on chronic eGFR changes lower than previously suspected [100], with the use of modern monitoring protocols, once daily lithium dosing and modest outpatient 12h serum levels (e.g. < 1.00 mEq/l), the risk of developing end-stage CKD attributable to lithium has been essentially eliminated in many countries [64, 65, 99]. (See Chapter 2 for a more complete discussion of renal issues related to lithium use.)

Although the potential effects of lithium on CKD risk demand routine monitoring, performing that task is relatively easy as laboratories report eGFR calculated from serum creatinine (and now cystatin C) values [101]. Moreover, changes in eGFR were typically a longer-term issue for the treating clinician, and not an immediate source of patient complaints. The more vexing clinical problem, and one that patients may notice early in therapy, is the development of polyuria (defined as 24h urinary output > 3 liters) [73]. Often patients will complain bitterly about the inconvenience of polyuria, but many clinicians appreciate that some underreport the functional impact of these problems, and actively query lithium treated patients about urinary frequency and thirst [66]. The goal of early recognition is to employ evidence based options for managing lithium related nephrogenic diabetes insipidus (NDI) such as amiloride, and forestall patient demands to discontinue lithium [68, 73]. The use of amiloride for lithium related NDI is well established, so statements that switching from lithium is the only option are simply untrue [68, 101, 102]. Unfortunately, the literature often recommends only one option for assessing the severity of a patient's concentration defect and for tracking changes to an intervention: the 24h urine collection [101]. While the gold standard for quantifying urine output [67], the impracticality of obtaining a valid 24h urine collection in many circumstances can preclude its use as a diagnostic tool and as a tool to track urine osmolality during amiloride treatment. Fortunately, a solution to this problem was provided a decade ago by the ambitious work of a group in Ireland who subjected a cohort of 179 lithium treated patients to a battery of subjective and laboratory tests, including the 24h urine collection [67]. This comprehensive study yielded two important clinical conclusions: (1) the 24h FIR is a useful method for office screening and for patients to easily monitor changes in polyuria; (2) EMUO is a valid method for estimating NDI severity [67]. How these are utilized is discussed extensively in Chapter 2, but the important message is that ongoing research has provided answers to help manage these important adverse effects, and that lithium related NDI should now be viewed as a problem with well-defined monitoring tools and a treatment pathway.

The pharmacological management of mental disorders for women of childbearing age demands nuanced and individualized decisions based not only on the literature, but on the prior history of stability with and without certain medications, and, importantly, patient values [69, 103]. The greatest area of concern is always 1st trimester exposure, and the impact of any medication on organogenesis. For lithium, the early focus was on cardiovascular malformations broadly, and Ebstein's anomaly specifically, based on spontaneous reports [80]. Unfortunately, the nature of these data led to risk estimates that were wildly inaccurate (e.g. 400-fold higher risk), but that continued to be cited in the absence of more systematic analyses [29]. As in other areas of research, more advanced statistical methods using propensity score matching and covariate balancing have been developed to analyze data sets retrospectively and remove many of the biases inherent to prescribing practices and to confounding factors in the population receiving a particular treatment [104]. Employing these robust statistical techniques, we can now estimate that the maximal increased risk for any cardiovascular malformation from lithium exposure is 1.8-fold higher than in non-exposed infants, which generates a number needed to harm of **83** [29, 69]. (See Chapter 7.) Whether this risk is acceptable to any individual depends on all of the factors mentioned above, but knowledge of this revised estimate, and the method by which this adjusted risk ratio was calculated, should inform any discussion about risk:benefit considerations around 1st trimester lithium exposure. Absolutist statements that lithium always presents an unacceptable risk for cardiovascular malformations are indeed based on misconceptions rooted in outdated risk estimates and do a disservice to the many women who must remain on lithium to preserve psychiatric stability [29].

As the reproductive risk associated with lithium has been reevaluated, that related to VPA has been subjected to increased scrutiny due to the known high rates of congenital malformations and neural tube defects from 1st trimester exposure, combined with the increased risk for polycystic ovary syndrome (PCOS) [105]. The 2017 British Association for Psychopharmacology (BAP) consensus guidance on the use of psychotropic medication during preconception, pregnancy and the postpartum period notes that VPA exposure increases the risk for any major congenital malformation 3-fold, and for spina bifida 13-fold, a risk that is not mitigated by the use of folate [105]. It is for that reason the BAP included the following language regarding VPA (p. 527):

- There is a particular concern around the use of anticonvulsant mood stabilisers, such as valproate or carbamazepine, whose adverse effects may have occurred before confirmation of pregnancy.
- **Valproate is the only psychotropic contraindicated in women of childbearing potential when used for psychiatric indications, although even here there can be very rare exceptions.**

The European Medicines Agency (EMA) subsequently issued a statement on March 23, 2018, endorsing new measures to avoid VPA exposure in pregnancy related to these concerns (www.ema.europa.eu/en/documents/press-release/new-measures-avoid-valproate-exposure-pregnancy-endorsed_en.pdf). Such warnings were deemed necessary as 2018 audit data indicated that VPA prescribing in BD women of reproductive age continued to fall short of best practice in developed countries such as the UK, particularly with regard to provision of information regarding the risks associated with VPA exposure during pregnancy, and the need for contraception to manage such risks [70]. While acknowledging the complexity of managing BD, a panel of experts convened in March 2019 and issued recommendations on use of VPA in women of childbearing age, including [30]:

1. Bipolar disorder childbearing women treated with VPA must be managed on a personalized basis according to the clinical situation.
2. It is mandatory to stop VPA during pregnancy. The duration of the discontinuation/switch process depends on different clinical variables.
3. Lithium, lamotrigine, quetiapine, olanzapine or aripiprazole are good options for switch in stable BD patients in planned/unplanned pregnancy.

The impact of these and earlier recommendations was slowly seen in declining rates of VPA use among BD women of childbearing age (Figure 0.5) [106]; moreover, statements in the literature suggesting that VPA is a reasonable option for this patient population have come under strong attack by reproductive psychiatric specialists. One group from Johns Hopkins University (Baltimore, Maryland) stated that "reproductive psychiatry has shifted away from considering valproate as a 'reasonable alternative' in women of reproductive age and toward viewing valproate as a last resort, not justifiable unless it is the only option for treating severe illness"

[31]. Should any clinician choose to use VPA in women of reproductive potential they were advised to document: (1) why there are no acceptable alternatives to VPA for a particular patient; (2) that the patient is using a highly reliable method of birth control; (3) that there has been a discussion of VPA's risks for both the patient and fetus, especially the high rates of fetal valproate syndrome; and (4) that the patient has been recommended to take 4 mg of folic acid daily to reduce the risks of congenital malformations in an unplanned pregnancy [31]. Starting in 2023, the UK banned VPA in women under age 55 unless two independent consultants certified there were no options and the patient was enrolled in a pregnancy prevention program.

Figure 0.5 Declining use of valproic acid (VPA) in Scotland for female bipolar disorder patients aged 18–50 years compared with males aged 18–50 years [106]

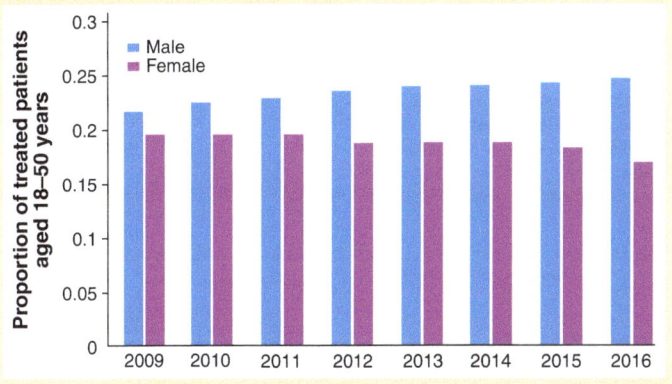

(Adapted from: L. M. Lyall, N. Penades and D. J. Smith [2019]. Changes in prescribing for bipolar disorder between 2009 and 2016: National-level data linkage study in Scotland. *Br J Psychiatry*, 215, 415–421.)

If the above concerns were not sufficiently sobering, the association between VPA exposure and PCOS became another important issue for managing bipolar women of childbearing age [71]. The primary features of PCOS include irregular menstrual cycles and hyperandrogenism (Figure 0.6), with insulin resistance also commonly seen as an independent finding, but one which is exacerbated by obesity [32]. The estimated PCOS prevalence worldwide was 6%–10% in 2016 [32], but a meta-analysis published that same year covering studies of VPA related reproductive and metabolic abnormalities in women with BD found that the risks of PCOS were almost 7-fold higher (OR 6.74), and the risk of hyperandrogenism 2-fold greater (OR 2.02) among VPA exposed patients [71].

Figure 0.6 Diagnosis of polycystic ovary syndrome (PCOS) [32]

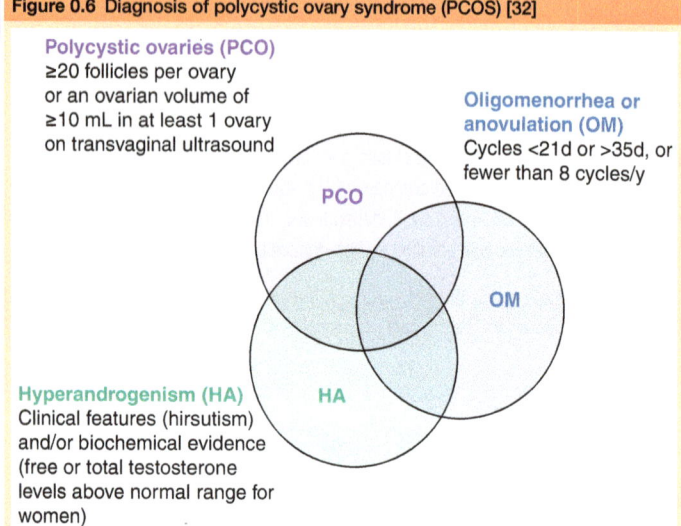

Polycystic ovaries (PCO)
≥20 follicles per ovary
or an ovarian volume of
≥10 mL in at least 1 ovary
on transvaginal ultrasound

Oligomenorrhea or anovulation (OM)
Cycles <21d or >35d, or
fewer than 8 cycles/y

PCO

OM

Hyperandrogenism (HA)
Clinical features (hirsutism)
and/or biochemical evidence
(free or total testosterone
levels above normal range for
women)

HA

(Adapted from: H. G. Huddleston and A. Dokras [2022]. Diagnosis and treatment of polycystic ovary syndrome. *JAMA*, 327, 274–275.)

While hypothyroidism is not among the 10 leading causes of lithium discontinuation, clinicians may cite a prior history of hypothyroidism as a reason to eschew lithium therapy, and still, occasionally, stop lithium in the face of rising TSH [73]. While perhaps less compelling to prescribers than fears surrounding renal and reproductive risks, the unfortunate persistence of lithium discontinuation for what is putatively a manageable problem is a source of consternation to mood disorder experts. Professor Michael Gitlin of the University California, Los Angeles School of Medicine has been publishing on lithium for nearly 40 years [107], and in his 2016 review on management strategies for adverse effects flatly stated: "The most important clinical rule is that hypothyroidism never justifies lithium discontinuation" [72]. While stopping lithium is not necessary to manage hypothyroidism, the effect of lithium on thyroid function is often reversible, and use of lithium is not associated with development of antithyroid antibodies [74–76]. The prevalence of overt hypothyroidism is in the range of 8%–19%, and easily screened for employing high sensitivity TSH levels that are obtainable at most laboratories [72].

Grade 1 subclinical hypothyroidism occurs when TSH levels are between the upper limit of the reference range (typically 4.5 or 5.0 mU/L) and 9.9 mU/L, and in the general population is rarely associated with somatic, cognitive or mood effects [108]. However, the threshold for thyroid supplementation may be different in BD patients as studies have shown that TSH levels that are otherwise in the upper limit of the normal range may be associated with more depressive relapse [77, 78]. A 2022 review noted that, since the use of thyroid extract was superseded by levothyroxine in the 1970s, "no major innovation has emerged for the treatment of hypothyroidism" [109]. The point is that most patients respond to L-thyroxine supplementation, although consultation with an endocrinologist may be helpful when cognitive and energy complaints persist that do not appear attributable to depressive mood symptoms [109].

 D **Conclusions**

Dissemination of new knowledge is central to dispelling outdated ideas regarding lithium and allowing patients access to its unique constellation of therapeutic properties. Professor Malhi's 2021 editorial on lithium mythology opens with a quote from former US President John F. Kennedy that aptly describes why certain ideas take root and are difficult to eradicate [41]:

> The great enemy of truth is very often not the lie – deliberate, contrived and dishonest – but the myth – persistent, persuasive and unrealistic. Too often we hold fast to the cliches of our forebears. We subject all facts to a prefabricated set of interpretations. We enjoy the comfort of opinion without the discomfort of thought.
> (Commencement address at Yale University, June 11, 1962)

As research continues to expand our frontiers about lithium's efficacy and tolerability profile, it is incumbent upon all mental health practitioners to reinforce new insights with colleagues, patients and caregivers, thereby changing the culture surrounding the use of lithium. Lessons from initiatives designed to stimulate clozapine prescribing are instructive in this regard – education can change attitudes.

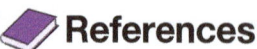 # References

1. De-Paula, V. J., Gattaz, W. F. and Forlenza, O. V. (2016). Long-term lithium treatment increases intracellular and extracellular brain-derived neurotrophic factor (BDNF) in cortical and hippocampal neurons at subtherapeutic concentrations. *Bipolar Disord*, 18, 692–695.

2. Harrison, P. J., Hall, N., Mould, A., et al. (2021). Cellular calcium in bipolar disorder: Systematic review and meta-analysis. *Mol Psychiatry*, 26, 4106–4116.

3. Athey, T. L., Ceritoglu, C., Tward, D. J., et al. (2021). A 7 Tesla amygdalar-hippocampal shape analysis of lithium response in bipolar disorder. *Front Psychiatry*, 12, 614010.

4. Haupt, M., Bahr, M. and Doeppner, T. R. (2021). Lithium beyond psychiatric indications: The reincarnation of a new old drug. *Neural Regen Res*, 16, 2383–2387.

5. Jones, G. H., Rong, C., Shariq, A. S., et al. (2021). Intracellular signaling cascades in bipolar disorder. *Curr Top Behav Neurosci*, 48, 101–132.

6. Keramatian, K., Su, W., Saraf, G., et al. (2021). Preservation of gray matter volume in early stage of bipolar disorder: A case for early intervention. *Can J Psychiatry*, 66, 139–146.

7. Lin, Y., Maihofer, A. X., Stapp, E., et al. (2021). Clinical predictors of non-response to lithium treatment in the Pharmacogenomics of Bipolar Disorder (PGBD) study. *Bipolar Disord*, 23, 821–831.

8. Osete, J. R., Akkouh, I. A., de Assis, D. R., et al. (2021). Lithium increases mitochondrial respiration in iPSC-derived neural precursor cells from lithium responders. *Mol Psychiatry*, 26, 6789–6805.

9. Puglisi-Allegra, S., Ruggieri, S. and Fornai, F. (2021). Translational evidence for lithium-induced brain plasticity and neuroprotection in the treatment of neuropsychiatric disorders. *Transl Psychiatry*, 11, 366.

10. Sanghani, H. R., Jagannath, A., Humberstone, T., et al. (2021). Patient fibroblast circadian rhythms predict lithium sensitivity in bipolar disorder. *Mol Psychiatry*, 26, 5252–5265.

11. Del' Guidice, T. and Beaulieu, J. M. (2015). Selective disruption of dopamine D2-receptors/beta-arrestin2 signaling by mood stabilizers. *J Recept Signal Transduct Res*, 35, 224–232.

12. Jia, S., Li, B., Huang, J., et al. (2018). Regulation of glycogen content in astrocytes via Cav-1/PTEN/AKT/GSK-3β pathway by three anti-bipolar drugs. *Neurochem Res*, 43, 1692–1701.

13. Rhee, T. G., Olfson, M., Nierenberg, A. A., et al. (2020). 20-year trends in the pharmacologic treatment of bipolar disorder by psychiatrists in outpatient care settings. *Am J Psychiatry*, 177, 706–715.

14. Rybakowski, J. K. (2018). Challenging the negative perception of lithium and optimizing its long-term administration. *Front Mol Neurosci*, 11, 1–8.

15. Kohler-Forsberg, O., Gasse, C., Hieronymus, F., et al. (2021). Pre-diagnostic and post-diagnostic psychopharmacological treatment of 16 288 patients with bipolar disorder. *Bipolar Disorders*, 23, 357–367.

16. Kushner, S. F., Khan, A., Lane, R., et al. (2006). Topiramate monotherapy in the management of acute mania: Results of four double-blind placebo-controlled trials. *Bipolar Disord*, 8, 15–27.

17. Carey, T. S., Williams, J. W., Jr., Oldham, J. M., et al. (2008). Gabapentin in the treatment of mental illness: The echo chamber of the case series. *J Psychiatr Res*, 14 Suppl. 1, 15–27.

18. Fullerton, C. A., Busch, A. B. and Frank, R. G. (2010). The rise and fall of gabapentin for bipolar disorder: A case study on off-label pharmaceutical diffusion. *Medical Care*, 48, 372–379.

19. Vasudev, A., Macritchie, K., Watson, S., et al. (2008). Oxcarbazepine in the maintenance treatment of bipolar disorder. *Cochrane Database Syst Rev*, CD005171.

20. Kishi, T., Ikuta, T., Matsuda, Y., et al. (2021). Mood stabilizers and/or antipsychotics for bipolar disorder in the maintenance phase: A systematic review and network meta-analysis of randomized controlled trials. *Mol Psychiatry*, 26, 4146–4157.

21. Wingård, L., Brandt, L., Bodén, R., et al. (2019). Monotherapy vs. combination therapy for post mania maintenance treatment: A population based cohort study. *Eur Neuropsychopharmacol*, 29, 691–700.

22. Velosa, J., Delgado, A., Finger, E., et al. (2020). Risk of dementia in bipolar disorder and the interplay of lithium: A systematic review and meta-analyses. *Acta Psychiatr Scand*, 141, 510–521.

23. Ballester, P. L., Romano, M. T., de Azevedo Cardoso, T., et al. (2022). Brain age in mood and psychotic disorders: A systematic review and meta-analysis. *Acta Psychiatr Scand*, 145, 42–55.

24. Beunders, A. J. M., Kemp, T., Korten, N. C. M., et al. (2021). Cognitive performance in older-age bipolar disorder: Investigating psychiatric characteristics, cardiovascular burden and psychotropic medication. *Acta Psychiatr Scand*, 144, 392–406.

25. Easter, R. E., Ryan, K. A., Estabrook, R., et al. (2022). Limited time-specific and longitudinal effects of depressive and manic symptoms on cognition in bipolar spectrum disorders. *Acta Psychiatr Scand*, 146, 430–441.

26. Chen, S., Underwood, B. R., Jones, P. B., et al. (2022). Association between lithium use and the incidence of dementia and its subtypes: a retrospective cohort study. *PLoS Med*, 19, e1003941.

27. Orsolini, L., Pompili, S. and Volpe, U. (2020). The "collateral side" of mood stabilizers: Safety and evidence-based strategies for managing side effects. *Expert Opin Drug Saf*, 19, 1461–1495.

28. Verdolini, N., Hidalgo-Mazzei, D., Del Matto, L., et al. (2021). Long-term treatment of bipolar disorder type I: A systematic and critical review of clinical guidelines with derived practice algorithms. *Bipolar Disord*, 23, 324–340.

29. Patorno, E., Huybrechts, K. F., Bateman, B. T., et al. (2017). Lithium use in pregnancy and the risk of cardiac malformations. *NEJM*, 376, 2245–2254.

30. Anmella, G., Pacchiarotti, I., Cubala, W. J., et al. (2019). Expert advice on the management of valproate in women with bipolar disorder at childbearing age. *Eur Neuropsychopharmacol*, 29, 1199–1212.

31. Leistikow, N., Smith, M. H., Payne, J. L., et al. (2021). Is valproate reasonable? *Am J Psychiatry*, 178, 99.

32. Huddleston, H. G. and Dokras, A. (2022). Diagnosis and treatment of polycystic ovary syndrome. *JAMA*, 327, 274–275.

33. Kan, A. C. O., Chan, J. K. N., Wong, C. S. M., et al. (2022). Psychotropic drug utilization patterns in pregnant women with bipolar disorder: A 16-year population-based cohort study. *Eur Neuropsychopharmacol*, 57, 75–85.

34. Judd, L. L., Akiskal, H. S., Schettler, P. J., et al. (2003). A prospective investigation of the natural history of the long-term weekly symptomatic status of bipolar II disorder. *Arch Gen Psychiatry*, 60, 261–269.

35. Amsterdam, J. D., Luo, L. and Shults, J. (2013). Efficacy and mood conversion rate during long-term fluoxetine v. lithium monotherapy in rapid- and non-rapid-cycling bipolar II disorder. *Br J Psychiatry*, 202, 301–306.

36. Amsterdam, J. D. and Kim, T. T. (2019). Prior antidepressant treatment trials may predict a greater risk of depressive relapse during antidepressant maintenance therapy. *J Clin Psychopharmacol*, 39, 344–350.

37. Yatham, L. N., Kennedy, S. H., Parikh, S. V., et al. (2018). Canadian Network for Mood and Anxiety Treatments (CANMAT) and International Society for Bipolar Disorders (ISBD) 2018 guidelines for the management of patients with bipolar disorder. *Bipolar Disord*, 20, 97–170.

38. Lintunen, J., Taipale, H., Tanskanen, A., et al. (2021). Long-term real-world effectiveness of pharmacotherapies for schizoaffective disorder. *Schizophr Bull*, 47, 1099–1107.

39. Rybakowski, J. (1972). [Effect of lithium on synaptic transmission in the central nervous system]. *Psychiatr Pol*, 6, 323–325.

40. Rybakowski, J. K. and Ferensztajn-Rochowiak, E. (2022). Mini-review: Anomalous association between lithium data and lithium use. *Neurosci Lett*, 777, 136590.

41. Malhi, G. S., Bell, E., Hamilton, A., et al. (2021). Lithium mythology. *Bipolar Disord*, 23, 7–10.

42. Malhi, G. S., Bell, E., Boyce, P., et al. (2020). Make lithium great again! *Bipolar Disord*, 22, 325–327.

43. Meyer, J. M. and Stahl, S. M. (2019). *The Clozapine Handbook* (Stahl's Handbooks). Cambridge: Cambridge University Press.

44. Winstanley, J., Young, A. H. and Jauhar, S. (2021). Back to basics – a UK perspective on "Make lithium great again" Malhi et al. *Bipolar Disord*, 23, 97–98.

45. Olfson, M., Gerhard, T., Crystal, S., et al. (2016). Clozapine for schizophrenia: State variation in evidence-based practice. *Psychiatr Serv*, 67, 152.

46. Bareis, N., Olfson, M., Wall, M., et al. (2022). Variation in psychotropic medication prescription for adults with schizophrenia in the United States. *Psychiatr Serv*, 73, 492–500.

47. Whiskey, E., Barnard, A., Oloyede, E., et al. (2021). An evaluation of the variation and underuse of clozapine in the United Kingdom. *Acta Psychiatr Scand*, 143, 339–347.

48. Sköld, M., Rolstad, S., Joas, E., et al. (2021). Regional lithium prescription rates and recurrence in bipolar disorder. *Int J Bipolar Disord*, 9, 18–27.

49. Carruthers, J., Radigan, M., Erlich, M. D., et al. (2016). An initiative to improve clozapine prescribing in New York State. *Psychiatr Serv*, 67, 369–371.

50. Bogers, J. P. A. M., Schulte, P. F. J., Van Dijk, D., et al. (2016). Clozapine underutilization in the treatment of schizophrenia. *J Clin Psychopharmacol*, 36, 109–111.

51. Schneck, C. D., Miklowitz, D. J., Calabrese, J. R., et al. (2004). Phenomenology of rapid-cycling bipolar disorder: data from the first 500 participants in the Systematic Treatment Enhancement Program. *Am J Psychiatry*, 161, 1902–1908.

52. Strawbridge, R., Kurana, S., Kerr-Gaffney, J., et al. (2022). A systematic review and meta-analysis of treatments for rapid cycling bipolar disorder. *Acta Psychiatr Scand*, 146, 290–311.

53. Fountoulakis, K. N., Tohen, M. and Zarate, C. A. (2022). Lithium treatment of bipolar disorder in adults: A systematic review of randomized trials and meta-analyses. *Eur Neuropsychopharmacol*, 54, 100–115.

54. Baldessarini, R. J., Tondo, L., Floris, G., et al. (2000). Effects of rapid cycling on response to lithium maintenance treatment in 360 bipolar I and II disorder patients. *J Affect Disord*, 61, 13–22.

55. Kemp, D. E., Gao, K., Ganocy, S. J., et al. (2009). A 6-month, double-blind, maintenance trial of lithium monotherapy versus the combination of lithium and divalproex for rapid-cycling bipolar disorder and co-occurring substance abuse or dependence. *J Clin Psychiatry*, 70, 113–121.

56. Young, R. C., Mulsant, B. H., Sajatovic, M., et al. (2017). GERI-BD: a randomized double-blind controlled trial of lithium and divalproex in the treatment of mania in older patients with bipolar disorder. *Am J Psychiatry*, 174, 1086–1093.

57. Rej, S., Yu, C., Shulman, K., et al. (2015). Medical comorbidity, acute medical care use in late-life bipolar disorder: A comparison of lithium, valproate, and other pharmacotherapies. *Gen Hosp Psychiatry*, 37, 528–532.

58. Rej, S., Abitbol, R., Looper, K., et al. (2013). Chronic renal failure in lithium-using geriatric patients: Effects of lithium continuation versus discontinuation – a 60-month retrospective study. *Int J Geriatr Psychiatry*, 28, 450–453.

59. Rej, S., Looper, K. and Segal, M. (2013). The effect of serum lithium levels on renal function in geriatric outpatients: A retrospective longitudinal study. *Drugs Aging*, 30, 409–415.

60. Rej, S., Li, B. W., Looper, K., et al. (2014). Renal function in geriatric psychiatry patients compared to non-psychiatric older adults: Effects of lithium use and other factors. *Aging Ment Health*, 18, 847–853.

61. Rej, S., Elie, D., Mucsi, I., et al. (2015). Chronic kidney disease in lithium-treated older adults: A review of epidemiology, mechanisms, and implications for the treatment of late-life mood disorders. *Drugs Aging*, 32, 31–42.

62. Juurlink, D. N., Mamdani, M. M., Kopp, A., et al. (2004). Drug-induced lithium toxicity in the elderly: A population-based study. *J Am Geriatr Soc*, 52, 794–798.

63. Rej, S., Shulman, K., Herrmann, N., et al. (2014). Prevalence and correlates of renal disease in older lithium users: A population-based study. *Am J Geriatr Psychiatry*, 22, 1075–1082.

64. Aiff, H., Attman, P.-O., Aurell, M., et al. (2014). The impact of modern treatment principles may have eliminated lithium-induced renal failure. *J Psychopharmacol*, 28, 151–154.

65. Castro, V. M., Roberson, A. M., McCoy, T. H., et al. (2016). Stratifying risk for renal insufficiency among lithium-treated patients: An electronic health record study. *Neuropsychopharmacology*, 41, 1138–1143.

66. Pradhan, B. K., Chakrabarti, S., Irpati, A. S., et al. (2011). Distress due to lithium-induced polyuria: Exploratory study. *Psychiatry Clin Neurosci*, 65, 386–388.

67. Kinahan, J. C., NiChorcorain, A., Cunningham, S., et al. (2015). Diagnostic accuracy of tests for polyuria in lithium-treated patients. *J Clin Psychopharmacol*, 35, 434–441.

68. Bedford, J. J., Weggery, S., Ellis, G., et al. (2008). Lithium-induced nephrogenic diabetes insipidus: renal effects of amiloride. *Clin J Am Soc Nephrol*, 3, 1324–1331.

69. Fornaro, M., Maritan, E., Ferranti, R., et al. (2020). Lithium exposure during pregnancy and the postpartum period: A systematic review and meta-analysis of safety and efficacy outcomes. *Am J Psychiatry*, 177, 76–92.

70. Paton, C., Cookson, J., Ferrier, I. N., et al. (2018). A UK clinical audit addressing the quality of prescribing of sodium valproate for bipolar disorder in women of childbearing age. *BMJ Open*, 8, e020450.

71. Zhang, L., Li, H., Li, S., et al. (2016). Reproductive and metabolic abnormalities in women taking valproate for bipolar disorder: A meta-analysis. *Eur J Obstet Gynecol Reprod Biol*, 202, 26–31.

72. Gitlin, M. (2016). Lithium side effects and toxicity: Prevalence and management strategies. *Int J Bipolar Disord*, 4, 27–36.

73. Öhlund, L., Ott, M., Oja, S., et al. (2018). Reasons for lithium discontinuation in men and women with bipolar disorder: A retrospective cohort study. *BMC Psychiatry*, 18, 37–46.

74. Kupka, R. W., Nolen, W. A., Post, R. M., et al. (2002). High rate of autoimmune thyroiditis in bipolar disorder: Lack of association with lithium exposure. *Biol Psychiatry*, 51, 305–311.

75. Kraszewska, A., Ziemnicka, K., Sowinski, J., et al. (2019). No connection between long-term lithium treatment and antithyroid antibodies. *Pharmacopsychiatry*, 52, 232–236.

76. Lieber, I., Ott, M., Öhlund, L., et al. (2020). Lithium-associated hypothyroidism and potential for reversibility after lithium discontinuation: Findings from the LiSIE retrospective cohort study. *J Psychopharmacol*, 34, 293–303.

77. Frye, M. A., Denicoff, K. D., Bryan, A. L., et al. (1999). Association between lower serum free T4 and greater mood instability and depression in lithium-maintained bipolar patients. *Am J Psychiatry*, 156, 1909–1914.

78. Frye, M. A., Yatham, L., Ketter, T. A., et al. (2009). Depressive relapse during lithium treatment associated with increased serum thyroid-stimulating hormone: results from two placebo-controlled bipolar I maintenance studies. *Acta Psychiatr Scand*, 120, 10–13.

79. Cole, D. P., Thase, M. E., Mallinger, A. G., et al. (2002). Slower treatment response in bipolar depression predicted by lower pretreatment thyroid function. *Am J Psychiatry*, 159, 116–121.

80. Meyer, J. M. (2022). Pharmacotherapy of psychosis and mania. In L. L. Brunton and B. C. Knollmann, eds., *Goodman & Gilman's The Pharmacological Basis of Therapeutics, 14th Edition*. Chicago: McGraw-Hill, pp. 357–384.

81. Allergan USA Inc. (2019). *Vraylar package insert.* Madison, NJ.

82. Berk, M., Daglas, R., Dandash, O., et al. (2017). Quetiapine v. lithium in the maintenance phase following a first episode of mania: Randomised controlled trial. *Br J Psychiatry*, 210, 413–421.

83. Post, R. M. (2018). Preventing the malignant transformation of bipolar disorder. *JAMA*, 319, 1197–1198.

84. Griffiths, K., Millgate, E., Egerton, A., et al. (2021). Demographic and clinical variables associated with response to clozapine in schizophrenia: A systematic review and meta-analysis. *Psychol Med*, 51, 376–386.

85. Kessing, L. V., Hansen, H. V., Hvenegaard, A., et al. (2013). Treatment in a specialised out-patient mood disorder clinic v. standard out-patient treatment in the early course of bipolar disorder: Randomised clinical trial. *Br J Psychiatry*, 202, 212–219.

86. Baldessarini, R. J., Tondo, L. and Vazquez, G. H. (2019). Pharmacological treatment of adult bipolar disorder. *Mol Psychiatry*, 24, 198–217.

87. Malhi, G. S., Bell, E., Boyce, P., et al. (2020). The 2020 Royal Australian and New Zealand College of Psychiatrists clinical practice guidelines for mood disorders: Bipolar disorder summary. *Bipolar Disord*, 22, 805–821.

88. McIntyre, R. S., Berk, M., Brietzke, E., et al. (2020). Bipolar disorders. *Lancet*, 396, 1841–1856.

89. Nunes, A., Ardau, R., Berghofer, A., et al. (2020). Prediction of lithium response using clinical data. *Acta Psychiatr Scand*, 141, 131–141.

90. Hui, T. P., Kandola, A., Shen, L., et al. (2019). A systematic review and meta-analysis of clinical predictors of lithium response in bipolar disorder. *Acta Psychiatr Scand*, 140, 94–115.

91. Grillault Laroche, D., Etain, B., Severus, E., et al. (2020). Socio-demographic and clinical predictors of outcome to long-term treatment with lithium in bipolar disorders: A systematic review of the contemporary literature and recommendations from the ISBD/IGSLI Task Force on treatment with lithium. *Int J Bipolar Disord*, 8, 1–13.

92. Calabrese, J. R., Shelton, M. D., Rapport, D. J., et al. (2005). A 20-month, double-blind, maintenance trial of lithium versus divalproex in rapid-cycling bipolar disorder. *Am J Psychiatry*, 162, 2152–2161.

93. Chen, T. K., Knicely, D. H. and Grams, M. E. (2019). Chronic kidney disease diagnosis and management: A review. *JAMA*, 322, 1294–1304.

94. Rej, S., Beaulieu, S., Segal, M., et al. (2014). Lithium dosing and serum concentrations across the age spectrum: From early adulthood to the tenth decade of life. *Drugs Aging*, 31, 911–916.

95. Rej, S., Segal, M., Low, N. C., et al. (2014). The McGill Geriatric Lithium-Induced Diabetes Insipidus Clinical Study (McGLIDICS). *Can J Psychiatry*, 59, 327–334.

96. Fotso Soh, J., Klil-Drori, S. and Rej, S. (2019). Using lithium in older age bipolar disorder: Special considerations. *Drugs Aging*, 36, 147–154.

97. Fagiolini, A., Chengappa, K. N., Soreca, I., et al. (2008). Bipolar disorder and the metabolic syndrome: Causal factors, psychiatric outcomes and economic burden. *CNS Drugs*, 22, 655–669.

98. Fagiolini, A., Forgione, R., Maccari, M., et al. (2013). Prevalence, chronicity, burden and borders of bipolar disorder. *J Affect Disord*, 148, 161–169.

99. Kessing, L. V., Gerds, T. A., Feldt-Rasmussen, B., et al. (2015). Use of lithium and anticonvulsants and the rate of chronic kidney disease: A nationwide population-based study. *JAMA Psychiatry*, 72, 1182–1191.

100. Clos, S., Rauchhaus, P., Severn, A., et al. (2015). Long-term effect of lithium maintenance therapy on estimated glomerular filtration rate in patients with affective disorders: A population-based cohort study. *Lancet Psychiatry*, 2, 1075–1083.

101. Schoot, T. S., Molmans, T. H. J., Grootens, K. P., et al. (2020). Systematic review and practical guideline for the prevention and management of the renal side effects of lithium therapy. *Eur Neuropsychopharmacol*, 31, 16–32.

102. Kortenoeven, M. L., Li, Y., Shaw, S., et al. (2009). Amiloride blocks lithium entry through the sodium channel thereby attenuating the resultant nephrogenic diabetes insipidus. *Kidney Int*, 76, 44–53.

103. Romaine, E. and McAllister-Williams, R. H. (2019). Guidelines on prescribing psychotropic medication during the perinatal period. *Br J Hosp Med (Lond)*, 80, 27–32.

104. Huybrechts, K. F., Hernandez-Diaz, S., Patorno, E., et al. (2016). Antipsychotic use in pregnancy and the risk for congenital malformations. *JAMA Psychiatry*, 73, 938–946.

105. McAllister-Williams, R. H., Baldwin, D. S., Cantwell, R., et al. (2017). British Association for Psychopharmacology consensus guidance on the use of psychotropic medication preconception, in pregnancy and postpartum 2017. *J Psychopharmacol*, 31, 519–552.

106 Lyall, L. M., Penades, N. and Smith, D. J. (2019). Changes in prescribing for bipolar disorder between 2009 and 2016: National-level data linkage study in Scotland. *Br J Psychiatry*, 215, 415–421.

107. Gitlin, M. J. and Jamison, K. R. (1984). Lithium clinics: Theory and practice. *Hosp Community Psychiatry*, 35, 363–368.

108. Biondi, B., Cappola, A. R. and Cooper, D. S. (2019). Subclinical hypothyroidism: A review. *JAMA*, 322, 153–160T.

109. Hegedüs, L., Bianco, A. C., Jonklaas, J., et al. (2022). Primary hypothyroidism and quality of life. *Nat Rev Endocrinol*, 18, 230–242.

1

The Efficacy Story

Acute Mania; Rapid Cycling Bipolar
Disorder; Bipolar II Disorder and Bipolar
Depression; Bipolar Disorder Prophylaxis,
Response Predictors; Unipolar Depression;
Suicidality; Aggressive or Impulsive
Behavior in Child/Adolescent Patients
with Conduct Disorder, in Borderline
Personality Disorder or in Patients with
Intellectual Disability; Neuroprotective
Properties; Elevation of Neutrophil Counts;
Mechanisms of Action

QUICK CHECK

PRINCIPLES

- Lithium is considered the gold standard for bipolar I disorder (BD-1) prophylaxis. Lithium monotherapy is effective in mania within the first seven days of treatment, and is no less effective than other mood stabilizer monotherapies for rapid cycling BD (RC-BD).

- Lithium remains an effective adjunctive option with antidepressants for unipolar major depressive disorder (MDD), but is not comparably effective as monotherapy for acute BD depression.

- Retrospective data indicate lithium reduces attempted and completed suicides, and reduces dementia incidence 50% among BD patients.

- Lithium has limited data for management of aggressive or impulsive behavior in child/adolescent patients with conduct disorder, in patients with borderline personality disorder or with intellectual disability, but can be considered in select circumstances.

- Lithium directly increases neutrophil counts by inducing production of granulocyte colony stimulating factor. This can be of clinical value in the management of clozapine treated patients.

- There are numerous intracellular pathways modulated by lithium therapy which explain its mood stabilizing and neuroprotective effects.

INTRODUCTION

WHAT TO KNOW: INTRODUCTION

- Lithium is considered the preferred maintenance mood stabilizer for any bipolar spectrum patient with a history of mania (e.g. bipolar I disorder; schizoaffective disorder, bipolar type [SAD-BT]). The role of lithium for bipolar II disorder depends on the need for mood stabilization.

- In real world studies, use of lithium, but not valproic acid, is associated with lower psychiatric hospitalization rates in bipolar disorder patients. Oxcarbazepine, topiramate and gabapentin have no effect on hospitalization risk.

- Retrospective studies provide compelling evidence for lithium's unique impact on risk for completed suicide, and for reduction in dementia risk with long-term use in older bipolar patients.

- Lithium is an effective adjunctive option for unipolar major depression.

As of this writing, every international bipolar disorder (BD) treatment guideline or major published review recommends lithium as the gold standard for acute and maintenance therapy in BD spectrum patients, especially those with a history of mania [1–4]. Lithium's acute antimanic properties and prophylactic effectiveness have been known for over 70 years, but the approval of second generation antipsychotics (SGAs) for BD-1 mania, BD depression and BD-1 maintenance (as monotherapy or adjunctive to mood stabilizers), and the increased use of anticonvulsant mood stabilizers such as divalproex (valproic acid or VPA), resulted in dramatic declines in lithium use over the past 20 years (Figure 1.1) [5]. These trends have stabilized, albeit at low levels, with a Finnish study noting that only 4.1% of newly diagnosed BD spectrum patients from 2016 to 2018 received lithium [5]. One epiphenomenon of low utilization is the loss of a shared cultural memory among mental health professionals regarding lithium's efficacy, leading to

Figure 1.1 20-year trends in use of mood stabilizing (MS) medications among newly diagnosed Finnish BD patients [5]

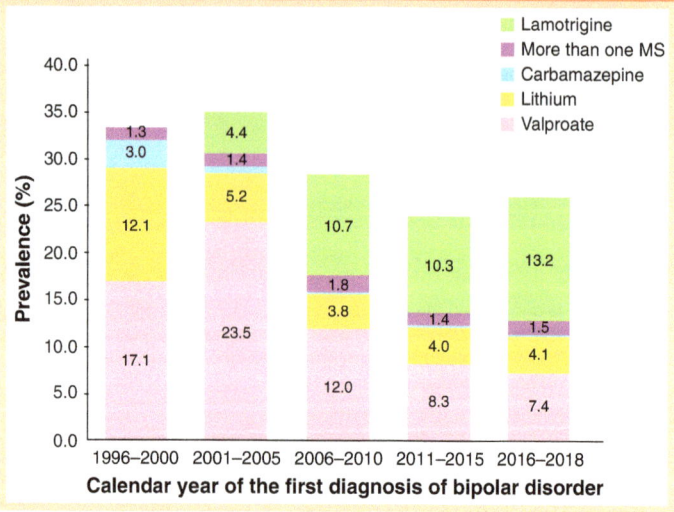

(Adapted from: J. Poranen, A. Koistinaho, A. Tanskanen, et al. [2022]. 20-year medication use trends in first-episode bipolar disorder. *Acta Psychiatr Scand*, 146, 583–593.)

erroneous conclusions that non-lithium therapies are equivalent, despite evidence to the contrary. Supporting the notion of lithium's overall superiority are papers that report real world outcomes among BD patients treated in an era when clinicians have access to an array of medication options including SGAs. One of the largest analyses examined rates of rehospitalization among 18,018 Finnish patients previously hospitalized for BD from 1996 to 2012 [6]. Although the data were not analyzed by BD subtype, the underlying assumption was that this population was predominantly BD-1, as other forms of BD have lower psychiatric hospitalization rates. The study used a within-individual analytic method in which each individual was used as his or her own control to examine hospitalization risk during periods on or off various treatments. Over a mean follow-up period of 7.2 years, 54.0% of the initial sample experienced a least one psychiatric rehospitalization. As noted in Table 1.1, lithium was the most effective mood stabilizer in preventing psychiatric rehospitalization, and carbamazepine also displayed efficacy, but this was not true for VPA or for any other anticonvulsant [6]. When outcomes were broken down by drug class, mood stabilizers were effective at reducing psychiatric rehospitalization risk while antipsychotics were not, and use of sedatives, benzodiazepines or antidepressants increased rehospitalization risk.

Table 1.1 A within-individual analysis of the association between use vs. no use of medications and the risk of psychiatric rehospitalization among Finnish BD patients previously hospitalized for bipolar disorder from 1996 to 2012 (n = 18,018) [6]

	Person-years	Fully adjusted HR (95% CI)	P value
Lithium	24815	0.78 (0.73–0.84)	< 0.001
Carbamazepine	5409	0.87 (0.77–0.98)	0.02
Gabapentin	541	0.96 (0.75–1.24)	0.76
Lamotrigine	12641	0.96 (0.89–1.04)	0.34
Oxcarbazepine	881	1.06 (0.84–1.33)	0.62
Topiramate	506	1.56 (1.21–2.00)	< 0.001 *
Valproate/divalproex	26091	0.99 (0.94–1.05)	0.80

* increased rehospitalization risk

(Adapted from: M. Lahteenvuo, A. Tanskanen, H. Taipale, et al. [2018]. Real-world effectiveness of pharmacologic treatments for the prevention of rehospitalization in a Finnish nationwide cohort of patients with bipolar disorder. *JAMA Psychiatry*, 75, 347–355.)

Few would dispute lithium's efficacy for acute mania, and a 2022 comprehensive meta-analysis on lithium treatment of adult BD noted that all of the placebo-controlled randomized clinical trials (RCTs) performed using modern study methodologies were positive, with onset of therapeutic effect by day 7 [4]. Despite the strength of this evidence, some clinicians lack familiarity with lithium loading or other means of rapidly starting lithium, and this can lead to relatively slow titrations and prolonged periods of subtherapeutic levels [7]. Any perceived lack of early efficacy in acute mania may partly be the product of the lithium initiation method [8, 9], but it is important to state that antipsychotics are extremely effective antimanic agents with faster onset than mood stabilizer monotherapy [9, 10]. Many first generation antipsychotics (FGAs) and SGAs have acute mania indications, some of which have injectable formulations that can be used for floridly manic patients who refuse oral mood stabilizers. Antipsychotics are indisputably an important part of acute mania management, and aripiprazole, olanzapine and injectable risperidone microspheres have indications as maintenance monotherapy in BD-1 adults; however, antipsychotics do not share lithium's impact on 2nd messenger systems, and failing to add lithium has clinical implications [11, 12]. As will be discussed in the section on lithium's mechanisms of action, stimulation of dopamine D_2 receptors by agonists (e.g. amphetamines) induces hyperlocomotion, a useful animal model for the psychomotor agitation of mania [13]. Dopamine D_2 receptor stimulation affects intracellular G-protein dependent pathways resulting in decreased cyclic AMP (cAMP) levels, but D_2 agonists also alter signaling in a non-G-protein pathway involving beta arrestin 2 (βArr2), increasing activity of glycogen synthase kinase 3-β (GSK3-β) and inducing hyperlocomotion [14]. Lithium robustly inhibits GSK3-β activity and markedly decreases D_2 agonist stimulated hyperlocomotion; moreover, lithium is an even more selective and potent inhibitor of GSK3-β activity than SGA antipsychotics [15]. Therefore, while certain features of mania will improve after antipsychotic administration, other untreated aspects can continue to drive positive psychotic symptoms, ongoing acts of impulsivity or mood instability [16]. This phenomenon was described by the Danish psychiatrist and lithium pioneer Mogens Schou in the sixth edition of his guide to lithium treatment: **"An experienced patient, who during previous manias had first tried a neuroleptic and then lithium, reported that during treatment with the former he felt as if the gas pedal and the brake were pressed down at the same time. With lithium it was as if the ignition had been switched off"** [17]. The differential effects of SGAs and lithium on mood stability are seen very clearly in long-term naturalistic outcomes of BD-1 patients after a manic episode. Follow-up data subsequent to 5713 hospitalizations for mania among Swedish BD-1 patients aged 18–75 (2006–2014) showed that those on SGA monotherapy experienced markedly higher rates of treatment failure than those on lithium, with medication switching and discontinuation the leading reasons for failure to persist with SGA monotherapy [18].

Despite the abundant RCT and retrospective data supporting lithium's effectiveness in BD-1, there is a surprising paucity of studies for other bipolar spectrum disorders such as BD-2, schizoaffective disorder, bipolar type (SAD-BT) and RC-BD patients [19–22]. As SAD-BT and BD-1 share the same liability for mania, it is often assumed that lithium's efficacy in BD-1 (acutely and prophylactically) should generalize to this related disorder. There are no data to suggest otherwise, but any statements about lithium's efficacy in SAD-BT patients rest largely on retrospective studies or older studies with methodological or definitional issues [21, 23].

In-Depth 1.2 Lithium in Schizophrenia Spectrum Patients

The limited prospective studies of lithium primarily involve schizophrenia, not SAD-BT, and a 2015 Cochrane review of trials where lithium was added adjunctively to antipsychotic therapy for schizophrenia (22 studies, total n = 763) found that most studies were small and methodologically weak. For nonaffective psychosis (i.e. schizophrenia), any evidence lithium is effective in augmenting antipsychotics was of low quality, and the effects were not significant when more prone-to-bias open RCTs were excluded [24]. However, a 2022 Finnish real world outcomes analysis of every individual hospitalized for schizophrenia during 1972–2014 (n = 61,889) found that use of adjunctive lithium, VPA or lamotrigine reduced risk of psychosis related rehospitalization by 12% during the follow-up period (1996–2017) [25]. That these effects were seen across several mood stabilizers with varying mechanisms of action suggests that a small subset of patients labeled with a schizophrenia diagnosis most likely have SAD-BT and therefore benefit from mood stabilization in a manner that patients with schizophrenia would not [16]. Employing this logic, a 2021 handbook on management of complex treatment resistant psychotic disorders suggests an empiric lithium trial in cases where the working diagnosis is schizophrenia, but SAD-BT is suspected based on history or clinical features [16]. Failure to improve with adjunctive lithium confirms the schizophrenia diagnosis, while substantial improvement demands a change in the working diagnosis to SAD-BT.

More research is clearly needed to examine lithium's efficacy for acute mania and mania prophylaxis in SAD-BT since these patients need mood stabilization for optimal symptom control [26]. Conversely, the clinical course of BD-2 dictates less dependence on mood stabilization to prevent hypomania/mania, and the lithium literature in this area is underdeveloped (Figure 1.2) [20, 27, 28]. The few prospective lithium trials in BD-2 focus exclusively on depressive symptomatology, with the limited data indicating modest efficacy for lithium as monotherapy [4]. There are also studies showing that BD-2 patients respond to and tolerate traditional antidepressant therapies (e.g. venlafaxine) without risk of hypomania induction [29]; nevertheless, lithium remains an important option for those BD-2 patients who do need mood stabilization and for whom non-lithium maintenance options such as lamotrigine have been insufficiently effective.

Figure 1.2 Proportion of time spent asymptomatic or with mood symptoms based on long-term weekly follow-up of BD-1 (n = 146, mean follow-up 12.8 years) and BD-2 (n = 86, mean follow-up 13.4 years) patients [27, 28]

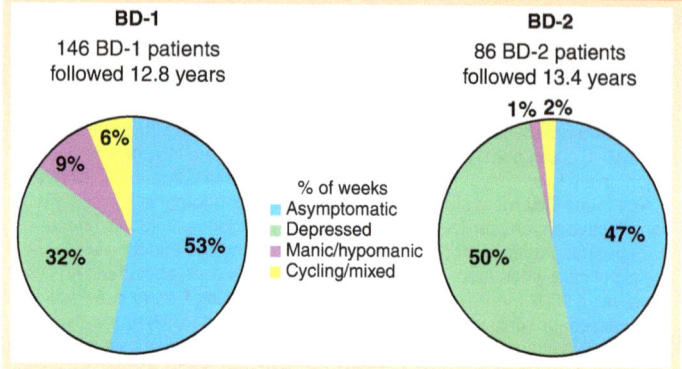

(Adapted from: L. L. Judd, H. S. Akiskal, P. J. Schettler, et al. [2002]. The long-term natural history of the weekly symptomatic status of bipolar I disorder. *Arch Gen Psychiatry*, 59, 530–537; L. L. Judd, H. S. Akiskal, P. J. Schettler, et al. (2003). A prospective investigation of the natural history of the long-term weekly symptomatic status of bipolar II disorder. *Arch Gen Psychiatry*, 60, 261–269.)

The exact place of lithium in the BD-2 algorithm is not easily answered with existing data, yet one area of the BD spectrum that has been addressed more successfully is the value of lithium for RC-BD patients [30, 31]. Extensive research into the clinical course of RC-BD has revealed that these patients respond poorly to any form of mood stabilizer monotherapy due to frequent depressive episodes of short duration [31]. Lithium is effective in preventing hypomania or mania in BD-1 or BD-2 patients with a history of rapid cycling, and lithium treated RC-BD patients do not spend a greater proportion of time ill than lithium treated BD patients without a history of rapid cycling [32]. The findings from multiple sources point to the fact that RC-BD patients will often need combination therapy, especially for management of recurrent major depressive episodes [31]. The few prospective studies in RC-BD show that lithium is not inferior to divalproex [33, 34], and therefore lithium remains the mood stabilizer of choice for RC-BD-1 patients, with the recognition that an adjunctive medication will almost certainly be needed for bipolar depression (e.g. certain SGAs for acute depressive symptoms, lamotrigine for maintenance) [31, 35].

In-Depth 1.3 Despite its Anti-Suicide Properties There are Limited Data for Lithium's Efficacy in Acute Bipolar Depression

Although there is a vigorous debate about the extent of lithium's anti-suicide properties [36], there is no high-quality evidence that lithium is an effective treatment for acute BD depression [4]. There is at least one study demonstrating that lithium monotherapy can reduce depressive recurrences during maintenance therapy of euthymic patients [37], but 10 of the 11 lithium monotherapy trials for acute BD depression were methodologically weak by modern standards. The one rigorous, prospective, double-blind, 8-week RCT randomized 802 depressed BD subjects (BD-1, n = 499; BD-2, n = 303) to one of 4 treatment arms: quetiapine 300 mg/d (n = 265), quetiapine 600 mg/d (n = 268), lithium 600–1800 mg/d (n = 136) or placebo (n = 133) [38]. This study did not find efficacy for lithium; there was no correlation between lithium serum levels and depression rating changes; and the lack of efficacy was true in study completers and in the subgroup with higher serum lithium levels (> 0.80 mEq/l) [4, 38]. Other agents with regulatory approval for acute BD depression are the treatments of choice (e.g. cariprazine, lumateperone, lurasidone, quetiapine, olanzapine/fluoxetine combination), with lamotrigine considered only for maintenance therapy to mitigate depressive relapse. (Lamotrigine's extended titration to eliminate Stevens–Johnson Syndrome risk prevents acute use for bipolar depression [39].)

The difficulty in using RCT results to prove that lithium has an impact on risk of completed suicide and possesses neuroprotective properties limits the robustness of conclusions for those applications [40]; however, it is worth noting the lack of compelling data to suggest greater effectiveness for other mood stabilizing agents in these areas, and the accumulation of findings from some (but not all) meta-analyses indicating that lithium has comparatively superior reduction vs. non-lithium therapy for dementia risk among older BD patients, and for reduction in serious suicide attempts and suicide mortality [4, 41–44]. Some of these data come from epidemiological studies in multiple countries that found a correlation between higher lithium levels in the municipal water supply and lower rates of suicide in certain geographic regions, as opposed to ones with comparable sociodemographic and psychiatric characteristics but lithium levels below the median [45–47]. The large number of studies reporting this finding across the Americas, Europe and Asia argue for a plausible association, with a significant caveat about the limitations of such retrospective analyses. Nonetheless, the weight of the evidence is sufficient for clinicians to consider lithium as the preferred agent for BD patients with a history of suicide attempts, despite the limitations of the RCT literature. The same logic also applies when treating older BD-1 patients: the findings of lithium's effect on dementia risk in BD patients are from retrospective analyses and not prospective RCTs; however, unlike suicidality, there are RCT data demonstrating neuroprotective properties among adults with mild cognitive impairment [48]. With that in mind, having a BD diagnosis is associated with a 3-fold increased risk for dementia, and a 2020 meta-analysis found that long-term lithium use was associated with a 50% reduction in dementia risk [44].

Lithium has been studied repeatedly for unipolar MDD, primarily as adjunctive therapy, but there is no consensus on lithium's place in the unipolar MDD treatment algorithm [49]. One issue is that certain SGA and glutamate based strategies (e.g. ketamine, esketamine) have double-blind placebo-controlled studies performed with patients on newer antidepressants, thus providing a certain level of confidence for the clinician that these findings will generalize to current practice settings. Unfortunately, much of the early lithium MDD research involved tricyclic antidepressants, and a 2019 meta-analysis found that the last placebo-controlled adjunctive lithium trial for unipolar MDD was published in 2003 [49]. Adjunctive lithium was also a treatment arm in a large sequential treatment algorithm study (STAR-D) for participants who failed two prior antidepressant treatments, but the results dampened the enthusiasm for lithium by finding that remission rates were modest for lithium and did not differ from the remission rate with triiodothyronine [50]. The authors commented that the lower side effect burden and ease of use for triiodothyronine augmentation suggest that it has slight advantages over lithium augmentation in unipolar MDD patients who failed several medication trials [50]. Nonetheless, despite the availability of SGA and glutamate based options that are effective and require less laboratory monitoring, a recent comparative review commented that adjunctive lithium was somewhat more effective and better tolerated than these other strategies for unipolar MDD, implying that lithium need not be relegated to the latter stages of the MDD treatment algorithm despite the limitations of the data [51].

The extent of lithium's anti-aggressive effects is another area where there are virtually no placebo-controlled prospective data, but a large volume of open-label, uncontrolled and retrospective studies, and several papers reporting a positive association between higher levels in drinking water and lower rates of violent crimes [52, 53]. While not a panacea, the paucity of options that convincingly decrease risk of completed suicide pose a reasonable argument for consideration of a lithium trial in suicidal BD patients as noted above [40]. A less convincing argument can be made for routine use of lithium to manage conduct disorder and aggression in non-bipolar children or adolescents [54, 55], for management of disruptive behaviors in intellectually disabled individuals [56, 57] or to manage impulsivity in borderline personality disorder [58]. There are more strongly evidence based treatments for some of these clinical scenarios (e.g. SGAs for irritability associated with autistic disorder), and the evidence for lithium (to the extent that any exists) is of low quality.

   Lithium has been studied for dozens of other clinical indications, both psychiatric and nonpsychiatric, some of which are no longer relevant, while others remain an important part of psychiatric practice. One example of the former is lithium's prophylactic use for patients with cluster headache. Early studies indicated lithium was efficacious, with subsequent research linking this to partial agonist activity at serotonin $5HT_{1B}$ receptors; however, lithium has been replaced by more effective options, including the potent $5HT_{1B}$ and $5HT_{1D}$ receptor agonist triptan class for abortive treatment, and by verapamil for prophylaxis [59, 60]. The last double-blind, placebo-controlled trial for cluster headache was performed in 1997, but was stopped after the 27th patient was enrolled when a planned interim analysis did not reach the prespecified efficacy signal to differentiate lithium from placebo [59]. Neutrophilia is a known consequence of lithium therapy, and one that should be communicated to all providers to avoid subjecting patients to an unnecessary work-up for occult infection or a hematological disorder. One current psychiatric application for this property is the use of lithium to support clozapine prescribing [61, 62]. Lithium directly stimulates neutrophil production by increasing the levels of granulocyte colony stimulating factor [63–65]. This is a niche but important use for lithium, and one that will likely persist until such time as a medication appears with clozapine's efficacy and without its neutropenia risk.

In-Depth 1.4 Lithium's Unique and Diverse Intracellular Mechanisms

That lithium is an agent with numerous and diverse properties is clear, leading to decades of research on lithium's numerous intracellular mechanisms of action (MOAs), specifically those activities that convey its mood stabilizing, neuroprotective and anti-aggression/anti-suicide properties [66–68]. One can practice psychiatric medicine effectively without understanding the biological hypotheses for lithium's effectiveness, but an appreciation of certain well-studied pathways, such as that leading to GSK3-β inhibition, can inform practice by providing a molecular basis for lithium's distinct spectrum of clinical activities. This preclinical research also sheds light on how agents with antimanic properties (e.g. antipsychotics, lithium, divalproex) are not necessarily interchangeable, why manic patients experience the effects of lithium and antipsychotics differently, and why SGA or divalproex monotherapy may not yield the same maintenance outcomes as lithium in BD-1 patients [18]. These are very relevant talking points with BD-1 patients who want to pursue SGA maintenance monotherapy due to concerns about lithium, or to avoid its monitoring burden. In an ideal world, there would be clinical predictors and biomarkers of treatment response for lithium and non-lithium therapies to inform treatment choices. While biomarker research is an exciting area of study, it is not yet at the stage of clinical application [69]. Translating some of the research on clinical predictors of lithium response into patient-level decisions can also be problematic. Many of the features associated with inadequate lithium response (e.g. substance use, RC-BD, chronic course, anxiety) are also shared with non-lithium therapies, but many of the papers lack comparative data to put those findings into context [69–75].

In the end, BD-1 is a difficult disorder to manage, and the finding that only 20% achieve durable remission on lithium monotherapy speaks more to the fact that a single mood stabilizing agent may be insufficient for many BD-1 patients, despite lithium's unique efficacy spectrum [74]. The consensus opinion that lithium is an unparalleled medication and the standard of care for BD-1 rests on the recognition that all treatments have limitations, yet lithium possesses comparative advantages that place it at the top of the treatment algorithm [3]. These relative advantages do not lie in the area of acute mania, BD-2 maintenance, acute bipolar depression or unipolar MDD antidepressant augmentation, but in BD-1 or SAD-BT maintenance, with the impact on suicide related deaths and dementia incidence as important differentiating factors. Those areas in particular where lithium presents a unique therapeutic option (e.g. reduced risk for completed suicide, reduction in dementia risk) are covered in greater length so clinicians can appreciate that conclusions about these properties rest primarily on retrospective analyses, despite attempts to study suicidality in RCTs [40]. There are areas of medicine where certain assertions appear true from the breadth and extent of the retrospective data, but not provably true without performing a large, long-term RCT whose sheer scope might not be economically feasible. Clinical decisions must be made using all of the effectiveness data, even those which are imperfect. After three-quarters of a century, the weight of the data supports the special role of lithium for treatment of mood disorders, especially BD spectrum patients with a history of mania or suicidality, and for older BD-1 individuals (Table 1.2).

Table 1.2 The place of lithium in treatment guidelines updated since 2018 [4]

	CANMAT/ ISBD 2018 [2]	WFSBP 2009–2018 [76–80]	RANCZP 2020 [81]	CINP 2017–2020 [82–84]	NICE 2020 [85]
Acute mania	1	3	1	2	1 *
Prophylaxis: any mood episode	1	1		1	1 *
Prophylaxis: mania	1	1	1	1	
Prophylaxis: depression	1	4		1	

* But not in primary care settings

(Adapted from: K. N. Fountoulakis, M. Tohen and C. A. Zarate [2022]. Lithium treatment of bipolar disorder in adults: a systematic review of randomized trials and meta-analyses. *Eur Neuropsychopharmacol*, 54, 100–115.)

A Acute Mania

WHAT TO KNOW: ACUTE MANIA

- In modern methodologically rigorous acute mania trials, lithium has comparable efficacy to the antipsychotic monotherapy options studied (aripiprazole, quetiapine) and also to divalproex/valproic acid. In clinical practice, lithium is rarely used as monotherapy for acute mania and is typically combined with an antipsychotic.
- Newer consensus recommendations suggest lithium levels in the range of 1.00–1.20 mEq/l for acute mania treatment. Higher levels are no longer employed due to the potential adverse renal impact of 12 h trough levels > 1.20 mEq/l, and other tolerability concerns.

Once early publications in 1949–1954 demonstrated lithium's acute antimanic properties [86], this was followed by papers noting robust prophylactic effectiveness, with reduction in mood relapses by as much as 90% in studies of various designs, including within-subject mirror-image studies utilizing periods on lithium or on placebo [87]. A 2022 meta-analysis and review of all adult BD trials noted that many of the early acute mania monotherapy studies were open-label, or possessed methodological issues in trial design or outcome reporting that prevent use of meta-analytic statistical methods. Among the 64 acute mania monotherapy studies examined, only five placebo-controlled trials published from 1994 to 2009 were of sufficient quality to merit inclusion in the review, all of which included other comparator arms (VPA, aripiprazole, quetiapine, topiramate) [4]. Based on change in the Young Mania Rating Scale (YMRS) total score, lithium monotherapy was clearly superior to placebo for acute mania at mean serum levels ranging from 0.76 to 1.20 mEq/l across those five trials. Superiority of lithium vs. placebo was also seen in the proportion of patients who achieved symptomatic response ($\geq$ 50% reduction in YMRS) or remission (YMRS $\leq$ 12) at study endpoint [4]. For acute mania, lithium was comparable in efficacy to monotherapy SGA options (aripiprazole, quetiapine) and to VPA, and more effective than topiramate, an anticonvulsant whose use as a mood stabilizer has been abandoned. The most common lithium initiation method was to commence with 900 mg/d in divided doses (typically 3 times per day) for the first few days, with flexible dosing from days 3–5 onward based on response and tolerability, while maintaining 12 h trough levels within a target range (e.g. 0.60–1.20 mEq/l, 0.60–1.40 mEq/l, etc.) [88–91]. With this dosing approach, efficacy was seen on average by day 7. These trials reported serum lithium level ranges and mean levels ($\pm$ a standard deviation), but lacked granular patient-level information to discern what proportion had subtherapeutic levels, and to what extent subtherapeutic levels depressed aggregate lithium response. There was also no exploration of response characteristics (e.g. continuous or categorical response) by serum lithium level [4].

Lithium and VPA are the most commonly used mood stabilizing agents as monotherapy, but their efficacy has not been adequately studied in patients diagnosed with mania or hypomania with mixed features using DSM-5 criteria [92]. The RCT literature on mixed BD states is composed exclusively of SGA trials. There are also no prospective RCT data for SAD-BT patients who present with acute mania, although BD-1 clinical trials report that lithium's antimanic activity exists in patients with and without psychosis [4]. Tolerability data indicate that lithium has more adverse effects than placebo (e.g. somnolence, tremor, gastrointestinal complaints) [4, 93], but a 2019 Cochrane review commented that adequate data on the incidence of adverse events vs. other agents were contained in too few studies to provide high certainty evidence of comparative tolerability [93]. It is worth noting that some acute mania studies allowed lithium levels as high as 1.40 mEq/l or 1.50 mEq/l, somewhat beyond the range used in current practice [88, 89].

In-Depth 1.5 The Evidence for Optimal Lithium Serum Levels in Acute Mania

Modern RCTs reinforce the observation from Cade's 1949 case series that lithium is effective for mania, but the omission of lithium level subanalyses in recent studies did not provide further insight with respect to optimal levels during acute treatment [94]. The absence of modern RCTs randomly assigning acutely manic subjects to target serum level ranges (e.g. 0.80–1.20 mEq/l vs. 1.00–1.20 mEq/l) and the lack of nuanced data from modern double-blind, placebo-controlled RCTs means that any recommended serum level minimum (e.g. ≥ 1.00 mEq/l) or suggested maximum level (e.g. 1.20 mEq/l) during acute mania treatment is not supported by high-quality data. Nevertheless, consensus recommendations for use of higher lithium levels during acute mania treatment are clearly supported by the older literature, but not as strongly as one might surmise [2, 83]. Achieving a serum level close to 1.00 mEq/l appears a reasonable inference from recent RCTs, while avoiding levels > 1.20 mEq/l is driven by three practical concerns: (1) lithium is rarely prescribed as monotherapy for acute mania, obviating to some extent the need to employ extremely high levels; (2) acute tolerability diminishes significantly at levels > 1.20 mEq/l, so patient exposure to higher levels increases the risk of adverse effects and lithium refusal; (3) evidence from a large retrospective outpatient study (n = 5751) published in 2016 indicated that a single lithium level exceeding 1.20 mEq/l was associated with increased risk of renal insufficiency (odds ratio 1.74, 95% CI 1.33–2.25) [95].

Supporting the common practice of lithium plus antipsychotic therapy for acute mania are the results of numerous trials showing the superiority of combination therapy over lithium monotherapy, with positive data specifically for haloperidol, asenapine, olanzapine, risperidone, quetiapine and carbamazepine [81]. Combined treatment also showed superiority over quetiapine monotherapy. The absence of prospective data on combined lithium plus divalproex therapy vs. either agent alone is a gap in the literature, but the few studies suggest additive benefit in acute mania consistent with the robust and comparable antimanic effect of each mood stabilizer as monotherapy [96]. It is for this reason that patients displaying an inadequate mania response despite a lithium level of 1.20 mEq/l and concurrent antipsychotic therapy should be considered candidates to receive an additional first line mood stabilizer for optimal mood control during the acute and maintenance phases of treatment [18, 81, 97]. The inability to load carbamazepine and its numerous kinetic interactions with antipsychotics place divalproex in the position as the adjunctive mood stabilizer of choice in these more challenging cases [12]. For clinicians with limited experience in using lithium for acute mania, the modern RCT data convincingly demonstrate that lithium is effective as monotherapy or in combination treatment, and that efficacy is seen within the first week even when an evidence based initiation or loading regimen is not employed (see Info Box 4.3) [7].

B   Rapid Cycling

WHAT TO KNOW: RAPID CYCLING

- The hallmark of rapid cycling bipolar disorder (RC-BD) is frequent depressive episodes of short duration. RC-BD patients will typically not respond completely to any mood stabilizer monotherapy and will require additional medications to manage recurrent bipolar depression.
- Lithium is equally effective in decreasing the time spent ill and the number of manic/hypomanic and major depressive episodes in RC-BD patients and non-RC-BD patients; however, RC-BD patients will experience higher numbers of depressive recurrences than non-RC-BD peers, despite having equivalent periods of time without mood episodes.
- The limited prospective data indicate that lithium is non-inferior to divalproex, and that the combination of divalproex and lithium is no more effective than lithium monotherapy.

As noted in the 2022 meta-analysis of adult lithium BD trials, "the widely believed concept among clinicians that divalproex is more effective than lithium in the long-term management of rapid-cycling BD was not supported" by the only clinical trial to examine this issue [33]. The current impression that lithium is not inferior to other mood stabilizers for RC-BD maintenance therapy is based on almost 50 years of research that characterized RC-BD as a difficult group to treat with any mood stabilizer monotherapy due to the frequency of depressive episodes [31]. As of 2022, leading BD experts comment about lithium: "It is equally efficacious in rapid and non-rapid cycling patients" [4].

The concept of rapid cycling is a relatively recent one in the world of BD, first elaborated in a 1974 paper [98]. The DSM-5-TR definition requires the presence of at least four mood episodes in the prior 12 months that meet criteria for mania, hypomania or major depression, excluding substance-induced episodes (e.g. due to stimulants, steroids, antidepressants) [99]. A 2004 paper provided one of the more complete characterizations of RC-BD patients by analyzing data from the first 500 subjects enrolled in a US National Institute of Mental Health (NIMH) study of BD depression (any BD subtype) for individuals age ≥ 15 years [100, 101]. This patient pool had a mean age of 41.7 years, with mean age of onset 17.5 years, and 59.4% were female. Of the 500 subjects, 483 could be classified as BD-1 or BD-2, and among the 456 individuals with data on episode frequency, 20% met DSM-IV criteria for rapid cycling in the prior 12 months [101]. As seen in Table 1.3, the prevalence of RC-BD was nearly identical in BD-1 and BD-2 patients, and

Table 1.3 The clinical course of rapid cycling bipolar disorder (RC-BD) in comparison with BD patients without a history of rapid cycling (n = 500) [101]

	BD-1	BD-2	Female	Male	BD-1 + substance use disorder	BD-2 + substance use disorder	Age of 1st manic or hypomanic episode	Age of 1st major depressive episode	Number of mood episodes in the prior year: mania or hypomania	Number of mood episodes in the prior year: major depression
RC-BD	20.0%	19.8%	23%	16%	41%	18%	18.8 ± 9.5	16.7 ± 8.7	9.0 ± 13.1	8.1 ± 11.5
Non-RC-BD	80.0%	80.2%	77%	84%	36%	36%	22.1 ± 10.0	20.0 ± 8.5	0.8 ± 0.9	1.1 ± 0.9

(Adapted from: C. D. Schneck, D. J. Miklowitz, J. R. Calabrese et al. [2004]. Phenomenology of rapid-cycling bipolar disorder: Data from the first 500 participants in the Systematic Treatment Enhancement Program. *Am J Psychiatry*, 161, 1902–1908.)

comparable when broken down by gender. Prior to treatment, RC-BD patients had 8-fold higher rates of mood episodes compared with those without rapid cycling, and this was equally true for mania/hypomania as for depressive episodes.

The putative association with lower lithium response rates was first noted in that 1974 paper, and this set the tone for years of misplaced conclusions about lithium's efficacy by reporting that 9 of 11 (82%) RC-BD patients experienced a mood relapse during follow-up, compared with 18 of 44 (41%) of non-RC-BD individuals [98]. The lack of a comparator arm was one limiting factor in placing the findings in the context of other therapeutic monotherapy options, and much of the subsequent literature was either naturalistic or consisted of post-hoc analyses of an RC-BD subgroup enrolled in other bipolar studies [31]. As of this writing, RC-BD remains understudied, with only six randomized, controlled prospective studies specifically for RC-BD, many of which are small, statistically underpowered or focus only on those with a specific mood state (e.g. depression) [102, 103].

In-Depth 1.6 Naturalistic Data Supporting Lithium's Efficacy in Rapid Cycling Bipolar Disorder (RC-BD)

By the year 2000, there was an inkling that any issues with lithium response in RC-BD lay in the phenomenology of the disorder itself, based on a study of naturalistic outcomes with lithium treatment in RC-BD and non-RC-BD adults [32]. The subjects of this analysis were 360 BD-1 or BD-2 adults followed from 1974 to 1998 in a Stanley Foundation Network study in Sardinia, which excluded from the analysis any individual who used other mood agents for 8 or more weeks at any time. The total sample had the following characteristics: BD-1: 60.6%; BD-2: 39.4%; 63.6% female. There was a mean of 8.83 ± 8.38 years of historical mood information available for the subjects prior to study entry, and a mean 4.49 ± 4.10 years of follow-up data on lithium [32]. Among the sample of 360 subjects, 15.6% had a lifetime RC-BD diagnosis based on ≥ 4 mood episodes in any year, with 30.4% averaging ≥ 4 mood episodes per year [32]. As seen in Table 1.4, clinical outcomes of the RC-BD and non-RC-BD groups on lithium were comparable, including the proportion of time spent ill, the annual rate of mania, the annual number of hospitalizations, and the percentage improvement in time spent ill [32]. Among all subjects, the percentage of time spent ill on lithium did not correlate with the pre-lithium cycling rate, and for the RC-BD cohort the percentage of time spent ill did not correlate with RC-BD status (i.e. the prior 12 months vs. historical), or pre-lithium mood episode frequency. For those with ≥ 3.5 episodes/year, $23.0 \pm 27.9\%$ of the time was spent ill on lithium compared with $18.6 \pm 22.7\%$ for those with fewer annual episodes (p = 0.762). However, lithium treated RC-BD patients had 3 times more depressive episodes per year, and fewer RC-BD patients had zero mood recurrences during follow-up compared with the non-RC-BD group (17.9% vs. 31.6%, p = 0.04).

Table 1.4 Comparison of RC-BD and non-RC-BD outcomes on lithium during routine long-term treatment [32]

	Rapid cycling (n = 56)	Non-rapid-cycling (n = 304)	P value
Years on lithium	4.96 ± 4.31	4.41 ± 4.07	NS
Mean serum lithium level (mEq/l)	0.596 ± 0.116	0.616 ± 0.143	NS
Hospitalizations per year	0.087 ± 0.351	0.073 ± 0.015	NS
Proportion of time ill (%)			
All episodes	21.2 ± 25.2	18.5 ± 22.6	NS
Manias	6.99 ± 10.5	8.04 ± 13.0	NS
Depressions	14.2 ± 17.2	10.5 ± 17.7	NS
Annual cycling rate			
All episodes	1.49 ± 1.94	0.73 ± 0.92	< 0.0001
Manias	0.49 ± 0.73	0.36 ± 0.55	NS
Depressions	1.00 ± 1.52	0.37 ± 0.60	< 0.0001
Subjects improved (%)			
No recurrences	17.9	31.6	0.04
Time ill improved ≥ 50%	66.1	60.5	NS
Time ill unimproved	16.1	25.4	NS
Percentage improvement (%)			
Episodes/year	56.5 ± 41.4	53.7 ± 43.0	NS
Manias/year	66.4 ± 42.5	63.1 ± 44.5	NS
Depressions/year	54.5 ± 42.8	54.6 ± 46.0	NS
Time ill in all episodes	61.4 ± 37.4	48.3 ± 41.6	NS
Time ill in manias	68.8 ± 39.6	64.0 ± 43.3	NS
Time ill in depressions	59.3 ± 39.1	57.9 ± 44.5	NS

(Adapted from: R. J. Baldessarini, L. Tondo, G. Floris, et al. [2000]. Effects of rapid cycling on response to lithium maintenance treatment in 360 bipolar I and II disorder patients. *J Affect Disord*, 61, 13–22.)

Nonetheless, well-designed prospective studies have provided the necessary comparative data to indicate that lithium is noninferior to divalproex monotherapy for RC-BD patients, and that the combination of lithium and divalproex is no more effective for these patients than lithium monotherapy. The first study was a 20-month, double-blind maintenance trial of lithium vs. divalproex in RC-BD disorder that enrolled 254 RC-BD adults with BD-1 or BD-2, with rapid cycling defined as a history of ≥ 4 episodes in the past 12 months, and at least one episode of mania or hypomania or a mixed episode in the 3 months prior to study entry [33]. Study exclusions included a prior history of combined lithium and divalproex use, history of intolerance to a lithium level 0.80 mEq/l or to a VPA level of 50 µg/ml, substance dependence criteria for alcohol or drugs in the prior 6 months, and patients who were on steroids or were pregnant or planning to become pregnant. The 2-phase study design included an open-label stabilization phase in which subjects were initially titrated on lithium to a target level of 0.80 mEq/l over 4–6 weeks, then divalproex was added to a target level of 50 µg/ml over 4–6 weeks. During this phase, 28% were lost due to poor adherence, 26% were lost due to symptom nonresponse (19% depression, 7% mania/hypomania/mixed), and 19% dropped out due to adverse effects. Subjects who maintained stability for 4 consecutive weeks were entered into the double-blind maintenance phase based on having a Hamilton Depression Scale (HAM-D$_{24}$) score ≤ 20, a YMRS score ≤ 12, and serum drug levels at or above the target levels. Only 24% (n = 60) met these criteria and were randomized to lithium or divalproex, stratified by BD-1 or BD-2 subtype [33]. As seen in Table 1.5, there were no-between group differences in

Table 1.5 Outcomes from the double-blind maintenance phase of a 20-month RC-BD trial [33]

	Lithium (n = 32)	Divalproex (n = 28)
Female	59%	43%
Bipolar 2	59%	61%
Mean age ± SD (years)	37.2 ± 9.0	37.0 ± 8.2
Mean dose and serum level	1359 mg; 0.92 mEq/l	1571 mg; 77 µg/ml
Dropouts		
Mood relapse	56%	50%
(Depression vs. Mania/Hypomania/ Mixed)	(34% vs. 22%)	(29% vs. 21%)
Substance use	16%	4%
Poor adherence	9%	11%
Other	3%	3%

(Adapted from: J. R. Calabrese, M. D. Shelton, D. J. Rapport, et al. [2005]. A 20-month, double-blind, maintenance trial of lithium versus divalproex in rapid-cycling bipolar disorder. *Am J Psychiatry*, 162, 2152–2161.)

time to treatment for a mood episode or time to discontinuation for any reason, nor was there any impact of BD-1 or BD-2 subtype diagnosis. The authors' conclusion is worth repeating verbatim: "The hypothesis that divalproex is more effective than lithium in the long-term management of rapid-cycling bipolar disorder is not supported by these data. Preliminary data suggest highly recurrent refractory depression may be the hallmark of rapid-cycling bipolar disorder" [33].

In-Depth 1.7 The Combination of Divalproex and Lithium is No More Effective than Lithium Monotherapy in RC-BD Patients with Substance Use Disorders

The second well-designed prospective RC-BD study was a 6-month, double-blind, maintenance trial of lithium monotherapy vs. the combination of lithium and divalproex in RC-BD patients with co-occurring substance abuse or dependence [34]. The exclusions and methods were identical to the prior 2-phase monotherapy RC-BD study with the only exception that subjects must have had alcohol, cocaine or cannabis abuse within the prior 3 months, or dependence within the prior 6 months by DSM-IV criteria. In the open-label stabilization phase 149 patients were enrolled, and 42% were lost due to poor adherence, 25% lost for inadequate symptom nonresponse (13% depression, 12% mania/hypomania/mixed), and 10% dropped out due to adverse effects. Only 21% (n = 31) of the sample met stability criteria and were subsequently randomized in the double-blind maintenance phase to lithium monotherapy or lithium and divalproex combination therapy, stratified by BD-1 or BD-2 subtype. This trial found no between-group differences in the time to treatment for a mood episode, time to discontinuation for any reason, nor was there any impact of BD-1 vs. BD-2 diagnosis (Table 1.6) [34]. While the small sample size in the double-blind phase increases the likelihood of type II error, this study illustrates the challenges in treating RC-BD patients with substance use comorbidity while providing controlled data suggesting that adding divalproex to lithium does not markedly enhance lithium's effectiveness in these patients.

Table 1.6 Data from the double-blind maintenance phase of a trial comparing lithium monotherapy vs. the combination of lithium and divalproex for RC-BD patients with co-occurring substance abuse or dependence [34]

	Lithium (n = 16)	Lithium + divalproex (n = 15)
Female	25%	40%
Bipolar 2	19%	13%
Mean age ± SD (years)	40.0 ± 10.6	37.1 ± 10.9
Mean dose and serum level	1440 mg; 0.88 mEq/l	Lithium: 1400 mg; 0.79 mEq/l Divalproex: 1583 mg; 67 µg/ml

Dropouts		
Mood relapse (Depression vs. Mania/Hypomania/Mixed)	56% (13% vs. 43%)	53% (13% vs. 40%)
Poor adherence	12%	13%
Other	12%	0%

(Adapted from: D. E. Kemp, K. Gao, S. J. Ganocy, et al. [2009]. A 6-month, double-blind, maintenance trial of lithium monotherapy versus the combination of lithium and divalproex for rapid-cycling bipolar disorder and co-occurring substance abuse or dependence. *J Clin Psychiatry*, 70, 113–121.)

One small maintenance study noted that adding carbamazepine to lithium may be more effective than lithium monotherapy in RC-BD patients, and a trial of quetiapine added to lithium or divalproex in RC-BD-1 patients found that these combinations were effective and well tolerated [4]. Given quetiapine's monotherapy indication for BD-1 and BD-2 depression, that result outlines a rational pharmacological approach to long-term RC-BD management, emphasizing the need to use combination therapy, and especially a combination with lithium that adds an agent to address the highly recurrent and difficult to treat depressive phases of the illness. That RC-BD is a predictor of inadequate response to lithium monotherapy can now be understood in the context of these trials – no monotherapy is likely to be effective in this population, but the available data indicate that lithium treated RC-BD patients will fare no worse than RC-BD patients on other monotherapies [31, 104].

 Acute Bipolar Depression and Bipolar II Disorder (BD-2)

WHAT TO KNOW: ACUTE BIPOLAR DEPRESSION AND BIPOLAR II DISORDER (BD-2)

- Lithium reduces depressive mood recurrence, but modern data do not strongly support its efficacy when used for acute bipolar depression.
- The treatment of BD-2 is nuanced. In those who require mood stabilization, lithium is the preferred agent at trough levels of 0.60–0.80 mEq/l, and possibly in the range of 0.40–0.60 mEq/l given tolerability concerns seen in a trial with a target lithium level of 0.80 mEq/l.
- Some BD-2 patients may not require a mood stabilizer and both tolerate and respond to traditional antidepressants.

Lithium possesses antidepressant properties, but the question is to what extent lithium is a proven effective option in acute BD depression. This is a question of relevance to the treatment of BD-1/SAD-BT and BD-2 patients for two reasons: (1) lithium utilization is so low across the BD spectrum that lithium emerges as an available adjunctive option to be considered for acutely depressed BD patients [5]; (2) when experiencing a mood episode, BD-2 patients spend a disproportionate amount of time depressed compared with that in hypomania or a mixed state, so any use of lithium is likely to be for an acute depressive episode (Figure 1.2) [27, 28]. Despite the extensive use of lithium during decades when no other mood stabilizing option existed, the 10 older studies of lithium monotherapy for acute bipolar depression were not conducted using modern RCT methods, thus limiting their interpretability [4]. There is a recent RCT published in 2010 that reported outcomes from a double-blind, 8-week trial which randomized 802 acutely depressed BD subjects (BD-1, n = 499; BD-2, n = 303) to one of 4 treatment arms: quetiapine 300 mg/d (n = 265), quetiapine 600 mg/d (n = 268), lithium 600–1800 mg/d (n = 136) or placebo (n = 133) [38]. The mean age was 42.2 years, and 59.3% of patients were female. While the efficacy results were positive for quetiapine, they were not for lithium treated subjects (mean serum level 0.61 mEq/l). As 34.9% of those in the lithium cohort had levels < 0.60 mEq/l, secondary analyses were performed for those with lithium levels > 0.80 mEq/l and for lithium treated study completers, but the findings were also negative, suggesting lithium is not effective for acute bipolar depression regardless of level or treatment duration [38]. Traditional antidepressants present a considerable risk when administered to BD-1 or SAD-BT patients due to possible switching into a hypomanic, mixed or manic episode [105], so other options are preferable for acute bipolar depression in those patients: cariprazine, lumateperone, lurasidone, and possibly quetiapine or the olanzapine/fluoxetine combination, although the latter two choices are eschewed due to significant weight gain, metabolic dysfunction and sedation [12, 106].

In-Depth 1.8 Bipolar II Depression and Antidepressant Use

The approach to BD-2 depression is qualitatively different than for BD-1/ SAD-BT patients as the risk of antidepressant related switching is lower, though not absent [105, 107]. Recent evidence for this assertion comes from two double-blind RCTs that examined the comparative efficacy of venlafaxine or sertraline vs. lithium in acute BD-2 depression. The first was a randomized, double-blind, 12-week study of adult outpatients in which lithium treated subjects (n = 64) experienced lower response rates than those randomized to venlafaxine (n = 65) (34.4% vs. 67.7% respectively;

p < 0.001), and lower remission rates (28.1% vs. 58.5% respectively; p < 0.001), with no significant between-group differences in the emergence of hypomania symptoms [29]. The second study was a 16-week, double-blind trial in which 142 adults with BD-2 depression were randomly assigned to lithium monotherapy (n = 49), sertraline monotherapy (n = 45) or combination treatment with lithium and sertraline (n = 48) [108]. The treatment response rate for the overall sample was 62.7% without significant between-group differences after accounting for dropouts. The lithium + sertraline combination cohort also experienced a significantly greater dropout rate than the monotherapy arms but without any efficacy benefit as measured by the extent of response or the time to response. Although 20 subjects (14%) did switch into hypomania, the switch rates did not differ between the 3 treatment arms even after accounting for dropouts, and no patient had a manic switch or was hospitalized for a switch [108]. From the limited data, one can conclude that BD-2 patients should consider options other than lithium for acute depression if unable to tolerate antidepressants due to switching. It is worth noting that two of the agents approved for BD-1 depression also have indications for BD-2 depression: quetiapine (monotherapy) and lumateperone (monotherapy or adjunctive to lithium or divalproex) [12].

A certain proportion of BD-2 patients will not tolerate traditional antidepressants due to the emergence of hypomania or a mixed state, and thus function best when chronically mood stabilized (see In-Depth 1.8); however, there are no double-blind BD-2 maintenance RCTs involving lithium, although there are two open-label studies. In one long-term study published in 1999, lithium and carbamazepine maintenance monotherapies were compared over 2.5 years in 57 patients with BD-2 or BD not otherwise specified (using DSM-IV terminology and criteria) [109]. This trial found no significant differences between lithium and carbamazepine in rates of mood recurrences, subclinical mood episodes, psychiatric hospitalizations, need for concomitant medications or severe adverse effects [109]. A 2021 single-blind 20-week study enrolled 44 subjects with newly diagnosed BD-2 and randomly assigned them to lithium (target serum level 0.80 mEq/l) or lamotrigine (target dose 200 mg/d) [22]. This study was terminated early due to greater rates of adverse effects in the lithium arm, although several subjects assigned to lamotrigine experienced psychosis. Analyses of study completer data for 28 participants suggested comparable efficacy of both medications [22]. Should lithium be used for BD-2 maintenance, strong consideration should be given to use of levels at the low end of the maintenance range (0.60–0.80 mEq/l), and possibly even to levels in the range of 0.40–0.60 mEq/l given the tolerability concerns raised in a BD-2 trial employing a target lithium level of 0.80 mEq/l [22].

In-Depth 1.9 Lithium Discontinuation and the Risk for Psychiatric Hospitalization in BD-1 vs. BD-2: A Retrospective Study

A Swedish group retrospectively examined psychiatric outcomes in 194 lithium treated individuals who had clinical data 2 years before and 2 years after lithium discontinuation, with the data broken down by BD subtype [21]. In the 2 years after lithium discontinuation, 51% of patients with BD-I/SAD-BT (n = 100) and 46% with BD-2 / other BD (n = 94) were on an alternative mood stabilizer. Using the primary outcome measure of psychiatric hospitalization, the BD-1/SAD-BT patient cohort experienced a significant increase in the percentage who were admitted and in total number of admissions, but the BD-2 /other BD cohort did not experience a significant change in those outcomes after lithium discontinuation [21]. Unfortunately, the use of psychiatric hospitalization as the only metric for mood recurrence obscures the extent and severity of mood relapses for the BD-2 group since they are less commonly hospitalized, so the true impact of lithium discontinuation on any BD-2 patient who requires mood stabilization is not easily quantifiable from the literature.

In-Depth 1.10 Newer Concerns About Lamotrigine's Safety

Lamotrigine lacks lithium's monitoring burdens and has therefore become a more popular option for BD patients in general over the past two decades, despite the fact that it is only approved for BD-1 maintenance [5]. Lamotrigine has its own safety concerns, including the risk of Stevens–Johnson Syndrome/toxic epidermal necrolysis, aseptic meningitis, hemophagocytic lymphohistiocytosis, and recent warnings issued in 2021 based on *in vitro* testing showing that it possesses class IB antiarrhythmic activity at therapeutic concentrations [110]. While QRS widening has not been observed in healthy individuals, the concern was that lamotrigine could slow ventricular conduction leading to arrhythmias and possible sudden death in patients with significant heart disease, including conduction system disorders, a history of ventricular arrhythmias, cardiac channelopathies (e.g. Brugada syndrome), ischemic heart disease or multiple coronary artery disease risk factors [110]. The clinical data informing this issue are limited as none of the 26 studies involving lamotrigine (n = 2326) examined risks in people with pre-existing cardiac conditions, so there is insufficient evidence to support or refute any association of lamotrigine with sudden death or ECG changes [111].

D **Bipolar Disorder Maintenance and Response Prediction**

WHAT TO KNOW: BIPOLAR DISORDER MAINTENANCE AND RESPONSE PREDICTION

- Randomized trials document lithium's efficacy for BD-1 maintenance, but modern studies often incorporate preferential responders to other agents (e.g. lamotrigine, quetiapine), limiting the ability to make comparative statements about lithium's efficacy.

- Real world data sets do support the concept that BD-1 patients have superior outcomes on lithium compared to monotherapy with an SGA or valproate.

- Certain clinical features such as substance use, personality disorder, illness chronicity, rapid cycling or inadequate social support limit response to treatment in general, and are not necessarily lithium specific. Patients with these clinical characteristics should not be deprived of a lithium trial because they are not "ideal candidates."

1 *Maintenance Studies*

The 2022 meta-analysis of adult lithium BD trials found 21 monotherapy maintenance studies, but the use of obsolete study designs and other methodological issues in older literature limited their analysis to 4 modern RCTs [4]. One of these studies was a negative study in which 372 adult BD-1 patients who met recovery criteria within 3 months of the onset of a manic episode were randomized to 12 months of maintenance treatment with divalproex, lithium or placebo in a 2:1:1 ratio [112]. Despite the larger sample size for the divalproex arm, the divalproex group did not differ significantly from the placebo group in time to any mood episode, and the same was true for the lithium cohort [112]. In 2003, two subsequent papers were published which separately reported positive outcomes from placebo-controlled 18-month maintenance studies of lamotrigine and lithium maintenance treatment in BD-1 patients who were recently manic/ hypomanic [113], or recently depressed [39]. As these were industry sponsored studies pursuing BD-1 maintenance indications for lamotrigine, patients began each study with an 8- to 16-week open-label phase during which lamotrigine was initiated and other psychotropics discontinued. Stable patients on lamotrigine monotherapy were subsequently randomized to lamotrigine (50, 200 or 400 mg/d if the most recent episode was depressed, 100–400 mg/d if the most recent episode was manic/hypomanic), lithium (0.80–1.10 mEq/l) or placebo as double-blind maintenance treatment for as long as 18 months. In the trial where the most recent mood episode was mania/hypomania, 349 patients entered the open-label phase, 175 met stabilization criteria and were randomized to lamotrigine (n = 59), lithium (n = 46) or placebo (n = 70) [113]. Although the study was performed in lamotrigine responders, both lamotrigine and lithium were superior to placebo at prolonging the time to intervention for any mood episode (lamotrigine vs. placebo, p = 0.02; lithium vs. placebo, p = 0.006). Lamotrigine was superior to placebo at prolonging the time to a depressive episode (p = 0.02), while lithium was superior to placebo at prolonging the time to a manic, hypomanic or mixed episode (p = 0.006) [113]. In the trial where the most recent mood episode was depression, 966 BD-1 patients entered the open-label phase, 463 met stabilization criteria and were randomized to lamotrigine (n = 221), lithium (n = 121) or placebo (n = 121) [39]. The time to intervention for any mood episode was statistically superior (p = 0.029) for both lamotrigine and lithium compared with placebo, and the median survival times were 200, 170, and 93 days, respectively. Lamotrigine was superior to placebo at prolonging the time to intervention for a depressive episode (p = 0.047), but the proportions of patients who were intervention-free for depression at 1 year were not significantly different between the three arms: lamotrigine 57%, lithium 46%, and placebo 45%. Lithium was statistically superior to placebo at prolonging the time to intervention for a manic or hypomanic episode (p = 0.026) [39].

There was also one trial involving continuation of quetiapine vs. switching to placebo or lithium for maintenance treatment of BD-1 patients [37]. That trial design involved stabilizing adult patients experiencing any recent mood episode (mania, mixed, depressive) on open-label quetiapine (300–800 mg/d) for 4–24 weeks, with those achieving stabilization then randomized in a double-blind manner to continue quetiapine or to switch to placebo or lithium (0.60–1.20 mEq/L) for up to 104 weeks [37]. Only 50% of the initial 2438 patients could be stabilized and randomized to double-blind treatment (n = 1172). Quetiapine and lithium significantly increased the time to recurrence of manic events (quetiapine HR 0.29; 95% CI 0.21–0.40; p < 0.0001; lithium HR 0.37; 95% CI 0.27–0.53; p < 0.0001) and depressive events (quetiapine HR 0.30; 95% CI 0.20–0.44; p < 0.0001; lithium HR 0.59; 95% CI 0.42–0.84; p < 0.004), compared with placebo [37]. That the study used a pool of patients who were quetiapine responders limits generalizability, as does the fact that 50% of the sample was lost during the stabilization phase. The indisputable fact is that quetiapine is better than placebo in BD-1 patients who respond to it as monotherapy, but in modern practice the use of quetiapine as BD-1 monotherapy is an unlikely scenario.

In-Depth 1.11 What Is Propensity Score Matching ?

As only one maintenance RCT provided an SGA comparator, and that study used quetiapine responders, clinicians might wonder whether there are any other data to provide relevant comparisons between lithium and maintenance SGA use, especially for BD-1 patients. Real world data sets present a naturalistic picture of medication outcomes, and modern statistical methods permit analyses that remove biases for or against prescribing a particular treatment by employing *propensity score matching.* (The details of this method are discussed extensively in Info Box 7.6, as is the use of propensity score matching in analyses of major congenital malformation rates with 1st trimester psychotropic exposure.) There are numerous reasons why clinicians choose a particular medication for a patient, but when retrospectively examining a set of new medication prescriptions, one can construct a statistical model based on the pattern of usage in that population that describes the likelihood a particular patient might have been prescribed a specific medication. From this logistic regression model, one can then take the characteristics of any individual subject and calculate what their *propensity* would have been to receive a specific treatment on a scale of 0 to 1.0. Essentially, this propensity score represents the probability that an individual would be assigned to a treatment based on their demographics and comorbidities present at that time [114]. Not uncommonly, two individuals can have identical propensity scores for receiving a treatment (e.g. lithium), yet one was given this medication and one was not. One can therefore match exposed and unexposed individuals by their propensity scores, and in doing so balance the treatment cohorts for their likelihood to have received a treatment in the manner that a prospective trial balances this likelihood (e.g. by using a 1:1:1 randomization scheme).

In-Depth 1.12 Lithium vs. Second Generation Antipsychotics for Maintenance Therapy in BD-1 Patients: Real World Outcomes Using Propensity Score Matching

Using a propensity score matched analysis, a population based cohort study was performed from electronic health records of 5089 UK BD patients prescribed lithium (n = 1505), VPA (n = 1173), olanzapine (n = 1366) or quetiapine (n = 1075) as monotherapy [115]. Treatment failure was defined as time to stopping medication or the need to add another mood stabilizer, antipsychotic, antidepressant or benzodiazepine. In unadjusted analyses, the duration of successful monotherapy was longest for lithium treated patients, with treatment failure not occurring in 75% of those prescribed lithium for 2.05 years (95% CI 1.63–2.51), vs. 1.13 years for olanzapine (95% CI: 1.00–1.31), 0.98 years for VPA (95% CI 0.84–1.18), and 0.76 years (95% CI 0.64–0.84) for quetiapine (Figure 1.3) [115]. Lithium's superiority remained in the propensity score matched analysis, and in sensitivity analyses where treatment failure was defined strictly as stopping the medication or adding a mood stabilizer or antipsychotic, or when treatment failure was restricted to more than 3 months after commencing the particular medication.

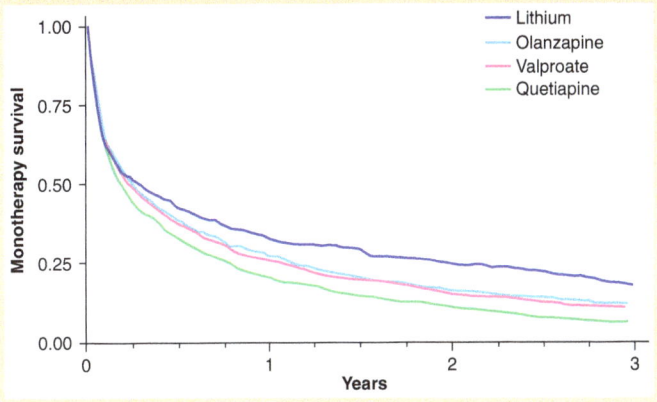

Figure 1.3 Time to treatment failure (defined as treatment discontinuation, or the need to add a mood stabilizer, antipsychotic, antidepressant or benzodiazepine) among 5089 British adults with BD prescribed lithium (n = 1505), valproate (n = 1173), olanzapine (n = 1366) or quetiapine (n = 1075) as monotherapy. [115]

(Adapted from: J. F. Hayes, L. Marston, K. Walters, et al. [2016]. Lithium vs. valproate vs. olanzapine vs. quetiapine as maintenance monotherapy for bipolar disorder: a population-based UK cohort study using electronic health records. *World Psychiatry*, 15, 53–58.)

Another method of defining treatment failure is rehospitalization, and this outcome was tracked in 18,018 Finnish patients previously hospitalized for BD, from 1996 to 2012 [6]. As mentioned in the chapter introduction, this study performed a within-individual analysis to examine hospitalization risk during periods on or off various treatments, with each patient serving as his or her own control. Over a mean follow-up of 7.2 years, lithium was the most effective mood stabilizer in preventing psychiatric rehospitalization (Table 1.1), but efficacy was not seen for VPA or for any anticonvulsant other than carbamazepine [6].

As many BD-1 patients are placed on SGAs during an acute manic/mixed episode, a Swedish group examined long-term naturalistic outcomes following a hospitalization for mania among those on monotherapy with a mood stabilizer or SGA, and for those on combination treatment [18]. This study used data from 3772 adults aged 18–75 with a primary diagnosis of a manic episode (ICD-10 F30.1–F30.9, and F31.1–F31.2) who were discharged from psychiatric inpatient care from July 1, 2006 to December 31, 2014. Compared with lithium monotherapy, VPA monotherapy had a higher rate of medication discontinuation, while all SGA monotherapies were associated with higher rates of all-cause treatment failure and failure due to medication switching (Figure 1.4) [18]. Speaking to the challenges in treating BD-1 patients, the risks for overall treatment failure were significantly lower for combination therapy, but only the combination of lithium + VPA + quetiapine was associated with a significantly lower rehospitalization risk during ongoing treatment compared with lithium monotherapy (AHR 0.57, 95% CI 0.32–0.99). Importantly, use of antidepressants in the prior year for these BD-1 patients increased risk of treatment failure (adjusted hazard ratio [AHR] 1.24, 95% CI 1.16–1.33), but use of a depot antipsychotic in combination lowered risk of treatment failure (AHR 0.79, 95% CI 0.68–0.93), as did a long index hospitalization exceeding 42 days (AHR 0.81, 95% CI 0.76–0.88) [18]. These real world studies

Figure 1.4 Time to treatment failure after hospitalization for mania among various treatment options for BD-1 using lithium (dark blue line) as the comparator treatment [18]

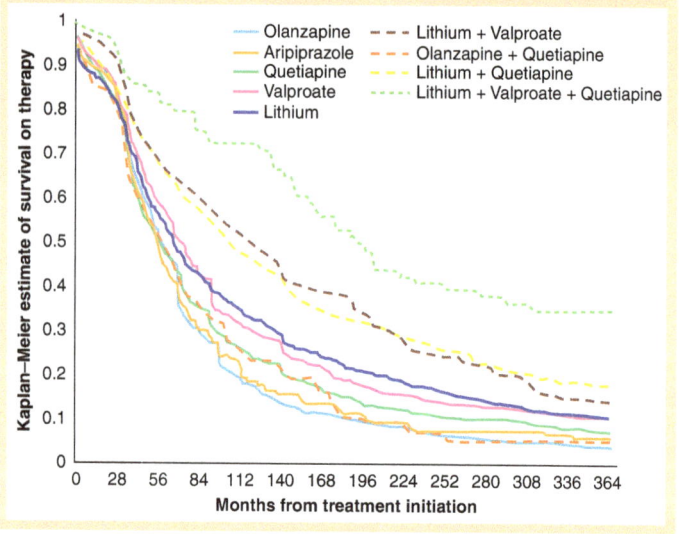

(Adapted from: L. Wingård, L. Brandt, R. Bodén, et al. [2019]. Monotherapy vs. combination therapy for post mania maintenance treatment: A population based cohort study. *Eur Neuropsychopharmacol*, 29, 691–700.)

from three different countries reinforce the notion that lithium is the preferred maintenance treatment for BD, especially for BD-1 patients, with clinical outcomes superior to SGA or VPA monotherapy using varying definitions of treatment failure.

In-Depth 1.13 Detailed Methods of the Swedish Study Examining Naturalistic Outcomes during Post-Mania Treatment with Psychotropic Monotherapy or Combinations [18]

Dementia, or those with schizophrenia or SAD-BT diagnoses, were excluded from the analysis, and patients hospitalized for mania multiple times were examined following each hospitalization, with hospitalizations for mania less than 7 days apart linked and counted as one episode. (Among the sample of 3772 patients, 1041 individuals contributed two or more hospitalizations.) After each hospitalization for mania, active treatment periods of lithium, VPA, olanzapine, quetiapine or aripiprazole, alone or in combination, were recorded. Each active treatment period was defined as starting on the day of a prescription fill of any of the medications, or the day of discharge if the patient filled a prescription during the index hospitalization. Patients who filled prescriptions of more than one drug within 2 weeks were considered to use combination therapy. Follow-up started on day 14 of the first active treatment period and ended after 365 days or upon the earliest of any of the following events: treatment failure, emigration, death or the end of the study period (December 31, 2014). In this study, treatment failure was defined as medication discontinuation or switching, or being readmitted to inpatient psychiatric care during an active treatment period. This study did not use propensity score matching but did examine an extensive list of covariates related to sociodemographic variables, severity of the index hospitalization, psychiatric history and comorbidities, history of self-harm and use of other psychotropics [18]. 17.6% of subjects were under 30 years of age, 24.5% were aged 30–44 years, and 57.9% were age 45 or older, and 57.1% of the sample was female. Most parameters were evenly distributed, but aripiprazole monotherapy patients were younger, while those with a first manic episode or who were naïve to antimanic drugs were overrepresented in the olanzapine group. The total follow-up time comprised 1773 patient-years, and treatment failure within 1 year was seen in 85.3% of patients. Of these, 2667 switched treatment, 1108 discontinued treatment and 1096 were rehospitalized despite ongoing treatment.

2 *The Search for Response Predictors*

As discussed extensively in Chapters 2 and 4, the perception of lithium's long-term renal risks has shifted significantly based on two realizations: (1) some of the risks for renal dysfunction were related to prior prescribing practices, such as use of high maintenance lithium levels and multiple daily dosing; and (2) the absence of systematic laboratory monitoring protocols [116]. Modern treatment guidelines emphasize regular monitoring and the use of more modest maintenance levels [117, 118], with the result that recent studies show that mean annual declines in estimated glomerular filtration rate (eGFR) are predicted primarily by medical comorbidities that increase chronic kidney disease (CKD) risk, exposure to nephrotoxic drugs and episodes of lithium toxicity, but not necessarily duration of lithium exposure [95, 119–121].

Nonetheless, concerns over lithium's safety were often a driver for studies that aimed to define "ideal" lithium candidates, with the goal of sparing individuals a lithium trial where the benefits might be outweighed by the risks. While the development of robust response predictors to drug therapy is the holy grail of psychiatric practice, a significant proportion of the lithium related clinical research was confined to monotherapy analyses, despite the recognition that many BD spectrum patients require combination therapy, especially to manage or prevent depressive episodes [18, 33, 74, 122]. Moreover, the finding that certain clinical features – such as substance use, personality disorder, illness chronicity, rapid cycling or inadequate social support – might negatively impact lithium response relates to aspects of BD patients that limit response to treatment in general, and are not necessarily lithium specific [1, 30, 74, 104, 123, 124]. Unfortunately, the absence of a comparator arm often paints a dismal portrait of the chances for lithium success [122]; however, as discussed in the section on RC-BD, when studies are designed to examine response in challenging patient cohorts, the picture that emerges is not lithium's lack of efficacy, but the limited efficacy of any monotherapy [33, 34, 125]. The presence of comorbidities that limit adherence with specific aspects of treatment (e.g. laboratory monitoring) will certainly factor into the decision to use lithium, yet current recommendations no longer focus on restricting lithium to ideal candidates for excellent monotherapy response, but on employing lithium as the preferred foundational mood stabilizer in any patient with a history of mania, and for BD-2 patients who require mood stabilization [81]. Alcohol use disorders, personality disorders, higher number of psychiatric admissions and rapid cycling are negative prognostic indicators of lithium monotherapy response, but patients should not be deprived of a lithium trial *a priori* due to the presence of these factors, especially where the data do not suggest superior outcomes for other medications in BD spectrum patients with these clinical features. Ideally, the database on clinical response predictors will enlarge over time to provide comparable analyses for divalproex and SGA monotherapies that mirror the approaches to predicting lithium monotherapy response.

In-Depth 1.14 Biomarker Studies of Lithium Response

Biomarker studies represent another important avenue of research that might provide insights into the biosignatures of lithium response and tolerability. Investigators are using a variety of avenues to tackle these issues, including polygenic risk scores, individual genetic markers, imaging findings, and novel methods such as the association between circadian rhythms in cultured patient neurons and lithium response [70, 73, 75]. One hopes that this research will mature sufficiently to provide robust predictors for a variety of mood stabilizing and other biological therapies employed in the management of BD, but at the present time we must rely on the evidence based indications for lithium to inform our decision to start lithium, especially given the extent of RCT and real world studies demonstrating comparative advantages over other medication options.

The role of treatment delay in lithium response is a subject of debate covered more extensively in Chapter 4. It is worth noting that examining longitudinal effects of any specific medication is challenging due to the episodic nature of BD and periods of spontaneous remission [126]. Nonetheless, a 2003 meta-analysis of 28 studies concluded that there was no association between treatment latency and lithium response [127], a finding echoed by a 2007 European study that noted treatment delay had little association with subsequent morbidity during mood stabilizer maintenance therapy [126]. A 2014 Danish analysis came to a different conclusion by examining psychiatric rehospitalization rates in a group of lithium treated BD-1 patients who, following a 6-month lithium stabilization period, continued on lithium as *monotherapy* [128]. Patients who started on lithium earlier (e.g. at the time of their first manic/mixed episode or psychiatric contact with BD-1 diagnosis) had lower rates of psychiatric rehospitalization during follow-up; however, generalizing this finding is difficult as BD-1 is not often treated with monotherapy, and clinicians have no *a priori* method of deciding who will be an excellent lithium monotherapy responder even with patients whose clinical features suggest greater likelihood of lithium response [128].

E Unipolar MDD

WHAT TO KNOW: ADJUNCTIVE LITHIUM FOR UNIPOLAR MDD

- The accumulated data indicate that lithium is an effective adjunctive option for inadequate responders to antidepressant therapy, with comparable response when added to tricyclic antidepressants or selective serotonin reuptake inhibitors.
- There are methodological concerns about older studies in this area, so the place of adjunctive lithium in the treatment algorithm of unipolar MDD, and the characteristics of preferential lithium responders, remains to be elucidated.

The RCT literature is sufficient to cement lithium's reputation for efficacy in acute mania and for BD prophylaxis, but there are areas where the presence of multiple RCTs has not eliminated controversy, and this is true for discussions about lithium's place in the unipolar MDD treatment algorithm [49]. A 2019 review of 12 controlled trials found that adjunctive lithium was superior to placebo for acute unipolar MDD when the data were pooled, but only 4 of the 12 individual studies were positive, the last of which was published in 1996 [49]. One concern is that the antidepressant was not optimized in many of the older studies prior to consideration of an adjunctive strategy with lithium [51]. Moreover, only two of the studies included more than 50 subjects, with the largest trial, a 2003 multicenter study that randomized 149 patients, finding no benefit at the week 6 endpoint for adjunctive lithium over placebo when added to clomipramine nonresponders [129]. Certain authors have postulated that lithium might appear more useful when added to less potent serotonin reuptake inhibitors (e.g. tricyclic antidepressants [TCAs]) based on the idea that lithium's potentiation of serotonergic neurotransmission might be less effective when added to a selective serotonin reuptake inhibitor (SSRI) [130]; however, the clinical trials data do not support this contention, as comparable response is seen in TCA and SSRI trials [131]. Although SGA augmentation is widespread due to perceived convenience, efficacy and safety advantages over lithium, a large 2020 propensity score matched study of 39,582 US adult unipolar MDD patients (mean age 44.5 years) who initiated augmentation with an SGA (n = 22,410; quetiapine 40%, risperidone 21%, aripiprazole 17%, olanzapine 16%) or with a second antidepressant (n = 17,172) noted increased mortality risk from SGA augmentation [132]. In this context, a 2021 review commented that adjunctive lithium was effective and might be better tolerated than SGA augmentation due to lithium's lack of D_2 related adverse effects (e.g. akathisia, parkinsonism), its limited effects on weight, and absence of any impact on serum glucose or lipid levels. Despite the paucity of recent RCTs, the authors implied that lithium is a relevant part of the unipolar MDD treatment algorithm [51]. Where lithium should fall within the current MDD treatment paradigm, and whether lithium's benefits accrue primarily to certain patients with mixed features or other BD characteristics, are important questions that hopefully will be addressed in future studies [49]. For the present, one must consider lithium as one of many viable adjunctive options for unipolar MDD therapy.

Suicidality

January 2022 saw publication of results from a multicenter trial conducted at 29 US Veterans Affairs (VA) hospitals with the goal of determining whether lithium augmentation of usual care for BD or unipolar MDD reduces rates of suicide related events in patients who survived a recent event [40]. The primary outcome was time to any suicide related event, defined as a suicide attempt, interrupted attempt, hospitalization specifically to prevent suicide, or death from suicide. Among the exclusion criteria were a diagnosis of schizophrenia, use of lithium within the prior 6 months, a history of lithium intolerance or ≥ 6 previous lifetime suicide attempts. The last criterion was chosen based on VA analyses showing that reattempts plateaued at 25% to 30% for those with ≥ 6 attempts, but none died from suicide within the next 2 years, so any association between suicidal behavior and risk of suicide death was attenuated in those individuals and this might blunt lithium's efficacy signal [40, 133]. Participants were randomized in a double-blind manner to receive extended-release lithium carbonate beginning at 600 mg/d or placebo, with a target level between 0.60 and 0.80 mEq/l. Placebo lithium levels were reported in that arm. If participants could not tolerate a dose needed to achieve the target level, they took their maximum tolerated dose, but that dose had to be at least 300 mg/d. The subjects were predominantly male (84.2%), mean age 42.8 ± 12.4 years, and 84.6% had unipolar MDD, 15.4% were diagnosed with BD, and the subject pool had high rates of posttraumatic stress disorder (59.7%), alcohol use disorders (48.4%) and other substance use disorders (36.4%) [40]. The important finding was that the trial was stopped for futility after 519 subjects were randomized due to the absence of significant between-group differences in repeated suicide related events (HR 1.10; 95% CI, 0.77–1.55). Mean treatment exposure was 6.7 ± 4.5 months for unipolar MDD subjects, 5.6 ± 4.6 months for the BD cohort, and mean lithium levels at 3 months were 0.46 ± 0.30 mEq/l for unipolar MDD patients and 0.54 ± 0.25 mEq/l for BD patients [40].

In-Depth 1.15 Discussion about the 2022 US VA Lithium Augmentation Trial for Suicidality

Following publication of the results, correspondence in the journal commented on certain aspects of the study, including: the fact that most of the subjects had unipolar MDD and lithium's anti-suicide effects may devolve more to BD patients; that mean treatment exposure was relatively brief (38.4 weeks) with only 56% of lithium treated subjects and 47% of placebo treated subjects retained for 1 year; and that there was evidence of functional unblinding as 68% of those on lithium correctly guessed their treatment assignment [36]. Moreover, the high rates of psychiatric comorbidity, and use of other medication or psychosocial treatments (which were not specified in the paper) might limit the chances of detecting any lithium effects on the outcome measures. In the end, while the goal of many RCTs is to examine the risk of completed suicide or serious attempts, the low frequency of suicide attempts and suicides even in large trials forces investigators to employ surrogate markers of risk (e.g. the need to intervene to avoid suicide, any self-injury), based on the assumption that they are comparable indicators of risk for completed suicide [36]. Unfortunately, that assumption, while reasonable, is "largely untested" according to one commentary, and this highlights a fundamental problem for this area of research: documenting that lithium decreases rates of completed suicide or serious suicide attempts might be impossible in the context of any RCT, as the sample sizes required and duration are beyond what is feasible [133]. Clinicians must, therefore, make treatment decisions based on the large body of retrospective data, while simultaneously acknowledging the limitations of this literature and the lack of comparable evidence of any type of suicide risk reduction for non-lithium therapies [41].

Lithium's effect on suicidal behavior had been known for decades through case series, clinical trials of variable quality, and numerous studies reporting an association between higher lithium levels in drinking water and decreased regional suicide rates [41, 134–139]. Despite this wealth of data, the extent of any risk reduction effect was not well quantified until the publication of two review papers in 2001 and 2006 by Professor Ross Baldessarini, a psychopharmacologist associated for decades with Harvard Medical School and McLean Hospital (Belmont, Massachusetts). As discussed in Info Box 1.1, the 2006 update covered 85,229 person-years of risk exposure from 31 papers providing data on attempted and completed suicides, after excluding 14 other studies that reported zero events in both the lithium and non-lithium arms [41]. The important finding was that the risk reduction appeared consistent across diagnostic categories with 5-fold higher risk in the non-lithium groups, and the effect of lithium was somewhat greater in BD patients compared with those with other major affective disorders. As noted in Table 1.7, the differential impact of BD diagnosis was seen for the primary outcome of attempted and completed suicide. A secondary analysis also examined the ratio of attempts to completed suicides, with higher values indicating reduced lethality of suicidal acts. Using this ratio, lethality decreased during lithium treatment by 2.5-fold across all studies, but the reduction was 2.9-fold when examined for BD patients specifically [41]. While the potential greater effect of lithium in those with a BD diagnosis was noted as one issue in the large VA study, another finding in the 2006 meta-analysis was that studies of shorter duration with mean length 1.41 years (primarily RCTs) saw lesser effects from lithium than those of longer duration (mean 7.77 years). From this finding, one might hypothesize that the anti-suicide impact of lithium might not be instantaneous, but one which accrues over months and years of exposure. This might partially explain the negative result in the VA study where mean treatment exposure was 38.4 weeks, compared with 18 months in the 2006 meta-analysis; however, if this is a biological reality, it might be impossible to test within the confines of an RCT as enormous sample sizes would be needed to retain sufficient numbers for an extended length of time. The 2006 meta-analysis contains limitations, particularly the absence of propensity score matching to balance out clinical features (e.g. history of prior suicide attempts as measured by emergency room visits or psychiatric hospitalizations) that influence real world prescribing practices. Nonetheless, the data indicate lithium has effects on risk for completed suicides, and attempts, not seen with non-lithium therapies.

 Info Box 1.1 The Impact of Lithium Therapy on Risk of Suicidal Acts, Attempted and Completed Suicide from a Meta-analysis of 31 Studies Comprising 85,229 Person-Years of Risk Exposure [41]

a. **Issue:** There was recognition that lithium might reduce the risk of completed suicides, but the extent was not well quantified in the literature prior to 2000. To address this, a large meta-analysis was published in 2001 and then updated in 2006 to cover all trials published through August 2005 [41]. The 2006 paper also performed analyses not previously explored, including the impact of lithium on attempted vs. completed suicide; the differential effects of lithium on BD vs. other major affective disorders; the impact of open clinical studies vs. RCT study design; and outcomes in studies with higher vs. lower quality ratings. Study quality was based on four factors: (1) the presence of subjects observed both with and without lithium treatment (1 point); (2) randomized treatment assignment and blind clinical assessments (1 or 2 points); (3) n ≥ 100 subjects per treatment arm (1 or 2 points); and (4) duration ≥ 1 year per treatment arm (1 or 2 points).

b. **Method:** For inclusion in the meta-analysis, the source papers must have provided data on attempted and completed suicides. From an initial pool of 45 studies, 14 were excluded from the final statistical calculations as being noninformative since they recorded zero events in both the lithium and non-lithium treatment arms [41].

c. **Results:** 31 papers comprising 85,229 person-years of risk exposure were analyzed. Subjects received lithium treatment on average for 18 months.

Table 1.7 The risk ratio (RR) of suicide related outcomes in non-lithium vs. lithium conditions

	Studies (n)	Risk ratio	RR 95% CI	p
1. All two-armed studies	31	4.91	3.82–6.31	< 0.0001
2. Omitting Goodwin et al. (2003)[a]	30	5.34	4.27–6.68	< 0.0001
3. Open clinical studies	26	3.41	2.61–4.46	< 0.0001
4. Randomized controlled trials	5	1.76	1.65–1.88	0.001
5. Suicides only	24	4.86	3.36–7.02	< 0.0001
6. Attempts only	17	4.98	3.56–6.96	< 0.0001
7. Bipolar disorder	14	5.34	3.59–7.93	< 0.0001
8. Major affective disorders (unipolar MDD, schizoaffective disorder)	17	4.66	3.43–6.33	< 0.0001
9. Quality score ≥ 50%	16	3.92	2.94–5.23	< 0.0001
10. Quality score < 50%	15	5.56	3.98–7.76	< 0.0001

[a] Results after the data from Goodwin et al. (2003) were omitted indicated that this very large study did not exert a misleading influence on the overall findings.

d. **Comments:** All of the RCTs had zero events in the lithium arm and were of much shorter duration than the open-label studies. Exposure times in studies rated as having higher quality (including RCTs) were 5.5 times shorter than in open-label clinical studies (1.41 ± 1.09 years vs. 7.77 ± 6.54 years).

e. Conclusions: Overall, there is significant consistency among the increased RR values for suicide attempts or completed suicides in non-lithium vs. lithium treated conditions across a variety of affective disorders, bearing in mind that real world prescribing patterns might result in preferential assignment of lithium treatment to those at highest risk, and thus potentially inflate RR estimates for non-lithium arms. The lower RR among higher-quality studies (RR 3.92) might be the product of removing biases in lower-quality studies. The lower RR in RCTs may also relate to the significantly shorter exposure duration compared with open-label studies, and possibly the impact of greater clinical scrutiny during RCTs than in routine clinical care (e.g. more frequent study visits and contact with study personnel) that might alter risk for all treatment arms.

As certain questions about lithium may be unanswerable by an RCT, subsequent investigators employed other analytic methods to examine its effects on suicidal behavior. As discussed in the section on maintenance treatment, a British group performed a propensity score matched, population based cohort study using electronic health records for 5089 UK BD patients prescribed lithium (n = 1505), VPA (n = 1173), olanzapine (n = 1366) or quetiapine (n = 1075) with an initial goal of examining the differential rates of treatment failure [115]. In a follow-up to that paper, the investigators performed a secondary analysis of this data set to examine lithium's comparative effects on self-harm, with the primary outcome defined as any emergency room or primary care visit for self-harm during the period of drug exposure and up to 3 months afterward [140]. The propensity score methods, subject exclusions and definitions of drug treatment periods were identical to the prior study. After propensity score adjustment and matching, the hazard ratio (HR) for the primary outcome of self-harm among the three non-lithium therapies combined (VPA, olanzapine, quetiapine) vs. lithium was 1.51 (95% CI 1.21–1.88) (Figure 1.5). The specific comparison between VPA and lithium yielded a slightly lower value (HR 1.31, 95% CI 1.01–1.70), although this result was also statistically significant [140]. The authors performed another analysis for the outcome of unintentional injury, and, after propensity score adjustment and matching, the HR for the three non-lithium therapies combined (VPA, olanzapine, quetiapine) vs. lithium was again significant (HR 1.19, 95% CI 1.01–1.41), as was the specific comparison between VPA and lithium (HR 1.34, 95% CI 1.09–1.65). Although this analysis might have captured behavior that was parasuicidal without suicidal intent, the use of propensity score matching mitigates some of the prescribing bias and supports the conclusions of lithium's superior impact on dimensions of suicidal behavior [140].

Figure 1.5 Cumulative self-harm rate among British BD patients aged ≥ 16 years prescribed monotherapy with lithium or non-lithium therapies (valproate, olanzapine or quetiapine) [140]

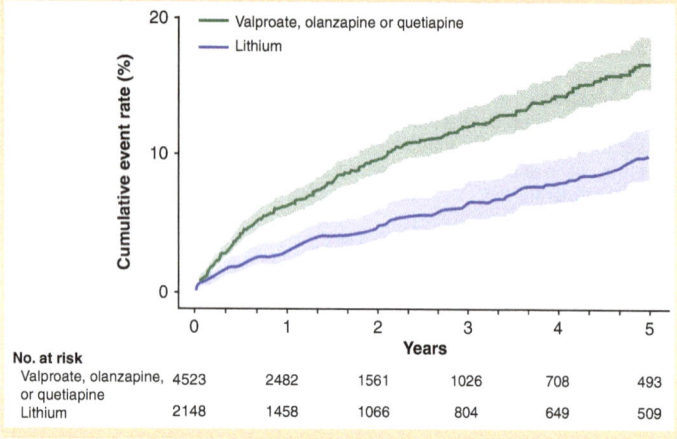

(Adapted from: J. F. Hayes, A. Pitman, L. Marston, et al. (2016). Self-harm, unintentional injury, and suicide in bipolar disorder during maintenance mood stabilizer treatment: A UK population-based electronic health records study. *JAMA Psychiatry*, 73, 630–637.)

Another approach to exploring lithium's relative effects vs. other treatments was employed in a within-individual 8-year study of suicidal behavior in BD patients on lithium or VPA treatment [141]. This study used the Swedish national registry of 51,535 BD patients followed from 2005 to 2013 receiving treatment with lithium or VPA to estimate the HR of suicide related events during treated periods compared with untreated periods [141]. In this large data set, there were 10,403 suicide related events that occurred in 4405 individuals [141]. The rate was significantly decreased by 14% during periods with lithium treatment (HR 0.86, 95% CI 0.78–0.95) but not during VPA exposure (HR 1.02, 95% CI 0.89–1.15), and this HR difference was statistically significant (p = 0.038). None of the sensitivity analyses showed any substantive difference from the main results, and analyses for the combination of lithium and VPA yielded no substantial difference from lithium alone, indicating a lack of benefit on suicidal behavior for VPA. Additionally, patients had an increased rate of suicidal behavior within 30 days of lithium discontinuation (HR 1.33, 95% CI 1.09–1.61) [141]. Another interesting finding was that the majority of suicidal events occurred in those with comorbid substance use (7976 events in 15,927 patients), and lithium use was also associated with reduced events even in this group (HR 0.84, 95% CI 0.75–0.94). The authors concluded that VPA offered no protective effect for suicide related events, and that there was a significant difference between lithium and VPA in the effects on suicidal behavior [141]. The paper also estimated that 12% (95% CI 4%–20%) of suicide related events could have been avoided if patients had taken lithium during the entire follow-up.

In-Depth 1.16 Detailed Methods of Swedish Registry Study on Lithium and Suicidality

Suicidal behavior was defined as attempted or completed suicide by specific diagnostic codes (ICD-10: X60–X84, Y10–Y34) that potentially included events with undetermined intent. A medication period was defined as a sequence of at least two prescriptions, with no more than 3 months (92 days) between any two consecutive prescriptions. Sensitivity analyses examined a number of parameters that might influence the outcome (the impact of year of diagnosis, use of concomitant medications, varying definitions of bipolar disorder, mixed vs. nonmixed episodes, starting lithium within 1 year of the initial BD diagnosis, varying definitions of suicidal events), but specifically addressed two crucial issues: bias in starting lithium due to recent suicidality, and whether monotherapy of either mood stabilizer was superior to the combination of lithium and VPA [141]. To test whether lithium use was biased toward those with a recent suicide history, the main analysis was repeated excluding periods containing a switch to lithium within 7, 14 or 30 days after a suicide attempt. To test the relative effects of mood stabilizer monotherapy or combinations, the main analysis was repeated by defining medication periods with lithium alone, VPA alone, and lithium plus VPA. As patients on lithium monotherapy might be different from patients who have switched between lithium and VPA, the analysis was repeated for the subgroup on lithium monotherapy [141].

All retrospective studies have limitations, and even the attempt to remove biases toward lithium use in the Swedish registry study might have been insufficient as clinicians might be influenced by suicidal events that occurred more than 30 days in the past, especially with a pattern of suicidal behavior or a serious past event. Nonetheless, this paper adds to other literature in this area pointing to an effect of lithium on risk of attempted or completed suicide, an effect not seen to the same extent with other mood stabilizers such as VPA. As discussed in Info Box 1.2, clinicians must be aware that these conclusions are based on retrospective analyses; however, in the absence of convincing data on suicidality reduction for any other medication used in BD, lithium remains unique among the options available to manage BD spectrum patients at risk for completed suicide, and possibly in those with unipolar MDD.

Info Box 1.2 Issues in Weighing Lithium's Anti-Suicide Effects

a. **What have we learned from retrospective analyses?** Bearing in mind the prescribing bias toward preferential use of lithium in patients with prior suicidal behavior [133], studies consistently find lower risk of completed suicides and suicide attempts among lithium users, without comparable effects for non-lithium therapies [41, 140, 141]. These effects from lithium may be greater among BD spectrum patients than in those with other disorders (e.g. unipolar MDD) [41]. As more retrospective studies employ propensity score matching to eliminate as much as possible prescribing biases, future analyses will hopefully yield more refined estimates of lithium's anti-suicide effects relative to other medications in real world usage [133].

b. **Limitations of the retrospective data:** There is no compelling evidence that lithium directly impacts suicidal ideation, with modest data to suggest an impact on all acts of self-harm and unintentional injury in BD spectrum patients [140]. The minimum duration necessary to achieve lithium's anti-suicidal effects is unknown, but 18 months or more of exposure may be required based on the smaller effect size seen in patients with shorter vs. longer periods of use in one large meta-analysis (1.41 ± 1.09 years vs. 7.77 ± 6.54 years) [41]. Clinicians should not assume the effect is instantaneous upon starting lithium.

c. **Randomized clinical trials (RCTs):** While evidence from RCTs is the gold standard for proving an efficacy claim, the infrequency of suicide attempts and completed suicides in prospective clinical trials has led to negative results when examining those outcomes. For this reason, most studies are forced to include additional surrogate measures of suicidal behavior (e.g. need for intervention to prevent suicide or self-harm), but those outcomes may not be comparable indicators of suicide risk [36]. Due to the low rates of suicide deaths or serious attempts, enormous sample sizes and an extended duration of follow-up would be necessary to study those particular outcomes in an RCT, and that presents an economic and feasibility barrier to such studies [133].

d. **Conclusions:** It might not be possible within the context of an RCT to prove that lithium reduces risk of suicide attempts and completed suicides, so clinicians must acknowledge the limitations of the data, but also the absence of robust data for any non-lithium therapy. Lithium should not be viewed as a panacea for all parasuicidal and suicidal behavior, but as a tool with significant value over the lifetime of a patient, especially those individuals with BD spectrum diagnoses who have a history of suicidality.

G Neuroprotection

WHAT TO KNOW: LITHIUM AND NEUROPROTECTION

- Bipolar spectrum patients have 3-fold higher risk for dementia. Lifestyle factors (e.g. smoking), cardiovascular comorbidity and mood relapses, especially episodes of mania and hypomania, all contribute to dementia risk.

- Use of lithium for at least 10 months in older bipolar patients reduces dementia risk by 23%, and longer-term use decreases this risk by 49%. There is no impact of non-lithium therapies on dementia risk.

- The neuroprotective properties of lithium were also evident in a 24-month trial of individuals without bipolar disorder who were diagnosed with mild cognitive impairment.

- Lithium's multiple neuroprotective mechanisms relate to decreases in intracellular inositol triphosphate (IP3) levels, inhibition of GSK3-β activity, and mitigation of telomere shortening.

1 *Clinical and Preclinical Evidence for Lithium's Neuroprotective Properties*

Lithium's neuroprotective properties have been studied for decades, with preclinical studies appearing more abundantly in the late 1990s that documented lithium's ability to limit the effects of ischemia, and to reduce apoptosis and excitotoxic cellular damage from a variety of toxic insults [142–145]. Animal stroke models proved especially useful for exploring the range of lithium's neuroprotective effects, as ischemic and hemorrhagic strokes present different forms of cellular injury and patterns of recovery [146]. In these studies, the neuroprotective effects of lithium were seen in the form of reduced infarct volume, reduced postischemic excitotoxicity, improved poststroke recovery, antiapoptotic effects, decreased expression of inflammatory markers, reduced oxidative stress, and activation of immune mediated responses involved in the restoration of blood–brain barrier integrity [146]. This array of early animal data on lithium's ability to reduce cellular injury from acute insults (e.g. ischemic, toxic) stimulated interest in lithium's long-term effects on neurodegenerative disorders, especially in transgenic mouse models of Alzheimer's disease [147, 148]. Preclinical animal findings are not always mirrored by human clinical outcomes, and, despite robust data from stroke models, the human data remain inconclusive regarding lithium's ability to limit damage or facilitate recovery following stroke [146, 149]. The opposite is true for lithium's impact on cognitive decline and dementia risk, with both retrospective and prospective studies illustrating this effect in patients with BD, and in those without mood disorders experiencing mild cognitive impairment (MCI) [44, 48, 150–154]. The majority of these data come from BD spectrum patients, but the estimated reduction in dementia incidence of 40%–50% across multiple studies presents one of the most convincing reasons for clinicians to master the use of lithium in older BD-1 patients (see Chapter 4), and to appreciate that the medical burden of lithium use in older BD-1 patients is not significantly different than for VPA (see Chapter 7) [155].

The other rationale for preferentially using lithium in older BD patients relates to the significantly higher dementia risk in this population, with mood relapses and disproportionate rates of smoking and cardiometabolic disorders contributing to this inflated figure [44]. A 2020 meta-analysis provided an estimate of dementia risk in BD patients by analyzing the odds of dementia vs. demographically matched controls in 10 studies that had adequate data for meta-analysis: 4 cohort studies (range of follow-up 3–17 years), and 6 studies with case-control designs. The total sample sizes were 6859 for the BD subjects and 487,966 for the controls. All but one of the studies indicated that a BD diagnosis increased dementia risk, and the pooled odds ratio indicated that this risk is 3-fold greater in BD patients compared with controls (OR 2.96, 95% CI 2.09–4.18, $p < 0.001$) [44]. There were two other findings of note: (1) The number of mood episodes in BD patients predicted dementia risk, with some studies suggesting that the risk was more attributable to periods of hypomania/mania than periods of depression [44]; (2) Dementia risk was greater for BD than for unipolar MDD patients based on a subset of studies that included both diagnostic groups, a finding consistent with data indicating a somewhat lower 1.65- to 2-fold increased risk for unipolar MDD [44].

In-Depth 1.17 The Impact of Manic and Hypomanic Episodes on Cognitive Decline

A 2020 publication provided confirmatory data on the effect of hypomania/ mania based on results of a prospective structural magnetic resonance imaging (MRI) study in BD patients and healthy control (HC) subjects. 206 subjects underwent imaging at baseline (123 BD, 83 HC) and 151 were available for repeat imaging 6 years later (90 BD patients, 61 HC) [156]. Over the 6 years of follow-up, BD patients showed abnormal cortical thinning of temporal cortices; moreover, those who experienced hypomanic or manic episodes showed abnormal thinning in inferior frontal cortices. Cortical changes did not differ between BD-1 and BD-2 subtypes – the effect was related to periods of hypomania or mania [156]. A 2021 study reinforced the differential effects of depression and hypomania/mania on brain function by combining demographic and illness history with results of a 13-part neuropsychological battery performed in 172 BD patients of mean age 66.0 years residing in Amsterdam, 56.4% with BD-1, and 43.6% BD-2 [157]. After controlling for age and education level, the final multivariable model explained 43.0% of the variance in composite cognitive score [157]. Two variables predicted relatively better cognitive performance, number of depressive episodes and onset at age ≥ 50 years, while five or more psychiatric admissions and use of benzodiazepines were associated with worse cognitive performance [157]. As BD-1 patients are disproportionately admitted for mania, this is another analysis demonstrating the cumulative deleterious effects of mania on cognition. It is worth noting that the association with the number of hypomanic/manic episodes fell just short of statistical significance ($p = 0.065$). Treatment related information was based on patient interview, so one hypothesis is that the number of prior psychiatric admissions is likely to be recalled more accurately in patients who are 66 years old than number of lifetime mood episodes.

In-Depth 1.18 Brain Age Gap in Bipolar Disorder vs. Unipolar Major Depression

The impact of hypomania or mania for the brain health of BD patients can also be explored by looking at brain aging in BD patients compared to those with unipolar MDD. In 2022, a meta-analysis was published comprising 18 studies which used neuroimaging data to calculate the *brain age gap* between psychiatric patients and age-matched controls [158]. As the three diagnostic groups consisted of patients diagnosed with schizophrenia, BD or unipolar MDD, one can compare the relative illness effects of these disorders on brain aging [158]. The random-effects model found a significantly increased neuroimaging-derived brain age gap relative to age-matched controls for all three cohorts, with schizophrenia having the largest gap (Δ 3.08 years; 95% CI 2.32–3.85 years; $p < 0.01$), followed by BD (Δ 1.93 years, 95% CI 0.53–3.34 years; $p < 0.01$) and then by unipolar MDD (Δ 1.12 years, 95% CI 0.41–1.83 years; $p < 0.01$) [158]. The clinical manifestation of accelerated brain aging found on imaging is also readily seen in neuropsychological performance. A cross-sectional trial compared the results of 113 BD-1 patients and 64 healthy adults aged 18–87 on measures of processing speed, attention, executive functioning and verbal fluency to explore the interrelationships of age, clinical variables and cognitive functioning [159]. In the linear regression models, BD-1 patients performed significantly worse than the comparison group on all neuropsychological measures [159]. Older age was also associated with poorer performance on Trails A in BD-1 patients but not in the healthy adults, further evidence of brain aging associated with the BD-1 diagnosis. It is important to appreciate that the effects of mood relapses on brain function, especially hypomania or mania, accrue over long periods of time. In minimally symptomatic stable BD outpatients, mood state at the time of neuropsychological testing and cognitive performance are generally unrelated, implying that any cognitive dysfunction seen at the time of testing is the product of longitudinal effects associated with the mood disorder [160]. This was confirmed by results of a large study of community dwelling BD adults (n = 773) with mean age 39.57 ± 13.61 years and a mean of 15.22 ± 2.19 years of education, whose baseline scores on the HAM-D and YMRS indicated full remission of mania and mild (subthreshold) depressive symptoms [160]. When the investigators compared neuropsychological battery results and mood assessments at baseline and after 1 year of follow-up, they found that baseline cognition significantly predicted cognitive ability after 1 year, with almost no influence from mood symptoms [160]. The authors concluded that any cognitive dysfunction seen in stable outpatients is not due to subtle mood symptoms at that time, but is either a trait effect of the BD diagnosis itself or a consequence of the disorder.

Multiple studies have examined lithium's cognitive effects in BD patients, but the 2020 meta-analysis that estimated BD dementia risk provided the most accurate assessment of this effect [44]. Five cohort studies and one case-control design were found that looked at the correlation between lithium exposure and dementia risk, but one of the cohort studies provided insufficient data for the meta-analysis. Most of the papers were rated as having good-quality designs using the Newcastle–Ottawa Quality Assessment Scale, and four of the five analyzable studies showed a preventative effect of lithium exposure on dementia risk. Overall, there were 6483 BD spectrum patients and 43,396 control individuals in the final analysis. As seen in Figure 1.6, lithium use in BD patients significantly and robustly reduced dementia risk by almost 50% (OR 0.51, 95% CI 0.36–0.72, p < 0.0001) [44].

Figure 1.6 Results from a 2020 meta-analysis of 6483 lithium treated bipolar disorder patients noting a 49% reduction in the risk of dementia [44]

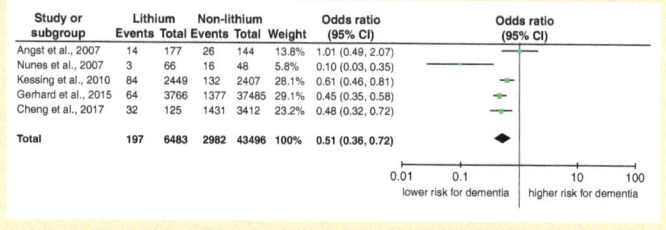

(Adapted from: J. Velosa, A. Delgado, E. Finger, et al. [2020]. Risk of dementia in bipolar disorder and the interplay of lithium: A systematic review and meta-analyses. *Acta Psychiatr Scand*, 141, 510–521.)

A cohort study appeared in the literature shortly after the 2020 meta-analysis was published providing further evidence for the robust association between lithium use and reduced dementia risk. The investigators used electronic clinical records of secondary care mental health services from the Cambridgeshire and Peterborough UK NHS Foundation to identify 548 lithium treated patients and 29,070 individuals not receiving lithium, mean age 73.9 years [154]. After controlling for sociodemographic factors, medications, other psychiatric and somatic comorbidities and smoking status, lithium use was associated with a 44% lower risk of any dementia diagnosis (HR 0.56, 95% CI 0.40–0.78, p = 0.0006), a 45% reduction for dementia of the Alzheimer type (HR 0.55, 95% CI 0.37–0.82), and a 64% reduction for vascular dementia (HR 0.36, 95% CI 0.1– 0.69) (Figure 1.7) [154]. In addition

Figure 1.7 Cumulative risk of dementia in lithium users (n = 548) vs. non-users (29,070) (mean 73.9 years) with at least 1 year of mental health follow-up during 2005–2019 at the Cambridgeshire and Peterborough NHS Foundation Trust [154]

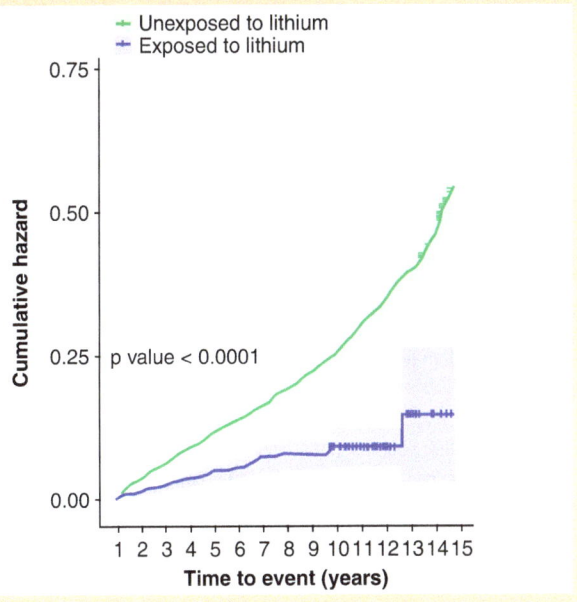

(Adapted from: S. Chen, B. R. Underwood, P. B. Jones, et al. [2022]. Association between lithium use and the incidence of dementia and its subtypes: A retrospective cohort study. *PLoS Med*, 19, e1003941.)

to finding that lithium reduces risk for the two most common forms of dementia, the UK analysis also noted that lithium's protective effect was seen within 1 year of exposure [154].

In-Depth 1.19 Lithium, but Not Anticonvulsant Mood Stabilizers, Reduces Dementia Risk: Evidence

The results of a large US cohort study that examined future dementia risk by duration of lithium use (0, 1–60, 61–300 and 301–365 days) in 6900 lithium treated BD patients age ≥ 50 years without a dementia diagnosis not only confirmed lithium's protective effect, but the absence of such effects from other mood stabilizers used as a control arm [161]. The data set employed for this analysis was a Medicaid extract for the years 2001–2004 from eight large US states, with anticonvulsants commonly used as mood stabilizers serving as the negative control (n = 20,778), and the results of both medication cohorts compared with the dementia incidence among 18,119 BD patients not on lithium or an anticonvulsant [161]. In this sample of mean age 60.4 years, 301–365 days of lithium exposure was associated with significantly reduced dementia risk (HR = 0.77, 95% CI 0.60–0.99) when compared with non-use of lithium. No corresponding association was observed for shorter lithium exposures (HR = 1.04, 95% CI 0.83–1.31 for 61–300 days; HR = 1.07, 95% CI 0.67–1.71 for 1–60 days) *or for any exposure to anticonvulsants* [161]. That as little as 10 months of lithium exposure can reduce dementia incidence in older BD patients by 23%, and that prolonged use reduces this risk by as much as 50%, places the onus on every clinician to justify withholding or discontinuing lithium in older BD patients who can comply with the necessary monitoring frequency based on their eGFR and CKD risk factors (Chapter 4). As reviewed in detail in Chapter 7, it is the unmonitored addition of a kinetically interacting medication that presents the greatest risk for lithium toxicity in older patients, not age itself [162, 163]. Moreover, it is CKD risk factors which have the more significant impact on eGFR trends in older adults, not lithium itself when it is prescribed according to modern dosing precepts and patients are not subjected to periods of lithium toxicity [119, 164].

There are other sources that support these findings, including one study of dementia incidence based on drinking water lithium levels [151], and numerous cross-sectional studies noting superior cognitive performance in BD patients on lithium vs. lithium non-users [150, 165–168]. As BD patients have 3-fold higher dementia risk than age-matched peers due to the combined effects of hypomania/mania and medical comorbidities, an intriguing question is to what extent lithium's neuroprotective effect might be seen in non-BD patients. The preclinical data from Alzheimer's disease models were considered compelling enough to pursue a prospective trial in 61 community-dwelling, healthy older adults with MCI (mean age 72.6 ± 4.8 years), randomized in a double-blind manner to lithium or placebo for 2 years, with an additional 24 months of single-blinded follow-up [48]. The target lithium level range was 0.25–0.50 mEq/l. Over the initial 24 months of the study, subjects in the placebo arm displayed cognitive and functional decline, while the lithium treated patients remained stable. Five subjects in the lithium group (16%) and nine in the placebo group (30%) converted from MCI to dementia during follow-up, but this fell just short of statistical significance for this difference ($p = 0.06$). Not only was lithium exposure associated with better performance on memory and attention tests after 24 months, there was also a significant increase in cerebrospinal fluid (CSF) amyloid-β peptide ($A\beta_{1-42}$) levels after 36 months among those with higher intracerebral $A\beta_{1-42}$ burden at baseline. The $A\beta_{1-42}$ fragment is the main component of amyloid plaques found in the brains of people with Alzheimer's disease, and these aggregates incite inflammatory changes that contribute to cellular damage and death. The finding of higher CSF $A\beta_{1-42}$ levels suggests that long-term lithium treatment promotes cerebral clearance of $A\beta_{1-42}$ [48]. While lithium has long been touted as a possible agent for patients with Alzheimer's disease [147–149, 169], MCI patients have greater preservation of cognitive function and lower amyloid plaque burden, and thus might be a more suitable target for future lithium trials. Hopefully, other investigators will replicate the results of the 24-month study in larger samples and thus establish lithium as an evidence based option to forestall MCI progression [149].

2 *Intracellular Mechanisms that Underlie Lithium's Neuroprotective Properties*

Lithium has numerous and complex interactions with intracellular pathways, each of which may contribute individually or synergistically to its neuroprotective effects (see Figure 1.8) [170]. Lithium's neuroprotective properties can thus be viewed on both the micro and macro level given that the effects are seen with *in vitro* and *in vivo* models of acute injury, as well as with chronic exposure in human beings with and without BD [171]. On the cellular level, lithium increases the production of nerve growth factors, mitigates the effects of inflammation and oxidative stress on mitochondrial function, and modulates autophagy and apoptosis [171]. As discussed below, lithium's mood stabilizing properties are especially ascribed to effects on pathways involving two primary targets: inositol monophosphatase (IMPase) and GSK3-β [67], with emerging evidence that the neuroprotective mechanisms in BD patients are the epiphenomenon of those same processes that maintain mood stability and limit episodes of hypomania and mania [171]. While certain aspects of research on lithium's neuroprotective properties and potential are still being developed, the clinical findings of reduced dementia risk in BD patients should provide sufficient impetus to consider lithium as the mood stabilizer of choice for older BD patients with a history of mania (e.g. BD-1, SAD-BT).

Figure 1.8 Multiple mechanisms that underlie lithium's neuroprotective effects [170]

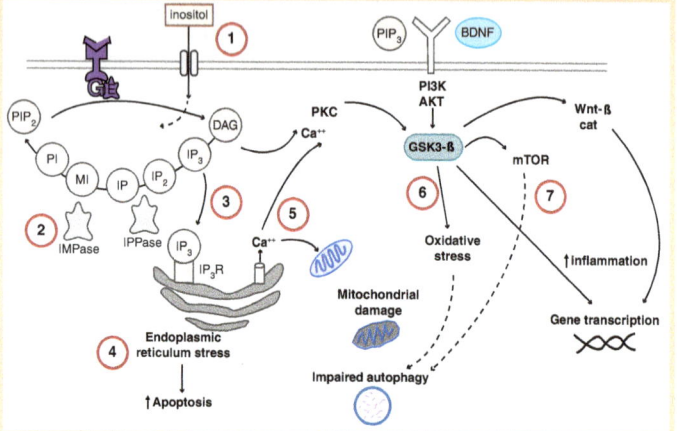

Legend

1. Inhibition of inositol reuptake
2. Depletion of intracellular inositol triphosphate (IP_3)
3. Decreased IP_3 levels minimize stimulation of endoplasmic reticulum (ER) calcium (Ca^{++}) release and downstream processes that induce mitochondrial damage
4. Impact on IP_3 levels also mitigates impaired stress related apoptosis regulation
5. Direct impact on Ca^{++} release from ER also lessens stimulation of protein kinase C (PKC) and its promotion of GSK3-β activity
6. Direct inhibition of GSK3-β activity, with the net result being less oxidative stress and less impaired autophagy
7. Direct inhibition of GSK3-β activity also promotes neurotrophic, neuroprotective and antioxidant gene expression

(Use under the terms of Common Creative License from S. Puglisi-Allegra, S. Ruggieri and F. Fornai [2021]. Translational evidence for lithium-induced brain plasticity and neuroprotection in the treatment of neuropsychiatric disorders. *Transl Psychiatry*, 11, 366.)

That lithium delays cognitive decline in non-BD patients with MCI is a convincing argument that some of its neuroprotective properties exist outside of the domain of any mood related impact, and that mood stabilization is the result of these homeostatic effects [67]. One neuroprotective effect recently identified that may not relate to mood stabilization is the impact of lithium on a marker of cellular aging: the telomere length [172]. Telomeres are stretches of TTAGGG nucleotide repeats at the ends of chromosomes, and these telomeric nucleotides protect coding DNA from being lost during replication by allowing portions of the telomeric sequence to be shed each time a cell divides; however, when the telomere shortens beyond a critical length, the cell loses its ability to divide [172]. As we age, this process of telomere shortening gradually limits the ability to replace older cells, setting the stage for age-related disease. Multiple studies thus indicate a strong association between genetic determinants of telomere length and the risk for age-related diseases and mortality [172]. Since 2013, papers have emerged documenting shorter telomere length in leukocytes of BD patients, although these findings are not seen in all studies [173, 174]. Similarly, there is a parallel literature describing a protective effect of lithium on telomere shortening that appears to correlate with duration of exposure [175, 176]. One recent example is a 2019 cross-sectional analysis of specimens from 384 BD patients which found that chronic lithium treatment was associated with longer telomeres compared with lithium non-users (p = 0.03) [172]. Moreover, polygenic risk scores associated with telomere length explained more of the variance in telomere length in lithium users compared with non-users, suggesting that lithium is promoting certain endogenous mechanisms that support telomere lengthening up to the genetically determined limit for that individual's telomere maintenance capacity [172]. One hypothesis for this telomere lengthening effect relates to evidence that lithium induces expression of telomere reverse transcriptase (TERT) [176]. Telomere shortening can be counteracted by the activation of telomerase, a complex consisting of telomerase RNA component, an RNA template used for telomere synthesis, and TERT, the catalytic subunit. The function of telomerase is to lengthen telomeres in the nucleus, preserving the integrity of end DNA sequences and promoting cellular repair and cellular survival [176]. Using leukocytes from 100 BD-1 patients and 100 healthy controls, investigators from the Karolinska Institute (Stockholm, Sweden) and the Mayo Clinic (Rochester) found that TERT expression was significantly and positively correlated with duration of lithium treatment in patients treated with lithium for ≥ 24 months; however, they did not find any significant effect of lithium on telomere length, nor did they find a significant difference in telomere length between BD-1 patients and controls [176]. From these data, the authors hypothesized that lithium related increases in TERT expression contribute to both mood stabilizing and neuroprotective properties by improving mitochondrial function and decreasing oxidative stress, but indicated that this is an area that deserves further study.

Aggressive or Impulsive Behavior in Child/Adolescent Patients with Conduct Disorder, Borderline Personality Disorder (BPD) and Intellectual Disability

 WHAT TO KNOW: IMPACT OF LITHIUM ON AGGRESSION AND IMPULSIVITY

- Most of the literature in this area is of poor quality or consists of single site trials that have not been replicated.

- The literature does not strongly support lithium's efficacy for conduct disorder, or for impulsive-behavioral dyscontrol in borderline personality disorder. There are somewhat more compelling data for management of disruptive behaviors in intellectually disabled individuals, but more effective options exist and should be tried initially.

- Any use of lithium to manage aggression or impulsivity in non-bipolar patients should be relegated to the latter stages of any algorithm, with lithium used at modest levels and withdrawn if robust effects are not seen after 1–2 months.

Animal models support the concept that lithium possesses anti-aggression properties [52], but this is an area where the human data are not compelling enough to justify routine clinical use. Nonetheless, suicide and aggression are conceptualized as having overlapping neurobiological bases, and one hypothesis for lithium's impact on suicide related mortality rests in its anti-aggression effects [52]. Supporting this idea are findings from epidemiological studies that correlate higher lithium levels in municipal drinking water supplies with lower regional rates of homicide and other violent crimes [53, 177–179]. Aggression is not a unitary concept, and studies among patients with severe mental disorders recognize three categories of acts: those due to uncontrolled psychosis or mania, those related to impulsivity, and those which are planned and engaged in to achieve an outcome such as intimidation or retribution (i.e. instrumental) [180–182]. In those without active psychosis or mania, any anti-aggressive effect of lithium is presumed related to decreased impulsivity, and this has been the basis for exploratory trials across a broad range of populations including some without obvious mental disorders (e.g. prisoners) [52]. Unfortunately, most of the literature in this area consists of open-label studies and case series, or individual double-blind, placebo-controlled trials that have not been replicated or that possessed methodological limitations. For example, the placebo-controlled literature on use of lithium for conduct disorder in children or adolescents consists of two trials, one of which employed unacceptably high mean lithium levels (1.20 mEq/l), and with no studies published since 2000 [183, 184]. A 2010 Cochrane review of pharmacological interventions for borderline personality disorder noted some beneficial effects with SGAs, mood stabilizers (lithium or divalproex) and dietary supplementation by omega-3 fatty acids, but mostly from single studies. Moreover, overall illness severity was not significantly influenced by any medication, and medications do not address the core borderline personality disorder symptoms of emptiness, identity disturbance and abandonment [185]. In addition to high dropout rates, variable study length, and widely divergent proportions of patients in psychotherapy (0–100%) or with comorbid mood disorders (0–100%), there are no long-term studies in borderline personality disorder, and most studies excluded patients with alcohol and substance use disorders, limiting the ability to generalize any findings to usual clinical practice [186]. A 2011 review did not include lithium among the list of agents proven useful to treat affective symptoms and impulsive-behavioral dyscontrol in borderline personality disorder patients [187], although a 2022 review comments that a mood stabilizer such as lithium or lamotrigine may be beneficial where family history suggests a genetic link to BD [58]. The idea that any benefit of lithium for impulsivity in borderline personality disorder relates to subtle forms of a BD diathesis in certain patients is based on the concept that there are qualitatively different types of affective variability in BD and borderline personality disorder individuals [188]. Patients with BD note more prolonged periods of raised or lowered affect, while those with borderline personality disorder report a higher frequency of transient affective variation. A conceptualization of these differences relates to divergent causes of affective variability: volatility, which leads to persistent changes in affect as seen in BD, and noise, which leads to transient changes as seen in borderline personality disorder. A 2022 prospective study showed that lithium is very effective for improving prolonged affective volatility, but is not generally effective in reducing affective noise for borderline personality disorder patients [188].

While the preclinical and available clinical data suggest some potential to manage conduct disorder and aggression in non-bipolar children or adolescents [54, 55], to lessen disruptive behaviors in intellectually disabled individuals, or to curtail impulsivity in borderline personality disorder, lithium's use should be relegated to the latter stages of any treatment algorithm for several reasons: there are more strongly evidence based treatments for certain clinical scenarios (dialectical behavioral therapy for borderline personality disorder, SGAs for irritability in autistic disorder), there are no long-term studies, and the evidence for lithium is generally uneven and of low quality. There are also safety concerns when high serum lithium levels (e.g. > 1.00 mEq/l) are employed [183], especially in patients with intellectual disability [56, 57, 189, 190]. Lithium can be used safely in intellectually disabled patients with careful monitoring [191], but clinicians should acknowledge the lack of methodologically strong controlled data for this patient population. Regardless of the application, certain aggressive or impulsive behaviors wax or wane based on dynamic factors [192], so any change associated with a lithium trial may be spurious. It is the clinician's responsibility to taper off lithium if the response has not been particularly robust, and to consider a taper after prolonged use where other interventions or factors may have contributed to a reduction in problematic behaviors [192]; moreover, as the benefits are largely unquantifiable, any clinician who uses lithium for these purposes must transparently communicate to patients and/or caregivers that the effect might be minimal, and employ prescribing and monitoring practices that emphasize patient safety. The use of lithium in these clinical situations is not inherently unreasonable once other options have been exhausted, but management of risk and periodic reassessment of efficacy are important guiding principles where the evidence base is limited.

Neutrophilia

WHAT TO KNOW: HOW LITHIUM INCREASES NEUTROPHIL COUNTS

- Lithium directly stimulates production of granulocyte colony stimulating factor (G-CSF), and thereby stimulates production of neutrophils. The concept that lithium only causes demargination of neutrophils in bone marrow reserves is incorrect.

- All clinicians should be aware that lithium may increase neutrophil counts starting 1–2 weeks after initiation to obviate any unnecessary work-up for occult sources of infection.

- Lithium has been used by hematologists to manage neutropenia since the 1970s, and by the psychiatric profession to manage neutropenia prior to or during clozapine therapy for over 30 years.

The association between lithium and neutrophilia has been known for over 50 years, and by 1978 it was shown that lithium-induced granulocytosis reflects enlargement of the total circulating neutrophil mass due to accelerated neutrophil production [63, 64]. Lithium's association with neutrophilia is occasionally misrepresented as the result of neutrophil demargination, but animal and human studies convincingly demonstrate that lithium exposure increases bone marrow organ cellularity, a fact proven in the 1970s and valued by hematologists to manage chemotherapy related neutropenia and to assist with stem cell mobilization prior to bone marrow transplantation [63, 64]. Multiple placebo-controlled trials reported lithium's effects for hematology uses in the 1970s and 1980s, and these findings led psychiatric providers to employ lithium for management of mild or moderate neutropenia during clozapine therapy, or to bolster low neutrophil counts prior to clozapine initiation [61, 62]. The underlying mechanism relates to lithium's ability to enhance production of granulocyte colony stimulating factor (G-CSF), and thereby stimulate proliferation of pluripotential stem cells resulting in increased bone marrow colony-forming units and bone marrow organ cellularity [65]. This effect occurs reproducibly in animal and human studies, and exhibits a dose dependency within the serum range of 0.30–1.00 mEq/l (0.30–1.00 mmol/l) [64]. Higher serum levels in animal models did not generate greater effects, and very high levels that would be toxic in humans (5.00 mEq/l or 5.00 mmol/l) cause bone marrow toxicity. At therapeutic doses of 900–1200 mg/day, the mean increase in absolute neutrophil count (ANC) averaged 88% in one small trial, and the effect was seen in the first week after lithium was initiated, although peak ANC values may not occur until week 2 or 3 [193]. This property also represents a unique advantage of lithium over VPA when managing clozapine treated patients who require mood stabilization since VPA is associated with a dose dependent risk for neutropenia [194]. A case–control study that examined risk factors for neutropenia during clozapine treatment (n = 272) found that concurrent use of VPA more than doubled the risk for neutropenia (OR 2.28, 95% CI 1.27–4.11, p = 0.006) [195]. While lithium induced neutrophilia can be exploited therapeutically, for the majority of patients it is an incidental laboratory finding of no consequence, but one that should be mentioned to patients and other health-care providers to avoid unnecessary alarm, and especially to obviate work-up for infection or for a hematological disorder.

J Lithium's Mechanisms of Action

Lithium's dense and interconnected cellular activities continue to be explored in an attempt to understand the biological underpinnings of BD and to develop novel treatments for this mood disorder [196–198]. Decades of research have established that lithium's mechanisms of action relate to modulation of signal transduction pathways, especially those regulated by inositol monophosphatase (IMPase) and GSK3-β, but also involving numerous other kinases and signaling proteins (e.g. protein kinase C [PKC], phospholipase A2, molecular target of rapamycin [mTOR], Wnt, ErbB, MAP kinase, and vascular endothelial growth factor [VEGF] pathways) [199, 200]. Certain mechanisms (e.g. GSK3-β inhibition) overlap with those of antipsychotics and mood stabilizers, but *in vitro* and *in vivo* research shows that lithium exhibits distinct properties via direct and indirect effects that result in comparatively greater GSK3-β inhibition [67]. These basic science findings have led to human trials probing the antimanic effects of IMPase inhibitors such as ebselen, an organoselenium compound developed as an antioxidant [201], and PKC inhibitors such as tamoxifen, a molecule primarily used as an estrogen receptor modulator [202]. The fact that lithium acts on numerous pathways simultaneously implies that it might be difficult to find any single molecule that replicates lithium's clinical profile, especially the combination of its mood stabilizing, anti-suicide and neuroprotective effects.

Part of lithium's uniqueness relates to it being a cation ion with similar ionic radius to magnesium (lithium 0.60 Å, magnesium 0.65 Å), thus allowing lithium to compete for binding sites at magnesium-dependent enzymes and other substrates [67]. Due to their similar radii, lithium's competition for low affinity magnesium binding sites is independent of the substrate; moreover, this type of interference is not seen with other Group I ions (e.g. potassium, sodium) as their larger size precludes interaction with the magnesium binding site [67]. The direct relevance of this finding for lithium's mood stabilizing properties can be seen with *in vitro* studies, especially those focused on lithium's core targets, IMPase and GSK3-β. In mammals, IMPase (and several other phosphomonoesterases) are magnesium dependent, and lithium thus inhibits IMPase activity by binding uncompetitively to one of its magnesium sites [67]. Lithium's direct inhibitory effect on GSK3-β also arises via competition at magnesium binding sites, with lithium binding resulting in impaired enzyme catalytic activity. It is difficult to predict the extent of lithium's *in vivo* direct inhibition of GSK3-β based on *in vitro* studies, as lithium's actions will depend on local conditions. Intracellular concentrations of free unbound magnesium range from 0.6 to 1.2 mmol/l, while lithium's ability to inhibit GSK3-β activity by 50% (IC_{50}) occurs at 2 mmol/l. By keeping cellular magnesium concentration low during *in vitro* assays, more magnesium binding sites are available, thus decreasing the IC_{50} for lithium's GSK3-β inhibition to under 0.8 mmol/l [67]. This artificial environment provides only limited guidance on the extent of lithium's GSK3-β inhibition during therapeutic use, but underscores the concept that lithium has direct effects on GSK3-β activity due to its ionic structure, a property that differentiates lithium from other psychotropics used for mood stabilization.

Many of lithium's actions are hypothesized to be downstream effects of IMPase inhibition and the central role played by the phosphophatidylinositol signaling pathway in regulating multiple cellular functions, including apoptosis and cell growth. Stimulation of certain G-protein coupled receptors results in activation of phospholipase C, an enzyme that hydrolyzes phosphatidylinositol biphosphate (PIP2) to produce diacylglycerol and inositol triphosphate (IP$_3$), both of which have 2nd messenger activities (Figure 1.9) [67]. It is worth noting that PIP2 is not only a precursor to these signaling molecules, it can also be phosphorylated to become PIP3, which is itself involved in cell movement, proliferation and apoptosis [67]. Among the two products of PIP2 hydrolysis, diacylglycerol activates several protein kinases such as PKC, while IP$_3$ induces release of calcium stores from endoplasmic reticulum into the cytoplasm. Both of these processes create

Figure 1.9 How lithium interacts with the phosphatidylinositol pathway by inhibiting the conversion of inositol triphosphate (IP$_3$) to free inositol [67]

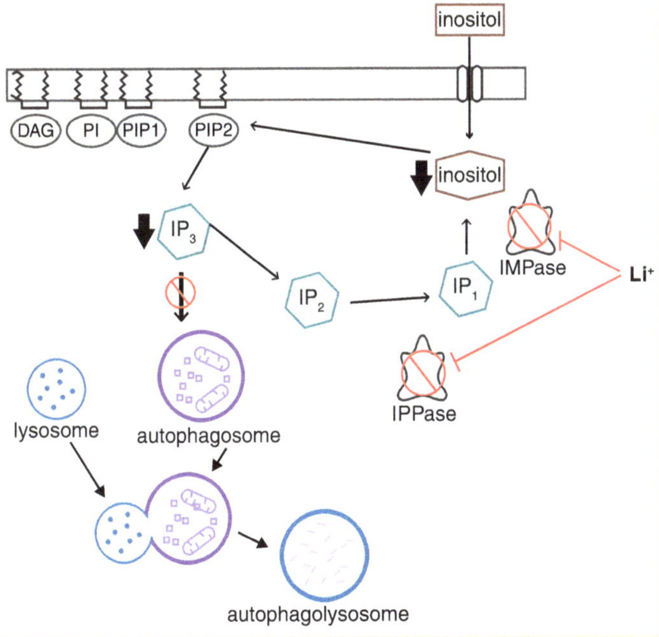

(Adapted from: L. Pasquali, C. L. Busceti, F. Fulceri, et al. [2010]. Intracellular pathways underlying the effects of lithium. *Behav Pharmacol*, 21, 473–492.)

significant downstream signals. At the neuronal level, the combined effects of diacylglycerol and IP_3 impinge on fundamental processes such as plasticity and long-term potentiation, and one regulator of PIP2 availability is the enzyme IMPase. This enzyme catalyzes the final step in converting IP_3 to produce PIP2 by dephosphorylating inositol 1-monophosphate to produce inorganic phosphate and inositol, the precursor to PIP2. Lithium inhibits both IMPase and inositol polyphosphate phosphatase (IPP) thereby reducing the intracellular availability of free inositol and limiting the formation of PIP2 and IP_3 [67]. Among the cellular processes highly correlated with these actions is autophagy, the normal process by which cells remove old or degraded elements via lysosomes. Animal models demonstrate that lithium related stimulation of autophagy counteracts those forces inducing neurodegeneration, and this may be crucial for lithium's effects on mood and cognition [67]. Another result of IPP inhibition is increased intracellular levels of inositol 1-monophosphate, the substrate of IMPase. Higher levels of inositol 1-monophosphate further reduce IMPase activity by limiting the amount of unbound enzyme available to catalyze inositol 1-monophosphate dephosphorylation. In addition to autophagy induction, multiple G-protein coupled receptor pathways are also regulated in a PIP2 dependent manner, including specific muscarinic cholinergic, serotonergic and dopaminergic receptors. These effects may also be part of lithium's mood related properties.

As mentioned in the Introduction, lithium moderates the downstream signal from dopamine D_2 receptor stimulation, and this is considered an important aspect of its antimanic actions [203, 204]. Activation of postsynaptic D_2 receptors by direct agonists or presynaptic dopamine releasing agents (e.g. amphetamine) induces effects on G-protein dependent and non-G-protein pathways (Figure 1.10), each of which moderate different behaviors. The hyperlocomotion induced by D_2 receptor agonists or amphetamines is associated with actions on a pathway that involves a scaffolding protein, β-arrestin2, and the net increase in GSK3-β activity. Binding of dopamine to D_2 (and other G-protein coupled receptors) recruits β-arrestin2 and supports formation of the stable complex of β-arrestin2, protein phosphatase 2A (PP2A) and the kinase Akt. Formation of this complex allows PP2A to phosphorylate and inactivate Akt. Inactivated Akt is no longer able to phosphorylate GSK3-β on its serine 9 residue, with the result that GSK3-β remains active. Not surprisingly, in blocking dopamine D_2 binding, antipsychotics inhibit β-arrestin2 recruitment and subsequent formation of the Akt/β-arrestin2/PP2A complex, thus allowing Akt to remain more active and inhibit GSK3-β [204, 205]. At concentrations that overlap with clinically effective serum levels (0.50–1.00 mEq/l), lithium destabilizes

Figure 1.10 How dopamine D2 receptor agonists recruit β-arrestin2, resulting in decreased Akt activity and increased GSK3-β activity, manifested as hyperlocomotion [13, 203, 204]

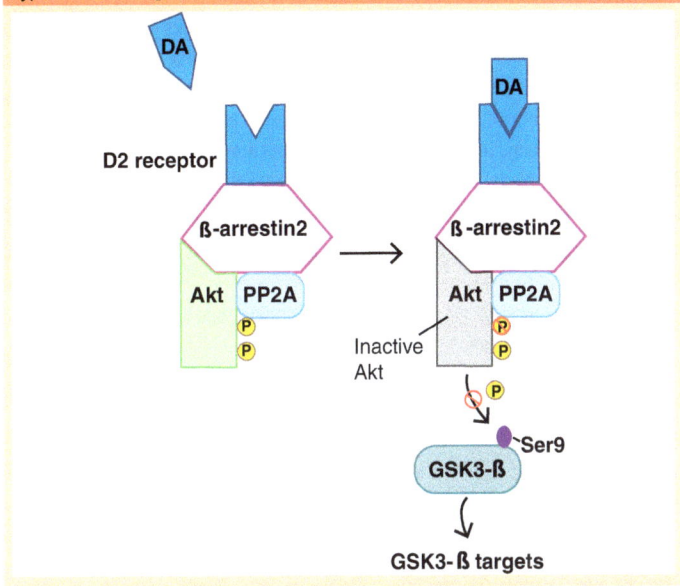

(Adapted from: J. M. Beaulieu, R. R. Gainetdinov and M. G. Caron (2009). Akt/GSK3 signaling in the action of psychotropic drugs. *Annu Rev Pharmacol Toxicol*, 49, 327–347; J. M. Beaulieu, T. Del'guidice, T. D. Sotnikova, et al. [2011]. Beyond cAMP: The regulation of Akt and GSK3 by dopamine receptors. *Front Mol Neurosci*, 4, 38.)

formation of the Akt/β-arrestin2/PP2A complex, leading to increased levels of activated Akt, and therefore greater inactivation of GSK3-β [13]. This destabilizing property, which indirectly reduces GSK3-β activity, is shared with lamotrigine and valproate, but what distinguishes lithium is its additional direct actions on GSK3-β through binding at the magnesium site [67]. The net result is greater GSK3-β inhibition, a factor that may be relevant to mood stabilization, but also to lithium's neuroprotective properties. Increased GSK3-β activity induces apoptosis in neurons, while decreasing GSK3-β activity either with lithium or other methods counteracts these effects. The protective properties from GSK3-β inhibition are in part mediated by effects on β-catenin. Inactive GSK3-β allows the active nonphosphorylated form of β-catenin to enter the nucleus, form a complex with the DNA-binding protein T-cell factor and activate transcription of a wide variety of genes, particularly growth promoting genes such as VEGF and other growth factors [67]. The more robust inhibition of GSK3-β activity by lithium than that by other mood stabilizers is postulated to be a contributing factor in lithium's neuroprotective effects (e.g. reduced dementia rates), clinical effects not seen with anticonvulsant mood stabilizers. Lithium indeed has complex actions that are still being understood, but the molecular evidence points to an array of actions that act synergistically to generate lithium's unique signature of clinical benefits.

Summary Points

a. Lithium has significant efficacy data for acute mania, and is considered the gold standard for maintenance treatment in patients with a history of mania (BD-1, SAD-BT). Older age or a history of rapid cycling are not reasons to eschew lithium – it is no less effective than other options. Lithium can be used for BD-2 patients who require mood stabilization, but is not demonstrably superior to other options.

b. Lithium's impact on suicide attempts and risk of completed suicide cannot be proven in the context of randomized clinical trials; however, the retrospective data are largely consistent that these are unique properties of lithium not seen to the same extent with other mood stabilizers. This effect may also be greater with BD spectrum patients than for other psychiatric diagnoses. Lithium does not have data supporting use for acute bipolar depression, but is effective as an adjunct to antidepressants for unipolar major depression. Lithium's prospective anti-aggression data are not of high quality and it is not routinely used to manage conduct disorder in children/adolescents, with limited data to support its value for impulsive behavior in those with intellectual disability or borderline personality disorder.

c. Lithium has extensive preclinical and clinical evidence demonstrating its neuroprotective properties. BD spectrum patients have 3-fold higher risk of dementia, and multiple studies indicate that use of lithium in older BD patients reduces this risk by 50%. This is one of the most compelling reasons to continue lithium therapy in older patients.

d. Lithium stimulates neutrophil production by increasing levels of granulocyte colony stimulating factor. Patients should be advised of this to avoid unnecessary medical work-up for other causes. This property is commonly exploited in the management of clozapine treated patients as a means to boost absolute neutrophil counts.

e. Lithium impacts numerous intracellular pathways, and these mechanisms differentially contribute to its mood stabilizing, anti-suicide and neuroprotective clinical profile. In animal models, lithium interferes with amphetamine induced hyperlocomotion from striatal dopamine D2 receptor stimulation by destabilizing β-arrestin2 complex formation and decreasing GSK3-β activity. This property is considered central to lithium's antimanic activity. No single medication replicates all of lithium's 2nd messenger effects and its clinical profile.

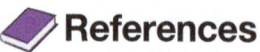 # References

1. Malhi, G. S., Gessler, D. and Outhred, T. (2017). The use of lithium for the treatment of bipolar disorder: Recommendations from clinical practice guidelines. *J Affect Disord*, 217, 266–280.

2. Yatham, L. N., Kennedy, S. H., Parikh, S. V., et al. (2018). Canadian Network for Mood and Anxiety Treatments (CANMAT) and International Society for Bipolar Disorders (ISBD) 2018 guidelines for the management of patients with bipolar disorder. *Bipolar Disord*, 20, 97–170.

3. McIntyre, R. S., Berk, M., Brietzke, E., et al. (2020). Bipolar disorders. *Lancet*, 396, 1841–1856.

4. Fountoulakis, K. N., Tohen, M. and Zarate, C. A. (2022). Lithium treatment of bipolar disorder in adults: A systematic review of randomized trials and meta-analyses. *Eur Neuropsychopharmacol*, 54, 100–115.

5. Poranen, J., Koistinaho, A., Tanskanen, A., et al. (2022). 20-year medication use trends in first-episode bipolar disorder. *Acta Psychiatr Scand*, 146, 583–593.

6. Lahteenvuo, M., Tanskanen, A., Taipale, H., et al. (2018). Real-world effectiveness of pharmacologic treatments for the prevention of rehospitalization in a Finnish nationwide cohort of patients with bipolar disorder. *JAMA Psychiatry*, 75, 347–355.

7. Kook, K. A., Stimmel, G. L., Wilkins, J. N., et al. (1985). Accuracy and safety of a priori lithium loading. *J Clin Psychiatry*, 46, 49–51.

8. Keck, P. E., Jr., McElroy, S. L. and Bennett, J. A. (2000). Pharmacologic loading in the treatment of acute mania. *Bipolar Disord*, 2, 42–46.

9. Cipriani, A., Barbui, C., Salanti, G., et al. (2005). Comparative efficacy and acceptability of antimanic drugs in acute mania: A multiple-treatments meta-analysis. *Lancet*, 378, 1306–1315.

10. Sun, A. Y., Woods, S., Findling, R. L., et al. (2019). Safety considerations in the psychopharmacology of pediatric bipolar disorder. *Expert Opin Drug Saf*, 18, 777–794.

11. Du, J., Quiroz, J., Yuan, P., et al. (2004). Bipolar disorder: Involvement of signaling cascades and AMPA receptor trafficking at synapses. *Neuron Glia Biol*, 1, 231–243.

12. Meyer, J. M. (2022). Pharmacotherapy of psychosis and mania. In L. L. Brunton and B. C. Knollmann, eds., *Goodman & Gilman's The Pharmacological Basis of Therapeutics, 14th Edition*. Chicago: McGraw-Hill, pp. 357–384.

13. Del' Guidice, T. and Beaulieu, J. M. (2015). Selective disruption of dopamine D2-receptors/ beta-arrestin2 signaling by mood stabilizers. *J Recept Signal Transduct Res*, 35, 224–232.

14. O'Brien, W. T., Huang, J., Buccafusca, R., et al. (2011). Glycogen synthase kinase-3 is essential for β-arrestin-2 complex formation and lithium-sensitive behaviors in mice. *J Clin Invest*, 121, 3756–3762.

15. Urs, N. M., Snyder, J. C., Jacobsen, J. P., et al. (2012). Deletion of GSK3β in D2 R-expressing neurons reveals distinct roles for β-arrestin signaling in antipsychotic and lithium action. *Proc Natl Acad Sci USA*, 109, 20732–20737.

16. Meyer, J. M. (2021). Approach to bipolar diathesis in schizophrenia spectrum patients. In M. A. Cummings and S. M. Stahl, eds., *Management of Complex Treatment-Resistant Psychotic Disorders* (Stahl's Handbooks). Cambridge: Cambridge University Press, pp. 42–50.

17. Schou, M. (2004). *Lithium Treatment of Mood Disorders* (6th edn.). Basle: S. Karger AG.

18. Wingård, L., Brandt, L., Bodén, R., et al. (2019). Monotherapy vs. combination therapy for post mania maintenance treatment: A population based cohort study. *Eur Neuropsychopharmacol*, 29, 691–700.

19. Tondo, L., Baldessarini, R. J. and Floris, G. (2001). Long-term clinical effectiveness of lithium maintenance treatment in types I and II bipolar disorders. *Br J Psychiatry Suppl*, 41, s184–190.

20. Chakrabarty, T., Hadjipavlou, G., Bond, D. J., et al. (2019). Bipolar II disorder in context: A review of its epidemiology, disability and economic burden. In G. Parker, ed., *Bipolar II Disorder: Modelling, Measuring and Managing* (3rd edn.). Cambridge: Cambridge University Press, pp. 49–59.

21. Öhlund, L., Ott, M., Bergqvist, M., et al. (2019). Clinical course and need for hospital admission after lithium discontinuation in patients with bipolar disorder type I or II: Mirror-image study based on the LiSIE retrospective cohort. *BJPsych Open*, 5, e101–112.

22. Parker, G., Ricciardi, T., Tavella, G., et al. (2021). A single-blind randomized comparison of lithium and lamotrigine as maintenance treatments for managing bipolar II disorder. *J Clin Psychopharmacol*, 41, 381–388.

23. Keck, P. E., Jr., McElroy, S. L., Strakowski, S. M., et al. (1994). Pharmacologic treatment of schizoaffective disorder. *Psychopharmacology (Berl)*, 114, 529–538.

24. Leucht, S., Helfer, B., Dold, M., et al. (2015). Lithium for schizophrenia. *Cochrane Database Syst Rev*, Cd003834.

25. Puranen, A., Koponen, M., Lahteenvuo, M., et al. (2022). Real-world effectiveness of mood stabilizer use in schizophrenia. *Acta Psychiatr Scand*, 147, 257–266.

26. Lintunen, J., Taipale, H., Tanskanen, A., et al. (2021). Long-term real-world effectiveness of pharmacotherapies for schizoaffective disorder. *Schizophr Bull*, 47, 1099–1107.

27. Judd, L. L., Akiskal, H. S., Schettler, P. J., et al. (2002). The long-term natural history of the weekly symptomatic status of bipolar I disorder. *Arch Gen Psychiatry*, 59, 530–537.

28. Judd, L. L., Akiskal, H. S., Schettler, P. J., et al. (2003). A prospective investigation of the natural history of the long-term weekly symptomatic status of bipolar II disorder. *Arch Gen Psychiatry*, 60, 261–269.

29. Amsterdam, J. D., Lorenzo-Luaces, L., Soeller, I., et al. (2016). Short-term venlafaxine v. lithium monotherapy for bipolar type II major depressive episodes: Effectiveness and mood conversion rate. *Br J Psychiatry*, 208, 359–365.

30. Hui, T. P., Kandola, A., Shen, L., et al. (2019). A systematic review and meta-analysis of clinical predictors of lithium response in bipolar disorder. *Acta Psychiatr Scand*, 140, 94–115.

31. Strawbridge, R., Kurana, S., Kerr-Gaffney, J., et al. (2022). A systematic review and meta-analysis of treatments for rapid cycling bipolar disorder. *Acta Psychiatr Scand*, 146, 290–311.

32. Baldessarini, R. J., Tondo, L., Floris, G., et al. (2000). Effects of rapid cycling on response to lithium maintenance treatment in 360 bipolar I and II disorder patients. *J Affect Disord*, 61, 13–22.

33. Calabrese, J. R., Shelton, M. D., Rapport, D. J., et al. (2005). A 20-month, double-blind, maintenance trial of lithium versus divalproex in rapid-cycling bipolar disorder. *Am J Psychiatry*, 162, 2152–2161.

34. Kemp, D. E., Gao, K., Ganocy, S. J., et al. (2009). A 6-month, double-blind, maintenance trial of lithium monotherapy versus the combination of lithium and divalproex for rapid-cycling bipolar disorder and co-occurring substance abuse or dependence. *J Clin Psychiatry*, 70, 113–121.

35. Zhihan, G., Fengli, S., Wangqiang, L., et al. (2022). Lamotrigine and lithium combination for treatment of rapid cycling bipolar disorder: Results from meta-analysis. *Front Psychiatry*, 13, 913051.

36. Baldessarini, R. J. and Tondo, L. (2021). Testing for antisuicidal effects of lithium treatment. *JAMA Psychiatry*, 79, 9–10.

37. Weisler, R. H., Nolen, W. A., Neijber, A., et al. (2011). Continuation of quetiapine versus switching to placebo or lithium for maintenance treatment of bipolar I disorder (Trial 144: A randomized controlled study). *J Clin Psychiatry*, 72, 1452–1464.

38. Young, A. H., McElroy, S. L., Bauer, M., et al. (2010). A double-blind, placebo-controlled study of quetiapine and lithium monotherapy in adults in the acute phase of bipolar depression (EMBOLDEN I). *J Clin Psychiatry*, 71, 150–162.

39. Calabrese, J. R., Bowden, C. L., Sachs, G., et al. (2003). A placebo-controlled 18-month trial of lamotrigine and lithium maintenance treatment in recently depressed patients with bipolar I disorder. *J Clin Psychiatry*, 64, 1013–1024.

40. Katz, I. R., Rogers, M. P., Lew, R., et al. (2022). Lithium treatment in the prevention of repeat suicide-related outcomes in veterans with major depression or bipolar disorder: A randomized clinical trial. *JAMA Psychiatry*, 79, 24–32.

41. Baldessarini, R. J., Tondo, L., Davis, P., et al. (2006). Decreased risk of suicides and attempts during long-term lithium treatment: A meta-analytic review. *Bipolar Disord*, 8, 625–639.

42. Smith, K. A. and Cipriani, A. (2017). Lithium and suicide in mood disorders: Updated meta-review of the scientific literature. *Bipolar Disord*, 19, 575–586.

43. Baldessarini, R. J., Tondo, L. and Vazquez, G. H. (2019). Pharmacological treatment of adult bipolar disorder. *Mol Psychiatry*, 24, 198–217.

44. Velosa, J., Delgado, A., Finger, E., et al. (2020). Risk of dementia in bipolar disorder and the interplay of lithium: A systematic review and meta-analyses. *Acta Psychiatr Scand*, 141, 510–521.

45. Barjasteh-Askari, F., Davoudi, M., Amini, H., et al. (2020). Relationship between suicide mortality and lithium in drinking water: A systematic review and meta-analysis. *J Affect Disord*, 264, 234–241.

46. Del Matto, L., Muscas, M., Murru, A., et al. (2020). Lithium and suicide prevention in mood disorders and in the general population: A systematic review. *Neurosci Biobehav Rev*, 116, 142–153.

47. Kugimiya, T., Ishii, N., Kohno, K., et al. (2021). Lithium in drinking water and suicide prevention: The largest nationwide epidemiological study from Japan. *Bipolar Disord*, 23, 33–40.

48. Forlenza, O. V., Radanovic, M., Talib, L. L., et al. (2019). Clinical and biological effects of long-term lithium treatment in older adults with amnestic mild cognitive impairment: Randomised clinical trial. *Br J Psychiatry*, 215, 668–674.

49. Undurraga, J., Sim, K., Tondo, L., et al. (2019). Lithium treatment for unipolar major depressive disorder: Systematic review. *J Psychopharmacol*, 33, 167–176.

50. Nierenberg, A. A., Fava, M., Trivedi, M. H., et al. (2006). A comparison of lithium and T(3) augmentation following two failed medication treatments for depression: A STAR*D report. *Am J Psychiatry*, 163, 1519–1530.

51. Vázquez, G. H., Bahji, A., Undurraga, J., et al. (2021). Efficacy and tolerability of combination treatments for major depression: Antidepressants plus second-generation antipsychotics vs. esketamine vs. lithium. *J Psychopharmacol*, 35, 890–900.

52. Muller-Oerlinghausen, B. and Lewitzka, U. (2010). Lithium reduces pathological aggression and suicidality: A mini-review. *Neuropsychobiology*, 62, 43–49.

53. Giotakos, O. (2018). Is violence in part a lithium deficiency state? *Pschiatriki*, 29, 264–270.

54. Masi, G., Milone, A., Manfredi, A., et al. (2009). Effectiveness of lithium in children and adolescents with conduct disorder: A retrospective naturalistic study. *CNS Drugs*, 23, 59–69.

55. Pringsheim, T., Hirsch, L., Gardner, D., et al. (2015). The pharmacological management of oppositional behaviour, conduct problems, and aggression in children and adolescents with attention-deficit hyperactivity disorder, oppositional defiant disorder, and conduct disorder: A systematic review and meta-analysis. Part 2: Antipsychotics and traditional mood stabilizers. *Can J Psychiatry*, 60, 52–61.

56. Deb, S., Chaplin, R., Sohanpal, S., et al. (2008). The effectiveness of mood stabilizers and antiepileptic medication for the management of behaviour problems in adults with intellectual disability: A systematic review. *J Intellect Disabil Res*, 52, 107–113.

57. Ji, N. Y. and Findling, R. L. (2016). Pharmacotherapy for mental health problems in people with intellectual disability. *Curr Opin Psychiatry*, 29, 103–125.

58. Stone, M. H. (2022). Borderline personality disorder: Clinical guidelines for treatment. *Psychodyn Psychiatry*, 50, 45–63.

59. Steiner, T. J., Hering, R., Couturier, E. G., et al. (1997). Double-blind placebo-controlled trial of lithium in episodic cluster headache. *Cephalalgia*, 17, 673–675.

60. Kwon, J. H., Han, J. Y., Choi, J. W., et al. (2022). Comparative impact of pharmacological therapies on cluster headache management: A systematic review and network meta-analysis. *J Clin Med*, 11, 1–20.

61. Mattai, A., Fung, L., Bakalar, J., et al. (2009). Adjunctive use of lithium carbonate for the management of neutropenia in clozapine-treated children. *Hum Psychopharmacol*, 24, 584–589.

62. Nykiel, S., Henderson, D., Bhide, G., et al. (2010). Lithium to allow clozapine prescribing in benign ethnic neutropenia. *Clin Schizophr Relat Psychoses*, 4, 138–140.

63. Rothstein, G., Clarkson, D. R., Larsen, W., et al. (1978). Effect of lithium on neutrophil mass and production. *N Engl J Med*, 298, 178–180.

64. Focosi, D., Azzara, A., Kast, R. E., et al. (2009). Lithium and hematology: Established and proposed uses. *J Leukoc Biol*, 85, 20–28.

65. Petrini, M. and Azzara, A. (2012). Lithium in the treatment of neutropenia. *Curr Opin Hematol*, 19, 52–57.

66. Phiel, C. J. and Klein, P. S. (2001). Molecular targets of lithium action. *Annu Rev Pharmacol Toxicol*, 41, 789–813.

67. Pasquali, L., Busceti, C. L., Fulceri, F., et al. (2010). Intracellular pathways underlying the effects of lithium. *Behav Pharmacol*, 21, 473–492.

68. Bellivier, F. and Marie-Claire, C. (2018). Molecular signatures of lithium treatment: Current knowledge. *Pharmacopsychiatry*, 51, 212–219.

69. Scott, J., Hidalgo-Mazzei, D., Strawbridge, R., et al. (2019). Prospective cohort study of early biosignatures of response to lithium in bipolar-I-disorders: Overview of the H2020-funded R-LiNK initiative. *Int J Bipolar Disord*, 7, 20.

70. Hou, L., Heilbronner, U., Degenhardt, F., et al. (2016). Genetic variants associated with response to lithium treatment in bipolar disorder: A genome-wide association study. *Lancet*, 387, 1085–1093.

71. Scott, J., Geoffroy, P. A., Sportiche, S., et al. (2017). Cross-validation of clinical characteristics and treatment patterns associated with phenotypes for lithium response defined by the Alda scale. *J Affect Disord*, 208, 62–67.

72. Scott, J., Etain, B. and Bellivier, F. (2018). Can an integrated science approach to precision medicine research improve lithium treatment in bipolar disorders? *Front Psychiatry*, 9, 360.

73. McCarthy, M. J., Wei, H., Nievergelt, C. M., et al. (2019). Chronotype and cellular circadian rhythms predict the clinical response to lithium maintenance treatment in patients with bipolar disorder. *Neuropsychopharmacology*, 44, 620–628.

74. Lin, Y., Maihofer, A. X., Stapp, E., et al. (2021). Clinical predictors of non-response to lithium treatment in the Pharmacogenomics of Bipolar Disorder (PGBD) study. *Bipolar Disord*, 23, 821–831.

75. Mishra, H. K., Ying, N. M., Luis, A., et al. (2021). Circadian rhythms in bipolar disorder patient-derived neurons predict lithium response: Preliminary studies. *Mol Psychiatry*, 26, 3383–3394.

76. Grunze, H., Vieta, E., Goodwin, G. M., et al. (2009). The World Federation of Societies of Biological Psychiatry (WFSBP) guidelines for the biological treatment of bipolar disorders: Update 2009 on the treatment of acute mania. *World J Biol Psychiatry*, 10, 85–116.

77. Grunze, H., Vieta, E., Goodwin, G. M., et al. (2010). The World Federation of Societies of Biological Psychiatry (WFSBP) guidelines for the biological treatment of bipolar disorders: Update 2010 on the treatment of acute bipolar depression. *World J Biol Psychiatry*, 11, 81–109.

78. Bauer, M., Pfennig, A., Severus, E., et al. (2013). World Federation of Societies of Biological Psychiatry (WFSBP) guidelines for biological treatment of unipolar depressive disorders, part 1: Update 2013 on the acute and continuation treatment of unipolar depressive disorders. *World J Biol Psychiatry*, 14, 334–385.

79. Grunze, H., Vieta, E., Goodwin, G. M., et al. (2013). The World Federation of Societies of Biological Psychiatry (WFSBP) guidelines for the biological treatment of bipolar disorders: Update 2012 on the long-term treatment of bipolar disorder. *World J Biol Psychiatry*, 14, 154–219.

80. Grunze, H., Vieta, E., Goodwin, G. M., et al. (2018). The World Federation of Societies of Biological Psychiatry (WFSBP) guidelines for the biological treatment of bipolar disorders: Acute and long-term treatment of mixed states in bipolar disorder. *World J Biol Psychiatry*, 19, 2–58.

81. Malhi, G. S., Bell, E., Bassett, D., et al. (2021). The 2020 Royal Australian and New Zealand College of Psychiatrists clinical practice guidelines for mood disorders. *Aust N Z J Psychiatry*, 55, 7–117.

82. Fountoulakis, K. N., Grunze, H., Vieta, E., et al. (2017). The International College of Neuro-Psychopharmacology (CINP) treatment guidelines for bipolar disorder in adults (CINP-BD-2017), Part 3: The clinical guidelines. *Int J Neuropsychopharmacol*, 20, 180–195.

83. Fountoulakis, K. N., Yatham, L., Grunze, H., et al. (2017). The International College of Neuro-Psychopharmacology (CINP) treatment guidelines for bipolar disorder in adults (CINP-BD-2017), Part 2: Review, grading of the evidence, and a precise algorithm. *Int J Neuropsychopharmacol*, 20, 121–179.

84. Fountoulakis, K. N., Yatham, L. N., Grunze, H., et al. (2020). The CINP guidelines on the definition and evidence-based interventions for treatment-resistant bipolar disorder. *Int J Neuropsychopharmacol*, 23, 230–256.

85. National Institute for Health and Care Excellence (2020). Bipolar disorder guidelines (NICE CG185): 2020 amendment: nice.org.uk/guidance/cg185.

86. Schou, M., Juel-Nielsen, N., Stromgren, E., et al. (1954). The treatment of manic psychoses by the administration of lithium salts. *J Neurol Neurosurg Psychiatry*, 17, 250–260.

87. Schou, M. (1999). The early European lithium studies. *Aust N Z J Psychiatry*, 33 Suppl., S39–47.

88. Bowden, C. L., Brugger, A. M., Swann, A. C., et al. (1994). Efficacy of divalproex vs lithium and placebo in the treatment of mania: The Depakote Mania Study Group. *JAMA*, 271, 918–924.

89. Bowden, C. L., Grunze, H., Mullen, J., et al. (2005). A randomized, double-blind, placebo-controlled efficacy and safety study of quetiapine or lithium as monotherapy for mania in bipolar disorder. *J Clin Psychiatry*, 66, 111–121.

90. Kushner, S. F., Khan, A., Lane, R., et al. (2006). Topiramate monotherapy in the management of acute mania: Results of four double-blind placebo-controlled trials. *Bipolar Disord*, 8, 15–27.

91. Keck, P. E., Orsulak, P. J., Cutler, A. J., et al. (2009). Aripiprazole monotherapy in the treatment of acute bipolar I mania: A randomized, double-blind, placebo- and lithium-controlled study. *J Affect Disord*, 112, 36–49.

92. Rosenblat, J. D. and McIntyre, R. S. (2017). Treatment of mixed features in bipolar disorder. *CNS Spectr*, 22, 141–146.

93. McKnight, R. F., de La Motte de Broons de Vauvert, S., Chesney, E., et al. (2019). Lithium for acute mania. *Cochrane Database Syst Rev*, 6, Cd004048.

94. Cade, J. F. J. (1949). Lithium salts in the treatment of psychotic excitement. *Medical J Aust*, 36, 349–351.

95. Castro, V. M., Roberson, A. M., McCoy, T. H., et al. (2016). Stratifying risk for renal insufficiency among lithium-treated patients: An electronic health record study. *Neuropsychopharmacology*, 41, 1138–1143.

96. Reischies, F. M., Hartikainen, J. and Berghöfer, A. (2002). Initial lithium and valproate combination therapy in acute mania. *Neuropsychobiology*, 46 Suppl. 1, 22–27.

97. Kishi, T., Ikuta, T., Matsuda, Y., et al. (2021). Mood stabilizers and/or antipsychotics for bipolar disorder in the maintenance phase: A systematic review and network meta-analysis of randomized controlled trials. *Mol Psychiatry*, 26, 4146–4157.

98. Dunner, D. L. and Fieve, R. R. (1974). Clinical factors in lithium carbonate prophylaxis failure. *Arch Gen Psychiatry*, 30, 229–233.

99. American Psychiatric Association (2022). *Diagnostic & Statistical Manual of Mental Disorders Fifth Edition –Text Revision*. Washington, DC: American Psychiatric Press, Inc.

100. Sachs, G. S., Thase, M. E., Otto, M. W., et al. (2003). Rationale, design, and methods of the Systematic Treatment Enhancement Program for bipolar disorder (STEP-BD). *Biol Psychiatry*, 53, 1028–1042.

101. Schneck, C. D., Miklowitz, D. J., Calabrese, J. R., et al. (2004). Phenomenology of rapid-cycling bipolar disorder: Data from the first 500 participants in the Systematic Treatment Enhancement Program. *Am J Psychiatry*, 161, 1902–1908.

102. Fountoulakis, K. N., Kontis, D., Gonda, X., et al. (2013). A systematic review of the evidence on the treatment of rapid cycling bipolar disorder. *Bipolar Disord*, 15, 115–137.

103. Kohler, S., Friedel, E. and Stamm, T. (2017). [Rapid cycling in bipolar disorders: Symptoms, background and treatment recommendations]. *Fortschr Neurol Psychiatr*, 85, 199–211.

104. Nunes, A., Ardau, R., Berghofer, A., et al. (2020). Prediction of lithium response using clinical data. *Acta Psychiatr Scand*, 141, 131–141.

105. Allain, N., Leven, C., Falissard, B., et al. (2017). Manic switches induced by antidepressants: An umbrella review comparing randomized controlled trials and observational studies. *Acta Psychiatr Scand*, 135, 106–116.

106. Doane, M. J., Bessonova, L., Friedler, H. S., et al. (2022). Weight gain and comorbidities associated with oral second-generation antipsychotics: Analysis of real-world data for patients with schizophrenia or bipolar I disorder. *BMC Psychiatry*, 22, 114–125.

107. Leverich, G. S., Altshuler, L. L., Frye, M. A., et al. (2006). Risk of switch in mood polarity to hypomania or mania in patients with bipolar depression during acute and continuation trials of venlafaxine, sertraline, and bupropion as adjuncts to mood stabilizers. *Am J Psychiatry*, 163, 232–239.

108. Altshuler, L. L., Sugar, C. A., McElroy, S. L., et al. (2017). Switch rates during acute treatment for bipolar II depression with lithium, sertraline, or the two combined: A randomized double-blind comparison. *Am J Psychiatry*, 174, 266–276.

109. Greil, W. and Kleindienst, N. (1999). Lithium versus carbamazepine in the maintenance treatment of bipolar II disorder and bipolar disorder not otherwise specified. *Int Clin Psychopharmacol*, 14, 283–285.

110. GlaxoSmithKline LLC (2022). *Lamictal package insert*. Research Triangle Park, NC.

111. Bunschoten, J. W., Husein, N., Devinsky, O., et al. (2022). Sudden death and cardiac arrythmia with lamotrigine: A rapid systematic review. *Neurology*, 98, e1748–e1760.

112. Bowden, C. L., Calabrese, J. R., McElroy, S. L., et al. (2000). A randomized, placebo-controlled 12-month trial of divalproex and lithium in treatment of outpatients with bipolar I disorder: Divalproex Maintenance Study Group. *Arch Gen Psychiatry*, 57, 481–489.

113. Bowden, C. L., Calabrese, J. R., Sachs, G., et al. (2003). A placebo-controlled 18-month trial of lamotrigine and lithium maintenance treatment in recently manic or hypomanic patients with bipolar I disorder. *Arch Gen Psychiatry*, 60, 392–400.

114. Deb, S., Austin, P. C., Tu, J. V., et al. (2016). A review of propensity-score methods and their use in cardiovascular research. *Can J Cardiol*, 32, 259–265.

115. Hayes, J. F., Marston, L., Walters, K., et al. (2016). Lithium vs. valproate vs. olanzapine vs. quetiapine as maintenance monotherapy for bipolar disorder: A population-based UK cohort study using electronic health records. *World Psychiatry*, 15, 53–58.

116. Aiff, H., Attman, P.-O., Aurell, M., et al. (2014). The impact of modern treatment principles may have eliminated lithium-induced renal failure. *J Psychopharmacol*, 28, 151–154.

117. Nolen, W. A., Licht, R. W., Young, A. H., et al. (2019). What is the optimal serum level for lithium in the maintenance treatment of bipolar disorder? A systematic review and recommendations from the ISBD/IGSLI Task Force on treatment with lithium. *Bipolar Disord*, 21, 394–409.

118. Schoot, T. S., Molmans, T. H. J., Grootens, K. P., et al. (2020). Systematic review and practical guideline for the prevention and management of the renal side effects of lithium therapy. *Eur Neuropsychopharmacol*, 31, 16–32.

119. Clos, S., Rauchhaus, P., Severn, A., et al. (2015). Long-term effect of lithium maintenance therapy on estimated glomerular filtration rate in patients with affective disorders: A population-based cohort study. *Lancet Psychiatry*, 2, 1075–1083.

120. Kessing, L. V., Gerds, T. A., Feldt-Rasmussen, B., et al. (2015). Use of lithium and anticonvulsants and the rate of chronic kidney disease: A nationwide population-based study. *JAMA Psychiatry*, 72, 1182–1191.

121. Fransson, F., Werneke, U., Harju, V., et al. (2022). Kidney function in patients with bipolar disorder with and without lithium treatment compared with the general population in northern Sweden: Results from the LiSIE and MONICA cohorts. *Lancet Psychiatry*, 9, 804–814.

122. Kessing, L. V., Hellmund, G. and Andersen, P. K. (2011). Predictors of excellent response to lithium: Results from a nationwide register-based study. *Int Clin Psychopharmacol*, 26, 323–328.

123. Grillault Laroche, D., Etain, B., Severus, E., et al. (2020). Socio-demographic and clinical predictors of outcome to long-term treatment with lithium in bipolar disorders: A systematic review of the contemporary literature and recommendations from the ISBD/IGSLI Task Force on treatment with lithium. *Int J Bipolar Disord*, 8, 1–13.

124. Scott, J., Bellivier, F., Manchia, M., et al. (2020). Can network analysis shed light on predictors of lithium response in bipolar I disorder? *Acta Psychiatr Scand*, 141, 522–533.

125. Calabrese, J. R., Suppes, T., Bowden, C. L., et al. (2000). A double-blind, placebo-controlled, prophylaxis study of lamotrigine in rapid-cycling bipolar disorder: Lamictal 614 Study Group. *J Clin Psychiatry*, 61, 841–850.

126. Baldessarini, R. J., Tondo, L., Baethge, C. J., et al. (2007). Effects of treatment latency on response to maintenance treatment in manic-depressive disorders. *Bipolar Disord*, 9, 386–393.

127. Bratti, I. M., Baldessarini, R. J., Baethge, C., et al. (2003). Pretreatment episode count and response to lithium treatment in manic-depressive illness. *Harv Rev Psychiatry*, 11, 245–256.

128. Kessing, L. V., Vradi, E. and Andersen, P. K. (2014). Starting lithium prophylaxis early v. late in bipolar disorder. *Br J Psychiatry*, 205, 214–220.

129. Januel, D., Poirier, M. F., D'Alche-Biree, F., et al. (2003). Multicenter double-blind randomized parallel-group clinical trial of efficacy of the combination clomipramine (150 mg/day) plus lithium carbonate (750 mg/day) versus clomipramine (150 mg/day) plus placebo in the treatment of unipolar major depression. *J Affect Disord*, 76, 191–200.

130. Chenu, F. and Bourin, M. (2006). Potentiation of antidepressant-like activity with lithium: Mechanism involved. *Curr Drug Targets*, 7, 159–163.

131. Nelson, J. C., Baumann, P., Delucchi, K., et al. (2014). A systematic review and meta-analysis of lithium augmentation of tricyclic and second generation antidepressants in major depression. *J Affect Disord*, 168, 269–275.

132. Gerhard, T., Stroup, T. S., Correll, C. U., et al. (2020). Mortality risk of antipsychotic augmentation for adult depression. *PLoS One*, 15, e0239206.

133. Katz, I. R., Ferguson, R. E. and Liang, M. H. (2022). Suicide risk and lithium-reply. *JAMA Psychiatry*, 79, 513–514.

134. Tondo, L., Hennen, J. and Baldessarini, R. J. (2001). Lower suicide risk with long-term lithium treatment in major affective illness: A meta-analysis. *Acta Psychiatr Scand*, 104, 163–172.

135. Vita, A., De Peri, L. and Sacchetti, E. (2015). Lithium in drinking water and suicide prevention: A review of the evidence. *Int Clin Psychopharmacol*, 30, 1–5.

136. Eyre-Watt, B., Mahendran, E., Suetani, S., et al. (2021). The association between lithium in drinking water and neuropsychiatric outcomes: A systematic review and meta-analysis from across 2678 regions containing 113 million people. *Aust N Z J Psychiatry*, 55, 139–152.

137. Araya, P., Martínez, C. and Barros, J. (2022). Lithium in drinking water as a public policy for suicide prevention: Relevance and considerations. *Front Public Health*, 10, 805774.

138. Kawada, T. (2022). Lithium in drinking water and suicide: A sex difference and dose-response relationship. *Bipolar Disord*, 24, 207–208.

139. Liaugaudaite, V., Raskauskiene, N., Naginiene, R., et al. (2022). Association between lithium levels in drinking water and suicide rates: Role of affective disorders. *J Affect Disord*, 298, 516–521.

140. Hayes, J. F., Pitman, A., Marston, L., et al. (2016). Self-harm, unintentional injury, and suicide in bipolar disorder during maintenance mood stabilizer treatment: A UK population-based electronic health records study. *JAMA Psychiatry*, 73, 630–637.

141. Song, J., Sjolander, A., Joas, E., et al. (2017). Suicidal behavior during lithium and valproate treatment: A within-individual 8-year prospective study of 50,000 patients with bipolar disorder. *Am J Psychiatry*, 174, 795–802.

142. Calabresi, P., Pisani, A., Mercuri, N. B., et al. (1993). Lithium treatment blocks long-term synaptic depression in the striatum. *Neuron*, 10, 955–962.

143. Nonaka, S. and Chuang, D. M. (1998). Neuroprotective effects of chronic lithium on focal cerebral ischemia in rats. *Neuroreport*, 9, 2081–2084.

144. Nonaka, S., Hough, C. J. and Chuang, D. M. (1998). Chronic lithium treatment robustly protects neurons in the central nervous system against excitotoxicity by inhibiting N-methyl-D-aspartate receptor-mediated calcium influx. *Proc Natl Acad Sci USA*, 95, 2642–2647.

145. Nonaka, S., Katsube, N. and Chuang, D. M. (1998). Lithium protects rat cerebellar granule cells against apoptosis induced by anticonvulsants, phenytoin and carbamazepine. *J Pharmacol Exp Ther*, 286, 539–547.

146. Almeida, O. P., Singulani, M. P., Ford, A. H., et al. (2022). Lithium and stroke recovery: A systematic review and meta-analysis of stroke models in rodents and human data. *Stroke*, 53, 2935–2944.

147. Nunes, M. A., Schowe, N. M., Monteiro-Silva, K. C., et al. (2015). Chronic microdose lithium treatment prevented memory loss and neurohistopathological changes in a transgenic mouse model of Alzheimer's disease. *PLoS One*, 10, e0142267.

148. Morris, G. and Berk, M. (2016). The putative use of lithium in Alzheimer's Disease. *Curr Alzheimer Res*, 13, 853–861.

149. Haupt, M., Bahr, M. and Doeppner, T. R. (2021). Lithium beyond psychiatric indications: The reincarnation of a new old drug. *Neural Regen Res*, 16, 2383–2387.

150. Rybakowski, J. K. (2016). Effect of lithium on neurocognitive functioning. *Curr Alzheimer Res*, 13, 887–893.

151. Kessing, L. V., Gerds, T. A., Knudsen, N. N., et al. (2017). Association of lithium in drinking water with the incidence of dementia. *JAMA Psychiatry*, 74, 1005–1010.

152. Parker, W. F., Gorges, R. J., Gao, Y. N., et al. (2018). Association between groundwater lithium and the diagnosis of bipolar disorder and dementia in the United States. *JAMA Psychiatry*, 75, 751–754.

153. Van Gestel, H., Franke, K., Petite, J., et al. (2019). Brain age in bipolar disorders: Effects of lithium treatment. *Aust N Z J Psychiatry*, 53, 1179–1188.

154. Chen, S., Underwood, B. R., Jones, P. B., et al. (2022). Association between lithium use and the incidence of dementia and its subtypes: A retrospective cohort study. *PLoS Med*, 19, e1003941.

155. Rej, S., Yu, C., Shulman, K., et al. (2015). Medical comorbidity, acute medical care use in late-life bipolar disorder: A comparison of lithium, valproate, and other pharmacotherapies. *Gen Hosp Psychiatry*, 37, 528–532.

156. Abé, C., Liberg, B., Song, J., et al. (2020). Longitudinal cortical thickness changes in bipolar disorder and the relationship to genetic risk, mania, and lithium use. *Biol Psychiatry*, 87, 271–281.

157. Beunders, A. J. M., Kemp, T., Korten, N. C. M., et al. (2021). Cognitive performance in older-age bipolar disorder: Investigating psychiatric characteristics, cardiovascular burden and psychotropic medication. *Acta Psychiatr Scand*, 144, 392–406.

158. Ballester, P. L., Romano, M. T., de Azevedo Cardoso, T., et al. (2022). Brain age in mood and psychotic disorders: A systematic review and meta-analysis. *Acta Psychiatr Scand*, 145, 42–55.

159. Lewandowski, K. E., Sperry, S. H., Malloy, M. C., et al. (2014). Age as a predictor of cognitive decline in bipolar disorder. *Am J Geriatr Psychiatry*, 22, 1462–1468.

160. Easter, R. E., Ryan, K. A., Estabrook, R., et al. (2022). Limited time-specific and longitudinal effects of depressive and manic symptoms on cognition in bipolar spectrum disorders. *Acta Psychiatr Scand*, 146, 430–441.

161. Gerhard, T., Devanand, D. P., Huang, C., et al. (2015). Lithium treatment and risk for dementia in adults with bipolar disorder: Population-based cohort study. *Br J Psychiatry*, 207, 46–51.

162. Juurlink, D. N., Mamdani, M. M., Kopp, A., et al. (2004). Drug-induced lithium toxicity in the elderly: A population-based study. *J Am Geriatr Soc*, 52, 794–798.

163. Heath, L. J., Billups, S. J., Gaughan, K. M., et al. (2018). Risk factors for utilization of acute care services for lithium toxicity. *Psychiatr Serv*, 69, 671–676.

164. Golic, M., Aiff, H., Attman, P. O., et al. (2021). Starting lithium in patients with compromised renal function – is it wise? *J Psychopharmacol*, 35, 190–197.

165. Wingo, A. P., Wingo, T. S., Harvey, P. D., et al. (2009). Effects of lithium on cognitive performance: A meta-analysis. *J Clin Psychiatry*, 70, 1588–1597.

166. Paterson, A. and Parker, G. (2017). Lithium and cognition in those with bipolar disorder. *Int Clin Psychopharmacol*, 32, 57–62.

167. Burdick, K. E., Millett, C. E., Russo, M., et al. (2020). The association between lithium use and neurocognitive performance in patients with bipolar disorder. *Neuropsychopharmacology*, 45, 1743–1749.

168. Forlenza, O. V., Hajek, T., Almeida, O. P., et al. (2022). Demographic and clinical characteristics of lithium-treated older adults with bipolar disorder. *Acta Psychiatr Scand*, 146, 442–455.

169. Patra, S. (2020). A salt for preventing Alzheimer's? Lithium seems to be! *Aust N Z J Psychiatry*, 54, 109–110.

170. Puglisi-Allegra, S., Ruggieri, S. and Fornai, F. (2021). Translational evidence for lithium-induced brain plasticity and neuroprotection in the treatment of neuropsychiatric disorders. *Transl Psychiatry*, 11, 366.

171. Ochoa, E. L. M. (2022). Lithium as a neuroprotective agent for bipolar disorder: An overview. *Cell Mol Neurobiol*, 42, 85–97.

172. Coutts, F., Palmos, A. B., Duarte, R. R. R., et al. (2019). The polygenic nature of telomere length and the anti-ageing properties of lithium. *Neuropsychopharmacology*, 44, 757–765.

173. Martinsson, L., Wei, Y., Xu, D., et al. (2013). Long-term lithium treatment in bipolar disorder is associated with longer leukocyte telomeres. *Transl Psychiatry*, 3, e261.

174. Powell, T. R., Dima, D., Frangou, S., et al. (2018). Telomere length and bipolar disorder. *Neuropsychopharmacology*, 43, 445–453.

175. Squassina, A., Pisanu, C., Congiu, D., et al. (2016). Leukocyte telomere length positively correlates with duration of lithium treatment in bipolar disorder patients. *Eur Neuropsychopharmacol*, 26, 1241–1247.

176. Lundberg, M., Biernacka, J. M., Lavebratt, C., et al. (2020). Expression of telomerase reverse transcriptase positively correlates with duration of lithium treatment in bipolar disorder. *Psychiatry Res*, 286, 112865.

177. Schrauzer, G. N. and Shrestha, K. P. (1990). Lithium in drinking water and the incidences of crimes, suicides, and arrests related to drug addictions. *Biol Trace Elem Res*, 25, 105–113.

178. Giotakos, O., Nisianakis, P., Tsouvelas, G., et al. (2013). Lithium in the public water supply and suicide mortality in Greece. *Biol Trace Elem Res*, 156, 376–379.

179. Giotakos, O., Tsouvelas, G., Nisianakis, P., et al. (2015). A negative association between lithium in drinking water and the incidences of homicides, in Greece. *Biol Trace Elem Res*, 164, 165–168.

180. Quanbeck, C. D., McDermott, B. E., Lam, J., et al. (2007). Categorization of aggressive acts committed by chronically assaultive state hospital patients. *Psychiatr Serv*, 58, 521–528.

181. Volavka, J. and Citrome, L. (2008). Heterogeneity of violence in schizophrenia and implications for long-term treatment. *International Journal of Clinical Practice*, 62, 1237–1245.

182. Brown, D., Larkin, F., Sengupta, S., et al. (2014). Clozapine: An effective treatment for seriously violent and psychopathic men with antisocial personality disorder in a UK high-security hospital. *CNS Spectr*, 19, 391–402.

183. Campbell, M., Adams, P. B., Small, A. M., et al. (1995). Lithium in hospitalized aggressive children with conduct disorder: A double-blind and placebo-controlled study. *J Am Acad Child Adolesc Psychiatry*, 34, 445–453.

184. Malone, R. P., Delaney, M. A., Luebbert, J. F., et al. (2000). A double-blind placebo-controlled study of lithium in hospitalized aggressive children and adolescents with conduct disorder. *Arch Gen Psychiatry*, 57, 649–654.

185. Stoffers, J., Völlm, B. A., Rücker, G., et al. (2010). Pharmacological interventions for borderline personality disorder. *Cochrane Database Syst Rev*, Cd005653.

186. Mercer, D., Douglass, A. B. and Links, P. S. (2009). Meta-analyses of mood stabilizers, antidepressants and antipsychotics in the treatment of borderline personality disorder: Effectiveness for depression and anger symptoms. *J Pers Disord*, 23, 156–174.

187. Bellino, S., Rinaldi, C., Bozzatello, P., et al. (2011). Pharmacotherapy of borderline personality disorder: A systematic review for publication purpose. *Curr Med Chem*, 18, 3322–3329.

188. Pulcu, E., Saunders, K. E. A., Harmer, C. J., et al. (2022). Using a generative model of affect to characterize affective variability and its response to treatment in bipolar disorder. *Proc Natl Acad Sci USA*, 119, e2202983119.

189. Janowsky, D. S., Soares, J., Hatch, J. P., et al. (2009). Lithium effect on renal glomerular function in individuals with intellectual disability. *J Clin Psychopharmacol*, 29, 296–299.

190. Janowsky, D. S., Buneviciute, J., Hu, Q., et al. (2011). Lithium-induced renal insufficiency – a longitudinal study of creatinine increases in intellectually disabled adults. *J Clin Psychopharmacol*, 31, 769–773.

191. Yuan, J., Song, J., Zhu, D., et al. (2018). Lithium treatment is safe in children with intellectual disability. *Front Mol Neurosci*, 11, 425.

192. Oliver-Africano, P., Dickens, S., Ahmed, Z., et al. (2010). Overcoming the barriers experienced in conducting a medication trial in adults with aggressive challenging behaviour and intellectual disabilities. *J Intellect Disabil Res*, 54, 17–25.

193. Ballin, A., Lehman, D., Sirota, P., et al. (1998). Increased number of peripheral blood CD34+ cells in lithium-treated patients. *Br J Haematol*, 100, 219–221.

194. Acharya, S. and Bussel, J. B. (2000). Hematologic toxicity of sodium valproate. *J Pediatr Hematol Oncol*, 22, 62–65.

195. Malik, S., Lally, J., Ajnakina, O., et al. (2018). Sodium valproate and clozapine induced neutropenia: A case control study using register data. *Schizophr Res*, 195, 267–273.

196. Jones, G. H., Rong, C., Shariq, A. S., et al. (2021). Intracellular signaling cascades in bipolar disorder. *Curr Top Behav Neurosci*, 48, 101–132.

197. Campbell, I. H., Campbell, H. and Smith, D. J. (2022). Insulin signaling as a therapeutic mechanism of lithium in bipolar disorder. *Transl Psychiatry*, 12, 350.

198. Tye, S. J., Borreggine, K., Price, J. B., et al. (2022). Dynamic insulin-stimulated mTOR/GSK3 signaling in peripheral immune cells: Preliminary evidence for an association with lithium response in bipolar disorder. *Bipolar Disord*, 24, 39–47.

199. Rapoport, S. I. (2014). Lithium and the other mood stabilizers effective in bipolar disorder target the rat brain arachidonic acid cascade. *ACS Chem Neurosci*, 5, 459–467.

200. Akkouh, I. A., Skrede, S., Holmgren, A., et al. (2020). Exploring lithium's transcriptional mechanisms of action in bipolar disorder: A multi-step study. *Neuropsychopharmacology*, 45, 947–955.

201. Sharpley, A. L., Williams, C., Holder, A. A., et al. (2020). A phase 2a randomised, double-blind, placebo-controlled, parallel-group, add-on clinical trial of ebselen (SPI-1005) as a novel treatment for mania or hypomania. *Psychopharmacology (Berl)*, 237, 3773–3782.

202. Valvassori, S. S., Cararo, J. H., Peper-Nascimento, J., et al. (2020). Protein kinase C isoforms as a target for manic-like behaviors and oxidative stress in a dopaminergic animal model of mania. *Prog Neuropsychopharmacol Biol Psychiatry*, 101, doi: 10.1016/j.pnpbp.2020.109940.

203. Beaulieu, J. M., Gainetdinov, R. R. and Caron, M. G. (2009). Akt/GSK3 signaling in the action of psychotropic drugs. *Annu Rev Pharmacol Toxicol*, 49, 327–347.

204. Beaulieu, J. M., Del'guidice, T., Sotnikova, T. D., et al. (2011). Beyond cAMP: The regulation of Akt and GSK3 by dopamine receptors. *Front Mol Neurosci*, 4, 38.

205. Beaulieu, J. M., Marion, S., Rodriguiz, R. M., et al. (2008). A beta-arrestin 2 signaling complex mediates lithium action on behavior. *Cell*, 132, 125–136.

2

Renal Handling of Lithium

Proximal and Distal Handling of Lithium;
The Staging of Chronic Kidney Disease;
Lithium Related Effects on Renal Function

QUICK CHECK

PRINCIPLES

- The impact of long-term lithium use on renal function is less than once assumed due to modern prescribing practices that lessen the risk of renal insufficiency (RI) (e.g. once daily dosing, maintaining outpatient 12 h trough levels < 1.00 mEq/l). Moreover, we have come to appreciate that the patient population for lithium therapy has a high prevalence of risk factors (e.g. hypertension, cardiometabolic disorders) that significantly contribute to RI risk, as can exposure to nephrotoxic medications (e.g. proton pump inhibitors, certain fibrates, nonsteroidal anti-inflammatory agents).

- Lithium is completely filtered in the glomerulus, and up to 80% is reabsorbed throughout the renal system. Understanding how lithium moves through the renal system is crucial to appreciating how circumstances (e.g. hyponatremia) or medications impact lithium clearance.

- Approximately 70% of total lithium reabsorption occurs in the proximal tubule by the sodium/hydrogen exchanger 3 (NHE3) where lithium competes with sodium for NHE3 uptake. Glomerular pathology due to lithium exposure manifesting as nephrotic syndrome is exceedingly rare, but proteinuria can occur due to systemic disorders (e.g. hypertension, diabetes mellitus) or other nephrotoxic medications.

- A smaller portion of lithium's reabsorption (20%) occurs in the collecting ducts where it enters principal cells through the epithelial sodium channel (ENaC). This is the site of lithium's greatest renal impact. As lithium readily enters these principal cells, its intracellular accumulation sets off a sequence of events that, in some patients, induces nephrogenic diabetes insipidus (NDI). Routine inquiry into patient fluid intake, combined with use of early morning urine osmolality (EMUO) to track concentrating ability, are important tools in assessing and managing polyuria complaints.

- Clinicians must be conversant in the criteria for chronic kidney disease (CKD) and the latest methods for quantifying renal parameters, including the new creatinine and cystatin C based estimated glomerular filtration rate (eGFR$_{cr-cys}$) formula that replaced the older race based eGFR equation.

- Aside from polyuria, rational monitoring for lithium related adverse effects involves routine eGFR measurement and the targeted use of the albumin-to-creatinine ratio (ACR) to track glomerular pathology arising from CKD risk factors such as hypertension and diabetes mellitus.

Introduction

WHAT TO KNOW: INTRODUCTION

- Bipolar spectrum patients have 3-fold increased risk for chronic kidney disease independent of lithium exposure, due to higher rates of cardiometabolic disorders. The independent effects of lithium on renal function in this population are more modest than previously appreciated.
- Prior practices that increased long-term risk for renal insufficiency (e.g. multiple daily lithium dosing, 12 h trough levels > 1.00 mEq/l) are no longer recommended.
- By understanding that ¾ of lithium reabsorption occurs in the glomerulus and proximal tubules, and that it competes with sodium for

reabsorption, the basis for many drug interactions and the effects of hyponatremia on lithium levels become clear.

- The fact that lithium readily enters collecting duct principal cells via the epithelial sodium channel (ENaC) underlies the pathophysiology of polyuria, and also explains why the diuretic amiloride is the medication of choice to manage polyuria: it is an ENaC blocking agent.

In a 1989 review entitled "Long-term treatment with lithium and renal function: A review and reappraisal," the pioneering Danish psychopharmacologist Mogens Schou concluded: "The fear of eventual kidney insufficiency as a result of long-term lithium treatment can be set at rest" [1]. Despite the certainty advanced by the preeminent authority on lithium at that time – the man responsible for all of the early data on lithium's efficacy and the first double-blind placebo-controlled trials – fear of lithium's long-term renal adverse effects remains a significant concern to clinicians, a concern that is often disproportionate to the emerging data in this area. In the 30 years since Schou published that review, it has become increasingly clear that long-term lithium treatment, *when overseen with modern monitoring principles*, should not result in severe renal insufficiency (RI) or renal failure using the eGFR based definitions of 15–29 ml/min and < 15 ml/min respectively [2]. Informing this new outlook on long-term RI risk is the literature documenting those practices that, in the past, substantially increased this risk, including multiple daily dosing, and allowing outpatient trough levels to exceed 1.00 or 1.20 mEq/l [3, 4]. Recent analyses have also noted that the primary diagnosis groups, those with bipolar disorder (BD) or schizoaffective disorder bipolar type (SAD-BT), are enriched with a high prevalence of cardiometabolic disorders, factors that by themselves increase RI risk 3-fold compared with the general population, independent of lithium exposure [5]. Retrospective studies of long-term lithium use have identified that significant predictors of eGFR trends during lithium treatment include age, baseline eGFR, medical comorbidities, exposure to nephrotoxic drugs, and episodes of lithium toxicity; however, duration of exposure to lithium by itself is not a significant predictor of eGFR decline [6]. To emphasize further that the impact of lithium on chronic eGFR changes may be less than previously suspected, *once important RI risk factors are included as covariates in statistical models*, a Scottish group performed a population based cohort study exploring eGFR changes in 305 patients (mean age 42.2 years) with mean lithium exposure 54.7 ± 42.1 months, compared with eGFR trends in demographically matched peers receiving treatment with valproate, quetiapine or olanzapine (n = 815) for comparable periods of time. The monthly eGFR decline attributable to lithium exposure amounted to only 0.02 ml/min after adjustment for the confounder risk variables noted above, a result that was not significant (p = 0.30) [6]. This finding is consistent with cross-sectional studies which note that the eGFR after a mean 7 years of lithium exposure was not significantly different than that in a matched non-lithium treated cohort, although those on lithium therapy did have lower urine osmolality (405 ± 164 mOsm/kg vs. 667 ± 174 mOsm/kg) [7].

Though the independent renal impact of lithium therapy is more modest than once assumed, there is no minimizing the fact that lithium exposure can be associated with short-term and long-term renal adverse effects. One need not be a nephrologist to prescribe lithium, but clinicians should understand how lithium moves through the renal system, the environmental and medication related factors which influence lithium clearance, and how lithium exposure induces polyuria. Lithium is the smallest metallic cation by molecular weight, and is completely filtered along with sodium in the glomerulus, with approximately 80% of the filtered lithium reabsorbed throughout the renal system [8]. Most of this reabsorption (70%) occurs in the glomerulus where lithium competes with sodium for the Na^+/H^+ exchanger-3 (NHE3) present on the apical surfaces of the epithelial cells [9]. From this basic appreciation of lithium's proximal renal clearance, it becomes clearer why medications or clinical states that diminish glomerular filtration by impacting renal blood flow (e.g. angiotensin converting enzyme inhibitors [ACEIs], angiotensin receptor II type 1 blockers [ARBs], nonsteroidal anti-inflammatory drugs [NSAIDs]) or which deplete sodium stores (e.g. ACEIs, ARBs, thiazide-type diuretics, loop diuretics in older patients) can result in supratherapeutic lithium levels [10]. While the glomerulus can be the site of kinetic issues, it is uncommonly the site of lithium related pathology, with only 36 reported cases of lithium induced proteinuria of sufficient severity to meet criteria for nephrotic syndrome (i.e. proteinuria > 3.5 g/24 h) [11].

Lithium's propensity to cause polyuria relates to its affinity for ENaC, present on collecting duct *principal cells* [12, 13]. ENaC is part of a superfamily of sodium selective channels including acid-sensing and degenerin ion channels, all of which have numerous physiological roles [14]. These various channels share a trimeric structure, with ENaC combining three of the four possible subunits (α, β, γ or β, γ, δ) to form the functioning channel. The β and γ subunits are essential for trafficking of the channel to the apical surface, while the α subunit (or in some cells the δ subunit) is the pore-forming component [15]. All ENaC isoforms that contain an α subunit exhibit 1.6-fold higher permeability for lithium than for sodium, and the form expressed in collecting duct cells is composed of an α, β and γ subunit [14]. It is worth noting that this ENaC isoform is also referred to as the amiloride-sensitive ENaC to differentiate it from variants in other tissues, and to reflect that the α subunit is required for amiloride sensitivity [14]. Lithium will readily enter these principal cells via ENaC, but lithium is a poor substrate for the ATP driven sodium/potassium pump (Na^+/H^+-ATPase) on the basal membrane, so transport out of principal cells must rely on the NHE1 isoform of the Na^+/H^+ exchanger. Basilar transport via NHE1 can be insufficient to compensate for the lithium entering via ENaC leading to intracellular accumulation and inhibition of various 2nd messenger intracellular pathways such as glycogen synthase kinase 3β (GSK3-β) [16]. In approximately 20% of patients this is manifested as insensitivity to antidiuretic hormone (ADH, also called vasopressin), downregulation of water absorbing aquaporin 2 (AQP2) channels on the apical surface, and the clinical syndrome of partial or complete NDI [10].

Trends in eGFR can be a vexing problem to clinicians during chronic treatment due to the impact of nephrotoxic medications, individual RI risk factors or lithium itself, yet patients disproportionately cite decreased urine concentrating ability, not decreased eGFR or other renal adverse effects, as a reason to stop lithium. Although the intracellular pathophysiology of lithium related NDI is complex, it rests on the simple fact that lithium outcompetes sodium for entry into collecting duct principal cells via ENaC. That fundamental principle defines the most evidence based strategy for managing NDI – use of the potassium sparing diuretic amiloride, an ENaC inhibitor, to block lithium's entry into these cells [12, 17]. (Management of polyuria with amiloride, and possible adjunctive use of acetazolamide, are covered in Chapter 5 [18].) The tools to track polyuria are very straightforward and easily mastered by clinicians, as are the eGFR criteria for the stages of CKD, the rationale for checking the ACR despite lithium's low risk for proteinuria, and the recent developments in calculating eGFR that dispense with problematic race based adjustments in older eGFR formulas [19, 20]. As will be discussed throughout this handbook, lithium has unique properties and efficacy advantages over non-lithium therapies. An understanding of the renal aspects of lithium therapy allows one to prescribe lithium in the safest and most tolerable manner, thereby maximizing patient acceptance and long-term retention on lithium treatment.

A 2018 retrospective analysis of all cases in Norrbotten, Sweden, involving bipolar or SAD-BT patients where maintenance lithium treatment was stopped (n = 561 episodes) found that nearly 4 times as many patients listed polyuria/diabetes insipidus (8.1%) as the adverse effect leading to their request for discontinuation compared with creatinine increase/lithium related nephropathy (2.1%) [21]. Polyuria ranked only below diarrhea (15.0%), tremor (10.2%), weight gain (8.7%) and emotional blunting (8.7%) among patient initiated reasons for ceasing lithium therapy. Given the importance of this complaint, it is incumbent upon clinicians to understand the sequence of events leading to NDI, and to be familiar with office based screening for NDI and the laboratory criteria for diagnosing NDI using early morning urine osmolality (EMUO) [10, 17, 22–23].

A How Lithium Moves Through and Affects Kidney Function: The Glomerulus and Loop of Henle

WHAT TO KNOW: MOVEMENT OF LITHIUM THROUGH THE PROXIMAL NEPHRON

- In the glomerulus and proximal tubules, lithium is reabsorbed via the Na^+/H^+ exchanger-3 (NHE3). Medications or physiological states that decrease serum sodium levels present a risk for lithium toxicity as lithium will be preferentially reabsorbed when sodium levels are low.

- Medications that diminish glomerular blood flow can decrease lithium clearance and potentially cause lithium toxicity if lithium levels are unmonitored and dosing adjustments not made.

- Only 10% of lithium is reabsorbed in the ascending thick loop of Henle via the $Na^+/K^+/2Cl^-$ cotransporter type 2 (NKCC2). Blocking this transporter with loop diuretics (e.g. furosemide) only presents a risk for lithium toxicity in elderly individuals.

1 Movement

The human kidney is composed of one million functional units called nephrons that perform filtration, reabsorption, secretion and excretion of various substances [24]. The nephron can be divided into two main components: the renal corpuscle, where plasma filtration occurs, and the renal tubule that carries away the filtered fluid (Figure 2.1). Importantly, the renal tubule is not simply a conduit to convey glomerular filtrate to the collecting duct system – the lining cells of each segment

Figure 2.1 How lithium moves through the kidney [8]

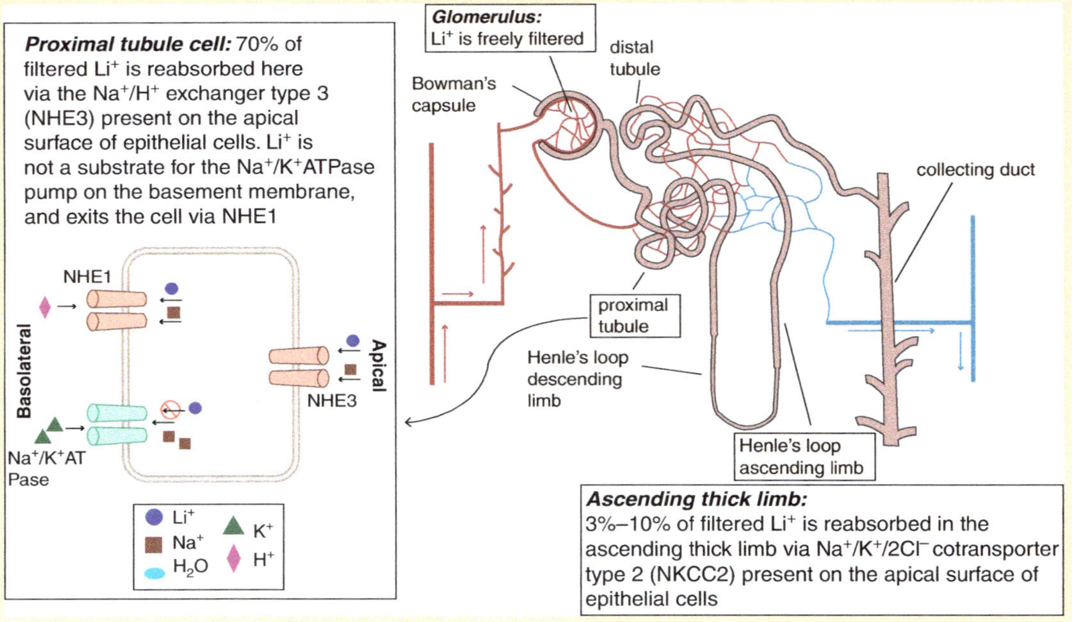

Glomerulus:
Li⁺ is freely filtered

collecting duct

distal
tubule

Bowman's
capsule

proximal
tubule

Henle's loop
descending
limb

Henle's loop
ascending limb

Ascending thick limb:
3%–10% of filtered Li^+ is reabsorbed in the
ascending thick limb via $Na^+/K^+/2Cl^-$ cotransporter
type 2 (NKCC2) present on the apical surface of
epithelial cells

Proximal tubule cell: 70% of
filtered Li^+ is reabsorbed here
via the Na^+/H^+ exchanger type 3
(NHE3) present on the apical
surface of epithelial cells. Li^+ is
not a substrate for the Na^+/K^+ ATPase
pump on the basement membrane,
and exits the cell via NHE1

Apical

NHE3

NHE1

Na^+/K^+ ATPase

Basolateral

Li^+ Na^+ H_2O K^+ H^+

(Adapted from: V. Bisogni, G. Rossitto, F. Reghin, et al. [2016]. Antihypertensive therapy in patients on chronic lithium treatment
for bipolar disorders. *J Hypertens*, 34, 20–28.)

perform specific reabsorptive and secretory functions that vary along the length of the tubule [8, 16, 25]. The renal tubule starts with the proximal convoluted tubule that emerges from Bowman's capsule, then proceeds through the descending and ascending limbs of the loop of Henle to the distal convoluted tubule and the connecting duct. Lithium exerts its greatest impact on renal function by entering the principal cells lining the collecting duct, and this will be discussed in detail in the next section [26, 27].

The renal corpuscle consists of the glomerulus, containing a network of capillaries known as the tuft, and Bowman's capsule [26]. Glomerular capillary endothelial cells have pores (fenestrae) that are 50–100 nm in diameter, big enough to permit the passage of fluid, blood plasma solutes and protein, but narrow enough to prevent filtration of platelets and red and white blood cells. Each glomerulus gets its blood supply directly from an afferent arteriole originating in the renal artery, and it is the hydrostatic pressure created by the smaller diameter of the exiting efferent arteriole (compared with the afferent arteriole) that provides additional force for filtering blood plasma of various solutes and water into the interior of Bowman's capsule [26]. Approximately 20% of plasma is filtered in the glomerulus during each passage through the kidney, with the remainder proceeding directly to the efferent arteriole and the general circulation. Bowman's capsule surrounds the glomerulus and is composed of two distinct layers: the inner visceral layer formed by specialized cells called podocytes, and an outer layer of squamous epithelium. The glomerular basement membrane is thicker than that found in other tissues (250–400 nm), and, due to its location between the glomerular capillaries and the podocytes, also serves as a barrier to proteins (e.g. albumin) (Table 2.1) [26]. The part of the podocyte in contact with the glomerular basement membrane is called a foot process or pedicle, and the space between adjacent pedicles contains slit diaphragms that allow the filtrate to flow into Bowman's capsule. Importantly, these openings are lined with negatively charged glycoproteins that repel the entry of negatively charged macromolecules such as albumin. The net result of this cellular architecture is selective permeability (also known as permselectivity) which creates the filtrate (tubular fluid) that moves into the proximal renal tubule [26].

Lithium is the lightest metal in Group I of the periodic table (molecular weight 6.94), followed by sodium (molecular weight 22.99) and then potassium (molecular weight 39.10). After being freely filtered in the glomerulus, most of lithium's reabsorption (70%) occurs in the proximal tubule where lithium competes with sodium for the Na^+/H^+ exchanger-3 (NHE3) present on the apical

Table 2.1 Permselectivity of substances in the glomerulus [28]

	Molecular weight (g/mol)	Ratio of the concentration in ultrafiltrate to the plasma concentration
Lithium	7	1.0
Sodium	23	1.0
Potassium	39	1.0
Water	18	1.0
Urea	60	1.0
Glucose	180	1.0
Inulin	5200	0.98
Hemoglobin	68,000	0.03
Serum albumin	69,000	<0.01

Note: Inulin is a small polysaccharide molecule used in laboratory studies of glomerular filtration since it is neither absorbed nor secreted by renal tubular cells (Adapted from: G. Giebisch, E. H. Windhager and P. S. Aronson [2017]. Glomerular filtration and renal blood flow. In W. F. Boron and E. L. Boulpaep, eds., *Medical Physiology: A Cellular and Molecular Approach* (3rd edn.). Philadelphia, PA: Elsevier, pp. 739–753.)

surfaces of these epithelial cells [9]. The delivery of lithium at the end of the proximal convoluted tubule exceeds that of sodium by approximately 14%, showing that lithium is reabsorbed to a slightly lower extent than sodium. While NHE3 transport mediates lithium uptake at the apical side of the cell, lithium efflux on the basal side of the cell is performed by the structurally related NHE1. NHE1 is expressed in the basolateral membrane of epithelial cells in most nephron segments, and is the primary route for lithium transport out of the cell [9]. Although a major route for basal sodium efflux is the Na^+/K^+-ATPase, this pump does not adequately transport lithium because of its low lithium affinity. (As discussed below, the Na^+/K^+-ATPase pump's low lithium affinity contributes to lithium's accumulation in collecting duct principal cells and the development of polyuria.) Prior to exiting the proximal nephron, another 3%–10% of filtered lithium is reabsorbed in the thick ascending limb of Henle, although this value may be as high as 20% in salt-depleted individuals [29–31]. Part of lithium's reabsorption in the thick ascending loop is via the $Na^+/K^+/2Cl^-$ cotransporter type 2 (NKCC2) present on the apical surface, a transporter which is inhibited by loop diuretics such as furosemide [8].

2 *Proximal Pathology*

WHAT TO KNOW: PROXIMAL RENAL PATHOLOGY

- The hallmark of glomerular pathology is albuminuria, and this can be induced by hypertension, diabetes mellitus and certain renal specific diseases.
- The monitoring test for albuminuria is the urine albumin-to-creatinine ratio (ACR), ideally performed on an early morning specimen.
- Lithium is only rarely associated with glomerular pathology. Monitoring ACR is important as the patient population who receives lithium has high rates of hypertension and diabetes.

The hallmark of glomerular pathology is albuminuria, a clinical finding which reflects impairment of the permselective barrier function that normally limits filtration of large molecules [32]. Increasing loss of albumin in the urine can be associated with renal dysfunction from a number of causes including hypertension, diabetes mellitus, advanced kidney disease of any etiology, and specific glomerular diseases from a variety of etiologies, both primary (e.g. genetic) and secondary (e.g. maladaptive responses to systemic disorders, viral, drug-induced) [32, 33]. As discussed in the section on monitoring and summarized in Info Box 2.7, the primary reason to monitor albuminuria periodically using the ACR is due to the high prevalence of cardiometabolic disorders in patients with serious mental illness (SMI) (e.g. schizophrenia spectrum disorders, BD), disorders that contribute to the development of CKD [10]. Therefore, the need to monitor ACR routinely for lithium treated patients exists for those with stage G2 or G3a CKD (eGFR 45–89 ml/min) but also for those with concurrent medical conditions associated with albuminuria regardless of eGFR. (The use of ACR to monitor the insidious onset of albuminuria from systemic illnesses such as hypertension or diabetes mellitus is reviewed in Section E and Info Box 2.7.)

In-Depth 2.2 Lithium Rarely Causes Proteinuria and Proximal Pathology

That the medical comorbidity seen in SMI populations is the primary reason for obtaining an ACR relates to the fact that lithium exposure is not a major contributor to glomerular pathology. Animal models indicate that lithium does not have a significant impact on the glomerular population [33] or on ultrastructural parameters [34, 35]. A 1-year chronic exposure study across 21 mouse strains found that all experienced increased evidence of NDI (e.g.

urine production and/or reduced urine osmolality), but in none of the strains was glomerular injury induced, and lithium exposure did not elevate urinary ACR [36]. Moreover, clinical studies also show no difference in ACR values between bipolar lithium users and age-matched bipolar patients who are non-lithium users, even among those with mean lithium exposure of 110 months (range 25–240 months) [7].

There are, however, rare cases of severe proteinuria during lithium treatment manifesting as nephrotic syndrome (defined as proteinuria > 3.5 g/24 h), with only 36 cases reported as of 2021 [11]. Unlike patients whose albuminuria progresses slowly and insidiously from systemic causes (e.g. diabetes mellitus), patients with nephrotic syndrome come to immediate medical attention as they exhibit the classic signs and symptoms such as weight gain, fatigue, frothy urine (due to excess urinary protein) and pitting edema due to low serum albumin levels [11]. Among the 36 reported cases of lithium related nephrotic syndrome, the onset varied from months to decades after commencing lithium, and renal biopsy results from 32 cases indicated that the most common cause was minimal change disease (MCD) (n = 19), followed by focal segmental glomerulosclerosis (FSGS) (n = 10) and membranous nephropathy (MN) (n = 3) [11]. The cause of MCD is hypothesized to be from T-cell cytokine release, but does not involve antibody binding to glomerular structures. MCD is noted pathologically by loss of the epithelial cell foot processes (also known as podocyte footplate effacement), and is typically reversible upon discontinuation of the offending agent, at times combined with corticosteroid therapy [11]. MN shows clear evidence of an immune-mediated etiology with immune complexes binding to antigens on the glomerular basement membrane. Among the MCD and MN cases, 100% improved upon lithium discontinuation, with 91% going into complete remission over the next 12 months (most of which, 59%, occurred within 2 months of lithium cessation). The immediate response to lithium cessation suggests an association with exposure, and lithium discontinuation must be considered when renal biopsy findings in a nephrotic patient are consistent with MCD or MN.

In the 2021 case review, the subgroup with lack of improvement following lithium discontinuation had biopsies consistent with FSGS (n = 10). FSGS is the most common cause of nephrotic syndrome (35% of all cases worldwide), and comprises a diverse group of genetic and other etiologies (e.g. loss of renal mass, systemic disorders, viral, drug-induced) [33]. Accurate classification of FSGS into subcategories is important due to the prognostic significance, but typically requires electron microscopy and genetic testing since light microscopy may be insufficient to differentiate the subcategories. Given that FSGS is the predominant cause of nephrotic syndrome, that it often responds poorly to immunosuppressive therapy, and that lithium discontinuation in these 10 cases yielded no benefit in 4/10 patients suggests an underlying pathology unrelated to lithium exposure [11]. Nonetheless, given the generally poor prognosis of FSGS, lithium discontinuation should be performed with the hope that the patient may exhibit some partial response [11]. The reassuring finding from the 2021 review is that lithium related glomerular pathology causing severe proteinuria is exceedingly uncommon and is not a reason to avoid lithium therapy.

It should be noted that there are mouse and human data showing that long-term lithium exposure can be associated with proximal tubular atrophy and interstitial fibrosis, although the human findings are predominantly from biopsies of patients with severe or end-stage CKD treated from the 1960s–1980s, before the emphasis on modern practices that minimize renal injury, such as once daily dosing and limiting outpatient serum level excursions above 1.00 or 1.20 mEq/l [37, 38]. Amiloride is a diuretic that specifically blocks the entry of sodium and lithium into principal cells of the collecting duct through ENaC and is the primary method for managing lithium related NDI and polyuria [13]. Using an animal model of lithium induced chronic interstitial fibrosis, 5 months of amiloride therapy partially mitigated lithium induced NDI and limited the progression of lithium induced fibrosis [13]. These and other studies suggest that the development of interstitial fibrosis relates to increased lithium concentrations in the collecting duct principal cell. At sufficiently high intracellular concentrations, lithium exerts inhibitory effects on the kinase GSK3-β that results in disruption of multiple downstream pathways involved in cell cycle progression [9, 16]. One effect of GSK3-β inhibition is that principal cells become arrested in a certain phase of their cell cycle (G2) and overproduce transforming growth factor beta 1 (TGF-β1). Elevated intracellular levels of TGF-β1 subsequently induce fibrotic changes in the cells. Another consequence of principal cell GSK3-β inhibition leading to fibrosis is elevated levels of β-catenin, a protein involved in cell–cell adhesion and regulation of gene transcription [9]. Agents which interfere with β-catenin-mediated gene transcription strongly reduce interstitial fibrosis in mouse models of lithium induced renal injury [9]. The conclusion from this body of research is that, aside from those rare cases of glomerular pathology noted above, lithium's inhibitory impact on GSK3-β in collecting duct principal cells is the primary cause of the early and late features of lithium related renal dysfunction. *The exciting practical implication is that prescribers have readily identifiable signals for this effect in the form of clinical complaints of polyuria, and from urine osmolality values consistent with partial or complete NDI.*

B How Lithium Moves Through and Affects Kidney Function: The Collecting Ducts

WHAT TO KNOW: MOVEMENT OF LITHIUM THROUGH THE DISTAL NEPHRON AND RELATED PATHOLOGY

- 20% of lithium's reabsorption occurs in the collecting duct principal cells via ENaC.
- Lithium has 1.6-fold higher affinity for ENaC than does sodium, but lithium exits these cells relatively slowly resulting in intracellular accumulation.
- Lithium's initial effect on renal function relates to inhibition of cellular processes in principal cells leading to downregulation of water absorbing aquaporin 2 channel expression and vasopressin insensitivity. The clinical manifestation is impaired urine concentrating ability.

1 *Movement*

Approximately 20% of lithium's reabsorption occurs in the collecting duct, where lithium is taken up from the tubular fluid by the principal cells through ENaC present on the apical surface [9]. Tight junctions between the cells forces all cation transport to be mediated by transcellular pump or exchange processes. Lithium has 1.6-fold higher affinity for ENaC than does sodium [14], but, unlike sodium, it is a poor substrate for the Na^+/H^+-ATPase on the basal membrane of principal cells (Figure 2.2) [12, 17]. Basilar transport of lithium out of principal cells and into the interstitium is thus dependent on NHE1 [9].

2 *Collecting Duct Pathology*

Basilar transport via NHE1 can be insufficient to compensate for the amount of lithium entering via ENaC leading to its intracellular accumulation and inhibition of various 2nd messenger intracellular pathways involving GSK3-β, inositol, prostaglandin E2 (PGE2), cyclooxygenase 2 (COX2) and protein kinase A (PKA) [16]. Collecting duct principal cells express aquaporin 2 (AQP2) on their apical surface to absorb water from tubular fluid and thereby concentrate urine [16], while water transport across the basolateral membrane into the interstitium is mediated by aquaporin 3 (AQP3) and aquaporin 4 (AQP4) [40]. Lithium interactions with the inositol and PKC pathways inhibit production of cyclic adenosine monophosphate

Figure 2.2 Detailed view of collecting duct principal cells illustrating how lithium enters via the epithelial sodium channel (ENaC) [39]

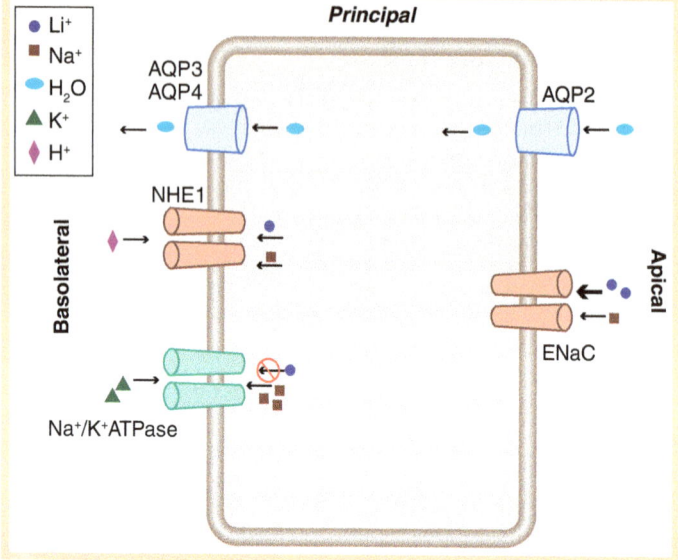

(Adapted from: J.-P. Grünfeld and B. C. Rossier [2009]. Lithium nephrotoxicity revisited. *Nat Rev Nephrol*, 5, 270–276.)

(cAMP) [16]. Low intracellular cAMP levels interfere with phosphorylation of protein kinase A (PKA), and this in turn results in less AQP2 phosphorylation. Phosphorylation of AQP2 by PKA and other kinases is crucial for appropriate movement of this protein channel to the apical membrane surface, so one effect of high intracellular lithium concentrations is decreased AQP2 channel density on the apical surface, and therefore decreased ability to reabsorb water [16]. As a consequence of GSK3-β inhibition, lithium also interferes with the nuclear factor of activated T cells 5 (NFAT5), a transcription factor that regulates expression of channels regulating osmolality (e.g. aquaporins) [16]. Lithium's inhibitory actions on NFAT5 activity are hypothesized to directly reduce AQP2 expression. Lastly, one feature of lithium related NDI is insensitivity of collecting duct principal cells to the actions of antidiuretic hormone (ADH, also called vasopressin). By its inhibitory actions on GSK3-β, lithium stimulates PGE2 production by COX2. PGE2 not only increases the breakdown of AQP2 channels, it also blocks the activity of ADH, further contributing to loss of AQP2 mediated functions [16]. ADH is produced in the hypothalamus in response to increased plasma osmolality and is secreted by the posterior pituitary. Binding of ADH to V2 receptors on collecting duct cells increases transcription of AQP2 channels and their insertion into the apical membrane, facilitating water absorption. Increased PGE2 production is thus another mechanism by which GSK3-β inhibition by lithium interferes with AQP2 density and urine concentrating ability [16].

In-Depth 2.3 Rates of Lithium-Induced Polyuria

The methods of screening for polyuria are discussed in Section 5, but the development of lithium related NDI is neither inevitable nor as prevalent as once feared. Though some sources cite rates as high as 73%, more recent data suggest that the prevalence of symptomatic polyuria is under 30% and perhaps < 20% [9, 10, 41, 42]. In one study of 45 geriatric patients (mean age 77.0 ± 7.83 years) with mean duration of lithium exposure 14.7 ± 11.5 years, the proportion with urine osmolality in the range of complete NDI (< 300 mOsm/kg) was 15.5% [42]. This was a sample of convenience, and the fact that these patients remained on lithium may reflect a survivor bias in favor of those not experiencing NDI, but these data are more reflective of recent lower estimates. This decrease in NDI incidence might possibly be a result of modern prescribing practices that reduce polyuria risk, especially once daily lithium dosing [43]. Given that entry of lithium into collecting duct cells via ENaC is a common mechanism underlying NDI and the rare late changes such as fibrosis, it is also not surprising that a practice which decreases polyuria risk (i.e. once daily dosing) is also associated with a 20% lower risk of renal insufficiency [4].

C   The Debate Concerning Lithium's Long-Term Impact on Renal Function

WHAT TO KNOW: LITHIUM'S LONG-TERM IMPACT ON RENAL FUNCTION

- The high rates of CKD in the lithium treated population is partly due to the relatively higher prevalence of cardiometabolic disorders. Lithium's independent impact on renal function is lower than previously estimated after controlling for CKD risk factors.

- With modern prescribing practices and monitoring, the rates of lithium related end-stage renal disease (ESRD) are extremely low.

- Renal microcysts are an uncommon sequela of uncontrolled lithium accumulation in collecting duct principal cells. There is no indication for routine MRI surveillance, but early use of the ENaC inhibitor amiloride may be important to minimize the risk of lithium related collecting duct pathology when polyuria complaints arise.

- Once daily lithium dosing, use of trough levels < 1.00 mEq/l, and prevention of trough level excursions > 1.20 mEq/l are all associated with lower risk of lithium related renal pathology.
- Clinicians should be knowledgeable about which non-lithium medications are associated with nephrotoxicity and work with other clinicians to minimize their use in lithium treated patients.

1 *How Much of the Risk of Renal Dysfunction Is Related to Bipolar Disorder?*

The focus on metabolic effects from second generation antipsychotics (SGAs) highlighted the high rates of medical comorbidity among SMI patients [44–46]. Of particular concern is the 2-fold greater prevalence of cardiometabolic disorders such as hypertension, metabolic syndrome and type 2 diabetes mellitus among SMI individuals, all of which combine with lifestyle factors (e.g. smoking, dietary habits, low activity levels) to create higher standardized mortality rates than for age-matched peers [46]. Moreover, despite the prevalence of comorbid health conditions, underutilization of nonpsychiatric medical care among SMI individuals also contributes to morbidity and mortality [8, 47]. Given the extent of medical comorbidity in the target population for lithium therapy, investigators have devised ways to examine to what extent the putative impact of lithium on renal function relates to what is termed confounding by indication: some of the effect may relate to the patients themselves, and to the prevalence of cardiometabolic disorders that increase risk for CKD [5].

2 *Long-Term Impact on Renal Function and Limited Association with End-Stage Renal Disease*

Although the patient pool exposed to lithium has higher rates of CKD risk factors, many lithium treated patients successfully take lithium for decades and only experience expected age-related declines in eGFR. To control for this type of confounding bias in longitudinal studies, investigators employed more sophisticated analyses of lithium's effect on eGFR that adjusted for age, baseline eGFR, medical comorbidities, use of nephrotoxic drugs, duration of lithium exposure, mean lithium levels and episodes of lithium toxicity, but also used a patient cohort with comparable psychiatric diagnoses exposed to other medications as the control group [6].

In-Depth 2.4 Understanding Confounding Bias: How a Danish Study Showed that Bipolar Disorder Itself Is Associated with 3-Fold Higher CKD Risk

To separate out any lithium effect from that inherent to a population with elevated CKD risk factors, investigators utilized the Danish health-care database records from 1994–2012 to examine the comparative prevalence of CKD between the general population and those with bipolar spectrum disorders, and then to look separately at CKD prevalence in BD patients (n = 10,591) exposed to lithium or anticonvulsants [5]. As shown in Table 2.2, the analysis created two cohorts: **Cohort 1**: a randomly selected general population adult sample of 1.5M individuals, enriched with all individuals prescribed lithium (n = 26,731) or anticonvulsants (n = 420,959) and anyone diagnosed with a single manic episode or BD by ICD-10 codes DF30–31.9 plus 38.00 (n = 10,591); **Cohort 2:** only those with BD (n = 10,591). Regardless of the CKD definition, those with BD had 3-fold higher CKD prevalence than the general population sample, evidence that this is a population with inherent risk for CKD. Importantly, the analysis of medication related risks found that both lithium and anticonvulsant exposure were equivalently associated with a 2-fold increased risk of possible or definite CKD in BD spectrum patients, supporting the contention that certain patient related risks may underlie the higher rates of CKD in these patients [5].

Observational studies such as this are subjected to biases, and these must be considered. Those patients on lithium have a higher likelihood of being diagnosed with CKD due to routine surveillance of renal function, so CKD rates may be increased due to detection bias. On the other hand, anticonvulsants have not been associated with CKD risk, so patients with decreased renal function might be more likely to receive an anticonvulsant, thus creating a confounding bias by enriching the pool of anticonvulsant users with patients having evidence of renal dysfunction. However, it was noted that the risk of CKD in the anticonvulsant group increased with the number of prescriptions in the same manner as those on lithium, suggesting a possible relationship with anticonvulsant exposure [5]. In discussing this issue, the authors point out that no such association with increased CKD risk was seen for antipsychotics or antidepressants in these bipolar patients, and caution that the biological mechanisms by which an anticonvulsant may induce renal dysfunction are speculative [5]. Despite all of this study's limitations, this analysis helped to highlight that some of the risk previously attributed to lithium may relate to confounding by indication: those most likely to receive lithium also have BD, and patients with BD are at increased risk for CKD.

Table 2.2 Danish study of chronic kidney disease (CKD) prevalence in the general population and in bipolar spectrum patients [5]

	Definite CKD	Possible CKD	End-stage CKD
Cohort 1 (n = 1,800,591): General Population			
Randomly selected sample of 1.5M individuals, plus all patients with a diagnosis of a single manic episode or bipolar disorder from 1994–2012 (n = 10,591), and all patients exposed to either lithium (n = 26,731) or anticonvulsants (n = 420,959). Note: Provides the rates of CKD, end-stage CKD regardless of indication for the medication used, and adjusted for age, sex, employment status, calendar year, a diagnosis of bipolar disorder, and use of all other kinds of medication.	0.80% (14,727)	1.0% (18,762)	0.2% (3407)
Cohort 2 (n = 10,591): Bipolar Disorder			
The subgroup of 10,591 with bipolar disorder diagnoses. Note: Provides the rates of CKD, end-stage CKD for bipolar disorder patients adjusted for age, sex, employment status, calendar year and use of all other kinds of medication.	2.6% (278)	3.0% (319)	0.6% (62)
Bipolar disorder subanalysis: CKD hazard ratios among those with high levels of medication use (≥ 60 prescriptions)			
Lithium	2.54	2.48	0.32
Anticonvulsants	2.30	1.97	2.06
Antipsychotics	1.27	1.30	0.74
Antidepressants	0.91	0.97	0.72

Outcome Definitions

a. **Definite CKD:** The first hospital contact with a diagnosis of CKD defined in a narrow way by the following ICD-10 codes: N18–N19.9 inclusive, plus N14.1, N14.2, N16.8, N25.1, N26 and N27.

b. **Possible CKD:** Detection bias may be more prevalent when CKD is the outcome measure but substantially less when end-stage CKD (dialysis or transplantation) is the outcome measure since almost all patients with end-stage illness will be diagnosed in Denmark and referred for dialysis or kidney transplantation. To asssess this bias, the investigators created a third broad definition of possible CKD for sensitivity analysis, using the ICD-10 codes: N18–N19.9 inclusive, plus N00, N01, N03, N04, N05, N06, N8.8, plus N14.1, N14.2, N16.8, N17, N25.1, N26 and N27.

c. **End-stage CKD:** Defined as irreversible end-stage CKD with either dialysis or transplantation.

In-Depth 2.5 An Early Study of Long-Term eGFR Changes in Lithium Treated Patients

An Israeli group published one of the earlier studies based on serum creatinine trends in 114 patients with bipolar, major depressive or schizoaffective disorder on lithium for 4–30 years from 1968 to 2000. These creatinine results were then compared with longitudinal changes in 94 age- and gender-matched general population subjects without SMI [48]. The lithium cohort started treatment at a mean age of 43.2 ± 12.1 years. Using the definition of renal insufficiency (RI) as serum creatinine ≥ 1.50 mg/dl, only 21% met RI criteria after a mean lithium exposure of 16.75 ± 7.89 years. Of the lithium treated individuals without RI, 79%, some with 30 years of exposure, remained comparable to the control group in the trajectory of age-related eGFR changes. RI was associated with episodes of lithium intoxication, medical comorbidity associated with CKD, and use of nephrotoxic medication, but not with gender, duration of lithium therapy, serum lithium concentration and cumulative lithium dose [48]. This study highlighted that most patients can remain on lithium for many years, and that some of the renal risk relates to lithium toxicity, or medication/disease related CKD risks; however, the use of general population subjects without SMI as a control group may have inflated the extent of lithium's effect on long-term renal function, since lithium treated patients typically have greater rates of CKD risk factors.

In-Depth 2.6 Comparing eGFR Changes in Bipolar Patients on Lithium or Non-Lithium Therapies

Clos and colleagues performed a population based cohort study of adults aged 18–65 years in Tayside, Scotland, newly started on lithium or other medications used for affective disorders (quetiapine, olanzapine and valproate) during 2000–2011 [6]. Patients had to have at least 6 months of exposure to lithium or any of the comparator drugs, and the study excluded those with prior exposure to lithium or one of the comparator drugs, those with a previous diagnosis of schizophrenia or other psychoses, those with glomerular disease, tubulointerstitial disease, CKD stages 4–5 at baseline, or a history of renal transplant. The mean age of the study sample was 42.2 years for the lithium group, and 40.9–43.0 years for the three comparator medications, and the baseline eGFR was 100.9 ± 15.6 ml/min for the lithium cohort, and 101.4 ± 17.2 ml/min in the combined comparator group. During a mean 55 ± 42 months exposure (n = 305), the average annual decline in eGFR (adjusted only for age, sex and baseline eGFR) was 1.3 ml/min in the lithium group, compared to 0.9 ml/min in the comparator group (n = 815). However, after adjustment for additional confounders such as medical comorbidity, high lithium levels (using several cutoffs), nephrotoxic medications or medications with known kinetic interactions with lithium, the estimated monthly decline in eGFR attributable to lithium exposure amounted to only 0.02 ml/min, a value not significantly different than that of the comparator group (p = 0.30) [6]. In a secondary analysis incorporating more covariates, the estimated annual decline in eGFR on lithium therapy was calculated as 1.00 ml/min [6]. This value is in line with a general population expected annual eGFR decrease of 1 ml/min per year [19], but does exceed the age-matched expected value of 0.80 ml/min cited in the UK at that time. Significant predictors of eGFR decline included baseline eGFR, age, medical comorbidities, use of nephrotoxic drugs and episodes of lithium toxicity (defined as any level > 0.80 mEq/l). Adding duration of lithium exposure or mean lithium serum level to the statistical model did not improve the model fit [6].

In-Depth 2.7 The Relationship of eGFR Changes to Age, Medical Comorbidity, Lithium Dose and Level

While lacking a comparator group, another analysis of lithium's long-term renal effects was performed in an international group of 312 bipolar adults of mean age 56 years (range 20–89 years), treated with lithium on average for 18 years (range 8–48 years). The goal was to examine the impact of baseline eGFR, age, medical comorbidity, lithium dose and levels [49]. Starting from a baseline eGFR of 94.2 ± 23.3 ml/min, these patients experienced a mean annual eGFR decline of 0.915%/year of treatment, corresponding to 0.86 ml/min per year [49]. The study found that more than age-expected eGFR declines did not appear until 6–10 years after starting lithium, and that predictors of accelerated declines included medical comorbidities (especially hypertension and diabetes mellitus), female gender, lower initial eGFR, duration of exposure and older age at lithium initiation [49]. While 18.1% of the sample recorded two or more eGFR values < 60 ml/min, no subjects experienced ESRD despite exposures exceeding 30 years in some instances.

The lack of ESRD noted in multiple papers published in the past decade is part of the reframing of renal risk related to lithium. The idea that lithium exposure might inevitably lead to stage G5 renal disease and need for dialysis or renal transplantation was called into question by various studies noting that lithium exposed individuals comprised a minute fraction of ESRD patients, with a 2000 paper stating that lithium related ESRD represented only 0.22% of all causes of ESRD in France [50], and Australia/New Zealand data from 2000 also finding that only 0.2% to 0.7% of all new ESRD cases for that year were due to lithium [16].

A 2014 paper analyzed the Swedish Renal Registry of patients on renal replacement therapy (RRT) (i.e. dialysis or renal transplantation) for two regions with total population 3M to identify individuals previously exposed to lithium [2]. Only 32 RRT patients were found for whom lithium treatment was the sole or main contributing cause of ESRD, and the starting year of lithium treatment for all of these 32 patients was between 1965 and 1980. No patient with ESRD in those areas of Sweden started lithium treatment later than 1980, the year that Sweden implemented a stricter lithium monitoring scheme which recommended serum creatinine and lithium levels every 3–4 months, and weight, blood pressure, thyroid indices, electrolytes, plasma glucose and serum calcium annually [2]. The same investigators subsequently analyzed serum lithium and creatinine levels for the years 1981–2010 from 4879 adult patients newly started on lithium on or after January 1, 1981, all of whom had at least 10 years of cumulative lithium treatment and normal creatinine levels when starting lithium [51]. Among the final sample (n = 630), only 5% developed CKD in the severe or very severe category, suggesting that the 1980 guidelines may have significantly reduced ESRD risk but not completely eliminated it due to the presence of CKD risks in this patient population [51].

To determine whether lack of adherence to monitoring guidelines may be one aspect of the small but persistent presence of lithium related ESRD cases, a retrospective review of 2841 Swedish patient records for the years 1981–2010 was performed, comprising 25,300 treatment-years of lithium exposure [52]. Over the span of those 30 years, most lithium levels (87%–94%) were within recommended range and the mean serum level decreased from 0.70 mEq/l in 1981 to 0.58 mEq/l in 2001, and remained stable through 2010 [52]. While adherence with recommended monitoring increased from 36% in 1981 to 68% in 2010, nearly one-third of patients were still not receiving acceptable monitoring as of 2010, a possible contributor to those rare cases of ESRD associated with lithium treatment. (The lower limit of eGFR where lithium should be discontinued is a subject of intense debate, and the nuances of this important issue are covered in Chapter 5, Section A, devoted to managing renal adverse effects.)

Given these low estimates of ESRD risk, Professor Ursula Werneke (Division of Psychiatry, Department of Clinical Sciences, Umeå University, Sweden) performed a decision analysis in 2012 using data from a systematic literature review to arrive at conclusions for two clinical questions: (1) Should one use lithium or an anticonvulsant at treatment initiation in patients with BD?; *and* (2) What are the risk:benefit considerations related to discontinuation of lithium in patients with CKD (defined as serum creatinine ≥ 1.7 mg/dl) after 20 years of lithium treatment? The point of this analysis was to examine the rates of 5 outcomes after 30 years of BD treatment: death from suicide, alive with stable or unstable BD, alive with or without ESRD [53]. Compounding the limitations inherent in any literature review, the authors did not examine outcomes from SGA use. They also used serum creatinine ≥ 1.70 mg/dl as the CKD definition instead of an eGFR based value, and this creatinine level in a 50-year-old male corresponds to an eGFR of 46 ml/min, at the lower limit of stage G3b CKD, while, for a 50-year-old female the eGFR would be 35 ml/min, at the lower end of stage G4 CKD. Nonetheless, this thought-provoking analysis laid bare the important inputs for any clinician: how to balance lithium's benefits on mood stability, and specifically the impact on risk of suicide related death, with its renal risk. Using the data available in 2012, Professor Werneke and colleagues found that, 20 years into treatment, lithium still remained the medication of choice for BD; moreover, even if CKD had occurred at this point (using their creatinine based definition), one should stop lithium only if the likelihood of progression to ESRD exceeded 41.3%, or if anticonvulsants always outperformed lithium for relapse prevention [53]. While SGAs were not part of the decision tree, these can be used adjunctively and equivalently with either lithium or anticonvulsants, and thus would balance out those two primary arms. The lack of data on suicide prevention for SGA monotherapy, and the emerging naturalistic data showing that BD-1 patients on SGA monotherapy have high rates of treatment failure compared with lithium monotherapy suggest that their analysis would remain unchanged even if SGA monotherapy was included as a treatment option [54].

3 *Association of Lithium Related Renal Dysfunction with Renal Cysts, and the Lack of Association with Renal Cancer*

As computed tomography, ultrasound and magnetic resonance imaging (MRI) became commonly used, literature emerged over the past 25 years noting an association between lithium exposure, renal dysfunction and the presence of renal microcysts (structures 1–2 mm in diameter) or macrocysts (> 2 mm), although the latter were less common and possibly not a unique marker of lithium related renal pathology [55–57]. To illustrate the last point, an ultrasound surveillance study of

120 bipolar patients detected macrocysts in 22% of long-term lithium users (n = 90, mean age 59 years, mean duration of lithium use 16 years), but also in 16% of an age- and gender-matched BD control group (n = 30, mean age 56 years) who had never taken lithium [57]. Duration of lithium exposure and age were not significantly different between lithium treated patients with or without macrocysts, but lithium treated patients with macrocysts had lower eGFR than those on lithium without macrocysts (66 ± 17 ml/min vs. 75 ± 15 ml/min, p = 0.035), and greater duration of BD [57]. MRI is much more sensitive than ultrasound for microcysts, and microcysts are not typically seen in other forms of renal disease, although the population prevalence is not well characterized [58]. Nonetheless, hypotheses emerged that microcyst development was a specific manifestation of pathology arising from excessive intracellular lithium levels in collecting duct principal cells, with macrocyst formation a late stage phenomenon arising from this or other etiologies [57]. This hypothesis appeared confirmed when microcysts in animal models of lithium induced renal dysfunction tested positive not only for the inhibited phosphorylated form of GSK3-β (reflecting lithium's effects), but also for the presence of AQP2 channels found in principal cells [16].

The MRI literature generally associates microcyst formation with longer-term lithium exposure and CKD [57, 59, 60], but some papers suggested that microcyst development may not necessarily correlate with impaired renal function, especially when arising during the earlier phases of lithium treatment [60]. Unfortunately, most publications involved small case series or reports of patients with numerous microcysts occurring in the context of advanced renal disease and medical comorbidities, thereby limiting conclusions regarding the time course of microcyst formation and its relationship to markers of renal dysfunction [58, 59]. The most detailed approach was pursued by the Parisian renal physiologist Dr. Nahib Tabizzadeh and a group of nephrologists and psychiatrists, who, from March 2015 to December 2020, screened 230 consecutive lithium treated adults referred for initial nephrology consultation at the Assistance Publique Hôpitaux de Paris. Of this sample, 217 remained on lithium, and had neither started dialysis nor undergone kidney transplantation, and consented to undergo a 5 h battery of clinical and laboratory measurements including the direct measurement of GFR (mGFR) using urinary clearance of ^{51}Cr-EDTA or ^{99}Tc-DTPA [44]. From the sample of 217 still on lithium, a subset of 99 underwent MRI examination for renal pathology. The MRI cohort had mean age 51 years, 62% were female, and had median lithium exposure of 5 years (range 2–14 years). MRI revealed that 51% had at least one microcyst, and a receiver operating characteristic curve analysis found that the presence of ≥ 5 microcysts was significantly associated with an mGFR < 45 ml/min (AUC 0.893, p < 0.001, sensitivity 80%, specificity 81%) [58]. Many long-term lithium exposed patients do not experience accelerated declines in GFR, and in this study low mGFR and longer lithium treatment duration were strongly correlated in patients with at least one microcyst, but not in the patients without microcysts [44]. This finding supports the concept that accelerated declines in eGFR and microcyst development are not inevitable consequences of long-term lithium exposure.

In-Depth 2.10 Should Imaging Be Used to Screen for Microcysts: Considerations

One question raised by the Parisian study [58] centered on whether MRI screening for microcysts might be a useful staging tool to manage the combined renal effects of exposure to lithium or nephrotoxic medications and medical comorbidity. Based on the fact that the strongest association with microcyst burden was only seen when mGFR was bordering on stage G3b CKD (45 ml/min), the use of MRI to detect microcysts as an early marker of renal pathology lacks sensitivity. Since microcysts arise from lithium's inhibitory effects on GSK3-β in collecting duct principal cells, an earlier signal of the process leading to microcyst formation might be the clinical complaint of polyuria or urine osmolality evidence of NDI. A 2018 review echoed similar sentiments in stating: "Whilst there has been growing interest in the use of non-invasive imaging, particularly MRI for visualization of microcystic disease, the utility of imaging for the routine clinical management of patients treated with long term lithium remains to be delineated. In addition, the significant impact on the patient's mental health also needs to be considered. For example, one would be less tempted to cease lithium in excellent lithium responders especially those who have not done well previously on other therapies, or whose illnesses have been severe or accompanied by risk to self or others" [61]. Further research may help illuminate whether and to what extent microcysts predict the trajectory of CKD; however, assuming a patient has sufficient renal function to remain on lithium, the finding of renal microcysts is not a reason to discontinue lithium.

Although microcysts are benign, in February 2015 the European Medicines Agency advised lithium manufacturers to alter their product warnings to note that long-term lithium exposure (> 10 years) may increase risk not only for microcysts, but also for malignancies such as oncocytomas and collecting duct renal carcinomas [62]. This advisory was seen as a reaction to a case series published in July 2014 (total n = 20) that inferred increased risk for such tumors [63, 64], but was surprising to many investigators since earlier studies found no effect of lithium on cancer risk, or possibly a protective effect in a dose dependent manner [65]. Moreover, in October 2014, members of the International Group for the Study of Lithium issued a vigorous response to the conclusions reached by authors of the July 2014 case series [64, 66]. Among the methodological shortcomings of that case series was the absence of a formal case-control design to calculate the odds ratio for these events accurately, failure to account for the effect of surveillance bias in lithium treated patients, and the use of national statistics based only on age and gender as the comparison group, ignoring the fact that lithium treated patients have a higher prevalence of medical comorbidities and lifestyle behaviors (e.g. smoking) that may influence cancer risk [66]. Nonetheless, the fact that lithium may induce microcyst formation and interstitial fibrosis long after entering collecting principal cells via ENaC led to speculation that lithium's untoward effects could theoretically occur in other ENaC expressing tissues such as the renal pelvis, ureter, bladder and urethra [62]. As these tissues differentially express the four ENaC subunits (α, β, γ and δ), it was hypothesized that, if there was a lithium effect at other sites in the urinary stream, it might only be seen in tissues expressing the ENaC isoform with an α subunit, since that form of ENaC has 1.6-fold higher permeability for lithium than for sodium. It was also hypothesized that this effect (if it existed) would not be seen in tissues expressing an ENaC isoform with the δ subunit in lieu of the α subunit, as that ENaC variant has 38% lower permeability for lithium than for sodium [14, 62].

Given the small samples in published case series, Professor Lars Kessing (Psychiatric Center Copenhagen, Rigshospitalet, University of Copenhagen) and colleagues performed a nationwide, population based longitudinal study (1995–2012) that included all lithium exposed patients (n = 24,272), all individuals with a diagnosis of BD (n = 9651), those exposed to anticonvulsants for any reason (n = 386,255) and a randomly selected sample of 1.5M adults from the Danish population [67]. The outcomes were hazard rate ratios (HRs) for malignant or benign renal upper tract tumors, adjusted for numerous covariates including concurrent medications, medical comorbidities, age, gender, calendar year and a diagnosis of BD. This methodologically rigorous analysis found that continued treatment with lithium was not associated with increased rates of malignant or benign renal upper tract tumors: HR for malignant or benign tumors: 0.67–1.18, p = 0.70; HR malignant tumors only: 0.61–1.34, p = 0.90; HR benign tumors only: 0.74–1.18, p = 0.70 [52]. This lack of association with increased risk for renal tract tumors was subsequently confirmed in multiple other studies [62, 68].

After Kessing's findings from the Danish population dispelled any notion that lithium might have oncogenic properties in the renal system, other investigators were inspired to study the association of lithium exposure and cancer risk of all types. A Swedish group performed a nationwide register study of incidence rate ratios (IRRs) for any cancer and specific cancers among BD adults aged 50–84 years diagnosed from July 2005 to December 2009 (n = 5442) compared with rates in the general population, stratified by lithium exposure [67]. The study found that there was no difference in overall cancer risk compared with the general population in BD patients on lithium treatment [IRR = 1.04, 95% CI 0.89–1.23] or BD patients without lithium treatment (IRR = 1.03, 95% CI 0.89–1.19). Interestingly, site specific cancer risk was significantly increased in BD patients not on lithium in three sites: the digestive organs (IRR = 1.47, 95% CI 1.12–1.93), respiratory system and intrathoracic organs (IRR = 1.72, 95% CI 1.11–2.66), and in the endocrine glands and related structures (IRR = 2.60, 95% CI 1.24–5.47), but the risk was not increased in lithium treated BD patients [69]. A Taiwanese group used their nationwide database to compare cancer incidence in adult BD patients exposed to lithium only, anticonvulsants only, or both agents during the years 1998–2009 after excluding those with < 1 year of drug exposure or pre-existing cancer diagnoses [70]. The median duration of medication exposure was 7.1 years for the lithium only group, 5.2 years for the anticonvulsant only group, and 7.5 years for the combined group. Compared with anticonvulsant only exposure, lithium exposure was associated with significantly lower cancer risk (HR = 0.74, 95% CI 0.55–0.97), and this risk declined in a dose dependent manner: the HR for those with the highest tertile of lithium exposure (> 810 mg/d) was 0.55 (95% CI 0.37–0.83) [68]. In 2021 an international collaborative team performed a systematic review and meta-analysis of the literature, with analyses based on outcomes of 2,606,187 individuals from five studies [71]. This comprehensive examination of the literature did not find an increased risk of cancer in BD patients on lithium, and even suggested a small but nonsignificant protective effect for any malignancy (RR = 0.94, 95% CI 0.72–1.22; p = 0.66] and urinary cancer (RR = 0.93, 95% CI 0.75–1.14; p = 0.48] [71].

4 *What are Prescribing Practices that Increase Risk for CKD?*

As increasingly sophisticated statistical methods separated risks related to lithium treatment from those inherent in lithium treated patients, a group in the Psychiatric and Neurodevelopmental Genetics Unit at Massachusetts General Hospital (MGH) and Harvard University sought to model the patient and treatment parameters associated with increased risk for renal insufficiency (RI), with RI defined by presence of ICD-9 code (ICD-9 586.*) or an eGFR < 60 ml/min [4]. Using electronic health records from a large New England health-care system (2006–2013), 1445 lithium treated adult patients with RI were identified and were matched by risk set sampling 1:3 with 4306 lithium-exposed adults without RI. An initial logistic regression model was created from a random two-thirds of the cohort, risk covariates adjusted to improve model fit, and the model retested in the remaining one-third of the sample. Demographic and patient related factors associated with increased RI risk were similar to those previously identified, including older age, female gender, smoking, hypertension and total medical comorbidity burden, and one novel finding: diagnosis of a schizophrenia spectrum disorder [4]. As both exposure to first-generation antipsychotics (FGAs) (but not SGAs) and a diagnosis of schizophrenia spectrum disorder were associated with RI risk, the authors speculated that these may be proxies of illness severity. The implication is that more severely mentally ill individuals may have suboptimal health outcomes of all types related to underutilization of medical services [47]. Despite modest duration of lithium exposure in the final sample (mean 501 days), after adjustment for all patient, demographic and other treatment related risk factors, there were two patterns of lithium treatment associated with significantly increased RI risk: use of lithium more than once daily, and having even one lithium level > 1.20 mEq/l.

In-Depth 2.12 Renal Benefits of Once Daily Lithium Dosing: The Debate

The debate over the renoprotective effect of once daily lithium dosing originated in the early 1980s with papers noting a greater degree of polyuria in patients receiving BID dosing compared with those on QHS dosing [43, 72]. It later became clear that polyuria is the earliest clinical manifestation of intracellular lithium accumulation in collecting duct principal cells and of the ensuing processes that combine with CKD risks to accelerate age-related eGFR declines. Unfortunately, the quality of the data differentiating the renal effects of single and multiple daily dosing was decidedly uneven. A 2013 review lamented that the available evidence was contradictory concerning whether once daily lithium administration reduced polyuria risk or severity; however, the authors stated that no trial demonstrates any loss of prophylactic efficacy or greater adverse effect burden associated with once daily dosing, and therefore endorsed this practice [73]. While not directly addressing the question of polyuria, the 2016 MGH case-control analysis provided the best evidence from a large methodologically sound study that once daily dosing reduces RI risk by 20% even with modest lithium exposure duration: OR 0.80 (95% CI 0.69–0.93; p = 0.003) [4]. There was also no difference in RI risk between standard or extended release lithium preparations.

The underlying reason for the association between once daily dosing and decreased renal dysfunction risk is unknown, but two plausible hypotheses are advanced. The first rests on the concept that many clinicians may unwittingly expose patients to more lithium when it is prescribed BID due to the distorting effect on morning trough values from divided dosages [49]. As shown in Table 2.3, when lithium is dosed BID the level obtained the next morning before the a.m. dose is markedly lower than a morning level obtained 12 h after QHS administration of *the same total daily dose* [74–76]. Therefore, patients on BID lithium will require 28% higher lithium doses to achieve comparable serum levels to QHS dosing. That lower doses are required to achieve the same 12 h trough level was confirmed by a study in which patients on BID, TID or QID lithium regimens were switched to QHS dosing; the dose needed to maintain a 12 h trough serum level of 0.80 mEq/l had to be decreased [77]. The other hypothesis is that prolonged higher trough lithium levels from divided daily dosing leads to a sufficiently high lithium concentration

Table 2.3 Differences in morning lithium levels when comparable daily doses are administered at bedtime (QHS) or twice daily (BID)

Study	Lithium level: QHS dosing (mEq/l)	Lithium level: BID dosing (mEq/l)
Amdisen [74]	1.37	1.07
Greil [75]	1.04	0.81
Swartz [76]	0.90	0.70
Mean level	1.10	0.86

Comments

a. **Kinetics:** Lithium has a peripheral half-life of 24 h on average and, by convention, dosing decisions are based on 12 h trough values obtained in the morning. When the dose is administered on a BID schedule, the morning level is a 12 h trough only for the evening portion of the dose – it is a 24 h trough for the dose ingested the prior morning.

b. **Converting patients on BID doses to QHS dosing:** When the comparable dose administered on a BID schedule is converted to a single QHS dose, the morning trough level will be 28% higher. Patients on BID dosing with levels thought to be at the high end of the maintenance therapeutic range may be overexposed to lithium and have trough levels that are supratherapeutic and potentially nephrotoxic. As there is no efficacy advantage from multiple daily dosing, those on BID dosing should be converted to single QHS dosing as soon as possible. (See Chapter 5 for management of adverse effects occasionally seen with larger single lithium doses.) After consolidation, the 12 h trough level is rechecked after 2 days on the new QHS dose, and the dose adjusted based on this new level. The 12 h trough is also used for patients on extended release lithium preparations.

c. **Clinical implication for patients remaining on BID doses:** Some patients may be wedded to BID dosing for a variety of reasons (e.g. historical stability and reluctance to change, prior episodes of adverse effects on single QHS doses). As the morning trough level would be 28% higher were the dose converted to a QHS schedule, **the maximum morning trough level on BID dosing should be 0.78 mEq/l, which would equate to 1.00 mEq/l if the dose were given QHS only**. If local guidelines suggest 0.80 mEq/l as the recommended maximum maintenance level, the corresponding BID level is 0.62 mEq/l.

in tubular fluid that enhances lithium's ability to outcompete sodium at ENaC (Figure 2.3). Although lithium has 1.6-fold higher ENaC affinity than does sodium, an extended period of lower lithium levels in tubular fluid after QHS dosing might lessen lithium's influx via ENaC for large portions of the day, thereby permitting its clearance from principal duct cells via NHE1. While both of these hypotheses are speculative, the MGH study provides a convincing reason to follow the advice from the 2013 review: as there is no demonstrable efficacy loss or greater adverse effect burden associated with once daily dosing, and once daily regimens decrease RI risk by 20%, this should be the norm. (As noted in Chapter 3, single doses should be QHS so that 12 h trough levels can easily be obtained the next morning. Administering lithium as a single noon or morning dose should be avoided due to the difficulty of obtaining 12 h trough serum levels.)

Figure 2.3 Serum levels from bedtime (QHS) dosing of standard lithium or twice daily (BID) dosing of an extended release formulation [43]

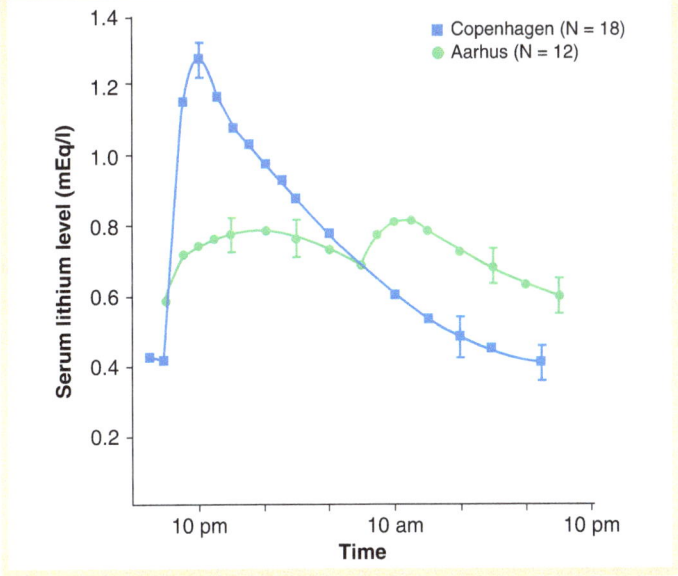

(Adapted from: M. Schou, A. Amdisen, K. Thomsen, et al. [1982]. Lithium treatment regimen and renal water handling: The significance of dosage pattern and tablet type examined through comparison of results from two clinics with different treatment regimens. *Psychopharmacology*, 77, 387–390.)

The MGH study also confirmed findings from a number of sources that episodes of high therapeutic outpatient lithium levels are a factor in RI risk, and that these levels are not necessarily in the "toxic" range (variably defined as > 1.50 mEq/l or higher). The emphasis on outpatient levels reflects two issues: (1) longitudinal studies are performed on outpatient databases; and (2) a single instance of an elevated outpatient level may reflect more chronic exposure, especially if there is no concomitant patient complaint or the level is not sufficiently high to warrant a laboratory alert. In the MGH study, lithium level data were available for 2650 subjects (926 cases, 1724 controls). In this subgroup, 285 cases and 299 controls had at least one level > 1.20 mEq/l prior to first recorded diagnosis of RI [4]. In adjusted regression models, presence of one level > 1.20 mEq/l was associated with a 72% increased RI risk (OR 1.72, 95% CI 1.38–2.14). To explore the impact of higher maximal lithium levels, data from the 115 cases and 106 controls who had at least one level > 1.50 mEq/L prior to first RI diagnosis were added to the model of RI risk as a separate indicator variable. With both indicator variables included (history of level > 1.20 mEq/l, history of level > 1.50 mEq/l), having experienced any lithium level > 1.20 mEq/l remained associated with higher risk – OR 1.74 (95% CI 1.33–2.25) – while history of a level > 1.50 mEq/l was not significant and did not improve the model fit. With the large sample size for this secondary analysis (n = 2650), the case-control design involving only lithium treated individuals, and advanced methods for handling covariates, the MGH data represent the strongest statement that maximal lithium outpatient levels should never exceed 1.20 mEq/l [4].

In-Depth 2.13 Any Supratherapeutic Lithium Level Increases Renal Insufficiency Risk: The Evidence

To document the ongoing renal impact from even one high serum lithium level, eGFR data on 699 lithium treated patients in the Norfolk, UK database were examined from baseline and after ≤ 3 months, 6 ± 3 months, and 12 ± 3 months of exposure to a lithium level within 1 of 3 ranges: 0.81–1.00 mEq/l (Group 2), 1.01–1.20 mEq/l (Group 3) or 1.21–2.00 mEq/l (Group 4). The reference group (Group 1) comprised patients whose lithium levels never exceeded 0.80 mEq/l [3]. Compared with Group 1, Groups 3 and 4 experienced significantly greater eGFR decreases in the first 3 months of treatment (p = 0.047 and p = 0.040). At the 6 (± 3) month time point, Group 4 eGFR values remained below baseline, but this result was not statistically significant (p = 0.298) [3]. As mentioned previously, a population based cohort study of adults aged 18–65 years was performed using a Tayside, Scotland database to examine trends and predictors of eGFR changes in patients newly started on lithium, with patients on other medications for affective disorders (quetiapine, olanzapine and valproate) used as a comparison group [6]. There were 305 lithium treated patients in the final analysis exposed to lithium for a mean of 55 ± 42 months. Significant predictors of eGFR decline included baseline eGFR, age, medical comorbidities, use of nephrotoxic drugs, and any episode in which the lithium level exceeded 0.80 mEq/l, while duration of lithium exposure or mean lithium serum level did not improve the model fit [6].

In-Depth 2.14 Managing Mean Lithium Levels to Lessen Renal Insufficiency Risk

As 2650 subjects in the MGH database study had lithium level data, 35% of whom met RI criteria, the investigators also examined to what extent mean levels influenced RI risk given the inconsistent findings in the literature. To perform this analysis, mean historical lithium levels were examined, but those values obtained within 90 days of the initial RI diagnosis were excluded, presumably because those levels may have been skewed by abrupt changes in renal function [4]. To allow for nonlinear effects, lithium levels were grouped in 0.2 mEq/l increments, and patients with mean levels < 0.60 mEq/l served as the reference cohort. In the fully adjusted models, the odds ratios for RI (vs. the reference cohort) by mean lithium level were: lithium level 0.60–0.80 mEq/l: OR 1.42 (95% CI 1.14–1.77); lithium level 0.80–1.00 mEq/l: OR 2.03 (95% CI 1.56–2.65); lithium level > 1.00 mEq/l: OR 2.20 (95% CI 1.43–3.38). Although the 95% confidence intervals for all three lithium ranges overlap, there is a trend towards level dependent risk, especially given that the mean duration of lithium exposure was only 501 days in this study. The field of BD research is increasingly recognizing that maintenance levels below 1.00 mEq/l may suit many patients, and in that vein the conclusions of a 2019 systematic review from a joint task force of the International Society for Bipolar Disorders and the International Study Group on the Treatment with Lithium are worth repeating (NB: units in mmol/l = mEq/l): "For adults with bipolar disorder there was consensus that the standard lithium serum level should be 0.60–0.80 mmol/l with the option to reduce it to 0.40–0.60 mmol/l in case of good response but poor tolerance or to increase it to 0.80–1.00 mmol/l in case of insufficient response and good tolerance" [78].

While management of medical comorbidity associated with renal impairment is important, clinicians must be mindful of the independent contribution of a variety of medications to renal dysfunction, as their persistent use may complicate one's ability to maintain patients on long-term lithium treatment [79]. (See Chapter 3 for management of lithium dosing when co-prescribed with medications that have significant kinetic interactions.) Although many of the agents in Table 2.4 are familiar due to their historical association with renal adverse effects, two types of medications, proton pump inhibitors [PPIs] and the fibrates bezafibrate and fenofibrate, deserve attention due to their widespread use, and the fact that their association with renal dysfunction is relatively recent [79]. Interstitial nephritis is an immune-mediated atypical kidney injury seen from a variety of medications, with the first reports of omeprazole associated nephritis appearing in 1992 [80, 81]. The risk attributable to PPIs as a class was not well quantified until more sophisticated analyses using propensity score matching were performed with large data sets. In one large US study, after adjusting for demographic, socioeconomic and clinical variables, PPI use was associated with a 50% increased risk of being diagnosed with CKD (HR, 1.50; 95% CI 1.14–1.96), and this association persisted when PPI users were compared directly with histamine H_2 receptor antagonist users (adjusted HR, 1.39; 95% CI 1.01–1.91) and with propensity score-matched non-users (HR, 1.76; 95% CI 1.13–2.74) [82]. The use of PPIs for extended periods without medical supervision is an area of concern, and a 2020 paper emphasized the need for deprescribing PPIs to lessen their renal impact, and to consider alternative treatments (e.g. histamine H_2 antagonists) for those with indications for chronic use [83]. The fibrates bezafibrate and fenofibrate have known associations with declines in eGFR, but it is unclear whether this represents a true nephrotoxic effect or an artifact from increased creatinine production [84–87]. As with PPIs, clinicians should be aware of these medication effects and alternative medication options for lithium treated patients where eGFR declines are concerning. For patients requiring a fibrate, gemfibrozil is an ideal alternative to bezafibrate and fenofibrate as studies have found that gemfibrozil lacks the renal adverse effects of the former two medications [88].

D **Renal Parameters Used in Lithium Monitoring**

WHAT TO KNOW: LABS USED TO MONITOR RENAL FUNCTION

- Clinicians should be conversant in the use of eGFR, early morning urine osmolality (EMUO), and the albumin-to-creatinine ratio (ACR) to monitor various aspects of renal function in lithium treated patients.
- Screening for polyuria initially involves direct patient inquiry and use of the 24 h fluid intake record (FIR). This will be supplemented by the EMUO when complaints arise.

Clinicians prescribing lithium routinely interact with nonpsychiatric medical professionals and must be conversant in the latest trends regarding renal function measurement, and with the significance of the three common laboratory measures

Table 2.4 Nephrotoxic medications used for chronic therapy [79, 85, 86, 88, 89]

Medication class	Mechanism for nephrotoxicity
Angiotensin converting enzyme (ACE) inhibitors (e.g. benazepril, enalapril, fosinopril, lisinopril, perindopril, ramipril, quinapril, trandolapril)	Interfere with production of angiotensin II from angiotensin I, thereby limiting angiotensin II induced constriction of the efferent renal arteriole and increased eGFR.
Angiotensin receptor II type 1 antagonists (e.g. azilsartan, irbesartan, losartan, olmesartan, telmisartan, valsartan)	Interfere with angiotensin II binding to angiotensin II type 1 receptors, thereby limiting angiotensin II induced constriction of the efferent renal arteriole and increased eGFR.
Calcineurin inibitors (cyclosporine > tacrolimus > sirolimus)	Vasoconstriction of afferent and efferent renal arterioles.
Diuretics: loop (e.g. bumetanide, furosemide)	Decreased renal perfusion due to volume depletion causing acute kidney injury.
Diuretics: thiazide-type (e.g. chlorthalidone, hydrochlorothiazide)	Decreased renal perfusion due to volume depletion causing acute kidney injury.
Fibrates (e.g. bezafibrate, fenofibrate, but not gemfibrozil)	Unclear. May increase creatinine production without impairing renal function. May also decrease renal blood flow by inhibiting prostaglandin production.
NSAID (aspirin, celecoxib, doclofenac, ibuprofen, indomethacin, ketoprofen, meloxicam, naproxen, piroxicam, sulindac)	Inhibitory effects on prostaglandins cause vasoconstriction of the afferent arteriole and reduced renal blood flow.
Proton pump inhibitors (e.g. lansoprazole, omeprazole, pantoprazole)	Acute interstitial nephritis from renal tubular deposition.
Reverse-transcriptase inhibitor (tenofovir)	Mitochondrial toxicity inducing acute tubular injury.
Statins (e.g. atorvastatin, cerivastatin, fluvastatin, lovastatin, rosuvastatin, simvastatin)	Myoglobin induced acute tubular necrosis secondary to rhabdomyolysis.

central to lithium monitoring: eGFR, EMUO and ACR. Familiarity with these laboratory parameters facilitates productive discussions with other clinicians (e.g. nephrology, internal medicine), and also informs how one conveys information on renal risk to patients and caregivers. Given the understanding that some of what was perceived as lithium's renal risk is related to inherent patient factors (e.g. medical comorbidity), and that development of ESRD is extremely rare, describing lithium monitoring as a means to prevent "renal failure" is inappropriate since the eGFR definition of kidney failure is stage G5 CKD, representing an eGFR < 15 ml/min [19]. Monitoring of eGFR, ACR and EMUO is part of a broad strategy to track intrinsic renal function changes in a population at higher risk for CKD, and optimize early detection of polyuria to possibly forestall long-term complications from GSK3-β inhibition in collecting duct principal cells [10, 19, 32].

1 *Estimated Glomerular Filtration Rate (eGFR)*

This measure represents the rate at which the glomerulus filters plasma to produce an ultrafiltrate, and is the best overall measure of renal function. As discussed in Info Box 2.1, GFR can be measured directly in animals and humans by infusing or injecting molecules with limited tubular secretion or reabsorption (mGFR), but as a screening tool this parameter is estimated as eGFR, with mGFR obtained only in very specific circumstances. For the past two decades, eGFR has supplanted the use of serum creatinine to track renal function since age and gender are important moderators of the relationship between creatinine and renal function [90]. The elimination of a race based coefficient from the eGFR equation is an important and very recent development (Info Box 2.2), with the new $eGFR_{cr-cys}$ equation utilizing age, gender and levels of serum creatinine and another protein, cystatin C. This new equation has superior performance across diverse populations compared with the older eGFR creatinine based equation ($eGFR_{cr}$) [20]. While that $eGFR_{cr}$ equation did have limitations, it was a vast improvement over the use of creatinine clearance (CL_{cr}) to estimate renal function. The exact definition of creatinine clearance is the volume of blood plasma cleared of creatinine per unit of time. The Cockcroft–Gault CL_{cr} formula was developed in 1976 from a sample of Canadian veterans, 96% of whom were white males, and later studies found that CL_{cr} exceeded GFR due to creatinine secretion in the tubules, with greater overestimation at lower GFR values [91, 92]. There is no modern use for CL_{cr}, although vestiges are found in old medication package inserts that refer to CL_{cr} in the section on renal dysfunction, with recent US drug labels using eGFR [93]. Cystatin C will increasingly be included as a reflexive order in all laboratory "renal panels" but may need to be ordered specifically until laboratories change the ordering system and their automated eGFR estimating equation to generate values from $eGFR_{cr-cys}$ when levels of creatinine and cystatin C are available. If the laboratory does not yet report $eGFR_{cr-cys}$ values using the 2021 CKD-EPI creatinine–cystatin equation, there are online calculators to provide a result using the patient age, gender, serum creatinine and cystatin C (www.kidney.org/professionals/KDOQI/gfr_calculator). Info Box 2.3 provides guidance on the use of $eGFR_{cr}$ in instances where cystatin C may not be readily available from the local laboratory, or the eGFR is expected to be so high that use of eGFR$_{cr}$ is unlikely to alter clinical care. The staging of CKD is based on eGFR and ACR, and stage is an important determinant of many decisions regarding the frequency of eGFR monitoring and the need to track ACR [19, 32]. The focus of renal monitoring and lithium prescribing practices is to minimize the risk that any patient will develop stage G3a CKD due to lithium itself, bearing in mind that the management of systemic illnesses (e.g. hypertension, diabetes mellitus) is often beyond the control of the lithium prescriber, and suboptimal control of these CKD risk factors may be the primary driver of accelerated eGFR declines.

 Info Box 2.1 Basic Concepts in Measuring Renal Function: The Estimated GFR (eGFR)

a. What is the glomerular filtration rate (GFR)?

The rate at which the glomerulus filters plasma to produce an ultrafiltrate. It is considered the best overall measure of renal function.

Creatinine clearance (CL$_{Cr}$) is the volume of blood plasma that is cleared of creatinine per unit of time. It approximates the GFR, but CL$_{Cr}$ values exceed GFR due to creatinine secretion in the tubules, with greater overestimation at lower GFR values [92]. Moreover, the Cockcroft–Gault CL$_{Cr}$ formula was developed in 1976 from a sample of Canadian veterans who were 96% white males [91]. CL$_{Cr}$ is not clinically used, although vestiges can be found in older medication package inserts that refer to CL$_{Cr}$ in the section on renal dysfunction [93]. eGFR is used in new package labeling in the US (2022 onwards).

b. How does one measure GFR and why is it usually estimated (eGFR)?

The measurement of GFR is performed using a renally cleared substance that is not protein bound, and is neither secreted nor reabsorbed in the tubules. Physiologist Homer W. Smith pioneered use of inulin in 1935 and it remains the gold standard for measured GFR (mGFR) [94]. Inulin is difficult to work with, so in modern practice other molecules are used for human mGFR: urinary clearance of iothalamate, plasma clearance of iohexol. Direct eGFR measurement in humans is performed only in certain clinical circumstances where the estimated GFR may be substantially in error, and/or a more accurate measurement will significantly change the management plan [19].

For routine screening, GFR is estimated based on the blood concentration of an endogenous filtration marker (creatinine or possibly other proteins). The level of any endogenous filtration marker is determined by GFR and physiologic processes other than GFR (non-GFR determinants). These non-GFR processes cannot be easily measured, but estimating equations include demographic and clinical variables as surrogates of the combined impact of all non-GFR determinants. In routine clinical practice, a calculated estimate of the GFR using the serum creatinine, age, gender, **and until recently race** (i.e. whether the individual is of African heritage), provided a value that could be used for the majority of patient situations and is referred to in the literature as eGFR$_{cr}$ to denote that it is derived from serum creatinine. (See Info Box 2.3 for a discussion of a new formula for eGFR that uses both creatinine and cystatin C values, and obviates the need for arbitrary use of race.)

c. What are normal GFR values?

Normal GFR values in healthy young adults are 100–125 ml/min per 1.73 m² of body surface area (BSA). GFR varies with hemodynamics, sympathetic tone, diet, time of the day, exercise, body size, pregnancy and drugs. Even in stable conditions, within-person variability of measured GFR (mGFR) is common and contributes to random measurement error. GFR is indexed by BSA because kidney size is proportional to body size.

d. What are the stages of kidney function using eGFR? [All units are ml/min/1.73 m²] [19]

- G1 (Normal)   eGFR ≥ 90
- G2 (Mildly decreased)   eGFR 60–89
- G3a (Mildly to moderately decreased)   eGFR 45–59
- G3b (Moderately to severely decreased)   eGFR 30–44
- G4 (Severely decreased)   eGFR 15–29
- G5 (Kidney failure)   eGFR < 15

Info Box 2.2 The Evolution of a Non-race Based eGFR Formula: eGFR$_{cr-cys}$

a. **Use of creatinine as the filtration marker**: Creatinine is a 113 dalton byproduct of creatine metabolism that is generated from muscle mass or diet, primarily from animal protein intake. It is freely filtered by the glomerulus and secreted by the renal tubules but not reabsorbed. Creatinine is also subject to some elimination by the gastrointestinal tract. Until recently, creatinine has been the preferred filtration marker for eGFR, and lab assays have been standardized since 2003 [19].

b. **The development of estimating equations** (e.g. the Chronic Kidney Disease Epidemiology Collaboration [**CKD-EPI**] and older Modification of Diet in Renal Disease Study [MDRD] equations) replaced the need for direct GFR measurement in clinical practice. The preferred eGFR equation in the US and Europe had been the CKD-EPI 2009 creatinine formula, based on large cohorts who underwent direct GFR measurement (e.g. by infusing iothalamate). It was more accurate than the earlier MDRD equation, particularly for eGFR values > 60 ml/min.

c. **Issue of race:** Investigators had found that Black race (as assigned) was independently associated with slightly higher GFR at the same serum creatinine for unknown reasons, despite extensive research into biological and environmental variables to explain this difference. The CKD-EPI equation incorporated a coefficient that increased $eGFR_{cr}$ in Blacks by 16% [95]. The older MDRD equation used a larger racial correction factor of 21% [96].

d. **Issues with race based $eGFR_{cr}$ formulas:**

i. Unlike other areas of medicine where ancestry provides insight into a known biological substrate (e.g. CYP 2D6 ultrarapid metabolizers from North Africa / the Middle East, sickle cell allele frequency in those from sub-Saharan Africa, HLA-B*1502 allele frequency in certain East Asian countries), extensive research has failed to explain the observed differences in mGFR values based on heritage.

ii. As a social construct, race is often applied in a nonstandardized manner, especially in those with mixed heritage where outward phenotype may play a significant role in the clinician assigned race [96, 97]. Given these and other societal issues regarding race, the use of one's heritage to guide clinical care is justified only if: "(1) the use confers substantial benefit; (2) the benefit cannot be achieved through other feasible approaches; (3) patients who reject race categorization are accommodated fairly; and (4) the use of race is transparent" [95]. The CKD-EPI eGFR equations fail criteria 3 and 4, and also criterion 1 since overestimating eGFR using a race based correction applied in a nonstandardized way may result in: decreased access to specialist care, renal disease education and kidney transplantation, while potentially preventing clinicians from modifying the use of certain medications due to the overestimated eGFR [96].

e. **Solution: Find an evidence based race-free eGFR alternative** [98, 99]: The National Kidney Foundation and the American Society of Nephrology established a task force to reassess inclusion of race in the estimation of eGFR, and this group suggested that the use of a second marker, **cystatin C,** might be useful [98]. Cystatin C is one of a family of cysteine protease inhibitors found in high concentrations in biological fluids, and expressed nearly ubiquitously in the body [98]. Importantly, cystatin C is less influenced by non-GFR determinants than creatinine in ambulatory patients [92]. Cystatin C is freely filtered at the glomerulus, is catabolized in the tubules with reabsorption of its metabolites, and undergoes some extrarenal elimination. **While $eGFR_{cys}$ is not more accurate than $eGFR_{cr}$, the combination $eGFR_{cr-cys}$ is more accurate than either marker when used alone for eGFR** [98].

f. **Development of the $eGFR_{cr-cys}$ equation:** The statistical model was developed on data sets previously used to create the current equations (development data sets): CKD-EPI 2009 for $eGFR_{cr}$ (10 studies, 8254 participants) and CKD-EPI 2012 for $eGFR_{cys}$ and $eGFR_{cr-cys}$ (13 studies, 5352 participants). For external validation, a new data set had to be used (CKD-EPI 2021), consisting of the CKD-EPI 2012 external validation data set and previously unused studies (12 studies [7 new], 4050 participants) (validation data set), to compare the performance of existing and new equations. Black participants made up 31.5% of the 2009 development data set, 39.7% of the 2012 development data set, and 14.3% of the 2021 validation data set [20].

g. **Benefits:** The new eGFR$_{cr-cys}$ equation had smaller differences in bias between race groups than the corresponding eGFR$_{cr}$ equation, with less effect on prevalence estimates for CKD and GFR stages [20]. It also performs better in situations with frail, sedentary or elderly patients, as low muscle mass and low activity levels induce less creatinine release from skeletal muscle and create a distorted impression of better renal function with the eGFR$_{cr}$ equation [100].

Info Box 2.3 Choosing an eGFR Formula: eGFR$_{cr}$ or the New 2021 CKD-EPI Creatinine–Cystatin eGFR$_{cr-cys}$

- **The ideal world:** In the near future, cystatin C will be provided routinely along with BUN and creatinine whenever a "renal function" panel is ordered from the laboratory. The new eGFR$_{cr-cys}$ formula will be used to calculate a result based on the patient's age, gender, serum creatinine and cystatin C values.

  Comment: Cystatin C has not been a commonly ordered test, so there has been a cost difference and slower turnaround than for creatinine. A 2020 paper examined worldwide test availability across all continents, and the difference in cost (normalized for the country's gross national income) between the assays for serum creatinine and for serum cystatin C. While serum creatinine was available in 100% of the 33 surveyed countries, cystatin C was only obtainable in 67%. Where available, the median cost was five times greater for serum cystatin C than for serum creatinine [101]. However, as with other tests that were initially more expensive (e.g. hemoglobin A1C), the cost dropped significantly over time due to increasing demand, economies of scale and technology improvements. The estimated cost for cystatin C (and availability) will steadily improve as the eGFR$_{cr-cys}$ formula is adopted as the new norm.

- **What should a clinician do?**

  a. **Where cystatin C is not available, use the CKD-EPI-2009 standard eGFR$_{cr}$ equation, but only record the result which omits the race based adjustment (often reported as 'non-African').**

    Rationale: The result from the CKD-EPI equation is still commonly reported in laboratories and relies only on creatinine. Using the result without the race adjustment regardless of heritage is adequate for many patients, but will generate a mean decrease in eGFR$_{cr}$ of 14.1 ml/min (13.7%) in Black adults. In the interest of safety during lithium treatment, it is preferable to underestimate eGFR rather than to overestimate with a race adjustment that is often applied idiosyncratically [20].

b. **Where cystatin C is available but the laboratory does not yet report eGFR results calculated from the new eGFR$_{cr-cys}$ equation, add cystatin C to the renal function or chemistry panel and use a smartphone app or website to calculate the eGFR using the 2021 CKD-EPI creatinine–cystatin equation.**

Rationale: Even when cystatin C becomes readily available, it will take time for laboratories to add this by default to the chemistry or renal function panels, and also to change the software to report results with the new 2021 CKD-EPI creatinine–cystatin eGFR$_{cr-cys}$ formula. Simply add cystatin C to one's routine laboratory orders until these changes occur, and find an electronic resource to perform this calculation using the reported serum creatinine and cystatin C values, the patient's age and gender. One such resource is: www.kidney.org/professionals/KDOQI/gfr_calculator.

2 *Early Morning Urine Osmolality (EMUO)*

The need to monitor carefully for evidence of polyuria is readily apparent for two reasons: it is a patient complaint that can lead to lithium discontinuation, and it is a marker for excessive lithium effects in collecting duct principal cells. One can obtain a urine osmolality at any time of the day from a spot specimen, but EMUO represents an ideal screening method for examining the kidney's ability to concentrate urine, since most individuals undergo a period of overnight water deprivation [22]. While the gold standard for calculating urine osmolality and quantifying the extent of polyuria is the 24 h urine collection, it can be impractical to obtain accurate adherence with the 24 h collection for inpatients and outpatients (Info Box 2.4); moreover, it is not feasible to order on a repeated basis as a tracking tool during amiloride titration for NDI. Laboratories may report a variety of normal ranges for urine osmolality, but there is a general consensus that EMUO values < 300 mOsm/kg represent NDI, while those in the range of 300–850 mOsm/kg are abnormal and consistent with partial NDI. Use of EMUO and urine osmolality from spot specimens during the day is also helpful in distinguishing psychogenic polydipsia from the polydipsia seen in lithium treated patients whose NDI is inadequately managed. Lastly, there are long-term age-related trends in urine osmolality, so establishing a pretreatment baseline in older patients can be helpful to ascertain to what extent future EMUO results might be related to factors other than lithium exposure [102]. (The combined use of EMUO and the 24 h FIR is discussed in Section 5 below.)

Basic Concepts in Measuring Renal Function: Assessing Polyuria and Urine Osmolality

a. **Urine osmolality:** The standard definition of polyuria is a urine volume > 3000 ml/24 h in adults, although patients may complain of urinary frequency with lower levels of urine output. Although the gold standard for quantifying polyuria is the 24 h urine collection, this is often problematic for busy outpatients, and at times impractical for more severely ill inpatients [22]. As a tool for assessing polyuria severity and for following response to treatment, early morning urine osmolality (EMUO) is much more feasible due to its ease of use. Urine is maximally concentrated in the morning after 12–14 h of fluid restriction, so EMUO is more sensitive than urine osmolality obtained at other times from a spot specimen.

- **Inpatient use of EMUO:** Ask the patient not to void in the morning until a specimen can be provided. For the convenience of the patient and staff, sample containers should be kept on the unit so a specimen can be provided at whatever time the patient arises in the morning.

- **Outpatient use of EMUO:** For convenience, a sample container should be given to the outpatient by office personnel (or the laboratory) to take home. The specimen is provided when the patient arises in the morning. The sample need not be delivered immediately to the laboratory, as urine osmolality results are stable when kept at room temperature for up to 5 days [103].

b. **Office screening:** At each visit, ask about excessive thirst and urination. To better quantify the extent of fluid intake needed to maintain homeostasis, the 24 h FIR is an evidence based screening tool. Every 6 months before the visit, or more often if amiloride is being used to manage polyuria, ask the patient to record their fluid intake for each 24 h period for 2 days and then average the result. In a dedicated polyuria assessment protocol with lithium treated patients, FIR values < 2000 ml/24 h were associated with a very low likelihood of polyuria (likelihood ratio [LR] = **0.18**), while an FIR > 3500 ml/24 h was associated with a very high likelihood (LR **6.1**) [22]. This is not a substitute for EMUO but is used to provide a screening tool that patients themselves can monitor.

c. **Staging of NDI using EMUO** (i.e. after 12–14 h water restriction)

Normal: > 850   mOsm/kg of H_2O

Partial NDI: 300–850 mOsm/kg of H_2O

NDI: < 300   mOsm/kg of H_2O

d. **Distinguishing NDI from psychogenic polydipsia:** Patients with lithium related NDI will drink as much water as is needed to maintain homeostasis. The evidence for this is that serum sodium and osmolality remain in the normal range unless the patient is deprived of adequate access to free water, in which case they become dehydrated and eventually hypernatremic. Importantly, patients with lithium related NDI do not experience fluctuations in weight throughout the day. Patients with psychogenic polydipsia are a subset of severely mentally ill patients typically with treatment resistant schizophrenia spectrum disorders who drink excessive quantities and therefore can gain 5 kg or more over short periods of time after water binges [104]. During water binge episodes, the serum sodium will also drop substantially, as will serum osmolality [105].

	Urine osmolality	Serum osmolality	Serum sodium	Marked diurnal weight changes
NDI	Low	Normal	Normal	Absent
Psychogenic polydipsia	Low	Low during periods of water intoxication	Low during periods of water intoxication	Present

Table 2.5 General population values by gender for spot urine osmolality from a large US study of subjects aged 12–80 (2009–2012) [102]

	Age 12–18	Age 19–50	Age 51–70	Age 71–80
Male	(n = 978)	(n = 2703)	(n = 1551)	(n = 713)
Mean BMI (kg/m²)	23.1	27.7	28.8	27.6
Mean eGFR (ml/min/1.73 m²)	135.8	102.3	81.5	62.5
Mean urine osm (mOsm/kg)	721	618	566	550
Female	(n = 882)	(n = 2849)	(n = 1526)	(n = 722)
Mean BMI (kg/m²)	22.9	27.6	28.7	27.7
Mean eGFR (ml/min/1.73 m²)	128.3	106.3	82.9	60.9
Mean urine osm (mOsm/kg)	621	522	455	456

BMI = body mass index; eGFR = estimated glomerular filtration rate

(Adapted from: J. D. Stookey [2019]. Analysis of 2009–2012 Nutrition Health and Examination Survey (NHANES) data to estimate the median water intake associated with meeting hydration criteria for individuals aged 12–80 in the US population. *Nutrients*, 11, 657–700.)

3   *Albumin-to-Creatinine Ratio (ACR)*

As mentioned frequently in this chapter, lithium is rarely associated with glomerular pathology that results in significant proteinuria [11]; however, lithium treated patients represent a group with a high prevalence of CKD risk factors (e.g. hypertension, diabetes mellitus) strongly associated with glomerular pathology [32]. The most sensitive and specific laboratory measure to track this problem is not a dipstick for urine protein or an estimate from urinalysis but the ACR (Info Box 2.5).

The ACR can be obtained from a spot urine specimen (Table 2.5); an early morning specimen is preferable but not as crucial as for urine osmolality. Many patients with SMI receive inadequate general medical care [47], so routine ACR monitoring by the mental health clinician when indicated can alert the patient and other providers that the ACR stage has progressed beyond A1, and that more attention must be focused on management of medical comorbidities related to CKD risk. The development of stage A2 albuminuria also serves as means to reinforce with patients and clinicians the concept that albuminuria is not a common lithium related adverse effect.

Info Box 2.5 Basic Concepts in Measuring Renal Function: Assessing the Urine Albumin-to-Creatinine Ratio (ACR)

a. What is the importance of albuminuria?

The loss of albumin into urine (albuminuria) reflects damage to the barrier functions of the glomerular capillary wall, and is thus an important marker of proximal renal dysfunction. Although lithium itself is rarely a cause of significant glomerular pathology and proteinuria [11], increases in albuminuria can be seen in the earlier stages of diabetes, hypertension and specific other causes of glomerular disease, or in the late stages of almost all causes of kidney disease regardless of the underlying etiology (inflammation, infiltration or fibrosis) [32].

b. How does one measure albuminuria?

Current guidelines recommend screening for albuminuria using the ACR calculated from a spot urine sample (although an early morning sample is preferred). The ACR test can be ordered as: **albumin/creatinine ratio (random urine)**. Asking outpatients not to void in the morning until a specimen can be provided at a lab is not practical. For convenience, a sample container should be given to the outpatient by office personnel (or the laboratory) to take home. The specimen is provided whenever the patient arises in the morning. The sample need not be delivered immediately to the laboratory, as ACR results are stable in specimens kept at room temperature for up to 7 days. If not available due to expense, one could use a urine protein-to-creatinine ratio or urine dipstick protein along with estimating equations to convert the results to ACR values; however, the accuracy of those methods is quite limited at low urinary protein concentrations [32].

c. What are the normal values and stages of albuminuria using ACR? [19]

Albuminuria staging from an early morning urine specimen:

- A1 (Normal to mildly increased)   ACR   < 30 mg/g
- A2 (Moderately increased)   ACR   30–300 mg/g
- A3 (Severely increased)   ACR   > 300 mg/g

4   *Staging Renal Dysfunction*

The staging of CKD is based on both eGFR and ACR values, with charts created to combine these results into risk categories (Info Box 2.6) [19, 32]. These categories not only provide prognostic information; ideally, they should drive improvements in medical care to change the trajectory of CKD progression. With respect to lithium prescribing, alterations in eGFR or ACR stages also inform the frequency of monitoring and when to obtain nephrology consultation (see Section E and Info Box 2.7). Most of the decision-making regarding the safety of continuing lithium will be based on eGFR, yet medical comorbidities may accelerate progression of ACR stages and complicate treatment. Documentation of CKD risk should always include the eGFR value itself, along with the eGFR and ACR stage. For example: CKD risk factors low, eGFR 71 ml/min, G2, A1. By noting the exact eGFR, clinicians will more easily associate the value with the appropriate eGFR stage, while including ACR information is a reminder that this patient population carries non-lithium related CKD risks that must be watched.

5   *Screening for and Diagnosis of NDI*

The early pathology from lithium exposure relates to excessive intracellular lithium levels in collecting duct principal cells, clinically manifested as changes in EMUO, polyuria complaints or both. Moreover, polyuria is an adverse effect that substantially increases the likelihood that a patient will discontinue lithium [21]. The prevalence of symptomatic polyuria is reported to be < 30% and perhaps < 20% [9, 10, 41, 42]; however, patients may underreport polyuria to clinicians. In one exploratory study, 56 BD patients on long-term lithium treatment underwent a 24 h urine collection and were interviewed about their experience with polyuria [41]. Polyuria (24 h urine volume > 3 liters) was found in 70% of subjects, but only 51% had complained about increased urinary frequency, and only 59% complained about the volume of urine, even though 90% noted that this adverse effect was distressing and often caused interference with work or daily routine [41]. Routine direct inquiry into the extent and impact of polyuria is crucial to developing patient rapport and for addressing the functional and renal sequelae of this problem.

CKD definition: An abnormality in kidney structure or function persisting > 3 months and including one or more of the following: (1) eGFR < 60 ml/min/1.73 m^2; (2) albuminuria (i.e. urine albumin ≥ 30 mg/24 h, or urine ACR ≥ 30 mg/g); (3) abnormalities in urine sediment, histology or imaging suggestive of kidney damage; (4) renal tubular disorders; or (5) history of kidney transplantation.

Risk categories using combined staging from eGFR and ACR values: These reflect risk of progression defined by a decline in the GFR category (accompanied by ≥ 25% decrease in eGFR from baseline) or a sustained decline in eGFR > 5 ml/min per year.

eGFR categories (units in ml/min/m^2)		Albuminuria categories		
		A1 < 30 mg/g (normal to mildly increased)	A2 30–300 mg/g (moderately increased)	A3 > 300 mg/g (severely increased)
G1 Normal or high	≥ 90			
G2 Mildly decreased	60–89			
G3a Mildly to moderately decreased	45–59			
G3b Moderately to severely decreased	30–44			
G4 Severely decreased	15–29			
G5 Kidney failure	< 15			

Green = low risk (if no other markers of kidney disease and no CKD)

Yellow = moderately increased risk

Orange = high risk

Red = very high risk

To address the question of which office and laboratory based screening tools most practically identify lithium related polyuria, investigators in Dublin, Ireland recruited 179 lithium treated patients from two centers to complete a battery of tests [22]. The subjects had mean age 57 ± 15 years, were 58% F, and had mean duration of lithium use 13 ± 10 years (range 0.3–47 years). Study subjects were asked to perform a 24 h urine collection and an EMUO; to complete multiple questionnaires on polyuria, polydipsia and nocturia; and also to perform a 24 h FIR. Dialysis patients are often asked to self-monitor fluid intake to prevent volume overload, but this was the first study to examine the correlation between 24 h FIR and polyuria measures in lithium treated patients [22]. Only 68% of the sample were able to perform the 24 h urine collection, and 79 subjects completed all of the assessments. The prevalence of polyuria (24 h urine volume > 3 liters) was 35% in this sample. As shown in Figure 2.4a, EMUO values did correlate with polyuria: an EMUO < 300 mOsm/kg was associated with almost a 4-fold increased risk of having polyuria (likelihood ratio [LR] 3.6), and all patients with polyuria had EMUO values under 600 mOsm/kg [22]. Nonetheless, the inconsistent relationship between EMUO and polyuria for individual patients implies that reliance on EMUO alone might overlook this problem in certain persons. The relationship between 24 h FIR and polyuria was also very instructive. Subjects with 24 h FIR values < 2000 ml had a very low likelihood of polyuria (LR 0.18), while those with 24 h FIR > 3500 ml had 6-fold higher risk (LR 6.1) (Figure 2.4b). As seen in Figure 2.4b, while there was a broad range of 24 h FIR values in those diagnosed with polyuria, those without polyuria rarely had fluid intake that exceeded 3 liters/24 h [22].

The results of the Dublin study reveal the need to ask routinely about polyuria at each visit, and more specifically to use the 24 h FIR as a tool that clinician and patient alike can employ to quantify the nature of this complaint, with periodic use of EMUO to provide additional information. When commencing lithium, all patients should be educated about the need to report polyuria complaints, and instructed to perform the 24 h FIR periodically. Since fluid intake may vary day to day, obtaining FIR results over 48 h (two separate 24 h days) and averaging the results may improve accuracy. Given both the ease and value of the 24 h FIR, this should be performed every 2 months during lithium titration and the first year of treatment, especially if routine inquiry reveals a polyuria complaint. As noted in Info Box 2.7, FIR frequency can be reduced to every 6 months over time. EMUO is the laboratory measure used to track response to amiloride treatment for NDI, but patients themselves can also measure their progress on amiloride as changes in 24 h FIR if desired [7, 23]. EMUO need not be obtained at baseline in all individuals,

Figures 2.4a and 2.4b The relationship between lithium related polyuria and early morning urine osmolality (EMUO) (Figure 2.4a) or the 24 h fluid intake record (FIR) (Figure 2.4b) [22]

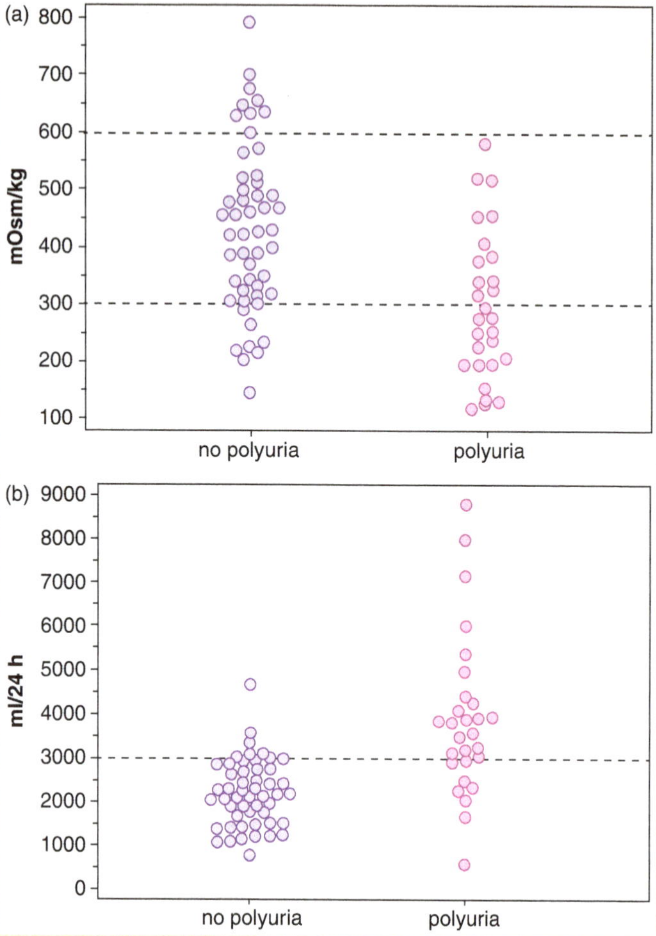

(Adapted from: J. C. Kinahan, A. NiChorcorain, S. Cunningham, et al. (2015). Diagnostic accuracy of tests for polyuria in lithium-treated patients. *J Clin Psychopharmacol*, 35, 434–441.)

but consideration should be given to a baseline EMUO in those > 50 years of age due to age-related declines in concentrating ability [102]. EMUO must be obtained every 6 months in those with polyuria/polydipsia complaints, in those on amiloride treatment, or in patients with an EMUO ≤ 850 mOsm/kg as verified by a repeat specimen. An EMUO every 3 months is reserved for increased or new complaints of polyuria, when titrating amiloride (or adjunctive acetazolamide) to manage polyuria, or for urine osmolality values < 300 mOsm/kg. To facilitate obtaining an accurate result, specimen cups should be given to outpatients in the office or by the laboratory so they can obtain the EMUO specimen in the morning upon arising. The specimen can be delivered at their leisure to the laboratory. No special storage is needed as the EMUO result will remain stable in specimens kept at room temperature for up to 5 days [103]. Monitoring polyuria is thus relatively easy, noninvasive and relies heavily on asking the patient about the problem and periodically totaling their 24 h fluid intake. The combination of 24 h FIR and EMUO thus represent powerful and inexpensive means to manage this important issue.

E A Proposed Renal Monitoring Scheme and the Rationale

WHAT TO KNOW: RENAL FUNCTION MONITORING

- A part of monitoring renal health involves periodic review of a patient's medical history to explore new or worsening CKD risk factors, and to look at the use of nephrotoxic medications.
- The frequency of eGFR monitoring depends on the CKD stage.
- Use of ACR depends on the CKD stage and presence of medical risks for albuminuria.
- 24 h FIR and EMUO are easy-to-use and effective tools to assess the extent of polyuria. 24 h urine collections are not necessary, and are inconvenient for the patient.

Nearly every country and international society has a suggested renal monitoring protocol during lithium therapy, and a 2018 international survey of 177 health-care professionals from 24 countries found that 74% of lithium prescribers follow an institutional protocol or published guideline [106]. The greatest recent change is the recognition that ACR should be obtained in those with CKD risks to detect proximal renal dysfunction from medical disorders, and that systematic inquiry for polyuria complaints and monitoring of urine osmolality deserve as much attention as eGFR [10]. In particular, it is now appreciated that lithium's entry into collecting duct principal cells via ENaC and the resultant GSK3-β inhibition are pivotal processes in lithium related kidney dysfunction. Moreover, as the earliest manifestation of this pathology is a urine concentration deficit, the monitoring scheme in Info Box 2.7 strongly emphasizes frequent early screening for NDI, and attentive EMUO monitoring when values slip into the abnormal range ≤ 850 mOsm/kg. Urine osmolality should exceed 850 mOsm/kg after 12–14 hours of water deprivation – **the inability of the kidney to perform this function adequately is a call to clinical action**. Nephrologists with expertise on the sequelae of high intracellular collecting duct lithium levels note that use of the ENaC-blocking diuretic amiloride is particularly effective when the concentrating deficit is mild to moderate [61], with experimental evidence demonstrating that amiloride can limit further progression of fibrosis in a rodent model [16]. Whether amiloride can prevent the long-term adverse effects of lithium is unknown, but there is intense interest in the question of whether amiloride should be used prophylactically in all lithium treated patients [39]. The recommendation for EMUO in lieu of 24 h urine collection is a conscious decision to use a method with superior feasibility, especially when repeated urine osmolality samples might be needed during amiloride titration. Moreover, in the Dublin polyuria study, all patients with polyuria had EMUO values under 600 mOsm/kg, and the combination of 24 h FIR with EMUO provided complementary information to assess the extent of the problem [22]. Lastly, there is no established benefit from obtaining routine MRI scans for microcystic disease, and no evidence that the performance of a renal biopsy changes clinical outcomes with lithium induced kidney dysfunction [61]. The need for any imaging, 24 h urine collection or renal biopsy is a decision to be made by a nephrologist, and typically will relate to the suspicion of other renal pathologies. Comfort with use of eGFR (especially the new eGFR$_{cr-cys}$ equation), ACR, 24 h FIR and EMUO provide all who prescribe lithium the essential tools to oversee the renal parameters of treatment.

Info Box 2.7 Routine Monitoring of Renal Parameters

a. Initial

   i. History: Note any prior personal or family history of renal dysfunction, and record risk factors for renal dysfunction (e.g. cardiovascular disease, dyslipidemia, metabolic syndrome or diabetes mellitus, hypertension, smoking). Note use of nephrotoxic medications or those with lithium interactions.

   ii. eGFR: Obtain a baseline eGFR to determine both the safety and feasibility of starting lithium. (See Chapter 4, Section B, for a discussion of the minimum acceptable eGFR for initiating lithium.)

Urinalysis is neither a sensitive nor specific screening tool for lithium related renal dysfunction. An early morning urine specimen osmolality (EMUO) is not necessary at baseline, but encouraged among older patients (age > 50 years) due to age-related declines in urine osmolality.

iii. **Albumin-to-creatinine ratio (ACR):** For those with a history of eGFR values < 90 ml/min, or risk factors for renal dysfunction (e.g. cardiovascular disease, metabolic syndrome or diabetes mellitus, hypertension, smoking), add an early morning urine specimen for albumin-to-creatinine ratio (ACR).

b. **Monitoring for the first 6 months of lithium treatment**

	6 weeks	3 months	18 weeks	6 months
eGFR (baseline eGFR ≥ 60 ml/min)	✓	✓		✓
eGFR (baseline eGFR 45–59 ml/min)	✓	✓	✓	✓
24 h FIR	✓	✓		✓
EMUO	✓	✓		✓
ACR		✓		✓

Notes

a. eGFR: After 6 months, monitoring frequency depends on CKD stage.

b. 24 h FIR: Ask the patient to record fluid intake for two separate days and average the result.

c. EMUO: Should also be added following a new complaint of polyuria/polydipsia.

d. ACR: At 3 months and 6 months for those with baseline eGFR < 90 ml/min **or** risk factors for renal dysfunction. After 6 months, the monitoring frequency depends on the ACR stage.

c. **Routine monitoring every 6 months during established lithium therapy**

i. Review medical history for renal dysfunction risk factors and use of nephrotoxic medications.

ii. eGFR

iii. 24 h FIR: Ask the patient to record fluid intake for two separate days and average the result.

iv. EMUO: For those with polyuria complaints, on stable amiloride treatment, or for patients whose most recent EMUO value is ≤ 850 mOsm/kg as verified by a repeat specimen.

v. ACR: For those with eGFR < 90 ml/min **or** risk factors for renal dysfunction as noted in the history.

d. Increase frequency of labs to every 3 months during established lithium therapy when one of the following are present: (higher-risk patients)

  i. eGFR value: When values are < 60 ml/min.

  ii. eGFR trends: Initial evidence of a decline in eGFR > 2 ml/min over 6 months or > 4 ml/min over 12 months as verified by a repeat specimen.

  iii. EMUO: For increased or new complaints of polyuria, when titrating amiloride (or adjunctive acetazolamide) to manage polyuria, or for urine osmolality values < 300 mOsm/kg.

  iv. ACR: If ACR has progressed from stage A1 to A2 as verified by a repeat specimen.

e. When to consult a nephrologist

  i. eGFR: Second decline in eGFR > 2 ml/min over 6 months or > 4 ml/min over 12 months as verified by a repeat specimen.

  ii. eGFR < 45 ml/min as verified by a repeat specimen.

  iii. ACR: Stage A3.

  iv. NDI (EMUO values < 300 mOsm/kg) unresponsive to maximal doses of amiloride (10 mg BID) plus adjunctive use of acetazolamide (up to 500 mg BID) for 6 weeks.

  v. Hematuria

Summary Points

a. Much of the renal risk attributed to lithium treatment relates to two factors: past practices that induced more renal dysfunction (e.g. multiple daily dosing, allowing 12 h trough maintenance levels to exceed 1.20 mEq/l); and CKD risks such as hypertension that are highly prevalent in the target patient population.

b. The standard laboratory measure of intrinsic renal function is the eGFR. Clinicians should understand CKD staging by eGFR, the new creatinine–cystatin C based eGFR formula, and the need to monitor albuminuria using the albumin-to-creatinine ratio (ACR). Lithium is not a common cause of proximal renal pathology manifested as proteinuria, but other CKD risk factors (e.g. hypertension, metabolic syndrome, diabetes mellitus) are associated with albuminuria.

c. Most of the filtered lithium is reabsorbed proximally in the glomerulus via the Na^+/H^+ exchanger-3 (NHE3) present on the apical surfaces of epithelial cells. States that induce hyponatremia thus present a risk for lithium toxicity as lithium will be preferentially absorbed via NHE3.

d. Clinicians should appreciate that lithium's primary site of early renal pathology is related to its entry into collecting duct principal cells via the ENaC. The clinical manifestation of this is a urinary concentration deficit, hence the importance of using early morning urine osmolality (EMUO) to screen for this problem routinely, along with regular inquiry about polyuria during office visits and use of the 24 h FIR to look for excessive fluid intake. The potassium sparing diuretic amiloride is a selective ENaC antagonist and the primary tool used to block lithium's entry into principal duct cells and thereby improve the kidney's urine concentrating ability.

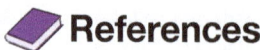

References

1. Schou, M. (1989). [Long-term treatment with lithium and renal function: A review and reappraisal. *Encephale*, 15, 437–442.

2. Aiff, H., Attman, P.-O., Aurell, M., et al. (2014). The impact of modern treatment principles may have eliminated lithium-induced renal failure. *J Psychopharmacol*, 28, 151–154.

3. Kirkham, E., Skinner, J., Anderson, T., et al. (2014). One lithium level > 1.0 mmol/L causes an acute decline in eGFR: Findings from a retrospective analysis of a monitoring database. *BMJ Open*, 4, e006020.

4. Castro, V. M., Roberson, A. M., McCoy, T. H., et al. (2016). Stratifying risk for renal insufficiency among lithium-treated patients: An electronic health record study. *Neuropsychopharmacol*, 41, 1138–1143.

5. Kessing, L. V., Gerds, T. A., Feldt-Rasmussen, B., et al. (2015). Use of lithium and anticonvulsants and the rate of chronic kidney disease: A nationwide population-based study. *JAMA Psychiatry*, 72, 1182–1191.

6. Clos, S., Rauchhaus, P., Severn, A., et al. (2015). Long-term effect of lithium maintenance therapy on estimated glomerular filtration rate in patients with affective disorders: A population-based cohort study. *Lancet Psychiatry*, 2, 1075–1083.

7. Dastych, M., Synek, O. and Gottwaldova, J. (2019). Impact of long-term lithium treatment on renal function in patients with bipolar disorder based on novel biomarkers. *J Clin Psychopharmacol*, 39, 238–242.

8. Bisogni, V., Rossitto, G., Reghin, F., et al. (2016). Antihypertensive therapy in patients on chronic lithium treatment for bipolar disorders. *J Hypertens*, 34, 20–28.

9. Alsady, M., Baumgarten, R., Deen, P. M., et al. (2016). Lithium in the kidney: Friend and foe? *J Am Soc Nephrol*, 27, 1587–1595.

10. Schoot, T. S., Molmans, T. H. J., Grootens, K. P., et al. (2020). Systematic review and practical guideline for the prevention and management of the renal side effects of lithium therapy. *Eur Neuropsychopharmacol*, 31, 16–32.

11. Łukawska, E., Frankiewicz, D., Izak, M., et al. (2021). Lithium toxicity and the kidney with special focus on nephrotic syndrome associated with the acute kidney injury: A case-based systematic analysis. *J Appl Toxicol*, 41, 1896–1909.

12. Kortenoeven, M. L., Li, Y., Shaw, S., et al. (2009). Amiloride blocks lithium entry through the sodium channel thereby attenuating the resultant nephrogenic diabetes insipidus. *Kidney Int*, 76, 44–53.

13. Kalita-De Croft, P., Bedford, J. J., Leader, J. P., et al. (2018). Amiloride modifies the progression of lithium-induced renal interstitial fibrosis. *Nephrology (Carlton)*, 23, 20–30.

14. Vallée, C., Howlin, B. and Lewis, R. (2021). Ion selectivity in the ENaC/DEG family: A systematic review with supporting analysis. *Int J Mol Sci*, 22. doi: 10.3390/ijms222010998.

15. Vandenbeuch, A. and Kinnamon, S. C. (2020). Is the amiloride-sensitive Na+ channel in taste cells really ENaC? *Chem Senses*, 45, 233–234.

16. Davis, J., Desmond, M. and Berk, M. (2018). Lithium and nephrotoxicity: Unravelling the complex pathophysiological threads of the lightest metal. *Nephrology (Carlton)*, 23, 897–903.

17. Bedford, J. J., Weggery, S., Ellis, G., et al. (2008). Lithium-induced nephrogenic diabetes insipidus: Renal effects of amiloride. *Clin J Am Soc Nephrol*, 3, 1324–1331.

18. Macau, R. A., da Silva, T. N., Silva, J. R., et al. (2018). Use of acetazolamide in lithium-induced nephrogenic diabetes insipidus: A case report. *Endocrinol Diabetes Metab Case Rep*, doi: 10.1530/EDM-17-0154.

19. Chen, T. K., Knicely, D. H. and Grams, M. E. (2019). Chronic kidney disease diagnosis and management: A review. *JAMA*, 322, 1294–1304.

20. Inker, L. A., Eneanya, N. D., Coresh, J., et al. (2021). New creatinine- and cystatin C-based equations to estimate GFR without race. *N Engl J Med*, 385, 1737–1749.

21. Öhlund, L., Ott, M., Oja, S., et al. (2018). Reasons for lithium discontinuation in men and women with bipolar disorder: A retrospective cohort study. *BMC Psychiatry*, 18, 37–46.

22. Kinahan, J. C., NiChorcorain, A., Cunningham, S., et al. (2015). Diagnostic accuracy of tests for polyuria in lithium-treated patients. *J Clin Psychopharmacol*, 35, 434–441.

23. Kinahan, J. C., Ni Chorcorain, A., Cunningham, S., et al. (2022). Managing polyuria during lithium treatment: A preliminary prospective observational study. *Ir J Psychol Med*, 39, 20–27.

24. Koomans, H. A., Boer, W. H. and Dorhout Mees, E. J. (1989). Evaluation of lithium clearance as a marker of proximal tubule sodium handling. *Kidney Int*, 36, 2–12.

25. Thomsen, K. and Shirley, D. G. (2006). A hypothesis linking sodium and lithium reabsorption in the distal nephron. *Nephrol Dial Transplant*, 21, 869–880.

26. Jackson, E. K. (2018). Drugs affecting renal excretory function. In L. L. Brunton, R. Hilal-Dandan and B. C. Knollmann, eds., *Goodman & Gilman's The Pharmacological Basis of Therapeutics*, 13th Edition. Chicago: McGraw-Hill, pp. 445–470.

27. Meyer, J. M. (2022). Pharmacotherapy of psychosis and mania. In L. L. Brunton and B. C. Knollmann, eds., *Goodman & Gilman's The Pharmacological Basis of Therapeutics*, 14th Edition. Chicago: McGraw-Hill, pp.357–384.

28. Giebisch, G., Windhager, E. H. and Aronson, P. S. (2017). Glomerular filtration and renal blood flow. In W. F. Boron and E. L. Boulpaep, eds., *Medical Physiology: A Cellular and Molecular Approach*, 3rd Edition. Philadelphia, PA: Elsevier, pp. 739–753.

29. Atherton, J. C., Doyle, A., Gee, A., et al. (1991). Lithium clearance: Modification by the loop of Henle in man. *J Physiol*, 437, 377–391.

30. Fransen, R., Boer, W. H., Boer, P., et al. (1993). Effects of furosemide or acetazolamide infusion on renal handling of lithium: A micropuncture study in rats. *Am J Physiol*, 264, R129–134.

31. Gimenez, I. (2006). Molecular mechanisms and regulation of furosemide-sensitive Na-K-Cl cotransporters. *Curr Opin Nephrol Hypertens*, 15, 517–523.

32. Levey, A. S., Grams, M. E. and Inker, L. A. (2022). Uses of GFR and albuminuria level in acute and chronic kidney disease. *N Engl J Med*, 386, 2120–2128.

33. De Vriese, A. S., Sethi, S., Nath, K. A., et al. (2018). Differentiating primary, genetic, and secondary FSGS in adults: A clinicopathologic approach. *J Am Soc Nephrol*, 29, 759–774.

34. Nyengaard, J. R., Bendtsen, T. F., Christensen, S., et al. (1994). The number and size of glomeruli in long-term lithium-induced nephropathy in rats. *Apmis*, 102, 59–66.

35. Min, G., Christensen, S., Marcussen, N., et al. (2000). Glomerular structure in lithium-induced chronic renal failure in rats. *Apmis*, 108, 652–662.

36. de Groot, T., Doty, R., Damen, L., et al. (2021). Genetic background determines renal response to chronic lithium treatment in female mice. *Physiol Genomics*, 53, 406–415.

37. Markowitz, G. S., Radhakrishnan, J., Kambham, N., et al. (2000). Lithium nephrotoxicity: A progressive combined glomerular and tubulointerstitial nephropathy. *J Am Soc Nephrol*, 11, 1439–1448.

38. Walker, R. J., Leader, J. P., Bedford, J. J., et al. (2013). Chronic interstitial fibrosis in the rat kidney induced by long-term (6-mo) exposure to lithium. *Am J Physiol Renal Physiol*, 304, F300–307.

39. Grünfeld, J.-P. and Rossier, B. C. (2009). Lithium nephrotoxicity revisited. *Nat Rev Nephrol*, 5, 270–276.

40. Kwon, T. H., Laursen, U. H., Marples, D., et al. (2000). Altered expression of renal AQPs and Na(+) transporters in rats with lithium-induced NDI. *Am J Physiol Renal Physiol*, 279, F552–564.

41. Pradhan, B. K., Chakrabarti, S., Irpati, A. S., et al. (2011). Distress due to lithium-induced polyuria: Exploratory study. *Psychiatry Clin Neurosci*, 65, 386–388.

42. Rej, S., Segal, M., Low, N. C., et al. (2014). The McGill Geriatric Lithium-Induced Diabetes Insipidus Clinical Study (McGLIDICS). *Can J Psychiatry*, 59, 327–334.

43. Schou, M., Amdisen, A., Thomsen, K., et al. (1982). Lithium treatment regimen and renal water handling: The significance of dosage pattern and tablet type examined through comparison of results from two clinics with different treatment regimens. *Psychopharmacology*, 77, 387–390.

44. Meyer, J. M. and Nasrallah, H. A., eds. (2009). *Medical Illness and Schizophrenia*, 2nd Edition. Washington, DC: American Psychiatric Press, Inc.

45. McElroy, S. L. and Keck, P. E., Jr. (2014). Metabolic syndrome in bipolar disorder: A review with a focus on bipolar depression. *J Clin Psychiatry*, 75, 46–61.

46. Hayes, J. F., Marston, L., Walters, K., et al. (2017). Mortality gap for people with bipolar disorder and schizophrenia: UK-based cohort study 2000–2014. *Br J Psychiatry*, 211, 175–181.

47. Lurie, I., Shoval, G., Hoshen, M., et al. (2021). The association of medical resource utilization with physical morbidity and premature mortality among patients with schizophrenia: An historical prospective population cohort study. *Schizophr Res*, 237, 62–68.

48. Lepkifker, E., Sverdlik, A., Iancu, I., et al. (2004). Renal insufficiency in long-term lithium treatment. *J Clin Psychiatry*, 63, 850–856.

49. Tondo, L., Abramowicz, M., Alda, M., et al. (2017). Long-term lithium treatment in bipolar disorder: Effects on glomerular filtration rate and other metabolic parameters. *Int J Bipolar Disord*, 5, 27.

50. Presne, C., Fakhouri, F., Noel, L. H., et al. (2003). Lithium-induced nephropathy: Rate of progression and prognostic factors. *Kidney Int*, 64, 585–592.

51. Aiff, H., Attman, P.-O., Aurell, M., et al. (2015). Effects of 10 to 30 years of lithium treatment on kidney function. *J Psychopharmacol*, 29, 608–614.

52. Golic, M., Aiff, H., Attman, P. O., et al. (2018). Compliance with the safety guidelines for long-term lithium treatment in Sweden. *J Psychopharmacol*, 32, 1104–1109.

53. Werneke, U., Ott, M., Renberg, E. S., et al. (2012). A decision analysis of long-term lithium treatment and the risk of renal failure. *Acta Psychiatr Scand*, 126, 186–197.

54. Wingård, L., Brandt, L., Bodén, R., et al. (2019). Monotherapy vs. combination therapy for post mania maintenance treatment: A population based cohort study. *Eur Neuropsychopharmacol*, 29, 691–700.

55. Tuazon, J., Casalino, D., Syed, E., et al. (2008). Lithium-associated kidney microcysts. *Scientific World Journal*, 8, 828–829.

56. Slaughter, A., Pandey, T. and Jambhekar, K. (2010). MRI findings in chronic lithium nephropathy: A case report. *J Radiol Case Rep*, 4, 15–21.

57. Jończyk-Potoczna, K., Abramowicz, M., Chłopocka-Woźniak, M., et al. (2016). Renal sonography in bipolar patients on long-term lithium treatment. *J Clin Ultrasound*, 44, 354–359.

58. Tabibzadeh, N., Faucon, A. L., Vidal-Petiot, E., et al. (2021). Determinants of kidney function and accuracy of kidney microcysts detection in patients treated with lithium salts for bipolar disorder. *Front Pharmacol*, 12, 1–12.

59. Golshayan, D., Nseir, G., Venetz, J. P., et al. (2012). MR imaging as a specific diagnostic tool for bilateral microcysts in chronic lithium nephropathy. *Kidney Int*, 81, 601.

60. Farshchian, N., Farnia, V., Aghaiani, M. R., et al. (2013). MRI findings and renal function in patients on lithium therapy. *Curr Drug Saf*, 8, 257–260.

61. Davis, J., Desmond, M. and Berk, M. (2018). Lithium and nephrotoxicity: A literature review of approaches to clinical management and risk stratification. *BMC Nephrol*, 19, 305.

62. Gahr, M., Wezel, F., Bolenz, C., et al. (2019). Lithium therapy associated with renal and upper and lower urinary tract tumors: Results from a retrospective single-center analysis. *J Clin Psychopharmacol*, 39, 530–532.

63. Rookmaaker, M. B., van Gerven, H. A., Goldschmeding, R., et al. (2012). Solid renal tumours of collecting duct origin in patients on chronic lithium therapy. *Clin Kidney J*, 5, 412–415.

64. Zaidan, M., Stucker, F., Stengel, B., et al. (2014). Increased risk of solid renal tumors in lithium-treated patients. *Kidney Int*, 86, 184–190.

65. Cohen, Y., Chetrit, A., Cohen, Y., et al. (1998). Cancer morbidity in psychiatric patients: Influence of lithium carbonate treatment. *Med Oncol*, 15, 32–36.

66. Licht, R. W., Grabenhenrich, L. B., Nielsen, R. E., et al. (2014). Lithium and renal tumors: A critical comment to the report by Zaidan et al. *Kidney Int*, 86, 857.

67. Kessing, L. V., Gerds, T. A., Feldt-Rasmussen, B., et al. (2015). Lithium and renal and upper urinary tract tumors – results from a nationwide population-based study. *Bipolar Disord*, 17, 805–813.

68. Pottegård, A., Hallas, J., Jensen, B. L., et al. (2016). Long-term lithium use and risk of renal and upper urinary tract cancers. *J Am Soc Nephrol*, 27, 249–255.

69. Martinsson, L., Westman, J., Hallgren, J., et al. (2016). Lithium treatment and cancer incidence in bipolar disorder. *Bipolar Disord*, 18, 33–40.

70. Huang, R. Y., Hsieh, K. P., Huang, W. W., et al. (2016). Use of lithium and cancer risk in patients with bipolar disorder: Population-based cohort study. *Br J Psychiatry*, 209, 393–399.

71. Anmella, G., Fico, G., Lotfaliany, M., et al. (2021). Risk of cancer in bipolar disorder and the potential role of lithium: International collaborative systematic review and meta-analyses. *Neurosci Biobehav Rev*, 126, 529–541.

72. Plenge, P., Mellerup, E. T., Bolwig, T. G., et al. (1982). Lithium treatment: Does the kidney prefer one daily dose instead of two? *Acta Psychiatr Scand*, 66, 121–128.

73. Carter, L., Zolezzi, M. and Lewczyk, A. (2013). An updated review of the optimal lithium dosage regimen for renal protection. *Can J Psychiatry*, 58, 595–600.

74. Amdisen, A. (1977). Serum level monitoring and clinical pharmacokinetics of lithium. *Clin Pharmacokinet*, 2, 73–92.

75. Greil, W. (1981). [Pharmacokinetics and toxicology of lithium]. *Bibl Psychiatr*, 161, 69–103.

76. Swartz, C. M. (1987). Correction of lithium levels for dose and blood sampling times. *J Clin Psychiatry*, 48, 60–64.

77. Kusalic, M. and Engelsmann, F. (1996). Renal reactions to changes of lithium dosage. *Neuropsychobiology*, 34, 113–116.

78. Nolen, W. A., Licht, R. W., Young, A. H., et al. (2019). What is the optimal serum level for lithium in the maintenance treatment of bipolar disorder? A systematic review and recommendations from the ISBD/IGSLI Task Force on treatment with lithium. *Bipolar Disord*, 21, 394–409.

79. Shaddock, R., Anderson, K. V. and Beyth, R. (2020). Renal repercussions of medications. *Prim Care*, 47, 691–702.

80. Ruffenach, S. J., Siskind, M. S. and Lien, Y. H. (1992). Acute interstitial nephritis due to omeprazole. *Am J Med*, 93, 472–473.

81. Wei, X., Yu, J., Xu, Z., et al. (2022). Incidence, pathogenesis, and management of proton pump inhibitor-induced nephrotoxicity. *Drug Saf*, 45, 703–712.

82. Lazarus, B., Chen, Y., Wilson, F. P., et al. (2016). Proton pump inhibitor use and the risk of chronic kidney disease. *JAMA Intern Med*, 176, 238–246.

83. Al-Aly, Z., Maddukuri, G. and Xie, Y. (2020). Proton pump inhibitors and the kidney: Implications of current evidence for clinical practice and when and how to deprescribe. *Am J Kidney Dis*, 75, 497–507.

84. Attridge, R. L., Frei, C. R., Ryan, L., et al. (2013). Fenofibrate-associated nephrotoxicity: A review of current evidence. *Am J Health Syst Pharm*, 70, 1219–1225.

85. Zingerman, B., Ziv, D., Feder Krengel, N., et al. (2020). Cessation of bezafibrate in patients with chronic kidney disease improves renal function. *Sci Rep*, 10, 19768.

86. Dohmen, K., Onohara, S. Y. and Harada, S. (2021). Effects of switching from fenofibrate to pemafibrate for asymptomatic primary biliary cholangitis. *Korean J Gastroenterol*, 78, 227–234.

87. Zhang, J., Ji, X., Dong, Z., et al. (2021). Impact of fenofibrate therapy on serum uric acid concentrations: A review and meta-analysis. *Endocr J*, 68, 829–837.

88. Broeders, N., Knoop, C., Antoine, M., et al. (2000). Fibrate-induced increase in blood urea and creatinine: Is gemfibrozil the only innocuous agent? *Nephrol Dial Transplant*, 15, 1993–1999.

89. Gray, M. P., Barreto, E. F., Schreier, D. J., et al. (2022). Consensus obtained for the nephrotoxic potential of 167 drugs in adult critically ill patients using a modified Delphi method. *Drug Saf*, 45, 389–398.

90. Morriss, R. and Benjamin, B. (2008). Lithium and eGFR: A new routinely available tool for the prevention of chronic kidney disease. *Br J Psychiatry*, 193, 93–95.

91. Cockcroft, D. W. and Gault, M. H. (1976). Prediction of creatinine clearance from serum creatinine. *Nephron*, 16, 31–41.

92. Inker, L. A. and Titan, S. (2021). Measurement and estimation of GFR for use in clinical practice: Core curriculum 2021. *Am J Kidney Dis*, 78, 736–749.

93. Meyer, J. M. and Stahl, S. M. (2021). *The Clinical Use of Antipsychotic Plasma Levels* (Stahl's Handbooks). New York: Cambridge University Press.

94. Shannon, J. A. and Smith, H. W. (1935). The excretion of inulin, xylose and urea by normal and phlorizinized man. *J Clin Invest*, 14, 393–401.

95. Eneanya, N. D., Yang, W. and Reese, P. P. (2019). Reconsidering the consequences of using race to estimate kidney function. *JAMA*, 322, 113–114.

96. Diao, J. A., Wu, G. J., Taylor, H. A., et al. (2021). Clinical implications of removing race from estimates of kidney function. *JAMA*, 325, 184–186.

97. Powe, N. R. (2020). Black kidney function matters: Use or misuse of race? *JAMA*, 324, 737–738.

98. Delgado, C., Baweja, M., Crews, D. C., et al. (2021). A unifying approach for GFR estimation: Recommendations of the NKF–ASN Task Force on Reassessing the Inclusion of Race in Diagnosing Kidney Disease. *Am J Kidney Dis*, 79, 268–288.e261.

99. Diao, J. A., Inker, L. A., Levey, A. S., et al. (2021). In search of a better equation – performance and equity in estimates of kidney function. *N Engl J Med*, 384, 396–399.

100. Shlipak, M. G., Inker, L. A. and Coresh, J. (2022). Serum cystatin C for estimation of GFR. *JAMA*, 328, 883–884.

101. Tummalapalli, S. L., Shlipak, M. G., Damster, S., et al. (2020). Availability and affordability of kidney health laboratory tests around the globe. *Am J Nephrol*, 51, 959–965.

102. Stookey, J. D. (2019). Analysis of 2009–2012 Nutrition Health and Examination Survey (NHANES) data to estimate the median water intake associated with meeting hydration criteria for individuals aged 12–80 in the US population. *Nutrients*, 11, 657–700.

103. Sureda-Vives, M., Morell-Garcia, D., Rubio-Alaejos, A., et al. (2017). Stability of serum, plasma and urine osmolality in different storage conditions: Relevance of temperature and centrifugation. *Clin Biochem*, 50, 772–776.

104. Meyer, J. M. and Stahl, S. M. (2019). *The Clozapine Handbook* (Stahl's Handbooks). Cambridge: Cambridge University Press.

105. Goldman, M. B. (2010). The assessment and treatment of water imbalance in patients with psychosis. *Clin Schizophr Relat Psychoses*, 4, 115–123.

106. Nederlof, M., Heerdink, E. R., Egberts, A. C. G., et al. (2018). Monitoring of patients treated with lithium for bipolar disorder: An international survey. *Int J Bipolar Disord*, 6, 12–20.

3

Clinical Pharmacokinetics
Principles Underlying Kinetic and Pharmacodynamic Drug Interactions; Clinically Relevant Drug Interactions and Their Management

 QUICK CHECK

 PRINCIPLES

- Lithium has a central nervous system half-life of at least 24 hours and is preferentially administered as a single bedtime dose. There is no efficacy advantage to multiple daily dosing but greater risk of renal dysfunction. Many patients tolerate standard lithium carbonate, although extended released preparations (also given as a single bedtime dose) can be used to lessen certain adverse effects (e.g. tremor, upper gastrointestinal cramping or nausea) but at the risk of possibly increasing others (e.g. diarrhea).

- Lithium has a peripheral half-life close to 24 hours, but by convention levels are obtained as 12 h trough levels in the morning. Administering lithium as a single dose at odd times (e.g. at 8 am, noon or 4 pm) will make levels obtained the next morning difficult to interpret.

- Multiple daily dosing distorts the trough level, as a significant portion of the dose will have been ingested 18–24 hours before the level was obtained.

- Use of test doses to predict maintenance doses, prediction formulas and loading are all possible considerations to improve on empiric titration (trial and error) and reduce the time to achieving therapeutic levels.

- Renal function is the basic determinant of lithium clearance. Those medications that impact renal blood flow or waste sodium are the primary concerns, although the list is modest. With careful attention to kinetic effects and level monitoring, there are very few medications that cannot be used with lithium.

- Sodium loss from sweating or gastrointestinal illness can induce lithium toxicity when patients hydrate themselves using free water *without electrolytes*. Temperature and strenuous exercise by themselves do not alter lithium clearance. High altitude and pregnancy do influence lithium clearance and require patient education and monitoring.

- At therapeutic levels, lithium has few pharmacodynamic interactions of consequence. Prior concerns about interactions with potent D_2 antagonists were probably an artifact of aggressive antipsychotic dosing in nearly all instances. There is no contraindication to prescribing lithium with any antipsychotic.

Introduction

WHAT TO KNOW: INTRODUCTION

- Historical recommendations to prescribe lithium multiple times per day are outdated, although this information persists in recent product labeling.
- Prescribing lithium once daily at bedtime allows one to obtain reliable 12 h trough values, and also minimizes the long-term risk for renal dysfunction incurred with multiple daily dosing.

As clinical psychopharmacology moves into the twenty-first century, there is an emphasis on rational prescribing practices informed by pharmacokinetic principles and clinical dictates. Publications note that certain oral medications which historically were dosed more than once per day (e.g. most antipsychotics including clozapine) have comparable efficacy with nightly (QHS) dosing for the majority of patients [1–3]. Consolidation of doses is important for patient convenience, and therefore is of importance to the clinician who appreciates that sustained response is highly correlated with oral medication adherence [4]. Even when medications are administered once daily, timing of the dose can influence the onset and severity of adverse effects [5]. There is convincing evidence that QHS antipsychotic dosing improves tolerability as peak central nervous system (CNS) levels that might exceed the tolerability threshold are achieved during sleep. Clinical data from the lurasidone pivotal studies dramatically illustrate this fact: in adult schizophrenia trials, the rate of akathisia for 120 mg given with a morning meal was 20.3%, compared with an akathisia rate of only 6.5% for 160 mg when dosed with an evening meal [6, 7]. Lithium's peripheral and CNS kinetics have been known for over 40 years and argue strongly for once daily dosing; however, like many psychotropics, lithium is a victim of historical dosing patterns that recommended multiple daily administration. Lithium gained its first US approval in April 1970, but modern package inserts still contain language suggesting twice or thrice daily dosing, wording that has changed little in the intervening 50 years despite significant updates to other sections devoted to safety, and despite data indicating that multiple daily dosing is associated with a short-term risk of polyuria and a 20% greater long-term risk for renal insufficiency [8–11]. As international experts have increasingly argued that an optimal maintenance trough level for many bipolar disorder (BD) patients is 0.60–0.80 mEq/l [12], an understanding of lithium's kinetics, and the subtle differences in maximum serum levels (C_{Max}) and time to maximal levels (T_{Max}) between standard and sustained release preparations, is crucial. Clinicians should also have familiarity with the small array of kinetically interacting medications, and those patient and environmental factors that affect lithium levels. The goal is to use kinetic principles to optimize efficacy and minimize adverse effects leading to discontinuation or morbidity. Lithium's efficacy in BD, its unique impact on suicide related mortality and its neuroprotective properties in older BD patients can only be realized by maintaining patients on therapy through kinetically informed rational prescribing.

A Peripheral and Central Nervous System Kinetics

WHAT TO KNOW: PERIPHERAL AND CENTRAL NERVOUS SYSTEM KINETICS

- At steady state, the peripheral half-life ($T_{1/2}$) in adults is 20–24 h and in the brain $T_{1/2}$ 28–48 h. There is no efficacy based reason to dose lithium other than once daily at bedtime in adults.

- Steady state for oral medications is reached after 5 half-lives. Trough levels should be obtained 12 h after the bedtime dose at steady state.

- Twice daily (BID) dosing distorts the trough level because half of the dose was ingested 24 h before the level is drawn the next morning. When a BID dose is converted to a single QHS dose, the 12 h trough level will increase by 28%.
- Sustained release preparations have similar $T_{1/2}$ to standard lithium, but a longer time to maximal levels (T_{Max}), which can mitigate upper gastrointestinal tract side effects such as nausea.
- Lithium citrate has similar kinetics to standard lithium.
- Every clinician should know this equivalence: 300 mg lithium carbonate = 56 mg of elemental lithium = 8 mEq of lithium ion.

The bioavailability of lithium is 80–100% irrespective of whether it is ingested in liquid or tablet form, or whether one uses a standard or sustained release preparation [13–16]. Lithium is rapidly absorbed in the upper gastrointestinal (GI) tract (jejunum and ileum) [17], with a time to maximal levels (T_{Max}) of 1–3 h for standard lithium preparations including lithium citrate, but a longer T_{Max} of 3–6 h for currently available sustained release forms (Info Box 3.1) [14, 15, 18, 19]. As discussed in Section A2 below, sustained release products also have a lower C_{Max}, a property that may be useful for patients with certain tolerability complaints, especially the 10–20% of patients who have nausea from rapid upper GI tract lithium absorption [20]. Food has interesting effects on lithium absorption and on adverse effects. While administering lithium with food does not substantially alter bioavailability, and the C_{Max} is higher with food intake of any composition (e.g. standard meal, high fat, high fat and high protein) [21], it has been known since 1975 that ingestion after a meal minimizes GI adverse effects, especially diarrhea related to rapid passage into the lower GI tract [22]. If use of a sustained release formulation does not resolve GI tolerability problems, ingestion of lithium after a meal should be tried, with the caveat that levels are ideally obtained 12 ± 2 h post-dose.

At steady state, the peripheral half-life ($T_{1/2}$) in adults is 20–24 h and in the brain $T_{1/2}$ 28–48 h [23, 24]. Given the long central nervous system (CNS) $T_{1/2}$ and the concerns that multiple daily dosing is associated with increased renal adverse effects and decreased adherence, lithium administration during maintenance treatment should be at bedtime (QHS) [8, 9, 23]. Bedtime dosing also permits obtaining 12 h trough values more easily [16]. Levels are best drawn at steady state to provide the most accurate picture of lithium exposure; with a peripheral $T_{1/2}$ close to 24 h, steady state is seen in 5 half-lives, or 5 days (Info Box 3.2) [25].

3

Lithium: Peripheral and CNS Kinetics, and Essential Facts

a. Peripheral kinetics [23]

 i. Peripheral T_{Max}: standard 1–3 h; sustained release 4–12 h (varies by preparation, most currently available forms are 3–6 h) [26]

 ii. Peripheral $T_{1/2}$: 20–24 h at steady state

 iii. Effects of food: does not alter bioavailability but sufficiently slows absorption to lessen upper and lower GI side effects (nausea, cramping, diarrhea) [22, 21]

b. CNS kinetics

 i. CNS T_{Max}: delayed approximately 3 h from the serum T_{Max} [27, 28]

 ii. CNS $T_{1/2}$: 28–48 h at steady state [24]

 iii. Brain-to-serum (BTS) ratio: steady state brain levels correlate with serum levels. 12 h post-dose brain levels are 50% lower than serum levels [29]. Factors influencing the BTS ratio:

  i. Dosing: single dosing is associated with a higher BTS ratio than BID dosing: 0.61 ± 0.12 vs. 0.37 ± 0.07 [30]

  ii. Age: the BTS ratio correlation appears significant in younger patients, but older age may blunt this association [31–33]

  iii. Mood state and unknown patient variables may also influence lithium CNS penetration and distribution [24, 29]

c. Essential facts

Atomic weight: 6.94

Equivalence: 8 mEq = 56 mg of elemental lithium = 300 mg lithium carbonate

Note: lithium citrate is often available in a concentration of 8 mEq/5 ml

Example 1: A clinician wishes to switch a nonadherent inpatient from lithium carbonate 900 mg QHS to lithium citrate, but the computerized pharmacy ordering package lists the lithium citrate concentration as follows: 8 mEq/5 ml. What is the equivalent dose of lithium citrate to 900 mg of lithium carbonate?

Answer: With the conversion above, 900 mg of lithium carbonate = 24 mEq of lithium, so the appropriate dose would be 24 mEq (or 15 ml).

Example 2: A patient purchases lithium orotate on the internet due to the belief that this salt has special kinetic and efficacy properties. The tablets are sold based on the dose of elemental lithium and contain 5 mg. The patient uses this on a PRN basis to manage stress and consumes on average four tablets per day. What would be the equivalent dose of lithium carbonate?

Answer: 20 mg of elemental lithium is 20/56 or 35.7% of the amount of lithium contained in a 300 mg dose of lithium carbonate. 300 x 35.7% = 107.4 mg of lithium carbonate.

Why 5 Half-Lives Equals Steady State: The Example of Lithium, Assuming a Peripheral $T_{1/2}$ of 24 h

	1st dose	2nd dose	3rd dose	4th dose	5th dose	Total
24 hours	50%	–	–	–	–	50%
48 hours	25%	50%	–	–	–	75%
72 hours	12.5%	25%	50%	–	–	87.5%
96 hours	6.25%	12.5%	25%	50%	–	93.75%
120 hours	3.125%	6.25%	12.5%	25%	50%	96.875%

Different forms of lithium are prescribed using different units, so it is important to know how to convert from milliequivalents (mEq) to milligrams (mg) of lithium carbonate or other lithium containing products. For monovalent ions such as lithium (Li^+) and sodium (Na^+), the units of mEq are the same as millimoles (mmol) (although for a divalent ion such as calcium [Ca^{++}] 1 mmol = 2 mEq). Lithium citrate is provided in a concentration typically described as 8 mEq/5 ml. By understanding that 8 mEq provides an equivalent lithium dose to 300 mg of lithium carbonate, one can easily switch between formulations. Moreover, lithium sulfate is available in some countries, with doses expressed both in mmol and the mg quantity of elemental lithium per tablet (e.g. a 6 mmol tablet = 42 mg elemental lithium) [34]. Since lithium is the active ingredient in all of these preparations, it is relatively easy to calculate the amount of elemental lithium for any product. To find mg from mEq one simply multiplies by lithium's atomic weight (approximately 7.0), so 8 mEq = 56 mg of lithium. Similarly, 300 mg of lithium carbonate contains 56 mg of lithium, a value that can be verified by calculating the lithium component of Li_2CO_3: the molecular mass of the carbonate salt is 73.89 g/mol of which 13.8 g/mol (i.e. 18.68%) is from lithium. 300 mg x 18.68% yields 56 mg of lithium content in 300 mg of lithium carbonate.

Performing these calculations with salts other than lithium citrate or carbonate is increasingly important thanks to the handiwork of Hans Alfred Nieper, a deceased German psychiatrist best known for his specious claims that various supplements, including the orotate salts of calcium, magnesium and lithium, could cure multiple sclerosis, cancer, atherosclerotic heart disease, alcoholism and many other disorders [35–37]. Orotate is a pyrimidine compound produced in mitochondria as a step in uridine synthesis, one of the components of ribonucleic acid. Nieper harbored many incorrect beliefs about orotate salts, but research in the 1970s and in 2023 confirmed greater tissue penetration for lithium orotate compared to other salts for any given peripheral level. While this may achieve more pronounced CNS effects, there is also the potential for greater renal dysfunction [38–40]. [Note: other lithium salts such as lithium salicylate and lithium lactate possess different kinetics than lithium carbonate in rat models, but the clinical significance in humans is unknown [41].] Despite the lack of human data establishing a safe therapeutic serum level range for lithium orotate, it can be purchased freely on the internet. The most common form of lithium orotate is a 120 mg tablet or capsule that contains 5 mg of elemental lithium, but strengths ranging from 1 mg to 20 mg of elemental lithium are available. As outlined in Info Box 3.1, a patient who freely consumes lithium orotate may expose themselves to substantial systemic exposure, with cases of lithium toxicity noted in the literature [42, 43].

In-Depth 3.1 Lithium Brain Kinetics

Clinicians use peripheral levels to monitor lithium exposure, and animal studies performed 50 years ago documented a significant association between serum and brain lithium levels [44]; however, the advent of magnetic resonance spectroscopy (MRS) has allowed researchers to quantify brain levels of the stable lithium isotope [7]Li in patients on lithium, study its brain kinetics, and delineate the relationship between CNS and peripheral levels in humans [27, 45]. The earliest MRS human studies were performed 30 years ago and noted that the brain T_{Max} was delayed approximately 3 h from the serum T_{Max} [27, 28], that steady state brain levels significantly correlated with serum levels [32, 46], and that the brain-to-serum (BTS) ratio averaged 0.50, meaning that brain levels are 50% lower than serum levels (Figure 3.1) [29]. This research also uncovered marked interindividual differences in brain lithium penetration, with age emerging as one possible factor in some, but not all, studies [31–33]. However, differences in BTS among patients of comparable age led investigators to posit that other biological variables influence lithium CNS transport, a topic that remains an important area of research [24]. Differences in the expression or function of lithium transport mechanisms may be a crucial variable influencing likelihood of response, with one MRS study finding a significant association between central and peripheral lithium levels among patients with bipolar depression who were remitters ($r = 0.7$, $p = 0.004$), but not in those who failed to achieve remission ($r = -0.12$, $p = 0.76$) [33]. Lithium's CNS distribution is not uniform, and MRS studies using powerful 7 Tesla magnets are able to perform high-quality, 3-dimensional mapping of lithium levels throughout the brain [47]. These studies confirm the nonuniform nature of lithium brain levels, and preferential accumulation in the left hippocampus [48]. While not at the stage of clinical application, such research will vastly improve our understanding of variations in regional CNS lithium levels and distribution to better explain interindividual differences in tolerability, mood disorder efficacy, and possibly the neuroprotective response to lithium therapy [47].

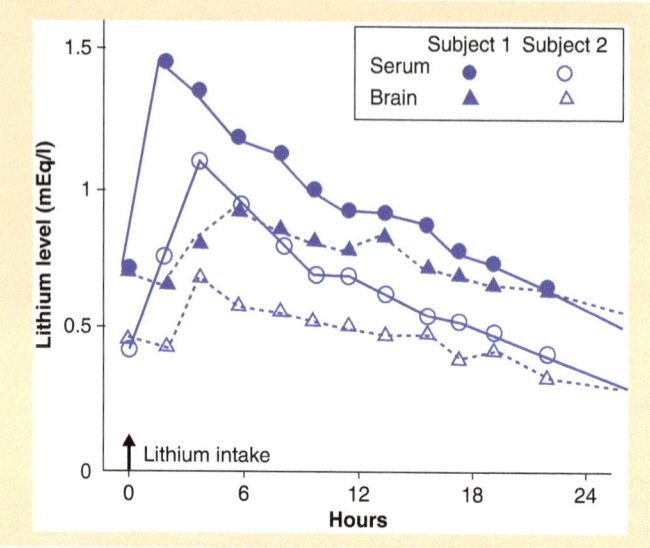

Figure 3.1 Comparative lithium kinetics in serum vs. those in the brain as determined by ⁷Li magnetic resonance spectroscopy [28]

(Adapted from: P. Plenge, A. Stensgaard, H. V. Jensen, et al. [1994]. 24-hour lithium concentration in human brain studied by Li-7 magnetic resonance spectroscopy. *Biol Psychiatry*, 36, 511–516.)

1 *Prescribing Factors Influencing Trough Levels: Multiple Daily Dosing and Timing of the Level*

Maintaining lithium levels within a certain range improves tolerability and minimizes renal impact [9, 12], and requires obtaining accurate and interpretable 12 h trough levels. Lithium is preferentially dosed QHS, and the bulk of the recent literature is built around use of the 12 h level as a standard measure of lithium exposure [16, 25]. When the time since last dose deviates significantly from the 12 h mark, it becomes challenging to impute what the 12 h value would have been. Table 3.1 provides data on lithium levels drawn ± 2 hours from the 12 h mark, showing that within this time frame the 2 h differential will alter lithium levels by 0.08 mEq/l on average [23]. However, individual patients are not average. As shown in Figure 3.2, while the lithium decay curve remains mostly linear even when ± 4 h from the 12 h mark, the extent of the difference from the 12 h trough value varied considerably between these seven individuals [49]. Patient education is important to reinforce the need for levels to be obtained as close as practicably possible to the 12 h mark; moreover, prescribing lithium once daily at odd times such as 8 am or noon means that trough levels drawn the next morning will be 24 h or 20 h respectively, and largely uninterpretable.

Table 3.1 Effect of time since last dose on the trough lithium level [23]

Time since last dose	10 h	12 h	14 h
Serum level (mEq/l)	1.28	1.20	1.12

Figure 3.2 Individual differences in lithium kinetics (n = 7) [49]

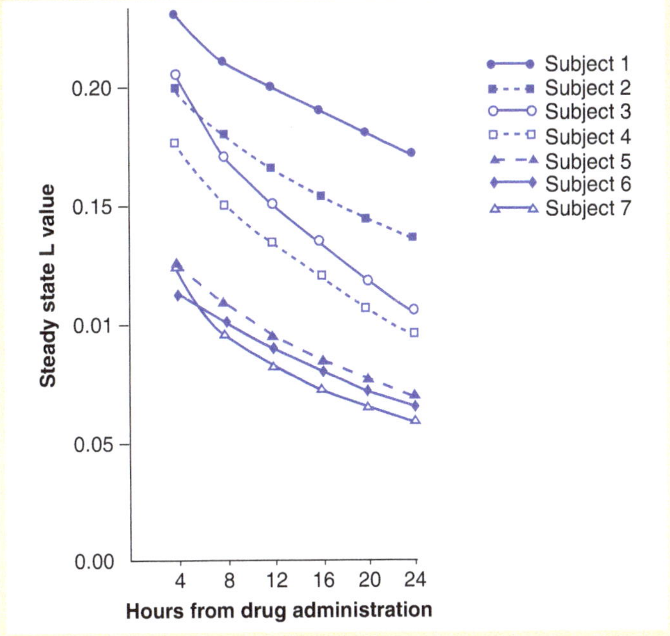
Subject 1
Subject 2
Subject 3
Subject 4
Subject 5
Subject 6
Subject 7
0.20
0.15
0.01
0.05
0.00
Steady state L value
4
8
12
16
20
24
Hours from drug administration

(Adapted from: P. E. Bergner, K. Berniker, T. B. Cooper, et al. [1973]. Lithium kinetics in man: Effect of variation in dosage pattern. *Br J Psychiatry*, 49, 328–339.)

The one variable completely under the control of the clinician is the decision to administer lithium as a single QHS dose. There has been a healthy debate over the past 40 years regarding why multiple daily dosing is associated with more renal dysfunction [8, 9, 50, 51]. One plausible hypothesis is that patients on BID dosing are simply exposed to more lithium due to the distorting effect on trough values when half of the dose is administered 24 h before the level is drawn (Table 3.2) [51]. Another possibility is that QHS dosing generates lower lithium levels throughout the day (Figure 3.3), thus diminishing lithium's entry into collecting duct principal cells via the epithelial sodium channel (ENaC), and allowing lithium to be cleared more effectively from these cells [50].

Table 3.2 Differences in morning lithium levels when comparable daily doses are administered at bedtime (QHS) or twice daily (BID)

Study	Lithium level: QHS dosing (mEq/l)	Lithium level: BID dosing (mEq/l)
Amdisen [52]	1.37	1.07
Greil [53]	1.04	0.81
Swartz [54]	0.90	0.70
Mean level	1.10	0.86

Comments

a. **Kinetics:** When the dose is administered on a BID schedule, the morning level is a 12 h trough only for the evening portion of the dose – it is a 24 h trough for the dose ingested the prior morning.

b. **Converting patients on BID doses to QHS dosing:** When a dose administered on a BID schedule is converted to a single QHS dose, the morning trough level will be 28% higher. Patients on BID dosing with levels thought to be in the high end of the maintenance therapeutic range may be overexposed to lithium and have trough levels that are supratherapeutic and potentially nephrotoxic. As there is no efficacy advantage from multiple daily dosing, those on BID dosing should be converted to single QHS dosing whenever possible. (See Chapter 5 for management of gastrointestinal adverse effects seen with larger single lithium doses.) After consolidation, the 12 h trough level is rechecked after 48 h on the QHS dose and the dose adjusted based on this new level. The 12 h trough is also used for patients on extended release lithium preparations.

c. **Clinical implication for patients remaining on BID doses:** Some patients may be wedded to BID dosing for a variety of reasons (e.g. historical stability and reluctance to change, prior episodes of gastrointestinal adverse effects on single QHS doses). As the morning trough level would be 28% higher were the dose converted to a QHS schedule, **the maximum morning trough level on BID dosing should be 0.78 mEq/l, which would equate to 1.00 mEq/l if the dose were given QHS only.** If local guidelines suggest 0.80 mEq/l as the recommended maximum maintenance level, the corresponding BID level is 0.62 mEq/l.

Figure 3.3 Serum levels from bedtime (QHS) dosing of standard lithium or twice daily (BID) dosing of an extended release formulation [55].

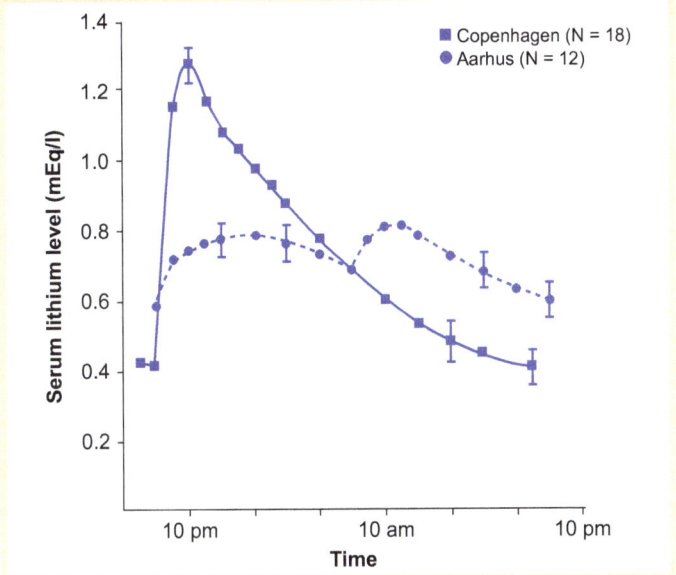

(Adapted from: M. Schou, A. Amdisen, K. Thomsen, et al. [1982]. Lithium treatment regimen and renal water handling: The significance of dosage pattern and tablet type examined through comparison of results from two clinics with different treatment regimens. *Psychopharmacology*, 77, 387–390.)

Advocates of single QHS lithium dosing note – in addition to possible renal advantages, improved adherence and more easily interpreted trough values – the absence of clinical data suggesting any loss of efficacy with once daily dosing, although stretching lithium administration to every other day does diminish response

[8, 56]. The persistence of multiple daily dosing is an artifact of prior prescribing recommendations from the 1960s, recommendations that were codified in lithium label information that has remained largely unchanged for over 50 years. Lithium was approved in the US on April 6, 1970, but the product labeling still reflects the original divided dosing strategies in common use at that time (Table 3.3) [11]. Information for an extended release formulation still states that, for "long-term control," the product can be administered BID or TID [10]. There are instances where divided dosing can be considered (e.g. pediatric patients), and one common use of split dosing is to lessen adverse effects (e.g. nausea) when starting lithium in acutely manic inpatients, since those individuals might balk at treatment if early tolerability issues arise. In the latter situation, the dose should be consolidated prior to discharge and adjusted based on the 12 h trough from QHS dosing. There are also clinical scenarios in which one feels compelled to move some lithium to the morning for tolerability reasons (e.g. nausea that does not improve over time and does not respond to use of a sustained release formulation or administering lithium with food), but in those circumstances the bulk of the dose should be QHS to minimize the distorting effects on the morning trough level if the dose were equally divided into a BID schedule (Info Box 3.3). Should evenly divided BID dosing be absolutely necessary, one can avoid lithium overexposure by adjusting the trough values mathematically. This is based on studies such as those in Table 3.3 indicating that the trough level will increase 28% when a BID dose is converted to a single QHS dose.

Although the current standard is to utilize serum lithium levels for routine monitoring, repeated phlebotomy during dose titration can be painful and also inconvenient for outpatients who must travel to a laboratory at a specific time in the morning. In the late 1970s and early 1980s, multiple investigators started to examine the concordance between salivary and serum levels, and early studies reported a poor correlation between the two [57–59]. However, subsequent research in 1982 showed that, by obtaining several baseline measures to establish the specific relationship for that patient, the expected correlation coefficient was quite high: ≥ 0.91 [60]. A 2017 study of 38 lithium treated patients found that single estimates showed a significant correlation ($r = 0.767$, $p < 0.001$) [61], but a 2021 paper utilized a larger sample of bipolar patients ($n = 75$) from whom repeated measurements were obtained for up to 18 months to find the optimal method that correlated serum and salivary lithium levels [62]. Levels from 169 passive drool samples were analyzed, and from these data a model was developed that adjusted for daily lithium dose, a diagnosis of diabetes mellitus (DM) and smoking. Using this model and the salivary lithium value, there was a strong correlation between predicted and observed serum lithium levels ($r = 0.70$). Importantly, use of the

Table 3.3 Outdated lithium dosing information still present in a 2020 US package insert [11]

Patient group	Starting dose	Dose titration	Acute goal		Maintenance goal	
			Serum level	Usual dose	Serum level	Usual dose
Adult and pediatric patients over 30 kg	300 mg three times daily	300 mg every 3 days	0.80 to 1.20 mEq/l	600 mg two to three times daily	0.80 to 1.00 mEq/l	300 to 600 mg two to three times daily
Pediatric patients 20–30 kg	300 mg twice daily	300 mg weekly		600 to 1500 mg in divided doses daily		600 to 1200 mg in divided doses daily

Info Box 3.3 Why Lithium Should Be Dosed Once Daily at Night

Concept 1 Many of the studies correlating serum lithium levels and response drew conclusions from 12 h post-dose data.

Rationale

a. In both inpatient and outpatient settings, obtaining samples in the morning is much more feasible than at other times during the day. Although the peripheral $T_{1/2}$ of lithium is closer to 24 h, the 12 h trough became the *de facto* standard due to convenience.

b. As a large portion of recent efficacy and safety data rely on conclusions from 12 h trough results, it is difficult for clinicians to interpret lithium levels drawn on samples obtained at nonstandard times (i.e. 18 h or 24 h after the last dose [as seen with qnoon or QAM dosing], or when morning levels are drawn in patients on twice daily dosing where half of the dose will have been administered 24 h previously.

Concept 2 There is no therapeutic advantage to multiple daily dosing [8]. In those uncommon instances where BID dosing is necessary (e.g. a patient who has reached their maximum tolerated bedtime lithium dose), the bulk of the dose should be given as close to bedtime as possible so that the 12 h trough level will not be as greatly distorted by having a large proportion of the medication (e.g. 50%) administered 24 hours previously.

Rationale

a. Lithium has a central nervous system (CNS) half-life and effects that persist ≥ 24 hours. Once daily dosing has the same effectiveness as multiple daily doses.

b. There are over 40 years of data substantiating that multiple daily lithium dosing incurs greater risk of renal dysfunction in the short term (e.g. greater urinary volume) [8, 50, 55] and over longer-term exposure (greater risk of renal insufficiency) [6, 7, 9].

mean intrasubject ratio from three prior observations more robustly predicted serum lithium levels (predicted vs. observed r = 0.90) [62]. The authors concluded that use of saliva appears quite feasible for lithium monitoring, and that the findings from their study will hopefully open new avenues for development of a point-of-care (POC) device to use in the clinic or at home. Use of POC devices is an exciting topic in psychiatry based on the successful implementation of a POC fingerstick device by a US manufacturer (www.athelas.com) to measure absolute neutrophil counts in clozapine treated patients [63, 64], and ongoing development of a POC fingerstick device for antipsychotic levels by another US company (www.saladax.com) [64]. While still in early stages, most of the research is focused on POC measurement of lithium levels from whole blood obtained from a fingerstick [65, 66], although there is considerable interest in wearable sensors based on electrochemical detection of lithium in sweat, or interstitial levels sensed with microneedle technology [67, 68]. It is hoped that rapid advances in these and other technologies (e.g. optical sensors) will obviate the need for phlebotomy based lithium levels, thereby removing an important patient barrier to lithium treatment [66].

2 *Lithium Citrate, and Standard vs. Sustained Release Kinetics*

Lithium citrate is a liquid formulation used since 1950 which has comparable kinetics to tablet or capsule lithium preparations manufactured in the past 30 years [15, 69]. Any kinetic differences between citrate and standard lithium are subtle, with the liquid having a 10% higher C_{Max} but levels identical to those from tablets at 2 h post-dose [15]. Lithium citrate is typically flavored with raspberry to improve palatability, but it can be dissolved in other liquids if desired, with the package insert making no comment about lack of compatibility; however, there is one report on undetectable levels when mixed with apple juice [70]. Liquid forms of antipsychotics are often used on inpatient units, and lithium citrate will precipitate when added to solutions of haloperidol, trifluoperazine and chlorpromazine [71], but not when mixed with risperidone solution [72].

In the 1970s a number of sustained release lithium preparations appeared that possessed a longer T_{Max} than standard lithium (by design) and a lower C_{Max}, with the idea that delaying and decreasing lithium's release might mitigate upper GI tract adverse effects (e.g. nausea), and perhaps lessen other tolerability complaints [73]. The T_{Max} of currently available sustained release tablets or capsules is 3–6 hours (Figure 3.4) after it became evident that extremely long T_{Max} times (e.g. 12 h) might limit upper GI absorption but incur greater rates of diarrhea due to ion delivery in the lower GI tract (Figure 3.5) [73]. Although the early kinetics differ between standard and sustained release forms, 12 h trough values do not differ when both are dosed QHS (Figure 3.4) [19]. Regardless of whether one uses lithium citrate, standard lithium or an extended release tablet, the medication is ideally administered as a single QHS dose and levels obtained as 12 h trough values.

Figure 3.4 Single-dose kinetic curves for two lithium carbonate sustained release formulations with a T_{Max} of 5 h compared with standard lithium carbonate (n = 12 for each) [19]

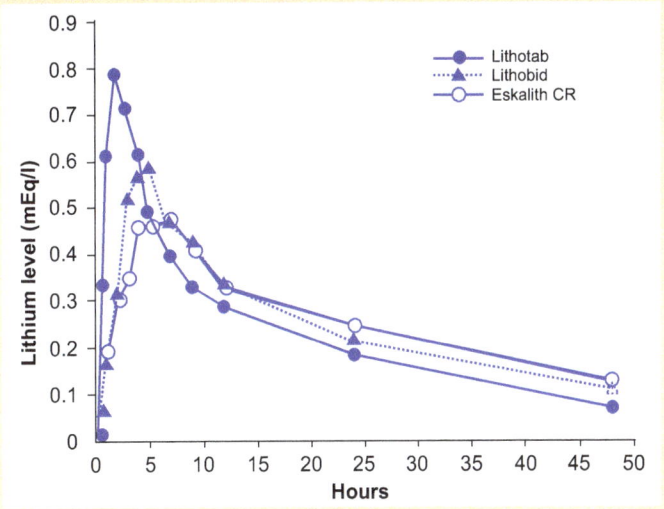

(Adapted from: C. K. Kirkwood, S. K. Wilson, P. E. Hayes, et al. [1994]. Single-dose bioavailability of two extended-release lithium carbonate products. *Am J Hosp Pharm*, 51, 486–489.)

B Methods for Lithium Dose Prediction

WHAT TO KNOW: DOSE PREDICTION

- There is a well-known method for estimating maintenance dose requirements based on a 24 h level after a 600 mg test dose. The output is the sum of all relevant clinical and physiological factors that influence lithium clearance in that patient.

- The test dose method obviates the need for complex calculations involving multiple variables (eGFR, use of kinetically interacting medications, gender, age, etc.).

For over 50 years, investigators have sought to develop lithium dose prediction models with two goals in mind: minimizing extended periods spent at subtherapeutic levels, especially when treating acutely manic inpatients; and lessening the patient burden of repeated level testing when clinicians employ an empirical "trial-and-error method" [75]. One early strategy developed in 1973 by Tom Cooper at Rockland State Hospital in New York estimated the daily dose needed to achieve a level in the range of 0.60–1.20 mEq/l from the 24 h level after a single 600 mg lithium test dose (Table 3.4) [76]. As many variables influence lithium's $T_{1/2}$ (e.g. eGFR, use of concurrent medications, comorbid medical illnesses), the simplicity of this method is that the sum of all these inputs is reflected in the 24 h post-dose level. Although the utility of the Cooper method was confirmed by four

Figure 3.5 Kinetic curve of a lithium carbonate sustained release formulation with an unusually long T_{Max} of 12 h compared with standard lithium carbonate [74]

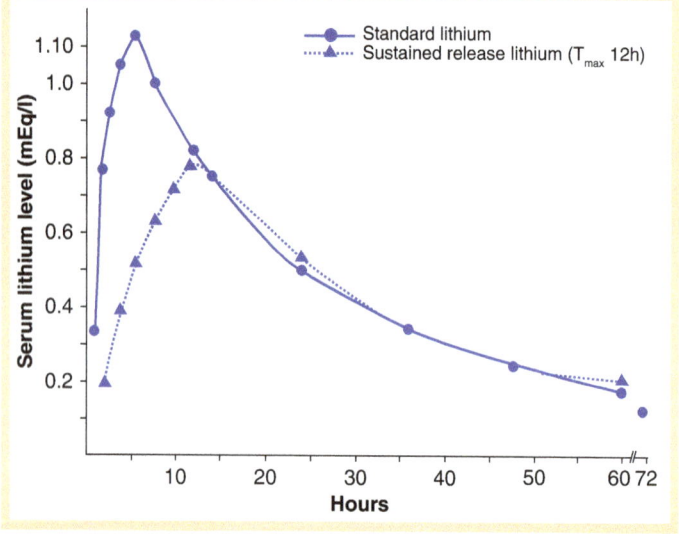

Comment

Sustained release lithium preparations with unusually long T_{Max} values (i.e. > 6 h) are not available in most countries due to the association with lower gastrointestinal adverse effects (e.g. diarrhea) [18].

(Adapted from: D. P. Thornhill [1978]. Pharmacokinetics of ordinary and sustained-release lithium carbonate in manic patients after acute dosage. *Eur J Clin Pharmacol*, 14, 267–271.)

subsequent papers over the ensuing 11 years [75, 77–79], one small study (n = 13) in 1981 noted that 4/13 did not achieve levels in the predicted range [80]. While the 1981 study did not invalidate the Cooper model, numerous variations of test dose methods appeared in the literature, some more rigorously derived than others, creating a somewhat confusing picture for clinicians. Perhaps the only drawback from the Cooper test dose method is that dosing recommendations in 1973 commonly employed multiple daily dosing, so all the recommended regimens are divided into 2, 3 or 4 times per day administration (see Comments, Table 3.4). Use of baseline eGFR to screen out those who are not lithium candidates was also not a consideration at that time, but is a necessary consideration in modern practice.

 Table 3.4 The 1973 Cooper test dose method: the 24 h lithium level after a single 600 mg test dose predicts the daily dose needed for a maintenance 12 h serum level in the range of 0.60–1.20 mEq/l [76]

24 h serum lithium level after single 600 mg loading dose (mEq/l)	Daily dosage required
< 0.05	1200 mg TID
0.05–0.09	900 mg TID
0.10–0.14	600 mg TID
0.15–0.19	300 mg QID
0.20–0.23	300 mg TID
0.24–0.30	300 mg BID
> 0.30	300 mg BID*

BID = twice per day; TID = thrice per day; QID = 4 times per day

* Cooper advises extreme caution if the 24 h level is > 0.30 mEq/l. Using modern monitoring methods, this group would likely not be lithium candidates due to baseline eGFR ≪ 60 ml/min.

Comments

1. **Drawback**: The recommended regimens are BID, TID or QID. The use of multiple daily doses for a few days on an inpatient unit is unlikely to induce any significant renal effects, but the daily dose will need to be consolidated before discharge, and a 12 h level obtained for dose adjustment.

2. **Dosage adjustment for single QHS dosing**: Kinetic studies indicate that multiple daily dosing distorts the morning trough level [52]. (See Chapter 4, Info Box 4.3, for estimated doses for QHS dosing, using calculations that assume a consolidated single dose QHS level will be at least 28% higher than levels on divided doses.)

In addition to the test dose method, *a priori* strategies were developed after retrospective chart reviews of hundreds of patients found that demographic and clinical variables such as age, weight, gender and inpatient status explained much of the variance in lithium clearance. One model was based on review of 548 charts, and the derived equation retrospectively applied to the outcomes from 390 patients: the mean difference between the estimated and the actual dose was 19 mg/day and the standard deviation was 325 mg/day [81]. Unfortunately, that equation was only studied prospectively in small trials, the largest of which enrolled 30 subjects, and did not consider the effects of renally acting medications influencing lithium clearance [82]. The absence of large-scale replication was a recurring theme in the 2013 review of 38 test dose or *a priori* predictive algorithms published in English, French or Dutch from 1966 to 2012 [83]. Although the predictive methods did shorten the time to therapeutic levels, the authors concluded: "The vast majority of predictive methods, however, show inconsistent or poor results or have not been replicated since their initial description" [83].

The tone of the 2013 review covering models for lithium dosing was decidedly nihilistic, yet other areas of medicine routinely use weight and other patient variables to predict medication dosing for agents with narrow therapeutic indices. Empiric lithium titration often introduces delays in achieving therapeutic levels, hence the clinical need to develop easily used predictive formulas employing a minimum amount of laboratory and demographic data. One important issue in early *a priori* predictive models was omission of any measure of renal function, or reliance on serum creatinine instead of creatinine clearance (CL_{Cr}) or eGFR, factors that may have hampered model performance. In 2018, a Japanese group addressed this issue in creating an *a priori* model derived from 132 samples in 82 subjects [84]. Variables used to develop the model included demographic factors, the last lithium level, time between the level and when the last dose was ingested, timing and frequency of lithium dosing, serum creatinine and concomitant medications [84]. An interesting aspect of model development was an estimation of the ratio of lithium clearance (CL_{Li}) to CL_{Cr}, while eschewing use of the more accurate eGFR as a measure of intrinsic renal function. Nonetheless, the model was subsequently examined in 30 randomly selected subjects with a finding of a large and significant correlation between observed and predicted lithium concentrations ($r = 0.781$, $p < 0.001$). Although this result has not been replicated, the authors reported that their model performed better than five of six previously published *a priori* predictive models [84].

In 2022, a Swedish group published the most advanced model to predict CL_{Li} and the daily lithium dose using data from lithium treated adult patients divided into two cohorts (cohort 1: n = 584; cohort 2: n = 1773), with genetic testing also performed to identify single nucleotide polymorphisms (SNPs) associated with age/gender corrected CL_{Li} [34]. The predictive models were developed independently within each cohort, and the other cohort used as a test sample. The total study population was 60.4% female, mean age 53.6 ± 14.7 years (range 17–89 years), mainly of European descent, all of whom were taking a minimum of 6 mEq per day (equivalent to 225 mg of lithium carbonate). In addition to age, gender, weight, height (to calculate body mass index [BMI]), lithium formulation, lithium dosing regimen, and use of medications that alter lithium clearance (e.g. diuretics, angiotensin converting enzyme inhibitors [ACEIs], angiotensin receptor II blockers [ARBs], nonsteroidal anti-inflammatory drugs [NSAIDs], etc.), 5627 data points were obtained for serum lithium concentration and serum creatinine (from which eGFR was calculated). The genome-wide association study (GWAS) analysis was derived from samples in 2190 subjects [34]. This is the largest study ever performed to develop a predictive model of CL_{Li} and the results confirmed that age, gender, eGFR, use of diuretics (except for potassium sparing agents), ACEIs and ARBs were all significant predictors of CL_{Li}, as was serum lithium level. Weight, height and BMI did not improve model fit, presumably due to the body surface adjustment derived from weight and height in the eGFR formula. Interestingly, a model which excluded serum lithium level significantly overestimated the daily lithium dose for patients with high serum lithium concentrations. The authors offer some hypotheses for this observed effect, including that exposure to lithium might cause physiological adaptations that alter its own clearance. Nonetheless, using serum lithium level as both an explanatory variable and in the dependent outcome is problematic from a statistical point of view; moreover, the reduced model performance without a prior lithium level limits accuracy when predicting dosing in new starts. The GWAS identified one SNP associated with CL_{Li}, and noted an association between a polygenic risk score using loci associated with eGFR, blood urea nitrogen (BUN) and BMI, but adding the genetic data did not improve model fit over an equation with the six clinical variables. The final model based on those six clinical predictors explained 61.4% of the variance in CL_{Li} in cohort 1 and 49.8% in cohort 2 [34]. To put the results into context, the explained variance in this model outperformed all other lithium prediction models except for one; moreover, this model performed better than all other models in terms of absolute accuracy. However, the mean error in predicting daily lithium intake was 6 mEq (equivalent to 225 mg of lithium carbonate), which the authors hope can be improved upon. That easily obtained clinical data are the only inputs into the model suggests that future analyses with large sample sizes and sophisticated statistical methods may yield a feasible predictive equation that can be used in lithium naïve and in lithium treated patients.

C Loading Lithium

WHAT TO KNOW: INTRODUCTION

- Prolonged slow lithium titration delays the time to clinical stability. While antipsychotics have antimanic properties, they lack lithium's numerous intracellular mechanisms that result in longer-term mood stability.
- In patients with an eGFR deemed acceptable to begin treatment, lithium can be safely loaded using a protocol developed in acutely manic adults. The total dose of 30 mg/kg is divided into three smaller doses of 10 mg/kg administered in the early evening using a sustained release preparation to minimize GI side effects.

One goal of test dose and predictive models is to reduce the delay in achieving therapeutic levels for acutely manic patients. A 2000 review on medication loading for acute mania commented that both humanitarian and economic reasons have spurred interest in mood stabilizer loading to rapidly reduce mania symptoms [85]. The feasibility of loading divalproex was established in 1999 by a double-blind study that randomized 59 acutely manic patients to either: divalproex with oral loading (n = 20); divalproex without loading (n = 20), starting at 250 mg TID on days 1–2 followed by standard dose titration on days 3–10; or lithium carbonate (n = 19) 300 mg TID on days 1–2 followed by standard dose titration on days 3–10. The loading protocol for divalproex was 30 mg/kg/day on days 1–2, followed by 20 mg/kg/day on days 3–10 [86]. By day 3 of the study, 84% of divalproex loaded subjects, but only 30% of nonloaded divalproex subjects, had serum valproate (VPA) levels > 50 µg/ml. None of the lithium treated patients had a serum lithium level > 0.80 mEq/l at day 3, providing more evidence that trial-and-error dosing is perhaps not the optimal method for initiating lithium [86].

While many clinicians are familiar with the 30 mg/kg divalproex loading regimen, lithium loading studies have also been performed, and, interestingly, the daily dose administered in the first 24 h is also 30 mg/kg [87, 88]. An important aspect of lithium loading is that GI adverse effects, especially nausea, become problematic with high initial doses, and that use of a sustained release preparation can mitigate this. The extent of this problem can be seen from data in two publications. One was a small (n = 9) study of lithium loading published in 1992 by a group of Israeli investigators whose goal was to spare acutely manic adults from the need to be exposed to first generation antipsychotics [89]. As noted in Table 3.5, there was no explicit loading formula, just a clinical estimate based on age, weight and prior patient experience with lithium tolerability. Despite the heroic dosages used on day 1, trough levels were within the acceptable range for acute mania. The paper does not indicate whether a sustained released form of lithium was used, but 4/9 patients developed nausea and 1/9 developed diarrhea, implicating a standard release form of lithium. A more explicit dosing formula of 30 mg/kg was incorporated into hospital guidelines for Auckland, NZ issued in 2000, but with a maximum daily dose of 2000 mg [88]. This weight based loading dose was chosen after an internal review of patients treated with loading (n = 12) vs. usual lithium titration (n = 15) found a faster time to therapeutic levels and a significantly shorter length of stay for loading: **20.2 ± 7.11 days** vs. usual titration **39.9 ± 24.2** days (p = 0.011). A 2008 follow-up paper examined clinical outcomes in 93 manic adults admitted to two Auckland psychiatric inpatient units in 2001 and who were started on lithium or VPA within 72 h of admission [88]. While more than four times as many loaded patients achieved therapeutic levels of either mood stabilizer by day 3 (27.9% load vs. 6.0% nonload), standard release lithium was administered resulting in adverse effect rates significantly higher in the loading group (63.6%) than in the usual titration group (38.7%) (p = 0.05), primarily due to GI adverse effects (diarrhea and nausea) and tremor [88].

What is somewhat perplexing is that both of these protocols completely overlooked a well-designed loading study published in 1985 in the *Journal of Clinical Psychiatry* that used divided loading doses of sustained release lithium to minimize adverse effects [87]. A group of Doctorates of Pharmacy at two hospitals in Los Angeles developed a 30 mg/kg loading formula predicted to achieve 12 h trough levels in the range of 0.90–1.10 mEq/l (Info Box 3.4). Critical to the success of their approach was to administer lithium in three divided doses (4 pm, 6 pm and 8 pm), and to use a sustained release preparation to minimize GI side effects such as nausea [87]. The study subjects were 38 manic inpatients (20 male/18 female), mean age 36.2 ± 2.95 years, mean weight 70.1 ± 3.50 kg, with CL_{cr} ranging from 46 to 128 ml/min. Using the 30 mg/kg formula, the loading dose range for female subjects was 1200–2400 mg, while that for the male subjects was 1800–3000 mg. Serum levels the following morning were within the acceptable range for 34/38 subjects (89.5%):

Males	12 h levels range: 0.58–1.10 mEq/l.	Mean Error: 0.16 ± 0.09 mEq/l.
Females	12 h levels range: 0.45–1.40 mEq/l.	Mean Error: 0.28 ± 0.14 mEq/l.

Only four subjects had levels beyond that predicted by the 30 mg/kg loading formula (1.28–1.40 mEq/l), three of whom were obese women. Despite maximal doses of 2400–3000 mg, there were no study dropouts and no patient experienced any

Table 3.5 Results of an exploratory lithium monotherapy loading trial (n = 9) [89]

	Clinical global impression – severity (mean ± SD)	Lithium dose (mg) (mean ± SD)	Lithium level (mEq/L) (mean ± SD)
Day 1 (baseline)	5.8 ± 0.8	3467 ± 634	1.01 ± 0.29
Day 2	5.6 ± 1.1	2267 ± 450	1.06 ± 0.43
Day 3	4.5 ± 1.2	1936 ± 468	1.28 ± 0.44
Day 7	3.7 ± 1.5	1725 ± 549	0.92 ± 0.17
Day 14 *(n = 8)**	1.6 ± 0.8	1680 ± 469	0.76 ± 0.27
Day 21 *(n = 8)**	1.3 ± 0.8	1800 ± 600	0.86 ± 0.39

Comments

1. All patients (6 female, 3 male; mean age 42 years) had a prior history of mania with median length of bipolar illness 5 years. The investigators did not employ a specific formula but estimated the day 1 dose from factors such as age, body size and past history of lithium tolerance. Doses were reduced daily based on levels drawn 8–12 h post-dose on days 1–3, and weekly thereafter.

2. The results in the table are for the final sample of 8; one individual was dropped from the analysis at day 14 after failing to respond to lithium monotherapy during the first week.

3. The authors did not specify whether a standard or extended release lithium preparation was used, but the pattern of adverse effects suggests standard lithium: nausea n = 4; diarrhea n = 1.

adverse effects during the loading procedure (nausea, diarrhea or other GI distress, neuromuscular or CNS effects) or in the 12 h afterwards [87]. Remarkably, this study was not cited in the Israeli or New Zealand papers, nor in the 2000 review of loading strategies for acute mania [85, 88, 89]. Unfortunately, this protocol was never replicated, although the dosing formula of 30 mg/kg is exactly that used in the Auckland guidelines. What this protocol does not define is the choice of maintenance dose to use starting the next evening. While this will necessitate clinical estimation of the QHS dose and a follow-up level in 4–5 days, at least the patient is proceeding from a point close to the serum level goal. Nonetheless, the results of this paper are compelling, and it is worth speculating whether elimination of individuals with unacceptably low renal function (CL_{Cr} in one subject was 46 ml/min) might further reduce the incidence of high post-loading levels. The important clinical conclusion from this thoughtfully designed protocol is that clinicians can consider abandoning gradual titration methods that result in prolonged subtherapeutic levels, especially on inpatient units where daily lithium level monitoring is eminently feasible and tolerability issues can be rapidly addressed. A 2017 review of 13 treatment guidelines from around the world found that only 4 provided a recommended lithium starting dose, and 3 of these suggested doses no greater than 400 mg without differentiating between acute inpatient or outpatient settings [25]. The use of lower starting doses is quite reasonable when there is no sense of urgency, but there are sufficient data to suggest that inpatients can tolerate higher starting dosages, and that this should be taken into account when treating acutely manic individuals in hospital settings.

Info Box 3.4 The Los Angeles County – USC Lithium Loading Protocol [87]

a. **Calculate the loading dose:** The total dose administered is 30 mg/kg.

b. **Consider a lower dose for obese females:** three of the four individuals with levels beyond that predicted by the loading formula (1.28–1.40 mEq/l) were obese women. A 20 mg/kg loading dose will minimize high trough values in those patients.

c. **Use a sustained release formulation for loading:** Critical to the loading protocol is the use of a sustained release lithium preparation for the loading doses to minimize side effects. In the loading study, no patient experienced any adverse effects (nausea, diarrhea or other GI distress, neuromuscular or CNS effects) during the loading procedure or in the 12 h afterwards [87].

d. **Administer the loading dose of lithium as three divided doses:** The doses should be given at 4 pm, 6 pm and 8 pm. The doses need not be exactly the same but should total 30 mg/kg.

   i. **Case** A 70 kg manic individual is deemed an acceptable lithium candidate and is to be started on lithium. The total loading dose is 30 mg/kg x 70 kg = 2100 mg. How should it be divided?

   ii. **Answer** Since many pharmacies may only stock sustained release lithium tablets or capsules in strengths of 300 mg or 450 mg, one option is: **4 pm – 900 mg; 6 pm – 600 mg; 8 pm – 600 mg.**

e. **Check the level:** Obtain a morning trough level the next day which will be 12 ± 2 h from the last evening dose.

f. **Adjust dosing:** Based on the morning trough level, adjust the lithium dose to obtain levels in the appropriate area of the therapeutic range (e.g. for acute mania, for maintenance). Either standard or sustained release preparations can be used, but dosing should be consolidated to QHS prior to discharge (for inpatients) or as soon as possible (for outpatients) with a repeat 12 h trough level ordered on QHS single dosing.

g. **Monitor eGFR:** Add a serum creatinine and cystatin C (if possible) for eGFR approximately 1 week after the loading procedure, and then repeat at week 6, month 3 and month 6 as with any new lithium start. (See Chapter 2, Info Box 2.3, for use of the new creatinine–cystatin C based eGFR formula, and Info Box 2.7 for renal monitoring of lithium treated patients.)

D Clinically Significant Kinetic Drug Interactions

WHAT TO KNOW: SIGNIFICANT KINETIC INTERACTIONS

- There are very few classes of medications with significant interactions. With a few minutes spent reviewing Table 3.6, every clinician should be able to prescribe lithium safely.

- Clinicians should communicate with other medical providers so that new use of a kinetically interacting medication can be immediately addressed, based on the extent of the interaction.

- Concomitant use of ACE inhibitors, ARBs, thiazides and furosemide can be safely managed by immediate lithium dose adjustment and use of follow-up levels on the combination. The only ACE inhibitor to avoid is lisinopril as it is 100% renally cleared and more likely to induce toxicity.

- Less than 5 days exposure to an NSAID in those with eGFR > 75 ml/min and baseline lithium levels < 0.80 mEq/l is unlikely to be clinically significant. More extended or chronic NSAID use in patients with high baseline levels ($\geq$ 0.80 mEq/l), an eGFR < 75 ml/min or in any patient receiving another higher-risk medication for kinetic interactions demands lithium level monitoring.

- SGLT2 and carbonic anhydrase inhibitors are two medication classes that lower lithium levels.

The prospect of pharmacokinetic interactions inducing supratherapeutic lithium levels and toxicity should not be minimized, but management of this issue is not as daunting as it might appear for one fundamental reason: the list of medications with significant kinetic effects is modest and comprises agents from a small number of pharmaceutical classes, very few of which are absolutely forbidden (e.g. lisinopril), although some are discouraged. In the vast majority of instances, the interacting medication is used on an ongoing basis for a chronic disorder (e.g. hypertension), so the period of biggest risk is when the two are combined and more

Table 3.6 Medications with kinetic interactions by class [91, 102]

Class	Magnitude of effect on lithium levels when used without other interacting medications	Management strategy [a,b] When added to lithium	Management strategy [a,b] When lithium is added
Angiotensin converting enzyme (ACE) inhibitors (e.g. benazepril, enalapril, fosinopril, lisinopril,[c] perindopril, ramipril, quinapril, trandolapril)	Increases levels on average by 36%, but can cause delayed toxicity after 3–5 weeks without lithium dosing adjustments or careful monitoring. (See note below about lisinopril.[c])	Decrease current lithium dose by 33%, check levels after 1 week, 3 weeks, 6 weeks and 12 weeks, or 1 week after any lithium or ACEI dosage change. In patients ≥ 60 years old, add serum sodium to routine monitoring.	Decrease proposed lithium dose by 33%, check levels after 1 week, 3 weeks, 6 weeks and 12 weeks, or 1 week after any lithium or ACEI dosage change. In patients ≥ 60 years old, add serum sodium to routine monitoring.
Angiotensin receptor II antagonists (e.g. azilsartan, irbesartan, losartan, olmesartan, telmisartan, valsartan)	Case reports of toxicity for most agents without lithium dosing adjustments or careful monitoring, but limited prospective data on mean effects.	Similar to ACE inhibitors.	Similar to ACE inhibitors.
Calcium channel blockers (dihydropyridines: amlodipine, clevidipine, felodipine, isradipine, levamlodipine, nicardipine, nifedipine, nimodipine, nisoldipine; non-hydropyridines: diltiazem, verapamil)	No significant effects.	No adjustments to current lithium dose.	No adjustments to proposed lithium dose.
Diuretics: carbonic anhydrase inhibitors (e.g. acetazolamide)	May reduce lithium levels due to 31% increased clearance.	No adjustments to current lithium dose. Check lithium level in 1 week and adjust dosage. Recheck level in 1 week.	No adjustments to proposed lithium dose, but may see lower levels than expected due to increased clearance. Check lithium levels after 1 week and 12 weeks.

Drug			
Diuretics: loop (e.g. bumetanide, furosemide)	In younger patients with normal renal function, effects are modest (11% or less increase in levels). Effects in older patients (especially with impaired renal function) are less well studied, but all reported cases of toxicity come from this cohort.	Patients < 60 years with eGFR > 60 ml/min: maintain current lithium dose and check lithium levels after 1 week. Patients ≥ 60 years or with eGFR ≤ 60 ml/min: decrease current lithium dose by 25%, and check levels and serum sodium after 1 week, 3 weeks, 6 weeks and 12 weeks.	Patients < 60 years with eGFR > 60 ml/min: no adjustments to proposed lithium dose and check lithium levels after 1 week. Patients ≥ 60 years: decrease proposed lithium dose by 25%, and check levels and serum sodium after 1 week, 3 weeks, 6 weeks and 12 weeks.
Diuretics: potassium sparing (e.g. amiloride, spironolactone, triamterene)	Limited effects.	No adjustments to current lithium dose. Check lithium level in 1 week and 12 weeks.	No adjustments to proposed lithium dose. Check lithium levels after 1 week and 12 weeks.
Diuretics: thiazide-type (e.g. chlorthalidone, hydrochlorothiazide)	Increases levels on average by 20–25%, but can cause toxicity without monitoring or dosing adjustments.	Decrease current lithium dose by 25%, and check levels after 1 week, 3 weeks, 6 weeks and 12 weeks, or 1 week after any lithium or diuretic dosage change. In patients ≥ 60 years old, add serum sodium to routine monitoring.	Decrease proposed lithium dose by 25%, and check levels after 1 week, 3 weeks, 6 weeks and 12 weeks, or 1 week after any lithium or diuretic dosage change. In patients ≥ 60 years old, add serum sodium to routine monitoring.
NSAID (aspirin, celecoxib, doclofenac, ibuprofen, indomethacin, ketoprofen, meloxicam, naproxen, piroxicam, sulindac)	≤ 5 day exposure in those with eGFR > 75 ml/min and baseline levels < 0.80 mEq/l unlikely to be clinically significant. More extended or chronic use in patients with high baseline levels (≥ 0.80 mEq/l), eGFR < 75 ml/min or in any patient receiving another higher-risk medication demands lithium level monitoring as increases up to 66.5% have been noted.	Time limited use (≤ 14 days): check levels after 1 week and only adjust lithium dose if levels are > 1.00 mEq/l. Resume prior lithium dose after NSAID discontinued. Extended or chronic use in patients with high baseline levels (≥ 0.80 mEq/l), eGFR < 75 ml/min or in any patient receiving another higher-risk medication: decrease current lithium dose by 25%, and check levels after 1 week, 3 weeks, 6 weeks and 12 weeks, or 1 week after any NSAID dosage change.	Consider eschewing lithium in those already on agents with significant kinetic interactions and with baseline eGFR < 75 ml/min. For other patients, decrease proposed lithium dose by 25%, and check levels after 1 week, 3 weeks, 6 weeks and 12 weeks.

Class	Magnitude of effect on lithium levels when used without other interacting medications	Management strategy [a, b]	
		When added to lithium	When lithium is added
Sodium–glucose cotransporter 2 (SGLT-2) inhibitors	May reduce lithium levels 63% due to increased clearance [103].	Check lithium level after 72 hours and adjust dosage. Recheck level in 1 week.[d]	No adjustments to proposed lithium dose, but may see markedly lower levels than expected due to increased clearance. Check lithium levels after 1 week, 12 weeks.[d]
Antibiotic: metronidazole	Rare case reports (n = 3). Kinetic interaction by unknown mechanism [104, 105].	A rare interaction best managed by warning lithium treated patients who start metronidazole to stop it immediately for central nervous system adverse effects, especially those which resemble lithium toxicity, and seek medical attention.	Metronidazole is not used chronically. If lithium must be started while on metronidazole, obtain a level after 1 week on both medications, and 1 week after completing the course of metronidazole.

Notes

[a] Lithium levels should always be rechecked 1 week after any dosage change.

[b] Two types of medications with significant interactions should not be used concurrently with lithium if avoidable. This includes combination products of ACEIs or ARBs with thiazides, these agents added independently, or use of a loop diuretic with agents that possess significant risk. The addition of an NSAID routinely for more than 3 days to other agents with significant risk also poses a hazard unless a lithium level is obtained.

[c] Lisinopril is the only ACE inhibitor that should be combined with lithium, for two reasons: (1) lisinopril is the only ACEI that is 100% renally cleared and thus will accumulate in those with subnormal renal function; (2) lisinopril has linear dose-dependent effects, so any decrement in renal function increases both the lisinopril level and its effects, leading to further decreases in lithium clearance and eventual lithium toxicity [94].

[d] Be vigilant for lithium toxicity if the SGLT-2 inhibitor is subsequently discontinued, as lithium levels may increase up to 3-fold. Inform the primary care provider or endocrinologist that they should notify you immediately if the SGLT-2 inhibitor is to be discontinued. The lithium dose should then be reduced by 50%, the level rechecked in 1 week, and further dosage adjustments made.

frequent lithium level monitoring is required, especially if one or both agents are being titrated. However, once a patient is on stable doses of both medications for months, an equilibrium has been reached and monitoring can gradually return to a schedule dictated by other factors (e.g. eGFR, risks for CKD, albumin-to-creatinine ratio; see Chapter 2, Info Box 2.7). The important safety principles are limited: avoid (if possible) using more than one agent with significant lithium kinetic effects concurrently (e.g. a combination product with an ACEI or ARB and a thiazide); recognize that certain medications may have limited effects in younger patients but warrant careful monitoring in patients > 60 years of age (e.g. loop diuretics such as furosemide); and appreciate that limited use of NSAIDs for 2–3 days is not the area of biggest concern, while chronic use, even with low-dose aspirin (ASA), can exert a measurable effect [90].

The easiest class of medications to master are the ACEIs and ARBs, both of which act to blunt agonist activity at the angiotensin II receptor type 1 [91]. Renin is a protein with enzymatic activity released by the kidneys in response to low vascular volume as sensed by decreased renal vascular perfusion pressure [91]. One function of renin is to convert the hepatically synthesized prohormone angiotensinogen into angiotensin I, and this is further cleaved into angiotensin II by angiotensin converting enzymes in pulmonary and other vascular beds. ACEIs block this last conversion step, while ARBs block the action of angiotensin II at its receptor site. The result of decreased angiotensin II activity is lower aldosterone levels and alterations in peripheral and renal hemodynamics that combine to decrease the reabsorption of sodium and water. As discussed in Chapter 2, lithium and sodium compete for proximal reabsorption at the Na^+/H^+-exchanger type 3 (NHE3), so increased sodium excretion can lead to a compensatory increase in lithium reabsorption, with a mean increase in lithium levels on average by 36% when ACEIs are added to existing lithium therapy [91, 92]. If no adjustments are made to lithium dosing, toxicity can occur, but this interaction is now widely established in a manner that was not true 20 years ago [93]. There is no compelling reason to avoid these useful classes of antihypertensive medications assuming all parties understand the need to adjust lithium dosing and recheck levels. The only medication in this group that should never be used is lisinopril as documented in the footnotes for Table 3.6 [94]. Any other ACEI or ARB can be used in lieu of lisinopril. With these concerns in mind, Table 3.6 outlines the need to decrease lithium doses initially by approximately 33% when an ACEI or ARB is added, to recheck levels until the patient is back to the pre-existing lithium level baseline, and also to check levels if the dose of the ACEI, ARB or lithium is changed. The biggest period of risk is shortly after combining the ACEI or ARB with lithium [93]. When adding lithium to a patient on an ACEI or an ARB, the proposed lithium dose (based on considerations of age, weight, eGFR, gender and clinical circumstances) should be 33% lower than one would typically employ until the extent of the kinetic effect is measured. As the risk for symptomatic hyponatremia from ACEIs or ARBs is higher among older individuals, serum sodium should be added to routine monitoring when lithium levels are checked in patients $\geq$ 60 years old [95].

Thiazide-type diuretics have been available since 1959, and the latest hypertension guidelines recommend them as first-line agents, with preferential use over ACEIs/ARBs in those with African heritage [96]. Given their long history and ubiquitous use, the interaction between thiazide diuretics and lithium has been known for 50 years, and was even studied by the famous Danish psychiatrist Mogens Schou [97, 98]. The thiazide-type diuretic family consists of the classical thiazide structures (e.g. hydrochlorothiazide [HCTZ]), and what are termed thiazide-like compounds, such as chlorthalidone, all of which share a common site of action at the Na^+/Cl^- electroneutral cotransporter (NCC) on the apical side of distal convoluted tubule epithelial cells [99]. By competing for the NCC chloride binding site, thiazide-type diuretics impair sodium transport in distal segments resulting in sodium wasting and water loss (Figure 3.6) [90]. Thiazide-type medications possess other mechanisms contributing to blood pressure reduction, including carbonic anhydrase inhibition by chlorthalidone and, to a lesser extent, by HCTZ, but it is this ongoing natriuresis that leads to a compensatory increase in proximal lithium reabsorption via NHE3 and the potential for lithium toxicity [100, 101]. However, the literature is also clear that, with careful monitoring, use of thiazide-type diuretics is not associated with undue risk of lithium toxicity. In 2004, a Canadian group published data on the risk of hospitalization for drug-induced lithium toxicity from a nested case-control study of 10,615 patients aged $\geq$ 66 years residing in Ontario during 1992–2001 [93]. There were 413 individuals admitted at least once for lithium toxicity in this age cohort and these subjects were matched with 4 lithium treated controls based on age and gender, with prescriptions examined for use of any diuretic, ACEI or NSAID before the index date (i.e. hospital admission for lithium toxicity) [93]. Thiazide-type diuretic exposure was not associated with increased relative risk (RR) of hospitalization during chronic use with lithium (RR 1.3; 95% CI 0.7–2.5), or among those newly initiated on thiazide treatment (RR 1.3; 95% CI 0.4–4.7). ACEIs were relatively new at the time and were associated with a markedly increased risk for lithium toxicity

Figure 3.6 Impact of antihypertensives on renal lithium clearance [91]

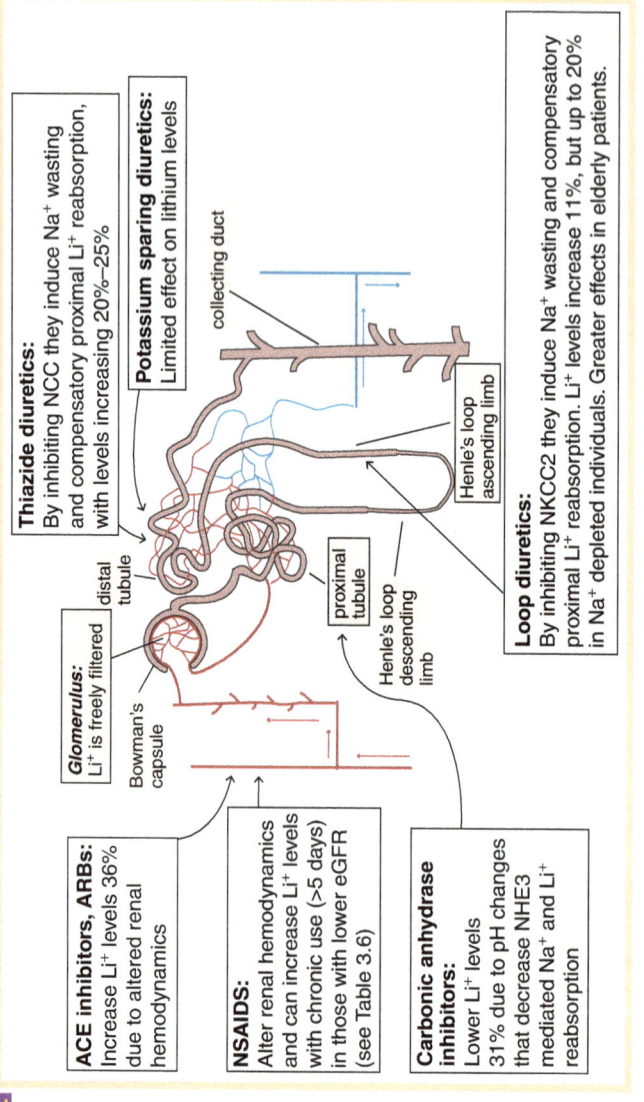

Thiazide diuretics:
By inhibiting NCC they induce Na⁺ wasting and compensatory proximal Li⁺ reabsorption, with levels increasing 20%–25%

Potassium sparing diuretics:
Limited effect on lithium levels

collecting duct

Henle's loop ascending limb

Loop diuretics:
By inhibiting NKCC2 they induce Na⁺ wasting and compensatory proximal Li⁺ reabsorption. Li⁺ levels increase 11%, but up to 20% in Na⁺ depleted individuals. Greater effects in elderly patients.

distal tubule

Glomerulus:
Li⁺ is freely filtered

proximal tubule

Henle's loop descending limb

Bowman's capsule

ACE inhibitors, ARBs:
Increase Li⁺ levels 36% due to altered renal hemodynamics

NSAIDS:
Alter renal hemodynamics and can increase Li⁺ levels with chronic use (>5 days) in those with lower eGFR (see Table 3.6)

Carbonic anhydrase inhibitors:
Lower Li⁺ levels 31% due to pH changes that decrease NHE3 mediated Na⁺ and Li⁺ reabsorption

(Adapted from: V. Bisogni, G. Rossitto, F. Reghin, et al. [2016]. Antihypertensive therapy in patients on chronic lithium treatment for bipolar disorders. *J Hypertens*, 34, 20–28.)

among new starts (RR 7.6; 95% CI 2.6–22.0), as was exposure to loop diuretics (RR 5.5; 95% CI 1.9–16.1), an unexpected finding discussed below [93]. In general, the mean increase in lithium levels from thiazide-type diuretics is in the range of 20–25%, so appropriate adjustments must be made to existing lithium therapy when a thiazide is added, or to lithium doses when starting lithium in a thiazide treated patient [102]. As the risk for symptomatic hyponatremia from thiazide-type diuretics is higher among older individuals, serum sodium should be added to routine monitoring when lithium levels are checked in patients $\geq$ 60 years old [101]. Nonetheless, the Ontario data provide reassurance that use of lithium in older patients on thiazide-type diuretics can be managed without undue risk when there is attentive monitoring of lithium levels.

As discussed in Chapter 2, prior to exiting the proximal nephron only a modest amount of filtered lithium is reabsorbed in the thick ascending limb of Henle (3–10%), although this value may be as high as 20% in salt-depleted individuals [106–108]. Part of lithium's reabsorption in the thick ascending loop is via the $Na^+/K^+/2Cl^-$ cotransporter type 2 (NKCC2) present on the apical surface, a transporter which is inhibited by loop diuretics such as furosemide [91]. As use of loop diuretics induces a certain amount of sodium and water loss, there was concern that lithium toxicity arising from sodium depletion would be seen to the same extent as with thiazide-type diuretics. Schou's 1968 study of lithium clearance among six healthy individuals given a single 600 mg lithium dose found a modest 11% reduction from furosemide pretreatment [109], but subsequent case reports emerged of lithium toxicity from concurrent loop diuretic use, all of which were in older individuals [102]. The Ontario, Canada study provided the first assessment of the relative risk among patients aged $\geq$ 66 years old (RR 5.5; 95% CI 1.9–16.1), and highlighted the need for assiduous monitoring and lithium dose adjustment when loop diuretics are used, but particularly in older individuals who appear to experience greater volume contraction and sodium depletion than do younger individuals [93].

Calcium channel blockers are another class of commonly used medications for hypertension with two major chemical groups: the dihydropyridine calcium channel blockers used primarily for hypertension (e.g. amlodipine and other -dipine medications); and those with other structures (e.g. diltiazem, verapamil) that may also be used for certain cardiac arrhythmias [91]. Despite widespread use over decades, there are only isolated case reports of adverse reactions to verapamil or diltiazem that likely represent idiosyncratic pharmacodynamic and not kinetic interactions with lithium [102, 110–113]. Among the dihydropyridines, there is one study which used lithium clearance as a measure of renal activity, and noted a 30% decrease after 12 weeks on nifedipine 40–80 mg/d [114]. As the dihydropyridines are also widely used and have been available for almost 30 years, the absence of case reports suggest that any impact is not clinically significant.

There are also certain classes of diuretics whose adverse impact on lithium clearance is clinically insignificant, although all patients commencing a combination with these agents deserve at least one repeat lithium level to confirm the lack of effect. Amiloride and potassium sparing diuretics (e.g. spironolactone, triamterene) are in this group, and amiloride is the medication with the most evidence for treating lithium related nephrogenic diabetes insipidus (NDI) [102, 115, 116]. As covered extensively in Chapter 2, lithium induces most of its renal effects by entering collecting duct principal cells via the apical ENaC, in part due to its 1.6-fold greater affinity than sodium for ENaC [117, 118]. The form of ENaC present in collecting duct cells is antagonized by amiloride, hence the rationale for its use in lithium treated patients whose urine osmolality dips into the abnormal range [115]. Moreover, amiloride induces modest sodium wasting and appears to have limited effects on lithium clearance when used for polyuria management [117, 119, 120]. Triamterene is also an ENaC inhibitor, but despite the fact that both triamterene and amiloride have been available since the 1960s there is limited literature on use of triamterene for lithium related NDI [121]. While triamterene itself is not associated with significant effects on lithium levels, the most common marketed form of triamterene is a combination with HCTZ due to the greater efficacy of the combination compared with thiazide monotherapy. Use of this combination product would incur all of the risks of any thiazide medication, as would the use of an amiloride–HCTZ combination agent [122, 123]. Spironolactone is an interesting medication: it is a potent aldosterone receptor antagonist and a moderate androgen receptor antagonist. The latter can complicate spironolactone's use in males as an antihypertensive due to risk of adverse effects such as gynecomastia and decreased libido [124]. Spironolactone has two mechanisms that contribute to its antihypertensive properties: antagonism of aldosterone mediated sodium–potassium exchange near the junction of the distal convoluted tubule; and antagonism of aldosterone-induced vasoconstriction in renal arterioles [124]. Spironolactone was one of the agents examined in Schou's 1968 study of six healthy individuals given a single 600 mg lithium dose. Pretreatment with spironolactone lowered lithium levels by 20% although the result was not statistically significant [109].

Another class of diuretics known as carbonic anhydrase inhibitors (e.g. acetazolamide) has been found to lower lithium levels, with the 1968 Schou study noting a 31% increase in lithium clearance, a finding that was statistically significant [102, 109]. The diuretic mechanism involves carbonic anhydrase inhibition in the renal proximal tubule. This enzyme catalyzes the breakdown of carbonic acid into carbon dioxide and water as shown: $HCO_3^- + H^+ \to H_2O + CO_2$. Inhibiting this enzyme induces local pH changes that decrease reabsorption of bicarbonate, chloride, sodium and lithium. Recall that lithium and sodium are reabsorbed via NHE3 by exchanging these cations for a proton (H^+) – the altered pH from carbonic anhydrase inhibition slows this process [91]. After finding that acetazolamide lowered lithium levels, Schou also examined bicarbonate infusion and noted an almost identical increase in lithium clearance of 27% [109]. The proximal pH alteration related to excessive bicarbonate exposure may explain certain cases in which clinicians experienced difficulties in achieving therapeutic lithium levels among outpatients who consumed large antacid doses [102]. It is the acetazolamide related increases in excretion of bicarbonate, sodium and chloride along with water which lowers blood pressure, with similar diuretic effects in the brain and eye that lead to decreased intracranial pressure and decreased intraocular pressure [125].

Acetazolamide thus has a number of uses including altitude sickness or idiopathic intracranial hypertension, glaucoma, epilepsy and essential tremor, but is not a commonly seen medication in clinical practice. It may, however, assume a greater use in management of NDI based on recent research findings. While amiloride is the preferred medication for lithium related NDI due its specific action on ENaC, there is a considerable literature on use of HCTZ for this same purpose [97, 99]. The explanation for the thiazide effect was unclear until research with mouse knockout models lacking the thiazide-sensitive NCC found that HCTZ also reduced lithium induced polyuria in these animals [99]. As NCC is the primary target for thiazide-type medications, it was postulated that a secondary property, carbonic anhydrase inhibition, mediated thiazide effects on lithium induced NDI in NCC knockouts [99, 126]. Thiazides were derived from carbonic anhydrase inhibitors, and subsequent studies with acetazolamide confirmed that carbonic anhydrase inhibition is an effective mechanism for lithium induced NDI, comparable to the effects of an amiloride/thiazide combination regimen but without the thiazide related risks for hyperkalemia, hyponatremia and increased lithium levels [126–128]. Several case reports emerged shortly thereafter noting clinical response to acetazolamide in lithium related NDI, often in patients who failed to respond to amiloride or HCTZ but who improved when acetazolamide was added [129, 130]. While there are limited data from human studies, these case reports and animal data suggest another option for lithium related NDI not responding to amiloride [126]. (See Chapter 5 for discussion of NDI management and adjunctive use of acetazolamide.)

There are two other classes of diuretics worth noting: osmotic diuretics (e.g. mannitol) and caffeine. Mannitol is commonly used to treat elevated intracranial pressure, and thus will induce a marked diuresis that substantially lowers lithium levels [102]. During such circumstances, the need to continue lithium must be considered, and the treatment team must also be informed that the patient may already possess a pre-existing urine concentration deficit, so serum osmolality and serum sodium may need to be monitored very carefully, even after forced diuresis, to prevent severe dehydration and hypernatremia [131]. Caffeine induced diuresis can lower lithium levels as noted by studies and case reports, including one where excessive diet cola consumption was the culprit [132]. Discontinuation of caffeine will subsequently be associated with an increase in lithium levels [133, 134]. In a controlled study of 11 subjects who were heavy coffee drinkers (mean 5.3 ± 0.7 cups per day, estimated caffeine content 70–120 mg/cup), 2 weeks of a caffeine free diet generated a mean 24% increase in lithium levels (along with high rates of caffeine withdrawal symptoms) [134]. With more modest consumption, the effect is presumed smaller, but the clinical point is to consider the impact of heavy caffeine use on lithium clearance, and the impact of significant changes in heavy caffeine consumption.

Nonsteroidal anti-inflammatory drugs (NSAIDs) represent the class of medications that engender the most confusion, partly due to the sporadic and uncontrolled nature of their use. By inhibiting prostaglandin synthesis, all of these agents alter renal hemodynamics and can potentially decrease lithium clearance. Whether the effect is clinically relevant depends on the chronicity of exposure, baseline lithium level, baseline renal function, and use of other medications with kinetic effects on lithium disposition. For example, a study of naproxen 220 mg TID for 5 days on lithium levels in 12 male volunteers (mean age 28 years) receiving lithium 600 mg/d found the impact negligible and indistinguishable from that of acetaminophen [135]. With normal renal function, modest baseline lithium levels (mean 0.40 ± 0.05 mEq/l) and a limited exposure of 5 days, there is unlikely to be a safety concern with any NSAID. However, there are sufficient reports of interactions with all NSAIDs, including aspirin, to warrant some form of lithium level monitoring during chronic or extended use, with the extent of concern based on the expected exposure duration, lithium level and eGFR, and presence of other medications that interact kinetically with lithium [90, 136]. The recommendations in Table 3.6 represent one approach to synthesizing these considerations, and thereby manage potential NSAID related risks while not subjecting patients in lower-risk situations to excessive worry and excessive monitoring. Patients in the highest-risk situation due to a trough level ≥ 0.80 mEq/l, an eGFR below the midpoint of stage G2 CKD (< 75 ml/min), and use of other medications with kinetic interactions must be counseled to use alternatives whenever possible (e.g. acetaminophen or paracetamol); moreover, if NSAID use is unavoidable for more than very short durations (e.g. 2–3 days), patients can be instructed to discuss with you a pretreatment lithium dose decrease of 25% with a follow-up level after 1 week, especially where access to an emergency room may be difficult should lithium toxicity develop. The Ontario, Canada study examining hospitalization for lithium toxicity in patients aged ≥ 66 years old found that NSAID use did not increase risk with new or ongoing prescriptions; however, only 7.1% of the sample were on NSAIDs, suggesting a selection bias towards those individuals who, despite their age, may have possessed lower risks for lithium toxicity and thus were acceptable NSAID candidates [93].

One kinetic interaction with lithium relates to use of a newer class of DM medication: the sodium–glucose cotransporter 2 (SGLT-2) inhibitors. SGLT-2 is a high capacity transporter which utilizes a sodium gradient created by the ATP driven Na^+/K^+ pump to move glucose from the apical surface of proximal tubule epithelial cells [137]. Glucose is freely filtered in the glomerulus, but over 90% of the glucose initially filtered is reabsorbed by SGLT-2 in the early convoluted segment of the proximal tubules [137]. Reabsorption of most of the remaining filtered glucose is mediated by the structurally related SGLT-1 [137]. SGLT-2 inhibitors have been approved for over a decade and are widely prescribed for several adult indications including: reducing the risk of cardiovascular death and hospitalization associated with heart failure, reducing the risk of cardiovascular death in patients with type 2 DM and cardiovascular disease, and for improving glycemic control in those with type 2 DM [138]. Despite multiple indications, it was not until 2020 that a case report emerged of a potential interaction in the form of a patient treated with empagliflozin whose 63% drop in lithium levels suggested an SGLT-2 inhibitor mediated effect on lithium excretion [103]. The single case involved an obese patient with a trough lithium level of 1.1 mEq/l on 1350 mg/d who was newly diagnosed with type 2 DM during a psychiatric hospitalization for mania [103]. Empagliflozin, an SGLT-2 inhibitor, was titrated to 25 mg QAM, but within 72 hours the 12 h trough lithium level had decreased to 0.4 mEq/l, a result that was confirmed the following morning. Empagliflozin was discontinued, the patient's hyperglycemia temporarily managed with routine QHS insulin, and 6 days later the trough lithium level was back to the pre-SGLT-2 inhibitor baseline. As the finding was unexpected and not documented in the literature, the patient was willing to undergo an empagliflozin rechallenge. Within 48 hours of resuming empagliflozin 25 mg QAM, the lithium level dropped to 0.5 mEq/l. The mean decrease in serum lithium levels during the two brief courses of empagliflozin therapy was 63%. Although this represents a single case, the robust effect upon rechallenge and the prompt return to baseline after empagliflozin discontinuation indicates an association with SGLT-2 inhibitor exposure. In the absence of contrary data that this case example represents a rare instance due to unknown patient factors, the potential SGLT-2 inhibitor interaction deserves significant attention as subtherapeutic levels might occur within 72 h of commencing the combination with lithium. Lithium level monitoring and dosage adjustment will also be necessary to prevent lithium toxicity when an SGLT-2 inhibitor is discontinued after co-treatment with lithium.

E | Other Factors Affecting Lithium Levels

WHAT TO KNOW: SIGNIFICANT KINETIC INTERACTIONS

- The most common scenario leading to lithium toxicity involves depletion of sodium stores by GI losses or excessive sweating *AND* failure to replace electrolyte losses. In these situations, patients must be instructed not to drink free water, but to manage their dehydration with a balanced over-the-counter electrolyte solution (available in packets or ready mixed) that replaces the lost sodium.

- High altitudes (≥ 3000 meters) decrease lithium clearance. Individuals who plan to spend 24 h or more must be counseled and a plan developed to mitigate lithium toxicity.

- Pregnancy involves a net increase in renal function which peaks in the 2nd trimester and slowly returns close to baseline over the 3rd trimester. Changes in lithium levels throughout pregnancy demand periodic monitoring and dosage adjustment.

- Patients undergoing bariatric surgery will have postoperative lithium levels increase 2-fold to 5-fold, regardless of the procedure type. This can be managed by reducing the dose by 50% immediately following surgery and checking the level 1 week after the surgery, with ongoing periodic levels and dosage adjustments over the first year as the patient loses weight.

Temporal factors can also alter lithium clearance, and the greatest effects are seen when patients are subjected to conditions associated with excessive sodium losses, including GI disorders with vomiting or diarrhea, or environmental situations that promote excessive sweating [139–142]. As discussed in the section above, any state that induces sodium depletion can potentially cause lithium toxicity as the relative paucity of sodium will cause lithium to be preferentially reabsorbed by

NHE3 in the proximal nephron [118, 143]. The season, the ambient temperature, sweating or strenuous exercise do not by themselves significantly impact lithium levels [141, 144, 145]. The scenario leading to lithium toxicity involves a dehydrated patient repleting losses from GI illness or heavy sweating with free water instead of with a balanced electrolyte solution [146]. While free water will restore vascular volume, it does not replace depleted sodium stores resulting in hyponatremia. The availability of electrolyte solutions initially geared for pediatric use during GI illnesses has broadened into a market with numerous products for adults who are ill or who experience significant exercise-related salt and water loss. The availability of these products is reinforced by messages from health-care providers on the need to replace both water and electrolytes with a solution that contains both. Patients commencing lithium therapy should be reminded that free water is not ideal during situations of extreme water and sodium loss, and educated about the need to use electrolyte replacement packets or ready-made electrolyte solutions (see Chapter 6 for more discussion). When persistent vomiting or diarrhea precludes acceptable oral intake for more than 12 h, patients should hold lithium for 24 h and contact their prescriber to provide guidance on resuming lithium or seeking medical attention if the GI illness does not improve. Once the patient is able to resume adequate oral intake, the usual lithium dose is restarted unless some other serious issue (e.g. acute kidney injury from severe dehydration) is detected in situations where the patient needed medical help. With a CNS $T_{1/2}$ of 28–48 h, a patient who holds their lithium for 24 h or even 48 h is unlikely to incur any psychiatric sequelae. After longer periods without lithium, the clinician may consider a modest loading procedure (e.g. two 10 mg/kg doses over 24 h) to hasten the time to therapeutic levels, with a follow-up level after 5 days on the prior stable dose.

Another mechanism leading to lithium toxicity relates to the effect of high altitude on renal hemodynamics resulting in decreased lithium clearance chronically and acutely. The acute effect was seen in the only prospective high altitude study in which healthy volunteers had levels on lithium 300 mg/d checked in Santiago, Chile (elevation 600 m) and then after 15 h in the Andes (elevation 4360 m) [147]. Chronic altitude exposure also decreased lithium clearance, although routine level monitoring mitigates any concerns from this and other kinetic issues [147]. The acute effect is what lithium treated patients need to be counseled on, with instructions about vigilance for signs of lithium toxicity appearing in the form of new or worsening adverse effects. There is one case report of a healthy 33-year-old female on lithium 900 mg/d who set out to ascend Mt. Whitney in California (altitude 4418 m) from sea level, with 1 day acclimatization at a midway point [148]. She developed symptoms of acute mountain sickness (headache, nausea), but also manifested evidence of increased CNS lithium levels with worsening of her lithium related tremor during the ascent. Ingestion of two 800 mg ibuprofen doses for headache was documented, but this brief NSAID exposure was unlikely to have created a significant kinetic effect – the altitude change seems the most probable explanation [148]. If patients who plan on high altitude exposure are concerned about this effect, one can discuss a possible modest dose reduction (e.g. 25–33%), starting 24 h prior to the trip. Since acetazolamide is used for acute mountain sickness, patients should also be educated that it will lower lithium levels if used persistently (e.g. when used for acute mountain sickness prophylaxis) [109].

Another temporal situation associated with altered renal hemodynamics and lithium clearance is pregnancy [149]. Fluid shifts during pregnancy induce a state of hyperfiltration (i.e. increased eGFR) clinically seen as a decrease in serum creatinine that reaches its nadir around week 18, and gradually increases in the 3rd trimester (Figure 3.7) [150]. Not surprisingly, changes in lithium levels parallel these eGFR trends, and these changes argue for more diligent serum level monitoring and dosage adjustment, especially if mood symptoms arise. In 2017, a Dutch group retrospectively examined 1101 lithium levels in 113 patients throughout the course of their pregnancy [149]. Lithium levels decreased on average 24% in the 1st trimester (95% CI -15% to -35%), and reached the lowest point in the 2nd trimester, 36% below the pre-pregnancy baseline (95% CI -27% to -47%) [149]. Levels increased modestly in the 3rd trimester but remained 21% below baseline (95% CI 13% to -30%), with a slight 9% increase in the postpartum period (95% CI +2% to

Figure 3.7 Changes in serum creatinine throughout the course of pregnancy [150]

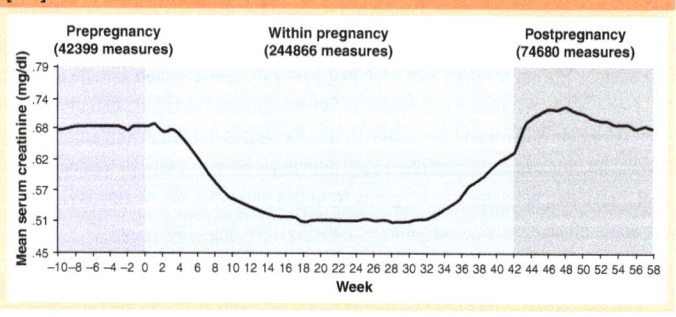

(Adapted from: Z. Harel, E. McArthur, M. Hladunewich, et al. [2019]. Serum creatinine levels before, during, and after pregnancy. *JAMA*, 321, 205–207.)

+15%). A Norwegian study noted a similar effect after examining 25 serum lithium levels from 14 pregnancies in 13 women, and compared these with 63 baseline levels from the same women [151]. Dose-adjusted serum concentrations in the 3rd trimester were significantly lower than baseline (-34%; 95% CI -44% to -23%, $p < 0.001$) [151]. This state of hyperfiltration is a unique feature of pregnancy, and neither use of oral contraceptives nor hormonal shifts during the menstrual cycle have any significant impact on lithium levels throughout the month [152].

The impact of the mood state on lithium levels was studied in prior decades, especially the relationship between mania and increased lithium clearance [153]. Hypotheses arose that an increase in total body water may occur during manic phases leading to dilution and reduced serum lithium levels, but these and other ideas were speculative and difficult to prove given the mental state of the subject population. As bipolar I disorder (BD-1) patients transition from mania to euthymia, lithium doses and levels are lowered into the preferred maintenance range of 0.60–0.80 mEq/l, so any putative impact of the manic state on lithium clearance will be compensated for once dosing is optimized for the maintenance phase of the illness [12]. During maintenance treatment, the greatest impact on longitudinal lithium levels is nonadherence. For adherent patients, changes in medications that kinetically interact with lithium and alterations in renal function are the primary suspects. Given this logic, any change in mood state, especially to the manic pole, should prompt a repeat 12 h trough level to rule out subtherapeutic levels related to nonadherence or kinetic factors, including the possible effects of the mood state itself, and a plan devised to restore levels to the therapeutic range for the particular mood state.

Obesity is a prevalent problem in those with serious mental illnesses, but having a psychiatric diagnosis is no longer considered a contraindication to surgical weight loss procedures, assuming a patient is deemed an appropriate candidate to follow all recommended treatment parameters [154, 155]. Bariatric surgery can impact the bioavailability of any orally administered medication, but the extent of the effect is quite variable and depends on the procedure and absorption characteristics of the medication. In the case of lithium, there are multiple changes to diet prior to and after surgery (e.g. low sodium diet), combined with alterations in body weight and composition that impact lithium clearance [156]. The net result is that postoperative lithium levels can increase 2-fold to 5-fold regardless of the type of bariatric procedure, a situation that can result in lithium toxicity [156–163]. A 2022 literature review of 11 cases found that occurrence of lithium toxicity ranged from 9 days to 6 months after surgery, with 8 of 11 cases having their onset within the first month after the bariatric procedure [156]. As bariatric surgery is scheduled in advance, it would seem prudent to mitigate this effect by lowering postoperative doses by 50% immediately following the procedure, and obtaining a level 1 week after the surgery. Lithium doses can then be adjusted to mirror the baseline level. Even after a period of lithium dosage adjustment, recent papers recommend rechecking the eGFR and lithium level weekly for the first 6 weeks, every 2 weeks through week 12, then tapering down to monthly levels as the patient approaches 6 months from the date of surgery [156]. As it may take 6–12 months to recover from bariatric surgery, consider monthly lithium level and eGFR monitoring during months 6–9 as the patient's body adapts to the rapid changes induced by the surgery, reducing to a bimonthly eGFR and lithium level through the end of the first year [162]. Bariatric surgery requires careful planning, so clinicians can use this planning stage to engage in discussions about postoperative lithium dosage adjustments and the need for regular level monitoring to minimize the risk of lithium toxicity.

 Lithium's Pharmacodynamic Interactions

WHAT TO KNOW: SIGNIFICANT PHARMACODYNAMIC INTERACTIONS

- Historical reports that use of lithium with a first generation antipsychotic (FGA) may induce neurotoxicity relates to excessively high antipsychotic dosages used in prior decades. A detailed review of these cases indicates that most of these patients manifested features of neuroleptic malignant syndrome.

- As FGAs are prescribed in much more modest dosages in modern practice, these cases have virtually disappeared from the literature. There is no contraindication to combining lithium with any antipsychotic.

- There are reports of lithium related exacerbation of Parkinson's disease motor symptoms, and rare reports of reversible drug-induced parkinsonism in older patients. The decision to continue lithium in these patients must be individualized and based on whether lithium's benefits (e.g. neuroprotection, mood stability, suicidality reduction) outweigh the motor effects.

Lithium has vanishingly few pharmacodynamic interactions of significance, with many associations raised in prior decades no longer supported by the literature. One example: rare cases of exaggerated reactions to lithium in patients on the calcium channel blockers verapamil or diltiazem, at times with altered mental states and psychosis, or bradycardia [110–113]. There is no obvious kinetic explanation for this interaction and no cases have been reported for over 20 years, leading one review paper to conclude that any CNS or cardiac interactions with diltiazem or verapamil are rare and idiosyncratic [102]. The implication is that no management strategy is necessary due to the rarity, and that these combinations are not unsafe given the paucity of cases after decades of widespread diltiazem and verapamil use. Any safety concerns about the verapamil–lithium combination were so insignificant that one group studied verapamil augmentation of lithium for mania treatment in 2008 [164]. On the other hand, lithium can potentiate the action of neuromuscular blockers through a hypothesized presynaptic mechanism [165]. The cases all appeared in the 1970s [166], with none for decades until one group from Japan published a case report in 2020. The authors of that case noted that the paralytic action of a modest rocuronium dose (50 mg) was markedly greater than expected after 1 hour in a lithium treated 64-year-old female, although the effect was reversible with sugammadex [167]. The absence of recent cases is likely related to modern practices involving more careful titration of neuromuscular blockers, routine evaluation of neuromuscular blockade with a nerve stimulation device prior to extubation, and use of reversal agents when neuromuscular blockade is more severe or persistent than expected [167].

One area of concern that has also subsided in recent years revolves around cases suggesting lithium can significantly potentiate D_2 antagonist actions leading to neurotoxicity. One of the frequently cited reports was a 1974 paper that documented altered mental status, rigidity and fever, among other clinical findings, in four inpatients receiving treatment with lithium and haloperidol, and concluded that their concurrent use must be the cause [168]. Using a modern retrospective lens all of these patients manifested core features of neuroleptic malignant syndrome, and the most likely etiology was use of aggressive haloperidol dosing (20–70 mg/d) starting from day 1 of hospitalization [169, 170]. These cases have virtually disappeared from the literature in the past two decades due to the use of second generation antipsychotics with less potent D_2 receptor blockade, combined with prescribing practices that emphasize use of low initial doses when using first generation agents [171]. Nonetheless, warnings about this interaction persist in the haloperidol product labeling: "A causal relationship between these events and the concomitant administration of lithium and haloperidol has not been established; however, patients receiving such combined therapy should be monitored closely for early evidence of neurological toxicity and treatment discontinued promptly if such signs appear" [172]. Admittedly, there are rare individuals who are very sensitive to the effects of D_2 antagonism, to which the addition of lithium may complicate the assignment of causality. A recent case of this type described a 75-year-old male admitted for mania who developed a temperature of 37.8 °C, resting tremor, rigidity, masked facies and generalized weakness 4 days after having risperidone 2 mg QHS added to lithium 450 mg BID [173]. While meeting many of the consensus neuroleptic malignant syndrome criteria, the creatinine kinase level was within the normal range and the lithium level was 1.47 mEq/l. As discussed earlier in this chapter (Table 3.2), a trough lithium level on BID dosing will be 28% higher with QHS dosing, so a level of 1.47 mEq/l on 450 mg BID would be 1.88 mEq/l on 900 mg QHS [173]. That lithium in the toxic range might complicate D_2 antagonism is possible, but it is hard to generalize from cases such as this. The one indisputable conclusion from the recent literature is that there is no contraindication to prescribing lithium with any antipsychotic.

Despite the statement above, there are cases of lithium causing a reversible impact on D_2 neurotransmission presenting as drug-induced parkinsonism (DIP), with the common demographic feature being older age [174–176]. Dopamine transporter (DaT) SPECT scanning was performed in nine cases to rule out primary Parkinson's disease, and in eight of nine patients the scans were normal [176]. This imaging finding, and the reversibility upon lithium discontinuation, indicates that any effect of lithium is transient, that lithium is not causing loss of dopaminergic neurons or some other neurodegenerative process, and that the incidence is extremely low even among older patients [176, 177]. It is worth noting that imaging studies of BD patients with parkinsonism suggest that a subset of this patient population (20%) may have a dopaminergic deficit, a finding that might explain the rare cases of lithium related parkinsonism [178]. Medium spiny neurons in the striatum receive serotonergic input, and medications that act as serotonin agonists directly or indirectly (e.g. selective serotonin reuptake inhibitors) can induce DIP, akathisia and other movement disorders [176, 179]. Lithium facilitates serotonin release in part by actions at the $5HT_{1B}$ autoreceptor [180], so any effect on dopamine neurotransmission likely occurs via serotonergic agonism in vulnerable patients, a mechanism also postulated to underlie the rare cases of lithium related myoclonus [176, 178, 181, 182]. Whether lithium offers any neuroprotective benefits in patients with primary Parkinson's disease is unknown, but the advantages of lithium (e.g. reduction in suicide mortality, mood stability, decreased dementia risk) outweigh the motor effects in most Parkinson's disease patients, especially since VPA is also associated with reports of DIP or exacerbation of motor symptoms in Parkinson's disease [164].

Summary Points

a. Lithium has a 24 h peripheral half-life and a CNS half-life of 28–48 h. There is no efficacy advantage from multiple daily dosing, but use of lithium more than once daily will distort morning trough levels and may result in excessive lithium exposure. Multiple daily dosing is also associated with greater risk for renal insufficiency.

b. Standard lithium carbonate and lithium citrate have a T_{Max} of 1–3 h, while that for sustained release preparations is 3–6 h. All of these formulations have similar 12 h trough values, and by convention lithium levels are obtained as a 12 h level following QHS dosing. Use of a sustained release preparation may help lessen upper GI side effects (e.g. nausea, cramping), as does administration of lithium with food. Food may also lessen diarrhea complaints.

c. Test dose and loading methods have been developed to hasten time to therapeutic levels, and should be considered for acutely manic inpatients.

d. There is a small list of medications that have kinetic interactions with lithium by impacting renal blood flow or inducing sodium wasting. Most can be safely used with more careful lithium level monitoring, often paired with lithium dose adjustments based on the expected extent of the interaction.

e. High altitude and pregnancy influence lithium clearance and require patient education and monitoring. Temperature and strenuous exercise by themselves do not alter lithium clearance unless patients hydrate themselves using free water without electrolytes and thus become sodium depleted. Patients should be educated to treat dehydration with balanced electrolyte solutions and not consume free water without electrolytes.

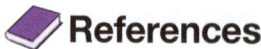

References

1. Takeuchi, H., Powell, V., Geisler, S., et al. (2016). Clozapine administration in clinical practice: Once-daily versus divided dosing. *Acta Psychiatr Scand*, 134, 234–240.

2. Meyer, J. M. and Stahl, S. M. (2019). *The Clozapine Handbook* (Stahl's Handbooks). Cambridge: Cambridge University Press.

3. Kitagawa, K., So, R., Nomura, N., et al. (2022). Clozapine once-daily versus divided dosing regimen: A cross-sectional study in Japan. *J Clin Psychopharmacol*, 42, 163–168.

4. Pfeiffer, P. N., Ganoczy, D. and Valenstein, M. (2008). Dosing frequency and adherence to antipsychotic medications. *Psychiatr Serv*, 59, 1207–1210.

5. Meyer, J. M. and Stahl, S. M. (2021). *The Clinical Use of Antipsychotic Plasma Levels* (Stahl's Handbooks). New York: Cambridge University Press.

6. Loebel, A., Cucchiaro, J., Sarma, K., et al. (2013). Efficacy and safety of lurasidone 80 mg/day and 160 mg/day in the treatment of schizophrenia: A randomized, double-blind, placebo- and active-controlled trial. *Schizophr Res*, 145, 101–109.

7. Hagi, K., Tadashi, N. and Pikalov, A. (2020). S5. Does the time of drug administration alter the adverse event risk of lurasidone? *Schizophr Bull*, 46, S31–32.

8. Carter, L., Zolezzi, M. and Lewczyk, A. (2013). An updated review of the optimal lithium dosage regimen for renal protection. *Can J Psychiatry*, 58, 595–600.

9. Castro, V. M., Roberson, A. M., McCoy, T. H., et al. (2016). Stratifying risk for renal insufficiency among lithium-treated patients: An electronic health record study. *Neuropsychopharmacology*, 41, 1138–1143.

10. ANI Pharmaceuticals Inc. (2020). *LithoBID package insert*. Baudette, MN.

11. Glenmark Pharmaceuticals Inc. (2020). *Lithium Carbonate capsule package insert*. Mahwah, NJ.

12. Nolen, W. A., Licht, R. W., Young, A. H., et al. (2019). What is the optimal serum level for lithium in the maintenance treatment of bipolar disorder? A systematic review and recommendations from the ISBD/IGSLI Task Force on treatment with lithium. *Bipolar Disord*, 21, 394–409.

13. Tyrer, S. P., Peat, M. A., Minty, P. S., et al. (1982). Bioavailability of lithium carbonate and lithium citrate: A comparison of two controlled-release preparations. *Pharmatherapeutica*, 3, 243–246.

14. Arancibia, A., Corvalan, F., Mella, F., et al. (1986). Absorption and disposition kinetics of lithium carbonate following administration of conventional and controlled release formulations. *Int J Clin Pharmacol Ther Toxicol*, 24, 240–245.

15. Guelen, P. J., Janssen, T. J., De Witte, T. C., et al. (1992). Bioavailability of lithium from lithium citrate syrup versus conventional lithium carbonate tablets. *Biopharm Drug Dispos*, 13, 503–511.

16. Grandjean, E. M. and Aubry, J.-M. (2009). Lithium: Updated human knowledge using an evidence-based approach. Part II: Clinical pharmacology and therapeutic monitoring. *CNS Drugs*, 23, 331–49.

17. Diamond, J. M., Ehrlich, B. E., Morawski, S. G., et al. (1983). Lithium absorption in tight and leaky segments of intestine. *J Membr Biol*, 72, 153–159.

18. Shelley, R. K. and Silverstone, T. (1986). Single dose pharmacokinetics of 5 formulations of lithium: A controlled comparison in healthy subjects. *Int Clin Psychopharmacol*, 1, 324–331.

19. Kirkwood, C. K., Wilson, S. K., Hayes, P. E., et al. (1994). Single-dose bioavailability of two extended-release lithium carbonate products. *Am J Hosp Pharm*, 51, 486–489.

20. Gitlin, M. (2016). Lithium side effects and toxicity: Prevalence and management strategies. *Int J Bipolar Disord*, 4, 27–36.

21. Gai, M. N., Thielemann, A. M. and Arancibia, A. (2000). Effect of three different diets on the bioavailability of a sustained release lithium carbonate matrix tablet. *Int J Clin Pharmacol Ther*, 38, 320–326.

22. Jeppsson, J. and Sjögren, J. (1975). The influence of food on side effects and absorption of lithium. *Acta Psychiatr Scand*, 51, 285–288.

23. Malhi, G. S. and Tanious, M. (2011). Optimal frequency of lithium administration in the treatment of bipolar disorder: Clinical and dosing considerations. *CNS Drugs*, 25, 289–298.

24. Luo, H., Chevillard, L., Bellivier, F., et al. (2021). The role of brain barriers in the neurokinetics and pharmacodynamics of lithium. *Pharmacol Res*, 166, 105480.

25. Malhi, G. S., Gessler, D. and Outhred, T. (2017). The use of lithium for the treatment of bipolar disorder: Recommendations from clinical practice guidelines. *J Affect Disord*, 217, 266–280.

26. Heim, W., Oelschlager, H., Kreuter, J., et al. (1994). Liberation of lithium from sustained release preparations: A comparison of seven registered brands. *Pharmacopsychiatry*, 27, 27–31.

27. Komoroski, R. A., Newton, J. E., Sprigg, J. R., et al. (1993). In vivo 7Li nuclear magnetic resonance study of lithium pharmacokinetics and chemical shift imaging in psychiatric patients. *Psychiatry Res*, 50, 67–76.

28. Plenge, P., Stensgaard, A., Jensen, H. V., et al. (1994). 24-hour lithium concentration in human brain studied by Li-7 magnetic resonance spectroscopy. *Biol Psychiatry*, 36, 511–516.

29. Soares, J. C., Boada, F. and Keshavan, M. S. (2000). Brain lithium measurements with (7) Li magnetic resonance spectroscopy (MRS): A literature review. *Eur Neuropsychopharmacol*, 10, 151–158.

30. Soares, J. C., Boada, F., Spencer, S., et al. (2001). Brain lithium concentrations in bipolar disorder patients: Preliminary (7)Li magnetic resonance studies at 3 T. *Biol Psychiatry*, 49, 437–443.

31. Moore, C. M., Demopulos, C. M., Henry, M. E., et al. (2002). Brain-to-serum lithium ratio and age: An in vivo magnetic resonance spectroscopy study. *Am J Psychiatry*, 159, 1240–1242.

32. Forester, B. P., Streeter, C. C., Berlow, Y. A., et al. (2009). Brain lithium levels and effects on cognition and mood in geriatric bipolar disorder: A lithium-7 magnetic resonance spectroscopy study. *Am J Geriatr Psychiatry*, 17, 13–23.

33. Machado-Vieira, R., Otaduy, M. C., Zanetti, M. V., et al. (2016). A selective association between central and peripheral lithium levels in remitters in bipolar depression: A 3 T-(7) Li magnetic resonance spectroscopy study. *Acta Psychiatr Scand*, 133, 214–220.

34. Millischer, V., Matheson, G. J., Bergen, S. E., et al. (2022). Improving lithium dose prediction using population pharmacokinetics and pharmacogenomics: A cohort genome-wide association study in Sweden. *Lancet Psychiatry*, 9, 447–457.

35. Nieper, H. A. (1967). A clinical study of the calcium transport substances Ca 1-d1 aspartate and Ca 2-aminoethanol phosphate as potent agents against autoimmunity and other anticytological aggressions: 2nd communication. *Agressologie*, 8, 395–406.

36. Nieper, H. A. (1973). The clinical applications of lithium orotate: A two years study. *Agressologie*, 14, 407–411.

37. Nieper, H. A. (1974). Capillarographic criteria on the effect of magnesium orotate, EPL substances and clofibrate on the elasticity of blood vessels. *Agressologie*, 15, 73–77.

38. Kling, M. A., Manowitz, P. and Pollack, I. W. (1978). Rat brain and serum lithium concentrations after acute injections of lithium carbonate and orotate. *J Pharm Pharmacol*, 30, 368–370.

39. Pacholko, A. G. and Bekar, L. K. (2023). Different pharmacokinetics of lithium orotate inform why it is more potent, effective, and less toxic than lithium carbonate in a mouse model of mania. *J Psychiatr Res*, 164, 192–201.

40. Smith, D. F. and Schou, M. (1979). Kidney function and lithium concentrations of rats given an injection of lithium orotate or lithium carbonate. *J Pharm Pharmacol*, 31, 161–163.

41. Smith, A. J., Kim, S. H., Tan, J., et al. (2014). Plasma and brain pharmacokinetics of previously unexplored lithium salts. *RSC Adv*, 4, 12362–12365.

42. Pauze, D. K. and Brooks, D. E. (2007). Lithium toxicity from an Internet dietary supplement. *J Med Toxicol*, 3, 61–62.

43. Balon, R. (2013). Possible dangers of a "nutritional supplement" lithium orotate. *Ann Clin Psychiatry*, 25, 71.

44. Ebadi, M. S., Simmons, V. J., Hendrickson, M. J., et al. (1974). Pharmacokinetics of lithium and its regional distribution in rat brain. *Eur J Pharmacol*, 27, 324–329.

45. Renshaw, P. F., Haselgrove, J. C., Bolinger, L., et al. (1986). Relaxation and imaging of lithium in vivo. *Magn Reson Imaging*, 4, 193–198.

46. Lee, J. H., Adler, C., Norris, M., et al. (2012). 4-T 7Li 3D MR spectroscopy imaging in the brains of bipolar disorder subjects. *Magn Reson Med*, 68, 363–368.

47. Mason, G. F. and Krystal, J. H. (2020). Mapping lithium in the brain: New 3-dimensional methodology reveals regional distribution in euthymic patients with bipolar disorder. *Biol Psychiatry*, 88, 367–368.

48. Stout, J., Hozer, F., Coste, A., et al. (2020). Accumulation of lithium in the hippocampus of patients with bipolar disorder: A lithium-7 magnetic resonance imaging study at 7 Tesla. *Biol Psychiatry*, 88, 426–433.

49. Bergner, P. E., Berniker, K., Cooper, T. B., et al. (1973). Lithium kinetics in man: Effect of variation in dosage pattern. *Br J Psychiatry*, 49, 328–339.

50. Plenge, P., Mellerup, E. T., Bolwig, T. G., et al. (1982). Lithium treatment: Does the kidney prefer one daily dose instead of two? *Acta Psychiatr Scand*, 66, 121–128.

51. Tondo, L., Abramowicz, M., Alda, M., et al. (2017). Long-term lithium treatment in bipolar disorder: Effects on glomerular filtration rate and other metabolic parameters. *Int J Bipolar Disord*, 5, 27.

52. Amdisen, A. (1977). Serum level monitoring and clinical pharmacokinetics of lithium. *Clin Pharmacokinet*, 2, 73–92.

53. Greil, W. (1981). [Pharmacokinetics and toxicology of lithium]. *Bibl Psychiatr*, 69–103.

54. Swartz, C. M. (1987). Correction of lithium levels for dose and blood sampling times. *J Clin Psychiatry*, 48, 60–64.

55. Schou, M., Amdisen, A., Thomsen, K., et al. (1982). Lithium treatment regimen and renal water handling: The significance of dosage pattern and tablet type examined through comparison of results from two clinics with different treatment regimens. *Psychopharmacology*, 77, 387–390.

56. Jensen, H. V., Plenge, P., Stensgaard, A., et al. (1996). Twelve-hour brain lithium concentration in lithium maintenance treatment of manic-depressive disorder: Daily versus alternate-day dosing schedule. *Psychopharmacology (Berl)*, 124, 275–278.

57. Davis, R. A., Taylor, M. A. and Abrams, R. (1978). Body fluid lithium measurements: Severity of illness and prediction of outcome. *Biol Psychiatry*, 13, 595–599.

58. Sims, A., White, A. C. and Garvey, K. (1978). Problems associated with the analysis and interpretation of saliva lithium. *Br J Psychiatry*, 132, 152–154.

59. Tyrer, S. P., Grof, P., Kalvar, M., et al. (1981). Estimation of lithium dose requirement by lithium clearance, serum lithium and saliva lithium following a loading dose of lithium carbonate. *Neuropsychobiology*, 7, 152–158.

60. Bowden, C. L., Houston, J. P., Shulman, R. S., et al. (1982). Clinical utility of salivary lithium concentration. *Int Pharmacopsychiatry*, 17, 104–113.

61. Murru, A., Torra, M., Callari, A., et al. (2017). A study on the bioequivalence of lithium and valproate salivary and blood levels in the treatment of bipolar disorder. *Eur Neuropsychopharmacol*, 27, 744–750.

62. Parkin, G. M., McCarthy, M. J., Thein, S. H., et al. (2021). Saliva testing as a means to monitor therapeutic lithium levels in patients with psychiatric disorders: Identification of clinical and environmental covariates, and their incorporation into a prediction model. *Bipolar Disord*, 23, 679–688.

63. Kelly, D., Glassman, M., Mackowick, M., et al. (2020). O9.1. Satisfaction with using a novel fingerstick for absolute neutrophil count (ANC) at the point of treatment in patients treated with clozapine. *Schizophr Bull*, 46, S20–S21.

64. Taylor, D., Atkins, M., Harland, R., et al. (2021). Point-of-care measurement of clozapine concentration using a finger-stick blood sample. *J Psychopharmacol*, 35, 279–283.

65. Komatsu, T., Maeki, M., Ishida, A., et al. (2020). Paper-based device for the facile colorimetric determination of lithium ions in human whole blood. *ACS Sens*, 5, 1287–1294.

66. Sheikh, M., Qassem, M., Triantis, I. F., et al. (2022). Advances in therapeutic monitoring of lithium in the management of bipolar disorder. *Sensors (Basel)*, 22, 736.

67. Criscuolo, F., Taurino, I., Carrara, S., et al. (2018). A novel electrochemical sensor for non-invasive monitoring of lithium levels in mood disorders. *Annu Int Conf IEEE Eng Med Biol Soc*, 2018, 3825–3828.

68. Sweilam, M. N., Varcoe, J. R. and Crean, C. (2018). Fabrication and optimization of fiber-based lithium sensor: A step toward wearable sensors for lithium drug monitoring in interstitial fluid. *ACS Sens*, 3, 1802–1810.

69. Roberts, E. L. (1950). A case of chronic mania treated with lithium citrate and terminating fatally. *Med J Aust*, 2, 261–262.

70. Awan, S., Abelleira, A., Khehra, L., et al. (2021). Undetectable serum lithium concentrations after coadministration of liquid lithium citrate and apple juice: A case report. *Ment Health Clin*, 11, 27–30.

71. Theesen, K. A., Wilson, J. E., Newton, D. W., et al. (1981). Compatibility of lithium citrate syrup with 10 neuroleptic solutions. *Am J Hosp Pharm*, 38, 1750–1753.

72. Park, S. H., Gill, M. A. and Dopheide, J. A. (2003). Visual compatibility of risperidone solution and lithium citrate syrup. *Am J Health Syst Pharm*, 60, 612–613.

73. Girardi, P., Brugnoli, R., Manfredi, G., et al. (2016). Lithium in bipolar disorder: Optimizing therapy using prolonged-release formulations. *Drugs R D*, 16, 293–302.

74. Thornhill, D. P. (1978). Pharmacokinetics of ordinary and sustained-release lithium carbonate in manic patients after acute dosage. *Eur J Clin Pharmacol*, 14, 267–271.

75. Fava, G. A., Molnar, G., Block, B., et al. (1984). The lithium loading dose method in a clinical setting. *Am J Psychiatry*, 141, 812–813.

76. Cooper, T. B., Bergner, P. E. and Simpson, G. M. (1973). The 24-hour serum lithium level as a prognosticator of dosage requirements. *Am J Psychiatry*, 130, 601–603.

77. Seifert, R., Bremkamp, H. and Junge, C. (1975). [Rationalized lithium adjustment by load-test (author's transl.)]. *Psychopharmacologia*, 43, 285–286.

78. Cooper, T. B. and Simpson, G. M. (1976). The 24-hour lithium level as a prognosticator of dosage requirements: A 2-year follow-up study. *Am J Psychiatry*, 133, 440–443.

79. Gengo, F., Timko, J., D'Antonio, J., et al. (1980). Prediction of dosage of lithium carbonate: Use of a standard predictive method. *J Clin Psychiatry*, 41, 319–320.

80. Naiman, I. F., Muniz, C. E., Stewart, R. B., et al. (1981). Practicality of a lithium dosing guide. *Am J Psychiatry*, 138, 1369–1371.

81. Zetin, M., Garber, D., De Antonio, M., et al. (1986). Prediction of lithium dose: A mathematical alternative to the test-dose method. *J Clin Psychiatry*, 47, 175–178.

82. Cummings, M. A., Haviland, M. G., Wareham, J. G., et al. (1993). A prospective clinical evaluation of an equation to predict daily lithium dose. *J Clin Psychiatry*, 54, 55–58.

83. Sienaert, P., Geeraerts, I. and Wyckaert, S. (2013). How to initiate lithium therapy: A systematic review of dose estimation and level prediction methods. *J Affect Disord*, 146, 15–33.

84. Yoshida, K., Uchida, H., Suzuki, T., et al. (2018). Prediction model of serum lithium concentrations. *Pharmacopsychiatry*, 51, 82–88.

85. Keck, P. E., Jr., McElroy, S. L. and Bennett, J. A. (2000). Pharmacologic loading in the treatment of acute mania. *Bipolar Disord*, 2, 42–46.

86. Hirschfeld, R. M., Allen, M. H., McEvoy, J. P., et al. (1999). Safety and tolerability of oral loading divalproex sodium in acutely manic bipolar patients. *J Clin Psychiatry*, 60, 815–818.

87. Kook, K. A., Stimmel, G. L., Wilkins, J. N., et al. (1985). Accuracy and safety of a priori lithium loading. *J Clin Psychiatry*, 46, 49–51.

88. Wheeler, A., Robinson, G. and Fraser, A. (2008). Mood stabilizer loading versus titration in acute mania: Audit of clinical practice. *Aust N Z J Psychiatry*, 42, 955–962.

89. Moscovich, D. G., Shapira, B., Lerer, B., et al. (1992). Rapid lithiumization in acute manic patients. *Hum Psychopharmacol*, 7, 343–345.

90. Scherf-Clavel, M., Treiber, S., Deckert, J., et al. (2020). Drug–drug interactions between lithium and cardiovascular as well as anti-inflammatory drugs. *Pharmacopsychiatry*, 53, 229–234.

91. Bisogni, V., Rossitto, G., Reghin, F., et al. (2016). Antihypertensive therapy in patients on chronic lithium treatment for bipolar disorders. *J Hypertens*, 34, 20–28.

92. Finley, P. R., O'Brien, J. G. and Coleman, R. W. (1996). Lithium and angiotensin-converting enzyme inhibitors: Evaluation of a potential interaction. *J Clin Psychopharmacol*, 16, 68–71.

93. Juurlink, D. N., Mamdani, M. M., Kopp, A., et al. (2004). Drug-induced lithium toxicity in the elderly: A population-based study. *J Am Geriatr Soc*, 52, 794–798.

94. Meyer, J. M., Dollarhide, A. and Tuan, I.-L. (2005). Lithium toxicity after switch from fosinopril to lisinopril. *Int Clin Psychopharmacol*, 20, 115–118.

95. Zhang, X. and Li, X. Y. (2020). Prevalence of hyponatremia among older inpatients in a general hospital. *Eur Geriatr Med*, 11, 685–692.

96. James, P. A., Oparil, S., Carter, B. L., et al. (2014). 2014 evidence-based guideline for the management of high blood pressure in adults: Report from the panel members appointed to the Eighth Joint National Committee (JNC 8). *JAMA*, 311, 507–520.

97. Thomsen, K. and Schou, M. (1973). The effect of prolonged administration of hydrochlorothiazide on the renal lithium clearance and the urine flow of ordinary rats and rats with diabetes insipidus. *Pharmakopsychiatr Neuropsychopharmakol*, 6, 264–269.

98. Petersen, V., Hvidt, S., Thomsen, K., et al. (1974). Effect of prolonged thiazide treatment on renal lithium clearance. *Br Med J*, 3, 143–145.

99. Sinke, A. P., Kortenoeven, M. L., de Groot, T., et al. (2014). Hydrochlorothiazide attenuates lithium-induced nephrogenic diabetes insipidus independently of the sodium-chloride cotransporter. *Am J Physiol Renal Physiol*, 306, F525–F533.

100. Solomon, J. G. (1980). Lithium toxicity precipitated by a diuretic. *Psychosomatics*, 21, 425, 429.

101. Filippone, E. J., Ruzieh, M. and Foy, A. (2020). Thiazide-associated hyponatremia: Clinical manifestations and pathophysiology. *Am J Kidney Dis*, 75, 256–264.

102. Finley, P. R. (2016). Drug interactions with lithium: An update. *Clin Pharmacokinet*, 55, 925–941.

103. Armstrong, G. P. (2020). Empagliflozin-mediated lithium excretion: A case study and clinical applications. *Am J Case Rep*, 21, e923311.

104. Teicher, M. H., Altesman, R. I., Cole, J. O., et al. (1987). Possible nephrotoxic interaction of lithium and metronidazole. *JAMA*, 257, 3365–3366.

105. Joos, A. A. (1998). [Pharmacologic interactions of antibiotics and psychotropic drugs]. *Psychiatr Prax*, 25, 57–60.

106. Atherton, J. C., Doyle, A., Gee, A., et al. (1991). Lithium clearance: Modification by the loop of Henle in man. *J Physiol*, 437, 377–391.

107. Fransen, R., Boer, W. H., Boer, P., et al. (1993). Effects of furosemide or acetazolamide infusion on renal handling of lithium: A micropuncture study in rats. *Am J Physiol*, 264, R129–134.

108. Gimenez, I. (2006). Molecular mechanisms and regulation of furosemide-sensitive Na-K-Cl cotransporters. *Curr Opin Nephrol Hypertens*, 15, 517–523.

109. Thomsen, K. and Schou, M. (1968). Renal lithium excretion in man. *Am J Physiol*, 215, 823–827.

110. Valdiserri, E. V. (1985). A possible interaction between lithium and diltiazem: Case report. *J Clin Psychiatry*, 46, 540–541.

111. Dubovsky, S. L., Franks, R. D. and Allen, S. (1987). Verapamil: A new antimanic drug with potential interactions with lithium. *J Clin Psychiatry*, 48, 371–372.

112. Price, W. A. and Shalley, J. E. (1987). Lithium–verapamil toxicity in the elderly. *J Am Geriatr Soc*, 35, 177–178.

113. Binder, E. F., Cayabyab, L., Ritchie, D. J., et al. (1991). Diltiazem-induced psychosis and a possible diltiazem–lithium interaction. *Arch Intern Med*, 151, 373–374.

114. Bruun, N. E., Ibsen, H., Skøtt, P., et al. (1988). Lithium clearance and renal tubular sodium handling during acute and long-term nifedipine treatment in essential hypertension. *Clin Sci (Lond)*, 75, 609–613.

115. Kortenoeven, M. L., Li, Y., Shaw, S., et al. (2009). Amiloride blocks lithium entry through the sodium channel thereby attenuating the resultant nephrogenic diabetes insipidus. *Kidney Int*, 76, 44–53.

116. Schoot, T. S., Molmans, T. H. J., Grootens, K. P., et al. (2020). Systematic review and practical guideline for the prevention and management of the renal side effects of lithium therapy. *Eur Neuropsychopharmacol*, 31, 16–32.

117. Bedford, J. J., Weggery, S., Ellis, G., et al. (2008). Lithium-induced nephrogenic diabetes insipidus: Renal effects of amiloride. *Clin J Am Soc Nephrol*, 3, 1324–1331.

118. Davis, J., Desmond, M. and Berk, M. (2018). Lithium and nephrotoxicity: A literature review of approaches to clinical management and risk stratification. *BMC Nephrol*, 19, 305.

119. Batlle, D. C., von Riotte, A. B., Gaviria, M., et al. (1985). Amelioration of polyuria by amiloride in patients receiving long-term lithium therapy. *NEJM*, 312, 408–414.

120. Kosten, T. R. and Forrest, J. N. (1986). Treatment of severe lithium-induced polyuria with amiloride. *Am J Psychiatry*, 143, 1563–1568.

121. Inoue, M., Nakai, K. and Mitsuiki, K. (2021). Triamterene in lithium-induced nephrogenic diabetes insipidus: A case report. *CEN Case Rep*, 10, 64–68.

122. Mehta, B. R. and Robinson, B. H. (1980). Lithium toxicity induced by triamterene-hydrochlorothiazide. *Postgrad Med J*, 56, 783–784.

123. Dorevitch, A. and Baruch, E. (1986). Lithium toxicity induced by combined amiloride HCl-hydrochlorothiazide administration. *Am J Psychiatry*, 143, 257–258.

124. Roush, G. C. and Sica, D. A. (2016). Diuretics for hypertension: A review and update. *Am J Hypertens*, 29, 1130–1137.

125. Supuran, C. T. (2016). Drug interaction considerations in the therapeutic use of carbonic anhydrase inhibitors. *Expert Opin Drug Metab Toxicol*, 12, 423–431.

126. Sands, J. M. (2016). Water, water everywhere: A new cause and a new treatment for nephrogenic diabetes insipidus. *J Am Soc Nephrol*, 27, 1872–1874.

127. de Groot, T., Sinke, A. P., Kortenoeven, M. L., et al. (2016). Acetazolamide attenuates lithium-induced nephrogenic diabetes insipidus. *J Am Soc Nephrol*, 27, 2082–2091.

128. de Groot, T., Doornebal, J., Christensen, B. M., et al. (2017). Lithium-induced NDI: Acetazolamide reduces polyuria but does not improve urine concentrating ability. *Am J Physiol Renal Physiol*, 313, F669–676.

129. Gordon, C. E., Vantzelfde, S. and Francis, J. M. (2016). Acetazolamide in lithium-induced nephrogenic diabetes insipidus. *N Engl J Med*, 375, 2008–2009.

130. Macau, R. A., da Silva, T. N., Silva, J. R., et al. (2018). Use of acetazolamide in lithium-induced nephrogenic diabetes insipidus: A case report. *Endocrinol Diabetes Metab Case Rep*, 2018, 17-0154.

131. Dabrowski, W., Siwicka-Gieroba, D., Robba, C., et al. (2021). Potentially detrimental effects of hyperosmolality in patients treated for traumatic brain injury. *J Clin Med*, 10, 4141.

132. Kralovec, K., Fartacek, R., Plöderl, M., et al. (2011). Low serum lithium associated with immoderate use of Coca-Cola Zero. *J Clin Psychopharmacol*, 31, 543–544.

133. Jefferson, J. W. (1988). Lithium tremor and caffeine intake: Two cases of drinking less and shaking more. *J Clin Psychiatry*, 49, 72–73.

134. Mester, R., Toren, P., Mizrachi, I., et al. (1995). Caffeine withdrawal increases lithium blood levels. *Biol Psychiatry*, 37, 348–350.

135. Levin, G. M., Grum, C. and Eisele, G. (1998). Effect of over-the-counter dosages of naproxen sodium and acetaminophen on plasma lithium concentrations in normal volunteers. *J Clin Psychopharmacol*, 18, 237–240.

136. Phelan, K. M., Mosholder, A. D. and Lu, S. (2003). Lithium interaction with the cyclooxygenase 2 inhibitors rofecoxib and celecoxib and other nonsteroidal anti-inflammatory drugs. *J Clin Psychiatry*, 64, 1328–1334.

137. Thomas, M. C. (2014). Renal effects of dapagliflozin in patients with type 2 diabetes. *Ther Adv Endocrinol Metab*, 5, 53–61.

138. Boehringer Ingelheim Pharmaceuticals Inc. (2022). *Jardiance package insert.* Ridgefield, CT 06877.

139. Pi, H. T. and Surawicz, F. G. (1978). Severe neurotoxicity and lithium therapy. *Clin Toxicol*, 13, 479–486.

140. Aref, M. A., El-Badramany, M., Hannora, N., et al. (1982). Lithium loss in sweat. *Psychosomatics*, 23, 407.

141. Jefferson, J. W., Greist, J. H., Clagnaz, P. J., et al. (1982). Effect of strenuous exercise on serum lithium level in man. *Am J Psychiatry*, 139, 1593–1595.

142. Grandjean, E. M. and Aubry, J.-M. (2009). Lithium: Updated human knowledge using an evidence-based approach. Part III: Clinical safety. *CNS Drugs*, 23, 397–418.

143. Davis, J., Desmond, M. and Berk, M. (2018). Lithium and nephrotoxicity: Unravelling the complex pathophysiological threads of the lightest metal. *Nephrology (Carlton)*, 23, 897–903.

144. Wilting, I., Fase, S., Martens, E. P., et al. (2007). The impact of environmental temperature on lithium serum levels. *Bipolar Disord*, 9, 603–608.

145. Cheng, S., Buckley, N. A., Siu, W., et al. (2020). Seasonal and temperature effect on serum lithium concentrations. *Aust N Z J Psychiatry*, 54, 282–287.

146. Merwick, A., Cooke, J., Neligan, A., et al. (2011). Acute neuropathy in setting of diarrhoeal illness and hyponatraemia due to lithium toxicity. *Clin Neurol Neurosurg*, 113, 923–924.

147. Arancibia, A., Paulos, C., Chavez, J., et al. (2003). Pharmacokinetics of lithium in healthy volunteers after exposure to high altitude. *Int J Clin Pharmacol Ther*, 41, 200–206.

148. Uber, A. and Twark, C. (2022). Symptom overlap of acute mountain sickness and lithium toxicity: A case report. *High Alt Med Biol*, 23, 291–293.

149. Wesseloo, R., Wierdsma, A. I., van Kamp, I. L., et al. (2017). Lithium dosing strategies during pregnancy and the postpartum period. *Br J Psychiatry*, 211, 31–36.

150. Harel, Z., McArthur, E., Hladunewich, M., et al. (2019). Serum creatinine levels before, during, and after pregnancy. *JAMA*, 321, 205–207.

151. Westin, A. A., Brekke, M., Molden, E., et al. (2017). Changes in drug disposition of lithium during pregnancy: A retrospective observational study of patient data from two routine therapeutic drug monitoring services in Norway. *BMJ Open*, 7, e015738.

152. Carmassi, C., Del Grande, C., Masci, I., et al. (2019). Lithium and valproate serum level fluctuations within the menstrual cycle: A systematic review. *Int Clin Psychopharmacol*, 34, 143–150.

153. Rittmannsberger, H. and Malsiner-Walli, G. (2013). Mood-dependent changes of serum lithium concentration in a rapid cycling patient maintained on stable doses of lithium carbonate. *Bipolar Disord*, 15, 333–337.

154. McElroy, S. L. and Keck, P. E., Jr. (2014). Metabolic syndrome in bipolar disorder: A review with a focus on bipolar depression. *J Clin Psychiatry*, 75, 46–61.

155. Godin, O., Leboyer, M., Belzeaux, R., et al. (2021). Non-alcoholic fatty liver disease in a sample of individuals with bipolar disorders: Results from the FACE-BD cohort. *Acta Psychiatr Scand*, 143, 82–91.

156. Ayub, S., Saboor, S., Usmani, S., et al. (2022). Lithium toxicity following Roux-en-Y gastric bypass: Mini review and illustrative case. *Ment Health Clin*, 12, 214–218.

157. Bingham, K. S., Thoma, J., Hawa, R., et al. (2016). Perioperative lithium use in bariatric surgery: A case series and literature review. *Psychosomatics*, 57, 638–644.

158. Musfeldt, D., Levinson, A., Nykiel, J., et al. (2016). Lithium toxicity after Roux-en-Y bariatric surgery. *BMJ Case Rep*, 2016, bcr2015214056.

159. Niessen, R., Sottiaux, T., Schillaci, A., et al. (2018). [Lithium toxicity after bariatric surgery]. *Rev Med Liege*, 73, 82–87.

160. Dahan, A., Porat, D., Azran, C., et al. (2019). Lithium toxicity with severe bradycardia post sleeve gastrectomy: A case report and review of the literature. *Obes Surg*, 29, 735–738.

161. Jamison, S. C. and Aheron, K. (2020). Lithium toxicity following bariatric surgery. *SAGE Open Med Case Rep*, 8, 2050313x20953000.

162. Lin, Y. H., Liu, S. W., Wu, H. L., et al. (2020). Lithium toxicity with prolonged neurologic sequelae following sleeve gastrectomy: A case report and review of literature. *Medicine (Baltimore)*, 99, e21122.

163. Marques, A. R., Alho, A., Martins, J. M., et al. (2021). Lithium intoxication after bariatric surgery: A case report. *Acta Med Port*, 34, 382–386.

164. Mallinger, A. G., Thase, M. E., Haskett, R., et al. (2008). Verapamil augmentation of lithium treatment improves outcome in mania unresponsive to lithium alone: Preliminary findings and a discussion of therapeutic mechanisms. *Bipolar Disord*, 10, 856–866.

165. Abdel-Zaher, A. O. (2000). The myoneural effects of lithium chloride on the nerve–muscle preparations of rats. Role of adenosine triphosphate-sensitive potassium channels. *Pharmacol Res*, 41, 163–178.

166. Jefferson, J. W. (1978). Lithium–pancuronium interaction. *Ann Intern Med*, 88, 577.

167. Kishimoto, N., Yoshikawa, H. and Seo, K. (2020). Potentiation of rocuronium bromide by lithium carbonate: A case report. *Anesth Prog*, 67, 146–150.

168. Cohen, W. J. and Cohen, N. H. (1974). Lithium carbonate, haloperidol, and irreversible brain damage. *JAMA*, 230, 1283–1287.

169. Gurrera, R. J., Caroff, S. N., Cohen, A., et al. (2011). An international consensus study of neuroleptic malignant syndrome diagnostic criteria using the Delphi method. *J Clin Psychiatry*, 72, 1222–1228.

170. Gurrera, R. J., Mortillaro, G., Velamoor, V., et al. (2017). A validation study of the International Consensus Diagnostic Criteria for neuroleptic malignant syndrome. *J Clin Psychopharmacol*, 37, 67–71.

171. Lieberman, J. A., Stroup, T. S., McEvoy, J. P., et al. (2005). Effectiveness of antipsychotic drugs in patients with chronic schizophrenia. *N Engl J Med*, 353, 1209–1223.

172. Mylan Pharmaceuticals Inc. (2019). *Haloperidol package insert*. Morgantown, WV.

173. Boora, K., Xu, J. and Hyatt, J. (2008). Encephalopathy with combined lithium–risperidone administration. *Acta Psychiatr Scand*, 117, 394–395; discussion 396.

174. Hermida, A. P., Janjua, A. U., Glass, O. M., et al. (2016). A case of lithium-induced parkinsonism presenting with typical motor symptoms of Parkinson's Disease in a bipolar patient. *Int Psychogeriatr*, 28, 2101–2104.

175. Marras, C., Herrmann, N., Fischer, H. D., et al. (2016). Lithium use in older adults is associated with increased prescribing of Parkinson medications. *Am J Geriatr Psychiatry*, 24, 301–309.

176. Friedman, J. H. (2020). Movement disorders induced by psychiatric drugs that do not block dopamine receptors. *Parkinsonism Relat Disord*, 79, 60–64.

177. Uwai, Y. and Nabekura, T. (2022). Relationship between lithium carbonate and the risk of Parkinson-like events in patients with bipolar disorders: A multivariate analysis using the Japanese adverse drug event report database. *Psychiatry Res*, 314, 114687.

178. Erro, R., Landolfi, A., D'Agostino, G., et al. (2021). Bipolar disorder and Parkinson's Disease: A (123)I-ioflupane dopamine transporter SPECT study. *Front Neurol*, 12, 652375.

179. Revet, A., Montastruc, F., Roussin, A., et al. (2020). Antidepressants and movement disorders: A postmarketing study in the world pharmacovigilance database. *BMC Psychiatry*, 20, 308.

180. Chenu, F. and Bourin, M. (2006). Potentiation of antidepressant-like activity with lithium: Mechanism involved. *Curr Drug Targets*, 7, 159–163.

181. Janssen, S., Bloem, B. R. and van de Warrenburg, B. P. (2017). The clinical heterogeneity of drug-induced myoclonus: An illustrated review. *J Neurol*, 264, 1559–1566.

182. Guttuso, T., Jr. (2019). High lithium levels in tobacco may account for reduced incidences of both Parkinson's disease and melanoma in smokers through enhanced β-catenin-mediated activity. *Med Hypotheses*, 131, 109302.

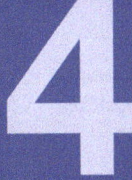

Lithium Initiation and Monitoring

Baseline Assessment; Loading and Initiation
Methods; Target Serum Levels; Monitoring
Intrinsic Renal Function with New $eGFR_{cr-cys}$
Formula; Office and Laboratory Methods for
Monitoring Polyuria; Monitoring Thyroid and
Parathyroid Function

QUICK CHECK

PRINCIPLES

- Despite educating patients about lithium's advantages and safety profile when dosed with modern prescribing principles, one must elicit a patient's thoughts about their illness, the need for any psychotropic medication and those about lithium itself, when commencing treatment. The same conversation should occur with new patients on existing lithium therapy. Consider Customized Adherence Enhancement (CAE) therapy for patients who struggle with lithium adherence.

- Many bipolar spectrum patients may need a 2nd medication to manage mania relapse or bipolar depression, so one need not search for an "ideal lithium monotherapy candidate" to commence lithium.

- Treatment algorithms often recommend a number of pre-treatment laboratory assessments and other measures (e.g. waist circumference, serum lipids) that relate to medical issues in the target population. The number of necessary items obtained before starting lithium is modest.

- As eGFR will be checked frequently during the early months of treatment, any patient with an eGFR $\geq$ 60 ml/min is a lithium candidate. In those patients with a *compelling indication for lithium* (e.g. prior failure of non-lithium therapies), a baseline eGFR in the range of 45–59 ml/min can be considered, albeit with vigilant eGFR monitoring.

- Clinicians should know how to load or initiate lithium more rapidly for management of inpatients with acute mania. In outpatient practice, the lower degree of urgency often allows a more leisurely titration.

- For bipolar spectrum patients, recent guidelines suggest a maintenance lithium level in the range of 0.60–0.80 mEq/l, with select patients needing a higher (0.80–1.00 mEq/l) or lower (0.40–0.60 mEq/l) range, depending on response and tolerability. Individuals over age 50 can have higher brain-to-serum lithium levels than younger patients and may respond to and better tolerate lower peripheral levels.

- Routine laboratory monitoring is not that complicated for most patients: lithium level, eGFR, serum calcium and thyroid stimulating hormone (TSH) every 6 months, with certain patients needing an early morning urine osmolality (EMUO) and/or urine albumin-to-creatinine ratio (ACR). Monitoring frequency depends primarily on eGFR and presence of medical comorbidity, not patient age. Obtaining a 24 h fluid intake record (FIR) every 6 months also helps early identification of polyuria and complements the information obtained from an EMUO.

Introduction

WHAT TO KNOW: INTRODUCTION

- An important aspect of lithium initiation is the need to elicit a patient's attitudes and beliefs about their diagnosis, the need for any medication that regulates mood, and specific thoughts about lithium.

- One key element in addressing medication related concerns involves communicating that you possess the clinical expertise to prescribe and monitor lithium treatment, and the willingness to address any issues that arise during treatment which interfere with adherence or which dissuade the patient from continuing lithium.

- Although a delay in initiating lithium may result in suboptimal symptom control, recent studies indicate that it does not lessen the likelihood of lithium response.

While the literature abundantly documents lithium's unique efficacy profile and the limitations of non-lithium therapies, starting a patient on lithium requires the complete array of one's clinical skills. One core ability relates to appropriate pharmacological use of lithium, including dosing, level monitoring, and management of drug interactions and adverse effects that lead to discontinuation [1]; however, it is facility in communicating with patients and eliciting their illness beliefs, their ideas about the need for any treatment, and their specific thoughts about lithium therapy that is crucial to minimizing nonadherence [2]. Nonadherence with oral medications is common in all chronic illnesses, as 50% of patients with hypertension or schizophrenia fail to meet any definition of adherence [3, 4]. A 1975 paper entitled "Why do patients with manic-depressive illness stop their lithium?" captured many of the common patient related non-somatic issues contributing to nonadherence (i.e. those not due to adverse effects) [5], and this list has changed very little 50 years later: inconvenience of daily medication, diminished need for lithium during periods of euthymia, a desire to persist in a hypomanic or even manic state (e.g. feeling more creative or productive, missing the elevated mood), comparative lack of efficacy for depressive episodes compared with significant impact on mania, or a wish not to be reminded of the illness itself [5]. Starting in the late 1970s, papers noted that clinicians overvalue certain aspects of lithium's efficacy and fail to appreciate that many patients, even lithium responders, do not like their mood being regulated by medication [6, 7]. A 2003 paper related that this disconnect between clinicians and patients, even lithium adherent patients, persists [8].

While lithium may have enjoyed a certain halo effect as a breakthrough medication once Australian and European psychiatrists reported its antimanic properties in the 1950s and 1960s [9, 10], this was followed by decades of papers highlighting safety concerns, and counterdetailing by manufacturers of anticonvulsant mood stabilizers and second generation antipsychotics (SGAs) that distorted clinician and public opinion about lithium's effectiveness and tolerability [11]. Moreover, patients, families and caregivers perform their own internet based research on sites with variable accuracy and with a variety of agendas, some of which are opposed to psychiatric medication of any type but couch this worldview in a format that disguises their bias [12]. Any conversation about commencing lithium ideally falls at the end of a process that begins by eliciting patient (and caregiver) notions surrounding psychiatric illness and treatment, mapping out the clinician's rationale for establishing the current working diagnosis, and providing evidence based reasons for choosing lithium among a range of options for their disorder [13]. Dr. Kay Redfield Jamison, a psychologist who documented her own struggles with bipolar I disorder (BD-1) and lithium adherence, commented in a 1979 paper that BD patients on lithium do appreciate the need to work on the psychological ramifications of BD in psychotherapy. In a study of factors contributing to nonadherence among 47 patients prescribed lithium (47% nonadherent, 53% adherent), Jamison found that 50% of patients considered psychotherapy to be "very important" in lithium adherence, compared with only 27% of clinicians, most of whom were actually psychotherapists [6]. The discussion about lithium is often an extended conversation that proceeds over many months and years, bolstered by the need to come to shared decisions regarding all aspects of treatment. The conclusion of a 2018 paper discussing interventions to improve medication nonadherence in BD is highly instructive: "The strategies that are adopted need to be patient specific, reflecting that nonadherence has no single cause, and chosen by the patient and clinician working together" [2].

From the clinician viewpoint, starting lithium in those with current mania or a history of mania (i.e. BD-1 and schizoaffective disorder, bipolar type [SAD-BT]) is imperative for optimal management and minimization of the morbidity from mood episodes (e.g. risk of rehospitalization, suicide and life disruption) [2, 14]. One important question has been whether treatment delays might be disease modifying and lessen the odds of lithium response [15]. For treatment resistant schizophrenia patients, commencing clozapine within 3 years of the timepoint when treatment resistance can be defined (e.g. verified failure of a second antipsychotic trial) improves the odds of response [16, 17]. No such signal was seen in the BD literature until 1999 when a group in Milan suggested that initiating lithium within the first 10 years of illness onset may predict better outcomes in BD and unipolar major depression [18]. This conclusion was based on an analysis of 270 patients with ≥ 4 years of follow-up on lithium, 179 of whom had a BD spectrum diagnosis, with 131 of the total sample having at least 8 years on lithium. The definition of response was a change in recurrence rates calculated as the ratio between the number of episodes over time (in months) between illness onset and starting lithium, and the number of episodes during lithium treatment [18]. After categorizing the sample into cohorts based on time from mood disorder diagnosis to starting lithium (very early, ≤ 5 years; early, 6–10 years; late, 11–20 years; very late, > 21 years), it was found that beginning lithium therapy within the first 10 years of illness onset predicted better preventive outcomes for major depression and BD patients, regardless of mood diagnosis [18]. One major limitation of this analysis was possible selection bias in those assigned to lithium, as those with the highest pre-lithium morbidity might also display the most robust early treatment response.

In-Depth 4.1 Early Studies Showing Lack of Association with Delay in Lithium Initiation and Response

In 2003, Baldessarini published outcomes from an analysis of 450 BD patients (BD-1, n = 293; BD-2, n = 157) with mean latency of 7.8 years before lithium, and an average of 9.0 mood episodes before various maintenance treatments were started that included, but were not restricted to, lithium [19]. During 4.2 years of follow-up, no measure of post-treatment morbidity related to treatment latency or to pretreatment episode count, including: percentage of time ill, episodes per year, proportion hospitalized, proportion without mood recurrences. Importantly, pretreatment morbidity was greater with shorter latency to maintenance therapy, and earlier treatment was associated with a larger relative reduction of morbidity. One explanation for this association is that the "sickest" patients were treated sooner and, due to their severity, also showed the greatest reduction in mood symptoms. The lack of association with treatment latency was also echoed by a meta-analysis published later in 2003 that examined 28 studies with data on latency and treatment outcomes [20]. A subsequent 2007 study by Baldessarini of 764 BD spectrum patients in two European centers also found that prior episode counts and treatment delay had little association with morbidity during mood stabilizer prophylaxis [21]. While confirming those negative associations in the literature, the authors commented that attempts to assess longitudinal treatment effects in BD patients are problematic due to the periodic nature of symptoms and spontaneous remission. Longer observation periods, even those without treatment, may potentially dilute the morbidity signal, particularly because medication interventions are commonly initiated after a mood episode when pretreatment morbidity is at its highest [21].

Given the problematic nature of analyses between latency and response, a Danish group led by Professor Lars Vedel Kessing (Copenhagen Affective Disorder Research Center in the Psychiatric Center Copenhagen, and faculty at University of Copenhagen, Health and Medical Sciences) used Danish registers to identify all patients with a diagnosis of BD in psychiatric hospital settings who were prescribed lithium during the period 1995–2012 in Denmark [15]. Although there was increased statistical power with the larger sample size (n = 4714), the analysis only looked at patients who, following a 6-month lithium stabilization period, continued lithium as *monotherapy*. The definition of response was also very specific: no need for psychiatric hospital admission. Early vs. late latency was defined in two ways: (a) patients with a diagnosis of a single manic episode / BD who started lithium following their first contact vs. patients who started lithium following later contacts; or (b) patients who started lithium following a diagnosis of a single manic or mixed episode vs. those who started lithium following a diagnosis of BD (i.e. implying at least two mood episodes). This analysis found that, regardless of the definition used, patients who started lithium early had significantly decreased rates of nonresponse: first vs. later initiation hazard ratio (HR) = 0.87, (95% CI 0.76–0.91); single manic/mixed episode vs. BD diagnosis, HR = 0.75 (95% CI 0.67–0.84) [15]. Although the HR values were adjusted for covariates that could influence the time to treatment and type of BD treatment, the authors did not have the ability to examine to what extent those who are prescribed lithium in Denmark might be prototypical lithium monotherapy responders (i.e. lower rates of rapid cycling or mood incongruent psychosis), a pattern of practice that may have influenced the outcome. Moreover, while lithium monotherapy is a laudable goal for BD-1 patients, many will need additional medications for treatment of or prophylaxis for mood episodes, especially depression, so the findings may not generalize to a population who does not fare as well on lithium monotherapy, but who may still benefit from lithium as part of their medication regimen.

While recent studies support the absence of a convincing association between lithium response and treatment latency, there is little doubt that patients suffer when untreated, and that early detection of BD is important to reduce morbidity and suicide risk [22]. In 2021, a German group published an analysis of 582 help-seeking adolescents and young adults (mean age 23.9 ± 0.6 years, 62% female) seen in a Dresden clinic from May 2009 to April 2018 who completed a diagnostic work-up that included various instruments designed to detect prodromal or at-risk BD states [23]. It has long been recognized that such help-seeking patient cohorts are enriched with individuals who later develop serious mental disorders such as schizophrenia and BD, so all adolescents and young adults who seek care warrant some form of ongoing monitoring, even if not presently manifesting those disorders. Among this sample, 4% met BD criteria and 21% fulfilled at-risk BD criteria based on having at least one of the following factors: family BD history (22%), history suggestive of hypomania or mania risk (44%) or variations in mood between periods with mild depression or increased activity (48%). The most common secondary risk factors were decreased psychosocial functioning (78%), lifetime diagnosis of depressive disorder (67%) and specific sleep/circadian rhythm disturbances (59%) [23]. Substance use was also very common in those identified as at-risk for BD (cannabis = 50%, alcohol = 33%), and even more prevalent in those diagnosed with BD (cannabis = 75%, alcohol = 40%) [23]. While this specialized clinic used instruments that are unfamiliar to most clinicians, their findings reinforce the concept that help-seeking adolescents or young adults with a BD family history and mood symptoms suggestive of a cyclic mood disorder should be engaged and followed up even if there is no present indication for medication. As BD predictive algorithms improve, it may be possible to determine whether at-risk patients benefit from medication. At that point, the extent to which a clinician can convince a minimally symptomatic individual with high likelihood of developing BD-1 to start any form of treatment may rest on the rapport developed during a period of watchful waiting while also providing supportive or other appropriate forms of psychotherapy. Over time, developing a therapeutic alliance with patients has been shown to positively influence adherence and clinical outcomes in serious mental illnesses such as schizophrenia, and this approach forms the basis of shared decision-making [24]. Medications such as lithium are tools employed to help patients reach their functional goals. The clinical knowledge of appropriate lithium monitoring and initiation strategies, use of target serum level ranges, and interventions to track and address adherence is not a body of secrets to be kept from patients, but facts to be shared in the effort to jointly address patient concerns and avoid pitfalls that may deprive them of the benefits of lithium treatment.

A   In Whom Should One Initiate Lithium?

WHAT TO KNOW: IN WHOM SHOULD LITHIUM BE INITIATED

- Any patient with a history of mania or mixed features is an ideal candidate for lithium. Moreover, those with BD-1 and SAD-BT diagnoses equivalently benefit from lithium as maintenance therapy.
- Decisions regarding lithium use in BD-2 patients are more nuanced and depend on the need for mood stabilization.
- Lithium remains an important medication for unipolar major depressive disorder (MDD) patients.

1 *Lithium in Bipolar Spectrum Disorders*

Among those with bipolar spectrum disorders (BD-1, BD-2, SAD-BT) patients with a history of mania or mixed episodes are obvious candidates for lithium, with a more nuanced case-by-case approach for BD-2 individuals. It is worth noting that the majority of the literature is built around lithium's efficacy for acute mania and mania prophylaxis in BD-1 (see Chapter 1). The prospective data from trials devoted to BD-2 and SAD-BT are so limited that these patient cohorts are often excluded from meta-analyses examining lithium's efficacy, or BD-2 is combined with BD-1 under the term "bipolar disorders" [25]. As discussed in Chapter 1, mirror image studies provide insight into lithium's benefits across the diagnostic spectrum by examining recurrence rates in BD-1, BD-2 and SAD-BT patients who stop lithium [26]. Using data from a Swedish observational study of lithium's efficacy and adverse effects in real world usage, 871 lithium treated individuals were identified from among those assigned bipolar spectrum diagnoses on at least two occasions in Norrbotten, Sweden. During the observational period, 54% of the cohort discontinued lithium, and 194 had clinical data two years before and two years after lithium discontinuation from 1997 to 2013 [26]. In the two years after lithium discontinuation, 51% of patients with BD-I/SAD-BT (n = 100) and 46% with BD-2/other BD (n = 94) were on an alternative mood stabilizer. Using the primary outcome measure of psychiatric hospitalization, the BD-1/SAD-BT patient cohort experienced a significant increase in the percentage who were admitted (18% while on lithium, 56% after discontinuation, p < 0.001), and in total number of admissions (33 vs. 130, p < 0.001). In this cohort, the overall increase in admissions was for mania and depression, and this occurred irrespective of lithium reinitiation, indicating a loss of stability that was not easily recaptured. The BD-2/other BD cohort did not experience a significant change in percent or total admissions after lithium discontinuation. While the use of hospitalization as the metric for recurrence might obscure the extent and severity of mood relapses in the BD-2 group, this data set substantiates that those with a history of mania or mixed features, regardless of BD-1 or SAD-BT diagnosis, have comparable benefits from lithium as maintenance therapy. What differentiates the SAD-BT group is the ongoing need for mood stabilizer and antipsychotic treatment to manage both components of their disorder. One of the few retrospective studies which addresses this issue looked at real world long-term outcomes in schizoaffective disorder patients using data in the Finnish (n = 7655) and Swedish (n = 7525) health registers [27]. While the analysis did not distinguish between those with SAD-BT and those with SAD depressed type, it still noted that mood stabilizers used in combination with antipsychotics were associated with a decreased risk of psychosis hospitalization compared with antipsychotic monotherapy (Finnish cohort HR 0.76, 95% CI 0.71–0.81; Swedish cohort HR 0.84, 0.78–0.90) [27].

While SAD-BT patients appear to do best with an antipsychotic + mood stabilizer combination, the approval of SGAs for BD-1 maintenance based on placebo-controlled trials raises the question of how patients in routine clinical practice fare on SGA monotherapy compared with other treatment options [28]. This is a topic of interest to clinicians and patients alike, as the SGA adverse effect profile and decreased need for monitoring may seem appealing, assuming that efficacy is acceptable. The absence of prospective long-term comparative data for SGAs vs. other treatments (i.e. > 1 year) again forces one to use naturalistic outcomes to inform treatment practice and patient recommendations. In 2019, a Swedish group examined data from 5713 hospitalizations for mania among 3772 adults with BD-1 (aged 18–75), from July 1, 2006 to December 3, 2014, to examine the time to treatment failure, with failure defined as medication discontinuation, switch or rehospitalization. As seen in Figure 4.1, those on SGA monotherapy had the shortest time to treatment failure of all treatments and combinations examined,

Figure 4.1 Time to treatment failure after hospitalization for mania among various treatment options for bipolar I disorder using lithium (dark blue line) as the comparator treatment [28]

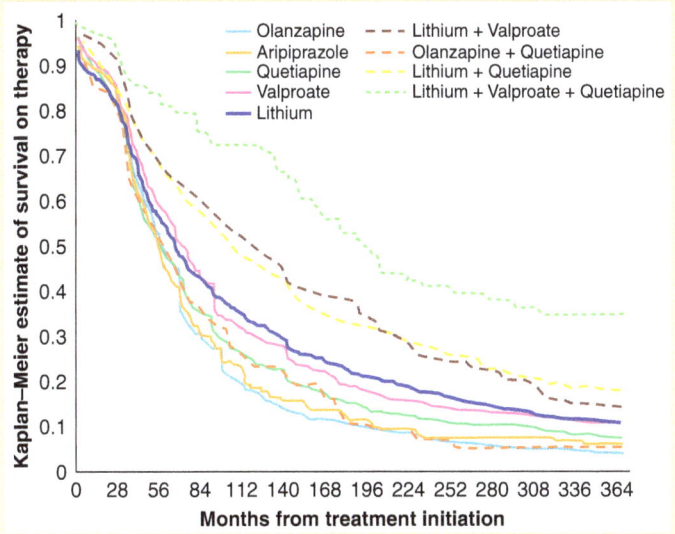

(Adapted from: L. Wingård, L. Brandt, R. Bodén, et al. [2019]. Monotherapy vs. combination therapy for post mania maintenance treatment: A population based cohort study. *Eur Neuropsychopharmacol*, 29, 691–700.)

and had a significantly higher risk of treatment failure compared with lithium monotherapy [28]. These results are sobering, and while certain SGAs lower the risk of BD relapse compared with placebo, in the world of clinical practice the point of comparison is not placebo, but agents such as lithium with extensive effectiveness data. Patients with BD-1 may reject any mood stabilizer for a variety of reasons, but in doing so must be apprised of the disadvantages with SGA monotherapy.

In-Depth 4.3 Detailed Methods in the 2019 Swedish Study Exploring Rates of Treatment Failure after a Hospitalization for Mania

Each period after a hospitalization for mania was analyzed separately. As BD-1 patients may be hospitalized repeatedly for manic episodes, those hospitalized for mania multiple times were included upon each hospitalization; however, hospitalizations for mania < 7 days apart were linked and counted as one episode. Patients with diagnoses of dementia, or those with schizophrenia or SAD-BT, were excluded to confine the analysis to BD-1 individuals. After each hospitalization for mania, active treatment periods of lithium, divalproex/valproate (VPA), olanzapine, quetiapine or aripiprazole, alone or in combinations, were recorded. Each active treatment period was defined as starting on the day of a prescription fill of any of the studied medications, or the day of discharge from the hospital if the patient filled a prescription during the hospitalization. If the hospitalization was > 4 weeks, only prescriptions during the last 4 weeks of the stay were considered. Patients who filled prescriptions for more than one drug within a time period of less than 2 weeks were considered to be on combination therapy. Follow-up started on day 14 of the first active treatment period and ended after 365 days or upon the earliest of any of the following events: treatment failure, emigration, death or the end of the study period (December 31, 2014). Medication discontinuation was defined as not having access to that treatment for 28 days or more. Patients who initiated combination therapy and subsequently stopped one drug while continuing the other were not considered to have discontinued their medication.

2 *Adjunctive Lithium in Unipolar Major Depressive Disorder*

Lithium is effective as an adjunct to antidepressants among inadequate responders with unipolar major depression, and it is also superior to placebo as monotherapy though not used in that manner in modern practice [29, 30]. The mixed quality of older studies is an issue when calculating the effect size for unipolar MDD adjunctive treatment [31], and study heterogeneity led a 2019 review to conclude that it remains uncertain whether lithium's efficacy for MDD occurs across the spectrum of unipolar patients, or if the benefits accrue preferentially to a subgroup with BD-like characteristics or mixed features [30]. These uncertainties, combined with safety and tolerability concerns surrounding lithium, present a dilemma when assigning lithium a place within the unipolar MDD treatment algorithm. Compounding this issue has been the lack of a consistent working definition of treatment resistance in the literature, with many trials of resistant individuals enrolling patients who have experienced only one antidepressant failure during the current depressive episode [32]. The nosology problem may have been resolved in 2022 when a group of 16 MDD experts employed the Delphi method to arrive at consensus definitions for treatment-resistant depression (TRD) and for partially responsive depression (PRD) to serve as operational criteria in future clinical studies [32]. Agreed upon criteria for TRD and PRD will improve the quality of upcoming studies, but for now the placement of lithium in the hierarchy of MDD biological therapies must rely on existing data and the clinician's judgment about relative safety concerns among adjunctive options.

In general, most unipolar MDD treatment algorithms start with antidepressant monotherapy (e.g. selective serotonin reuptake inhibitors, serotonin norepinephrine reuptake inhibitors, presynaptic alpha$_2$-adrenergic autoreceptor antagonists, etc.), with the decision to switch or augment driven by the perceived benefit and tolerability of the initial trial [33]. For cost and safety reasons, antidepressant combination therapy is often the next step in PRD, in part because it avoids tolerability concerns related to SGAs (movement disorders, metabolic adverse effects), or lithium. A 2022 review of 39 randomized clinical trials (n = 6751) found that combination antidepressant treatment was associated with improved treatment outcomes compared with monotherapy (standardized mean difference [SMD] = 0.31; 95% CI 0.19–0.44), with the strategy of combining a reuptake inhibitor with an alpha$_2$-adrenergic autoreceptor antagonist (e.g. mianserin, mirtazapine) superior to other combinations (SMD = 0.37; 95% CI 0.19–0.55) [34].

In-Depth 4.4 Tolerability Concerns During Adjunctive SGA Use in Unipolar MDD

In the last 15 years, SGAs have emerged as a popular evidence based option for persistent MDD symptoms despite antidepressant combinations, especially SGAs with low risk of metabolic adverse effects and sedation (e.g. the dopamine D$_2$ receptor partial agonist aripiprazole) [35]. However, the last 5 years have seen a tempering of enthusiasm for SGAs, in part due to recognition that even partial agonist antipsychotics carry a risk for tardive dyskinesia (TD) based on multiple case reports of mood disorder patients with no prior antipsychotic exposure who developed TD after SGA treatment [36, 37]. Unfortunately, following an acute 4 or 6 week adjunctive MDD trial, subsequent open-label extension studies rarely exceed 52 weeks, thus making it difficult to estimate the TD risk from aripiprazole or other SGAs approved for this indication [38–41]. While the risk may be small, the consistent reporting of TD cases in antipsychotic-naïve MDD patients newly exposed to an SGA demands that clinicians inform patients about TD risk even if unable to quantify the extent of such risk.

In-Depth 4.5 Emerging Concern about Mortality Risk and Adjunctive SGA Use in Adults of Age 25–64 Years Old with Unipolar MDD

Aside from risks of metabolic dysfunction and TD, another concern which recently emerged was a signal for increased mortality when SGAs are used for unipolar MDD. It has been known for nearly 20 years that all antipsychotics increase mortality at least 1.5-fold in dementia patients [42, 43], but this had not been described in other diagnostic groups until a 2020 retrospective analysis examined the relative mortality risk of SGAs vs. a 2nd antidepressant among nonelderly adults (aged 25–64 years) diagnosed with unipolar MDD, and receiving public insurance in the US via Medicaid (2001–2010) [44]. All eligible subjects for this study had to have uninterrupted Medicaid coverage during the 180 days preceding the index period, with this index period defined as when a patient initiated augmentation with an SGA or a 2nd antidepressant after ≥ 3 months of antidepressant monotherapy. Importantly, those with alternative SGA indications were excluded (e.g. schizophrenia, psychotic depression, autism, dementia or BD) [44]. The primary outcome measure was all-cause mortality, and the study used advanced analytic techniques such as propensity score matching, so that the SGA and 2nd antidepressant cohorts were both matched by the likelihood to have received an SGA prescription. In addition, the cohorts were balanced for other covariates of importance, and inverse probability of treatment weights assigned to each subject to compensate for underrepresentation or overrepresentation of certain types of individuals in each treatment group [45]. In the SGA cohort, 25,172 patients received an initial prescription, as did 19,129 in the 2nd antidepressant group. The mean age in this patient pool was 44.3 years, 78% were female, and 69% were white, non-Hispanic. The crude unadjusted death rate for the SGA group was 138.1 per 10,000 person-years, based on 105 deaths during 7601 person-years of follow-up, while that for the 2nd antidepressant cohort was 83.8 per 10,000 person-years, representing 48 deaths during 5727 person-years of follow-up. The adjusted hazard ratio (HR) calculations found that SGA use increased mortality by 45% (HR 1.45, 95% CI 1.02–2.06), or a risk difference of 37.7 per 10,000 person-years (95% CI 1.7–88.8). Given the inherent low mortality rate in a population of mean age 44.3 years, this risk difference corresponds to a number needed to harm (NNH) of 265. The adjusted HR was also consistent when restricted to natural deaths (HR = 1.58, 95% CI 1.02–2.45) or non-cancer deaths (HR = 1.65, 95% CI 1.05–2.60), and showed no dose-response effect. This NNH figure is quite large, and indicates that one would need to treat 265 MDD patients with an adjunctive SGA for 1 year before seeing one additional death compared with the addition of a second antidepressant.

While the study reporting increased mortality risk with SGA use has not been replicated, this is a safety concern worth following in the literature as it represents another adverse effect that may need to be added to the informed consent, alongside movement disorders and weight gain, when using SGAs as adjunctive MDD treatments. As with all clinical decisions, safety and tolerability issues, patient acuity, patient preferences and concerns, medical comorbidity and clinical course must be balanced by the strength of the efficacy evidence to arrive at a shared decision on any adjunctive strategy. While certain older strategies are not strongly supported by the literature (e.g. thyroid hormone or buspirone augmentation) [46, 47], lithium remains one of the evidence based adjunctive biological therapies for unipolar MDD along with SGAs, esketamine or ketamine, transcranial magnetic stimulation and electroconvulsive therapy [35].

3   *Is There Clinical or Biomarker Evidence for an "Ideal" Lithium Patient?*

Lithium is one of numerous options for patients with unipolar MDD, but for BD patients, especially those with BD-1, lithium is an essential part of the treatment armamentarium. As discussed at length in Chapter 2, concerns about lithium's long-term renal impact have moderated in recent years based on research showing that severe chronic kidney disease (CKD) is exceedingly rare, and that much of the CKD risk relates to medical comorbidity in the target population [48, 49]. Nonetheless, lithium's reputation in this area, combined with other adverse effects and the need for ongoing monitoring of renal and thyroid function, stimulated research into identification of the "ideal" lithium candidate among BD spectrum patients, with the goal of sparing those with low likelihood of response an unnecessary lithium trial. Broadly speaking, the psychiatric field has long sought clinical features or biomarkers that predict response to guide treatment choice, and this remains an active area of research for lithium in particular (Info Box 4.1) [50–52].

Info Box 4.1   Is There a Specific Candidate for Lithium Therapy?

a. **Current practice:** The general answer is "no," assuming the patient has adequate renal function by eGFR for commencing lithium treatment, and has a disorder with an evidence based use for lithium. There has been exhaustive research on clinical predictors of lithium response due to concerns about lithium's narrow therapeutic index, and with the goal of limiting lithium to those with an optimal profile for response. Why is this discussion less compelling than in prior years?

   i. There is increasing recognition of lithium's unique benefits (e.g. reduced suicide mortality, neuroprotection), and the limitations of anticonvulsant mood stabilizers (e.g. divalproex) and SGA monotherapy without mood stabilization [28].

ii. Data on the predictive value of family history, age of onset, polarity of first mood episode or pattern of mood episodes (e.g. mania–depression vs. depression–mania) is often not robust, and in many instances conflicting [53]. Mood stabilizer response among those with a history of rapid cycling (RC) is consistently poor due to frequent brief depressive episodes [54, 55]. From the limited retrospective and prospective studies, lithium fares no worse than anticonvulsant mood stabilizers in RC-BD patients [55, 56]. Analyses that note low lithium response in RC-BD often fail to place this into context – these patients will typically not attain mood stability on any mood stabilizer monotherapy, and will require additional medications, especially for depressive episodes [52, 53].

iii. **One repeated clinical finding over the past decade is that a history of migraine is a predictor of inadequate lithium response, especially control of hypomanic symptoms** [52, 57, 58]. Clinical studies since 2003 indicate that BD patients have 2–3 times higher migraine prevalence than the general population, with one study finding a gene locus associating with migraine risk in BD patients that is not a risk allele in non-BD migraneurs [59]. How this association translates to diminished lithium response is a subject of interest [58], but clinicians should be prepared to consider alternate or adjunctive therapies in migraine patients who do not respond adequately to lithium monotherapy.

iv. There is an enhanced understanding that some of the renal effects attributed to lithium relate to CKD risk factors in the patient population (e.g. hypertension, diabetes mellitus), and that the independent effect of lithium on eGFR trends is more modest than previously estimated [60]. Moreover, there is a growing sophistication about dosing practices that lessen risk for renal insufficiency, including use of lower maintenance levels for most patients (0.60–0.80 mEq/l) [61], once daily dosing [62], the need to adjust lithium dosing quickly in the presence of kinetic interactions [63, 64] and the need to prevent outpatient levels from ever exceeding 1.00 mEq/l, and especially 1.20 mEq/l [62].

b. **Future research:** There is no questioning the value of finding biomarkers for lithium response, assuming one also has equivalent data for other mood stabilizing molecules, and also assuming that an agreed upon definition of response can be operationalized [57, 65–68]. The search for genetic, imaging and clinical markers to guide clinical medication choices may also provide insights into which aspects of lithium's multiple mechanisms of action correlate with specific outcomes, and how this interacts with specific patient biotypes. This will not only facilitate targeted treatment, but perhaps inspire new directions in drug development.

One difficulty in implementing the results of lithium-specific clinical analyses is that most omit a comparison treatment to place the results in context. Often the features identified (e.g. comorbid substance use) are predictors of poor response to BD treatment in general [69], or represent subgroups (e.g. rapid cycling patients) for whom lithium effectively provides mania prophylaxis, but in whom any mood stabilizer monotherapy will be insufficient to manage recurrent brief depressive episodes [52, 54, 55, 74]. Ongoing biomarker studies are examining a variety of approaches such as polygenic risk scores, individual genetic markers, imaging findings, and circadian rhythms in cultured patient neurons to predict lithium response. One hopes that this research will mature sufficiently that robust predictors to a variety of mood stabilizing therapies can be applied in clinical practice [67, 68, 71]. At the present time, one must rely on evidence based indications to inform a decision to start lithium, especially where it provides comparative advantages vs. other options. Patients with an evidence based reason for lithium use, especially those with a history of mania, are lithium candidates and should not be deprived of a trial by the treating clinician unless there is a medical contraindication to commencing lithium. As noted in a 2020 comprehensive review of bipolar disorder: "Lithium is the gold standard mood-stabilising agent for the treatment of people with bipolar disorders" [72].

 B **What to Tell Patients, and the Value of Customized Adherence Enhancement (CAE)**

 WHAT TO KNOW: PATIENT COMMUNICATION AND EVIDENCE BASED ADHERENCE TREATMENT

- Developing a treatment alliance is the best tool to promote adherence, but developing this alliance demands an appreciation of the patient's perspective on their illness.

- Medication nonadherence should be discussed, along with the fact that many patients struggle with adherence. Conversations about adherence should revolve around specific issues likely to induce nonadherence in newly treated patients, or elicited from those patients who are continuing on lithium.

- CAE is one of the few evidence based therapies that improves adherence in BD patients. This easily delivered modular treatment specifically addresses the four most common reasons underlying nonadherence with all aspects of bipolar disorder pharmacotherapy.

The cornerstone of promoting adherence is treatment alliance, and the foundation for alliance is created by the time spent understanding the patient's worldview with regard to the illness itself, the use of medications in general and the role of lithium. Before any meaningful discussion can occur about interventions, it is important to delve into what the patient thinks is actually happening, especially with newly diagnosed patients, and how this is formulated by them. The formal term is the *cognitive representation of illness*, and this typically encapsulates five major themes: What is the nature of the problem?; What is the cause?; How long will it last and will it recur?; What effects will it have on me?; What can I do to make it go away or manage it? [13]. By understanding this cognitive representation of their illness, the clinician is also presented with a set of health beliefs that might impact treatment adherence (Figure 4.2). Importantly, one can then tailor education interventions to promote adherence based on these concerns or ideas about treatment.

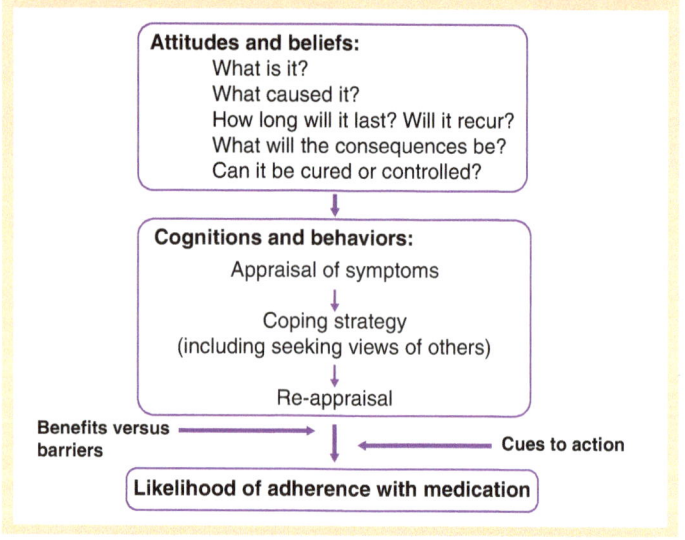

Figure 4.2 Diagrammatic representation showing that medication adherence is the product of individual processing and reassessing of illness attitudes and beliefs [13]

(Adapted from: J. Scott and M. J. Tacchi [2002]. A pilot study of concordance therapy for individuals with bipolar disorders who are non-adherent with lithium prophylaxis. *Bipolar Disord*, 4, 386–392.)

Nonadherence with lithium has been documented for over 50 years, but this mirrors a problem with oral medication adherence seen to varying degrees in all chronic illnesses [5]. Regardless of medication choice, nonadherence is common in BD, with particularly high rates of nonadherence and discontinuation in the first 6 months of treatment [73, 74]. A significant driver of future nonadherence is attitude towards the use of medications for psychiatric illness and towards lithium specifically. A 1983 Danish study of 140 lithium treated patients found that 25% perceived no advantage to taking lithium, other than possibly satisfying the demands of their family or clinician [7]. In 2007, an analysis of Danish data by Kessing covering all new lithium starts in adults from 1995 to 2000 (n = 14,277) found that the median time to discontinuation was 181.0 days (95% CI 135.7– 181.0), and that 25% stopped lithium within 45.2 days [75].

From these studies, it becomes quite obvious that assessing the patient's perspective on lithium must be performed early in treatment, even for patients who are new to you but have been on lithium for years, and their attitude quantified (if possible) with formal instruments such as the Lithium Attitudes Questionnaire (LAQ) [76]. That patients prescribed lithium might not fully accept the need for medication or might have negative feelings about adverse effects is not surprising, but a 2019 study of 76 BD patients on lithium for an average of 2 years noted that LAQ score was the single most significant predictor of self-reported adherence (p < 0.0001), and predicted 75% of the variance [77]. This study is consistent with decades of research that demonstrate a significant correlation between adherence and a patient's attitude toward lithium, and between adherence and the patient's level of disease and medication knowledge [78].

Given that knowledge and attitude are important predictors of adherence, any conversations about adherence should be folded into a broad approach to psychoeducation, with elements tailored toward specific issues likely to engender nonadherence in newly treated patients, or elicited from individuals continuing on lithium [2]. For those already on lithium, nonadherence should be normalized as something that all patients struggle with, and the extent of adherence quantified in some manner, such as the self-rated 8 item Medication Adherence Rating Scale [79]. Patients starting lithium for the first time and those with ongoing adherence issues should be enrolled in a psychoeducation program that places emphasis on addressing the specific reasons for nonadherence. Most programs fostering improved lithium adherence were tailored to BD-1 patients, given the significant impact of lithium discontinuation on mood recurrence [27, 80]. The content and implementation methods of adherence programs have evolved [81], but a 2018 systematic review of 40 studies on BD psychoeducation lamented that 70% of the research focused on group or family modalities, while only a few explored individual or internet based programs, and the results of those were inconsistent [82]. Nonetheless, group psychoeducation was associated with reduced stigma, improved adherence, higher maintenance lithium levels, reduced illness recurrence, decreased hospitalizations and shorter stay, and increased time to illness relapse. Family psychoeducation also reduced illness recurrence and hospitalization rates; improved caregiver self-efficacy, knowledge and sense of well-being; and decreased caregiver burden [82].

The lack of individually tailored evidence based programs designed to improve adherence among BD patients was recently addressed by Dr. Martha Sajatovic (holder of the Willard Brown Chair in Neurological Outcomes at University Hospitals Cleveland Medical Center, and the Rocco L. Motto Professorship in Child and Adolescent Psychiatry) who developed CAE, and then compared its impact on treatment adherence in a group of 184 BD adults randomized to CAE or a rigorous BD-specific educational program [83]. As noted in Table 4.1, the CAE modules cover four areas: increasing patient knowledge, improving skill at communicating with providers, enhancing motivations for treatment, and identifying issues with medication routines (e.g. unnecessary complexity). *Patients were assigned to specific modules based on their individual reasons for nonadherence* and each module was delivered in one-on-one sessions spaced 1 week apart, with a booster session 4 weeks after completion of the last session. At time of study entry, subjects missed a mean of $55.15\% \pm 28.22\%$ of prescribed BD drugs within the past week, and $48.01\% \pm 28.46\%$ in the past month. Study attrition was < 20%. Compared with those randomized to education only, individuals enrolled in CAE had significantly improved adherence after 6 months (as measured by the Tablets Routine Questionnaire) in the preceding week ($p = 0.001$) and in the past month ($p = 0.048$) [83]. With this robust response for oral medication adherence, trials of CAE to improve long-acting injectable antipsychotic adherence in BD patients were performed, and these also showed a significant reduction in nonadherence [84, 85]. CAE thus represents the most evidence based approach to improving nonadherence in BD patients, with demonstrated superiority to psychoeducation alone. It also reinforces the concept that reasons for nonadherence are unique to each individual, and these must be elucidated before CAE or any other adherence measures can be implemented.

Table 4.1 Module elements of Customized Adherence Enhancement for bipolar disorder patients [83]

Element	Rationale	Module content
1. Psychoeducation on medication treatment	Psychoeducation approaches BD as a biological disorder that can be managed by appropriate medication treatments in conjunction with non-somatic coping strategies. Psychoeducation has been noted to improve medication adherence.	This module uses a modified Life Goals Program. The module consists of 3 individual units including: (1) basic information about BD, its neurobiological underpinnings, and information on mania and depression; (2) a focus on medication management, identifying the purpose of medication, reviewing good and bad effects of medication; and (3) following discussion of functional impact of symptoms, the interventionist and individual with BD collaboratively develop a personal symptom profile for the individual's own episodes of depression and mania, as well as their early warning signs of impending relapse.
2. Modified Motivational Enhancement Therapy (MET)	MET is an evidence based psychosocial intervention for individuals with dual diagnosis.	This 2-unit module helps individuals understand the effects of substance abuse on their BD in general, and on their adherence to medication specifically. Individuals are encouraged to access personal motivation to change their substance use, making it more likely that they will be adherent to their medication regimen. The module consists of a guided assessment of individual substance use/abuse followed by modified MET that addresses adherence specifically within the context of substance abuse.
3. Communication with providers	Using principles from collaborative care, this module focuses on improving communication with providers from a patient-focused, patient-directed approach.	Individuals with BD are supported in examining and exploring key components of treatment planning with their provider, including expectations for medication response, and feared/experienced medication side effects. Key critical issues include understanding of differential burden of medication related effects, and how these effects might be prioritized for discussion with a clinician. This 2-unit module also provides information on commonly utilized psychotropic agents.

Element	Rationale	Module content
4. Medication routines	Complex medication regimens may interfere with daily activities and adherence.	This 2-unit module focuses on assisting individuals to modify treatment regimens as appropriate, and facilitates discussion with providers. Using principles from interpersonal and social rhythm therapy for BD, a key activity is to outline and review the individual's daily routine with respect to medication-taking and problem-solving regarding common barriers. This module emphasizes the use of prompts/reminders and self-monitoring/self-regulation to maximize and maintain adherence. A key activity in this module is a review of medication-taking patterns, including examination of when, where and how medications are taken.

(Adapted from: M. Sajatovic, C. Tatsuoka, K. A. Cassidy, et al. [2018]. A 6-month, prospective, randomized controlled trial of Customized Adherence Enhancement versus bipolar-specific educational control in poorly adherent individuals with bipolar disorder. *J Clin Psychiatry*, 79, 17m12036.)

One demographic factor not covered by the initial CAE research was the child and adolescent BD population, a group with developmental issues that influence their approach to mental illness and treatment in a manner not seen with adults. A significant fraction of BD spectrum patients have their disease onset before age 25, and a 2010 paper used data from six international sites to calculate the median age of onset for BD-1 (n = 1089) at 24.3 years, and for BD-2 (n = 476) at 30.1 years (Figure 4.3) [86]. Moreover, the proportion with onset before age 20 appeared close to 11% when combining BD-1 and BD-2 patients. A 2022 comprehensive review of median age of onset for mental disorders used data from 192 epidemiological studies comprising 708,561 individuals to provide more exact estimates of illness onset with a variety of age cutpoints [87]. Among the eligible protocols, 40 studies had data sets that addressed bipolar spectrum disorders, and in these studies the median age of onset was 33 years (25th percentile 22 years; 75th percentile 49 years), with peak age of onset at 19.5 years [87]. Importantly, 13.7% were diagnosed by age 18, and 32.0% were diagnosed by age 25 [87]. Self-stigma related to the diagnosis can be daunting to younger individuals establishing their identity, but the relationship to adherence and the impact of maturity have not been extensively studied. In 2020, researchers at the National Institute of Mental Health reanalyzed data from the CAE study of 184 nonadherent BD patients to explore differences in medication adherence, psychiatric symptom severity and internalized stigma levels in adults younger than age 55, or those aged 55 and older [88]. The investigators found that the older cohort was less anxious and depressed compared with the younger group, while the younger group rated higher on self-stigma. Another interesting finding of relevance to age is that the older individuals randomized to psychoeducation only, but not to CAE, appeared to do less well with medication adherence over time than younger individuals. Although this analysis did not specifically focus on children and adolescents, the fact that adults in their 30s and 40s struggle with self-stigma highlights the need to discuss this issue with all patients in treatment. Given the unique cognitive and developmental issues for juvenile onset BD, CAE is now being tailored to adolescents and young adults, with a clinical trial having commenced in 2022 [89].

Figure 4.3. 2010 estimate of median age of onset for bipolar I and II disorders across 6 international sites [86]

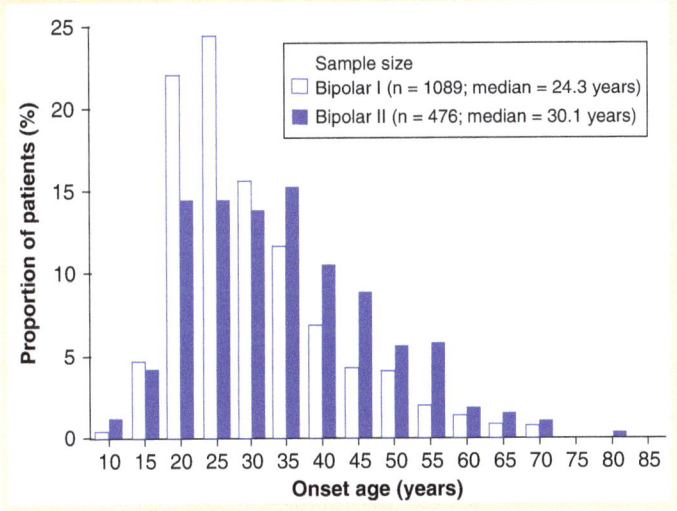

(Adapted from: R. J. Baldessarini, L. Bolzani, N. Cruz, et al. [2010]. Onset-age of bipolar disorders at six international sites. *J Affect Disord*, 121, 143–146.)

The discussions with a patient starting lithium should not only cover medication specific issues, but, as alluded to above, delve into the patient's ideas about the psychiatric diagnosis, its implications and the role of medications (Table 4.2). Despite attempts to outline one's rationale for arriving at a specific diagnosis and treatment plan, a patient may reject the diagnosis or the need for medications. The predominant theme in these conversations should be one's openness to hearing the patient's perspectives and to being as flexible as is clinically practicable in reaching shared decisions. In some instances, patient requests are untenable (e.g. remove all psychotropic medications in someone with a recent episode of mania), but providing options when possible is important. As noted in one 12-week switch study for nonadherent BD patients, providing a medication alternative to the agent deemed to be the key offender in weight gain led to a marked improvement in adherence [90]. At study baseline, 48.6% of prescribed BD medication was missed in the prior week, but this dropped to 25.3% (p = 0.002) at study endpoint [90]. These conversations must also involve family members or caregivers to incorporate their perspectives and concerns, and to offer the option of family psychoeducation, an intervention with proven benefit as noted in the 2018 review of controlled BD psychoeducation trials [82]. The tone of the lithium discussions should emphasize its benefits in general, but specifically how this might apply to the individual, and why these benefits outweigh the monitoring burdens and adverse effects of treatment. In covering common adverse effects as part of informed consent, one should emphasize the willingness to hear about adverse effects as soon as they arise, one's expertise in managing these issues, and the modern perspective on important outcomes such as renal dysfunction. When talking about adherence, it is important to normalize that nonadherence is common in chronic disorders such as BD or hypertension [3], that lithium is only effective above a minimum serum level threshold, and that part of routine level monitoring is for safety reasons but also to help detect problems with nonadherence so appropriate interventions that promote adherence can be implemented (e.g. pill boxes, text reminders, CAE, etc.).

In-Depth 4.6 How Often and Why Do Patients Stop Lithium?

Despite a clinician's best efforts, some patients will discontinue lithium, although the reasons vary somewhat depending on the underlying diagnosis [1]. A retrospective analysis of 873 new lithium starts in Norrbotten, Sweden, from 1997 to 2013, found that 54% subsequently discontinued lithium, with some patients reporting more than one reason. Adverse effects were the most frequent cause (62%), followed by psychiatric reasons (44%) and other physical reasons interfering with lithium treatment (12%). The influence of diagnosis was seen in both the rates of, and reasons for, stopping lithium. Patients with BD-2 or unspecified BD were three times as likely to discontinue lithium for lack of effectiveness (p < 0.001). Overall, patients with BD-1 or SAD-BT were more likely to discontinue lithium than those with BD-2 or unspecified BD (p < 0.01), and those with BD-1 or SAD-BT were also more likely to refuse medication (p < 0.01). Interestingly, women and men stopped lithium at equal rates, but women were twice as likely to consult a doctor before doing so (p < 0.01). BD-2 patients spend 50% of the time in periods of depression [91], so discontinuing lithium for lack of efficacy is not an indictment of clinical practice, just an acknowledgment that lithium's antidepressant actions may not be sufficiently robust for all BD patients, and of the fact that limited options for bipolar depression before 2013 may have impelled clinicians to try lithium for BD-2 depression. There are reasons why certain BD-2 patients should be placed on lithium, but demonstrating to the patient that you have a grasp of all the treatment options for various evidence based lithium uses, including newer agents (e.g. lumateperone for BD-1 or BD-2 depression), will hopefully inspire confidence that you can work together to address adverse effects or lack of efficacy regardless of the medication regimen. In the end, one wants to avoid unfortunate situations documented in the literature where patients felt that lithium monitoring was inadequate, that options to try lithium were not provided or decision-making was rushed [92].

Table 4.2 Areas of focus during patient/caregiver discussions about lithium

	Educational points	Patient perspectives to elicit
Diagnosis	• Outline the rationale for the current working diagnosis and how diagnoses may be revised over time based on course, medication response and additional history • Discuss whether any uncertainty exists about the diagnosis (e.g. BD-1 vs. BD-2; BD-1 with psychotic features vs. SAD-BT) • Provide prognostic information	• Acceptance or rejection of diagnosis • Meaning of diagnosis based on personal knowledge, and concerns about stigma • Implications of diagnosis for lifetime goals
Lithium as core medication	• Outline a clinical rationale for the choice of lithium • Discuss lithium's benefits and advantages vs. other mood stabilizers or medication in general, and also how this applies to their diagnosis and history • Inform about the possible need for other medications to address or provide prophylaxis for mood symptoms, or medications to manage adverse effects • Review the need for laboratory monitoring, and why this is not unique to lithium • Discuss alternatives to lithium, and their risks, benefits and limitations	• Feelings about medications to manage mood symptoms • Meaning of and beliefs about being on lithium, and stigma related to lithium (as compared with other medications) • Preferences about type of medication, dosing frequency and route of administration (e.g. long-acting injectable antipsychotic vs. daily pill taking)

	Educational points	Patient perspectives to elicit
Importance of adherence	• Normalize that oral medication nonadherence is common among all chronic disorders • Review the reasons why lithium must be taken daily (i.e. kinetics and efficacy) • Mention the minimum effective serum levels and target-level range • Review how to handle missed doses [93], or what to do with significant GI illnesses resulting in vomiting or diarrhea (see Chapter 6) [94] • Review the consequences of relapse due to nonadherence, and how this may interfere with a patient's functional goals • Note one's openness to medication simplification	• Feelings about daily pill taking (i.e. inconvenience, daily reminder of their illness) • Frustration with complex oral regimens • Concerns about phlebotomy (fears, inconvenience) • Beliefs about stopping medication during periods of wellness
Side effects	• Emphasize the need to communicate side effects early so they can be addressed (even if this occurs between appointments) and your willingness to act on these issues expeditiously • Note that steps can be taken to manage adverse effects and improve tolerability • Discuss that some adverse effects may be seen earlier (e.g. tremor, weight gain, polydipsia/polyuria, skin reactions), and some may appear over time (e.g. hair loss, hypothyroidism, polydipsia/polyuria) • Outline modern concepts about renal risks and current approaches to mitigate these risks (e.g. lower target levels than in the past, eGFR monitoring, management of other CKD risks such as hypertension)	• Address concerns and fears about renal issues • Address concerns and fears about other side effects of specific concern (e.g. weight gain)
Drug interactions	• Emphasize that most interactions are manageable • Reinforce the need to communicate when new routine medications are added from certain classes, and to ask if unsure about an interaction with lithium • Provide realistic guidelines for use of NSAIDs	• Address any concerns about current medications or new medications

C **What is the Baseline Work-Up and What is an Acceptable eGFR for Starting Lithium?**

 WHAT TO KNOW: INTRODUCTION

- There is no consensus on the baseline work-up, but the number of essential baseline laboratory and clinical measures to obtain is surprisingly modest. However, local guidelines may require a more extensive work-up.

- In addition to eGFR, TSH and serum, clinicians should be familiar with the need to obtain a urine albumin-to-creatinine ratio (ACR), early morning urine osmolality (EMUO) or an ECG in some circumstances.

- There is no consensus opinion on the minimum eGFR for starting lithium. Based on recent studies of renal outcomes during lithium therapy, the following guidelines are suggested:

  - for any patient with an evidence based indication for lithium:
    minimum eGFR ≥ 60 ml/min

  - for any patient with a *compelling indication* for lithium:
    minimum eGFR ≥ 45 ml/min

The basic requirements for a baseline pretreatment work-up are not necessarily onerous and are outlined in Table 4.3. There is no universal agreement on this issue, with various groups incorporating extensive laboratory measures intended to detect common medical comorbidities in BD and SAD-BT patients (e.g. cardiometabolic dysfunction), but which are not absolutely necessary to start the first dose of lithium. In 2017, Professor Gin Malhi (Psychiatry Chair at The University of Sydney, Executive and Clinical Director of the CADE Clinic at the Northern Clinical School and Head of the Academic Department of Psychiatry at the Royal North Shore Hospital) reviewed BD treatment guidelines from 13 societies and national organizations, and created a synthesis of their recommendations that form the basis for the items in Table 4.3 [95]. Among laboratory measures, there is universal agreement that TSH, serum calcium and renal function should be obtained. As noted in Chapter 2, the latter is best tracked using eGFR$_{cr-cys}$ derived from serum creatinine and cystatin C values, although one can use eGFR$_{cr}$ if necessary. The core items highlighted in Table 4.3 are generally congruent with Malhi's 2017 synthesis, but with a few differences. As nearly all patients will have blood pressure (BP) measured at some point, BP has been added to detect untreated hypertension and the subsequent need to use a medication class that has kinetic interactions with lithium. Untreated hypertension should not forestall commencing lithium, but it should foster communication with the primary care provider regarding choice of antihypertensives, especially to avoid use of certain agents (e.g. lisinopril) contraindicated with lithium [64, 96]. The use of waist circumference is also not included due to its poor reproducibility in routine clinical practice [97]. Body mass index correlates highly with the central obesity criterion of metabolic syndrome and is subject to much less user error. Due to the high prevalence of CKD risks in the target population, early morning urine ACR is suggested in those eGFR below stage G1 (i.e. < 90 l/min) or who have CKD risks. Lithium only rarely induces glomerular pathology and proteinuria, but albuminuria is not uncommon with hypertension or cardiometabolic disease. Obtaining a baseline assessment of albuminuria severity in those at higher risk is helpful to identify a pre-existing problem, and to forestall complaints from other providers who might blame lithium for the patient's proteinuria despite the presence of medical comorbidities that better explain this problem [98, 99]. An EMUO is not mandatory prior to starting lithium, but may be useful to obtain in older individuals so that age-related declines in EMUO are not mistaken for a lithium effect on renal concentrating ability [100].

Table 4.3 Baseline Work-Up

Measure	Rationale	Response to abnormal results
History	To note personal or family history of renal dysfunction, or risk factors for CKD (e.g. cardiovascular disease, dyslipidemia, metabolic syndrome, diabetes mellitus, hypertension, smoking). To record use of nephrotoxic medications or medications having significant kinetic interactions with lithium.	Medical comorbidity and CKD risk factors are common in patients with serious mental disorders. Their presence does not disqualify a patient from a lithium trial (see Info Box 4.3).
Weight, BMI	Lithium may induce weight gain, and this effect will be additive with that from antipsychotic therapy and other psychotropics (e.g. divalproex/valproate).	Establishes baseline.
Blood pressure	Rule out untreated hypertension, a significant CKD risk factor.	Refer for treatment. Not a reason to delay lithium, but must follow-up if a medication is added due to interactions between certain antihypertensives and lithium.

Measure	Rationale	Response to abnormal results
TSH	Baseline is necessary due to lithium's effect on thyroid function.	Refer for treatment. Hypothyroidism is not a reason to delay lithium, but treatment should start as lithium commences, with follow-up to adjust the dose of L-thyroxine. Endocrinology consultation (even if informal) is helpful for undiagnosed hyperthyroidism to determine which laboratory assessments are needed prior to lithium therapy.
Chemistry panel	Rule out undiagnosed electrolyte disturbances, document serum calcium, and check eGFR. As noted in Chapter 2, one may need to add cystatin C as a separate order until laboratories routinely include this as part of the renal function panel, and calculate $eGFR_{cr-cys}$. If cystatin C is not available, the $eGFR_{cr}$ is based on the serum creatinine (see Chapter 2, Info Box 2.3).	Appropriate work-up depending on the electrolyte abnormality found (e.g. hyponatremia, hypercalcemia, hyperkalemia). Baseline eGFR is necessary to determine the monitoring frequency (see Info Box 4.3).
Pregnancy test	For women of reproductive age.	Rule out undetected pregnancy.
Urine ACR (if indicated)	Indication: early morning urine specimen for ACR in those with a history of eGFR < 90 ml/min, or risk factors for renal dysfunction (e.g. cardiovascular disease, metabolic syndrome, diabetes mellitus, hypertension, smoking) to detect baseline glomerular disease in those at risk.	Stages A2 (30–300 mg/g) or A3 (> 300 mg/g) should be referred to nephrology for evaluation and consultation prior to starting lithium.
ECG (if indicated)	Indication: consider in patients > 40 years old, especially with cardiac risk factors, to rule out untreated conduction abnormalities or other cardiac disease. Not mandatory for patients ≤ 40 years old, but often required by certain institutional or regional protocols. Strongly consider if the patient has a history of arrhythmia, other cardiac disease, recurrent syncope or near syncopal episodes, family history of sudden death before the age of 45 or Brugada syndrome.	Cardiology consultation for abnormal findings, or when the patient has a history of arrhythmia, other cardiac disease, recurrent syncope or near syncopal episodes, or family history of sudden death or Brugada syndrome.

Measure	Rationale	Response to abnormal results
EMUO *	Not necessary at baseline, but EMUO encouraged among older patients (age > 50 years) due to age-related declines in urine osmolality.	Establishes a baseline urine osmolality to help track lithium related changes.
Complete blood count (CBC)*	Absolute neutrophil count (ANC) to define the patient's baseline, as lithium increases the ANC due to its effects on granulocyte colony stimulating factor (G-CSF) production.	Appropriate work-up depending on the abnormality found (e.g. differentiating low ANC due to medications such as divalproex, or due to benign neutropenia).
A1C *	Rule out untreated diabetes mellitus (DM) or prediabetes, both of which are significant CKD risk factors.	A1C values ≥ 6.5% are diagnostic of diabetes. In those with known DM, values > 7.0% represent less than ideal control and need to be addressed. Undiagnosed or undertreated DM should be addressed, but need not delay lithium treatment.
Lipid panel *	Rule out untreated dyslipidemia, a significant CKD risk factor.	Significant abnormalities must be addressed, but need not delay lithium treatment.

* Optional, but may be useful to serve as a baseline prior to treatment.

In-Depth 4.7 Starting Lithium With eGFR < 60 ml/min: New Data Indicating Stable Renal Function over 6–8 Years in 50% of These Patients [101]

Clinicians have great concern about starting lithium in patients with subnormal baseline renal function, and justifiably so [101]. Many papers discuss the sequelae of continuing or stopping lithium as eGFR drops below 60 ml/min [102, 103], but those decisions are also informed by the history of lithium response, the trajectory of eGFR decline, and whether suitable alternatives exist for that patient. Initiating lithium with low baseline eGFR raises a different set of concerns: will the patient derive much long-term benefit from lithium, and will starting lithium in a patient with CKD related comorbidities cause an accelerated progression to stage G3b–G5 CKD (eGFR 0–44 ml/min)? In lithium continuers, CKD risks (e.g. diabetes mellitus, hypertension) clearly contribute to patients experiencing more than age-related eGFR decreases over 4–30 years of treatment [104], but there were limited systematic data about CKD progression among new starts with comorbidities and subnormal eGFR until 2021, when Dr. Mihaela Golic (Department of Psychiatry and Neurochemistry, Institute of Neuroscience and Physiology, Sahlgrenska Academy, University of Gothenburg, Gothenburg, Sweden) led a group of investigators who scoured the laboratory database of Sahlgrenska University Hospital from 1981–2017 to find an appropriate sample for analysis. Employing a cohort study design, 83 patients with high serum creatinine prior to lithium were matched by gender, age when initiating lithium, and duration of lithium treatment to 83 individuals with a normal creatinine when starting lithium [101].

Prior to commencing lithium, the low eGFR and reference groups had mean age of 61.2 ± 15.1 years and 60.9 ± 14.8 years respectively, and mean eGFR of 48 ± 14 ml/min and 80 ± 16 ml/min respectively. After a duration of 7.9 years on lithium for both groups, the annual eGFR decline in the low eGFR group was 1.1 ml/min, a rate that was not significantly different than the 1.5 ml/min annual decline in the reference cohort; however, due to their lower starting eGFR, by the end of the observation period 48% of the low eGFR group progressed to stage G4–G5 CKD (eGFR < 30 ml/min), compared with only 10% of the reference group. A secondary analysis was performed within the low baseline eGFR cohort to examine differences between the 48% who progressed to stage G4–G5 CKD (progressors, n = 40) and the 52% (n = 43) of subjects who were nonprogressors. Prior to lithium exposure, the progressors were significantly older (67.4 ± 9.9 years vs. 55.5 ± 16.8 years), disproportionately female (72.5% vs. 51%) and had lower eGFR (42 ± 11 ml/min vs. 54 ± 15 ml/min) (p < 0.001 for each comparison) [101]. Progressors also had a greater burden of somatic illness (p < 0.012), and higher rates of diabetes mellitus (23% vs. 12%) and cardiovascular disorders (63% vs. 42%), although the difference for those specific causes did not reach statistical significance due to the small sample sizes involved. The only lithium related treatment factor that was significantly different between the two subgroups was the finding that 43% of progressors commenced treatment before 1981 (vs. 7% of nonprogressors, p < 0.001), and thus were exposed to lithium during a period prior to the implementation of modern lithium monitoring principles in Sweden [105].

The results of a 2021 Swedish study by Golic and colleagues showing that patients started with a mean eGFR of 54 ml/min might have limited eGFR declines over 7–8 years of treatment are instructive for clinicians wrestling with the decision to use lithium in cases where an indication for lithium treatment exists but the patient has low eGFR [101]. On the one hand, there are patients for whom the risk of stage G4–G5 CKD is extremely high. Given the morbidity and increased mortality associated with this level of renal dysfunction, the benefits of lithium may not outweigh the risks in those patients. However, the Golic study indicates that perhaps 50% of those with pretreatment eGFR under 60 ml/min may be able to persist on lithium for 6–8 years with limited eGFR declines. Unfortunately, while the need for a baseline measure of renal function is accepted practice, no eGFR threshold for starting lithium is mentioned in Malhi's 2017 review of 13 treatment guidelines [95]. Moreover, no minimum eGFR for starting lithium was noted in a 2018 survey of international monitoring recommendations from 24 countries [106]. As there is no consensus recommendation, the risk–benefit considerations outlined in Info Box 4.2 focus on whether the patient's history presents a *compelling indication* for lithium. A 2022 review of median age of onset for mental disorders estimates that 25% of bipolar spectrum individuals will be diagnosed after the age of 52, so the prospect of trying lithium in a newly diagnosed older BD patient with CKD risks and subnormal renal function is not a subject of idle speculation. There will also be patients with this level of CKD risk who have failed other treatments and have thus demonstrated the compelling need for lithium. For a newly diagnosed patient with BD-1 or SAD-BT, low eGFR and multiple CKD risks, initially trying other non-lithium therapies might be feasible; however, for a patient with that same renal risk profile who has failed other options, the compelling indication for lithium alters the risk–benefit assessment in favor of a lithium trial.

Prior to commencing lithium in these higher-risk patients, discussions with other stakeholders (e.g. primary care or other medical specialists, family, carers) should occur to ensure all are in agreement that this patient's psychiatric condition warrants this step, and to define a risk management strategy. The cornerstone of risk management is frequent and diligent eGFR monitoring, something that would be true for any lithium treated patient whose eGFR slips into the range of stage G3a CKD, 45–60 ml/min. As discussed in Info Box 4.4, it is suggested that higher-risk patients have eGFR checked every 6 weeks for the first 6 months after starting lithium, with subsequent monitoring frequency based on the eGFR. (See Info Box 4.4 for routine monitoring of higher-risk patients.) However, if the patient, the patient's other medical professionals, family or carers want the eGFR to be checked every 4 weeks for a few months, this is an eminently feasible request to facilitate a lithium trial for a patient who may have limited options.

 D | **Starting Lithium – Methods and Concerns**

WHAT TO KNOW: STARTING LITHIUM

- Clinicians should be familiar with the Cooper test dose method for estimating dosing requirements, and the Los Angeles County (LAC) – USC loading protocol.
- The goal of using evidence based initiation strategies in acute situations is to obviate prolonged titrations in manic inpatients. For less acute outpatients, slower titrations are reasonable.

4

Info Box 4.2 **What Is an Acceptable Starting eGFR?**

a. **There is a lack of guidance in systematic guidelines:** While the need for a baseline measure of renal function is accepted practice, no eGFR threshold is mentioned in Malhi's 2017 review of guidelines from 13 societies and national organizations worldwide [95]. Neither is a minimum eGFR for starting lithium noted in a survey of international monitoring recommendations from 24 countries [106]. Attempts have been made to generate algorithms which address this issue, but the last attempt was over 10 years ago, and contains certain assumptions about clinical course and treatment options that may no longer apply, especially for bipolar depression [107].

b. For any patient with an evidence based indication for lithium:
minimum eGFR ≥ 60 ml/min

Rationale

i. The Golic 2021 retrospective study illustrated that there are patients with mean age 55 who can start lithium with an eGFR of 54 ml/min and not exhibit significant annual eGFR declines over 6–8 years of treatment [101].

ii. The value of 60 ml/min represents the lower bound of stage G2 CKD, and is an easily remembered cutpoint often referred to as the limit of "normal" in many papers and laboratory reports.

c. For any patient with a *compelling indication* for lithium:
minimum eGFR ≥ 45 ml/min

Rationale

i. For patients who have failed prior lithium therapies, especially where some of lithium's putative advantages are relevant (e.g. reduction in suicide related mortality, 50% lower dementia risk in older BD patients), the risk–benefit assessment skews toward accepting more baseline risk since non-lithium therapies have not been sufficiently effective. Embedded in the acceptance of a lower baseline eGFR for these patients is the concern about depriving of lithium patients who lack therapeutic options [108].

ii. Every patient newly started on lithium receives more frequent monitoring during the first 6 months of treatment regardless of eGFR (see Info Box 4.4). To manage the renal risks in those starting with an eGFR in the range of stage G3a CKD (45–59 ml/min), especially in the presence of CKD risks due to advanced age and medical comorbidity, the eGFR will be monitored every 6 weeks during the first 6 months, with future monitoring dictated by the eGFR. The goal is to identity quickly those who are rapidly progressing to stage G3b CKD after starting lithium (eGFR 30–44 ml/min).

How quickly one initiates lithium depends largely on the clinical context. For modestly symptomatic BD outpatients with hypomania, or outpatients with unipolar MDD, gradually starting lithium is very appropriate, especially if the patient is apprehensive about adverse effects (see Info Box 4.3). The loading and test dose methods discussed in Chapter 3 are best reserved for situations where clinical urgency necessitates mood stabilizing a manic BD-1 or SAD-BT patient as soon as they are willing to take oral medication. Numerous antipsychotics have indications for mania and are available in acute injectable forms that can be used to manage the more florid neurovegetative symptoms of mania. However, antipsychotics do not have the same pharmacology as first-line mood stabilizers (e.g. lithium or VPA) on 2nd messenger intracellular pathways (see Chapter 1) [109, 110]. Antipsychotics improve the psychomotor symptoms of mania, but other untreated aspects of the mood disorder will continue to drive positive psychotic symptoms or ongoing acts of impulsivity [111]. This phenomenon was noted by the famous Danish psychiatrist and lithium researcher Mogens Schou, who described it eloquently in the 6th edition of his guide to lithium treatment: "An experienced patient, who during previous manias had first tried a neuroleptic and then lithium, reported that during treatment with the former he felt as if the gas pedal and the brake were pressed down at the same time. With lithium it was as if the ignition had been switched off" [112]. With that in mind, Info Box 4.3 summarizes methods of lithium initiation based on the clinical scenario, and the advantages or disadvantages of various strategies. As always, clinical flexibility in the approach is needed to balance out the necessities of clinical urgency and a patient's preferences, beliefs and concerns.

 Info Box 4.3 Methods and Considerations When Initiating Lithium for Patients Who Are Lithium Candidates

a. Gradual titration

i. Advantages: unlikely to incur tolerability issues, unlikely to have supratherapeutic levels.

ii. Disadvantages: prolongs the time to therapeutic serum levels.

iii. Optimal situation: initiation in outpatients with modest symptoms where a delay in reaching therapeutic levels is not critical, and when establishing rapport by minimizing adverse effects is important.

b. Test dose method to estimate maintenance lithium dose

i. Advantages: reduces the time to therapeutic serum levels.

ii. Disadvantages: the need to get a level at exactly 24 h post-dose and concerns about supratherapeutic levels when patients have low baseline eGFR, although the prediction model accounts for renal function.

iii. Optimal situation: initiation in manic inpatients where a delay in reaching therapeutic levels will prolong morbidity and length of hospitalization and where a lithium level can be obtained at exactly 24 h after the 600 mg test dose is administered.

The Cooper test dose method: Use the lithium level obtained 24 h after a single 600 mg test dose to predict the daily dose needed for a maintenance 12 h serum level in the range of 0.60–1.20 mEq/l [113].

24 h serum lithium level after single 600 mg loading dose (mEq/l)	Daily dosage required (original Cooper recommendation)	Daily dosage required[1] (QHS dosing and rounded to nearest 150 mg increment)
< 0.05	1200 mg TID	(See note below)[2]
0.05–0.09	900 mg TID	2250 mg
0.10–0.14	600 mg TID	1500 mg
0.15–0.19	300 mg QID	900 mg
0.20–0.23	300 mg TID	750 mg
0.24–0.30	300 mg BID	450 mg
> 0.30	300 mg BID[3]	Avoid lithium[3]

BID = twice per day; TID = thrice per day; QID = 4 times per day

1. Kinetic studies indicate that multiple daily dosing distorts the morning trough level as most of the dose is ingested » 12 h prior to the level being drawn (see Chapter 2, Table 2.3). When patients on BID dosing are administered the same daily total (mg) as a consolidated single QHS dose, the 12 h morning trough level will be at least 28% higher [114]. (TID dosing alters this only slightly more than BID dosing.) The calculated doses in this column are therefore lower than Cooper's original recommended doses.

2. Depending on the laboratory method used, these values may be below the limit of detection and should not be used for dose prediction. A value below the limit of detection may also represent nonadherence with the test dose method or extremely high eGFR and rapid lithium clearance. If the eGFR is > 90 ml/min, consider repeating the test dose; if this is not feasible and the patient is on no medications with significant kinetic interactions, consider a target initial dose of 1200 mg QHS with a follow-up level in 5 days.

3. Cooper advises extreme caution if the 24 h level is > 0.30 mEq/l. Using modern monitoring methods, this group would likely not be lithium candidates due to baseline eGFR « 45 ml/min.

c. Loading method – the LAC–USC protocol [115]

i. Advantages: reduces the time to therapeutic serum levels significantly.

ii. Disadvantages: theoretical concerns about tolerability or supratherapeutic levels.

iii. Optimal situation: initiation in manic inpatients where a delay in reaching therapeutic levels will prolong morbidity and length of hospitalization and where eGFR and morning lithium levels can be checked frequently.

The protocol: Total dose of 30 mg/kg is divided into three roughly equal doses of extended release lithium (to minimize GI side effects) given at 4 pm, 6 pm and 8 pm. The 12 h level is obtained the next morning and QHS dosing commences that night based on the level that morning [115]. (For more extensive discussion of this method, see Chapter 3, Info Box 3.4).

Considerations: Should be avoided in patients with eGFR < 60 ml/min as the dosing is weight based, not eGFR based. For extremely obese patients (BMI > 35 kg/m^2) or those with eGFR 60–74 ml/min, consider use of a 20 mg/kg loading dose (e.g. 10 mg/kg given at 4 pm and at 8 pm).

E   Monitoring

WHAT TO KNOW: LITHIUM MONITORING

- The frequency of lithium level and eGFR monitoring, and the need to obtain ACR and EMUO, depend on: whether this is a new start; current renal function; patient complaints of polyuria; and the presence of medical comorbidities associated with CKD risk.

- During routine treatment, serum calcium, TSH and blood pressure are obtained every 6 months. The frequency may change if abnormalities are detected or treatment initiated.

Every treatment guideline contains some form of monitoring protocol, including periodic lithium levels, certain vital signs (typically weight or BMI), renal parameters, TSH and serum calcium, with variations including electrolytes, waist circumference, parathyroid hormone (PTH) and even ECG [95]. The scheme suggested in Info Box 4.4 is informed by our current understanding that the earliest signal of renal dysfunction is a urine concentration deficit, as noted by complaints of thirst, polyuria or decreasing EMUO. The need for other office based and laboratory measures is an extension of the rationale for baseline monitoring discussed in Table 4.3. Local practice protocols may dictate certain measures be obtained for all patients (e.g. annual ECG), but in stable patients with eGFR ≥ 60 ml/min, every 6 month monitoring strikes the balance between the burdens of excessive laboratory testing and the needs to assure patient safety and track lithium adherence. A 2021 analysis of 46,555 lithium levels obtained in three UK centers from 3371 patients over 7 years found that, for levels within the range of 0.40–0.99 mEq/l, 90% of the results 3 months later remained in this range, as did 85% of the results drawn 6 months later [116]. Neither age nor duration of lithium therapy had any significant effect on lithium level stability; however, levels in the high therapeutic range (0.80–0.99 mEq/l) had a 10% risk of subsequent levels being ≥ 1.00 mEq/l, compared with only 2% for those with levels in the 0.40–0.79 mEq/l range [116]. The authors conclude that, for outpatients with maintenance levels < 0.80 mEq/l, checking levels every 6 months decreases the burden of frequent phlebotomy, but one might consider obtaining levels every 3 months in those who reside in the high end of the therapeutic range (0.80–0.99 mEq/l) to forestall supratherapeutic levels that incur greater renal insufficiency risk [62, 116, 117].

Info Box 4.4 Routine Monitoring

a. **Vital signs:** Weight at every visit with BMI calculated, blood pressure every 6 months.

b. **ECG**: A follow-up should be obtained once lithium is at steady state after initial titration (e.g. week 12) only in those who required an ECG upon lithium initiation (certain patients > 40 years old, younger patients with cardiac risk factors, or if required by institutional protocol). In those patients, an annual ECG may be required by local protocol or the presence of pre-existing abnormalities. An annual ECG is not recommended by most treatment guidelines for other patients [95].

c. **Serum calcium and TSH:** Every 6 months. As discussed in Chapter 5, an increase in the frequency or the need to add additional laboratory measures (e.g. ionized calcium, parathyroid hormone, T3, T4, free T4 index) will be dictated by the presence of abnormalities.

d. **Lithium level:**

   i. **New lithium starts:** A 12 h trough should be obtained approximately 1 week after any dosage change or introduction or removal of a medication having kinetic interactions with lithium. Through week 24 (6 months), the level should be obtained with the eGFR.

   ii. **Established therapy:** The 12 h trough level should be obtained with the eGFR, and the frequency dictated by the eGFR. For patients with low eGFR values, this may necessitate levels every 6 weeks. For those whose maintenance levels are in the range of 0.80–1.00 mEq/l, consider increasing the frequency of levels to every 3 months to minimize the occurrence of supratherapeutic levels that might incur risk for renal toxicity [62, 116, 117].

e. Renal:

i. Monitoring for the first 6 months of lithium treatment

	6 weeks	3 months	18 weeks	6 months
eGFR (baseline eGFR ≥ 60 ml/min)	X	X		X
eGFR (baseline eGFR 45–59 ml/min)	X	X	X	X
24 h FIR	X	X		X
EMUO	X	X		X
ACR		X		X

Notes

- eGFR: After 6 months the monitoring frequency depends on CKD stage.
- 24 h FIR: Ask the patient to record fluid intake for two separate days and average the result.
- EMUO: Should also be added following a new complaint of polyuria/polydipsia.
- ACR: At 3 months and 6 months for those with baseline eGFR < 90 ml/min **or** risk factors for renal dysfunction. After 6 months, the monitoring frequency depends on the ACR stage.

ii. Routine 6-month monitoring during established lithium therapy

1. Review medical history for renal dysfunction risk factors and use of nephrotoxic medications.

2. eGFR.

3. 24 h FIR: Ask the patient to record fluid intake for two separate days and average the result.

4. EMUO: For those with polyuria complaints, on stable amiloride treatment, or for patients whose most recent EMUO value is ≤ 850 mOsm/kg as verified by a repeat specimen.

5. ACR: For those with eGFR < 90 ml/min **or** risk factors for renal dysfunction as noted in e, subsection i, above.

iii. Increase frequency of labs to every 3 months during established lithium therapy when one of the following is present: (higher-risk patients)

1. eGFR value: When values are < 60 ml/min.

2. eGFR trends: Initial evidence of a decline in eGFR > 2 ml/min over 6 months or > 4 ml/min over 12 months as verified by a repeat specimen.

3. EMUO: For increased or new complaints of polyuria, when titrating amiloride (or adjunctive acetazolamide) to manage polyuria, or for urine osmolality values < 300 mOsm/kg.

4. ACR: If ACR has progressed from stage A1 to A2 as verified by a repeat specimen.

iv. When to consult a nephrologist

1. eGFR: Second decline in eGFR > 2 ml/min over 6 months or > 4 ml/min over 12 months as verified by a repeat specimen.

2. eGFR < 45 ml/min as verified by a repeat specimen.

3. ACR: Stage A3.

4. Nephrogenic diabetes insipidus (EMUO values < 300 mOsm/kg) unresponsive to maximal doses of amiloride (10 mg BID) plus adjunctive use of acetazolamide (up to 500 mg BID) for 6 weeks.

5. Hematuria.

 F | **Assessing Adherence**

WHAT TO KNOW: ASSESSING ADHERENCE

- One purpose of routine periodic lithium levels is to assess adherence. Adherence changes over time, so past patterns of excellent adherence are no guarantee of future adherence.

- For the sake of consistency and interpretability, levels should be obtained as 12 h troughs.

- Based on studies of serum level variation during extended treatment, a deviation of 30% or more in the 12 h trough serum lithium level from the mean baseline level is a useful indicator of nonadherence.

One of the primary reasons to obtain periodic lithium levels is to monitor medication adherence. As with any chronic disorder, oral medication nonadherence is very common with BD and SAD-BT. The various reasons for patient nonadherence were discussed earlier in this chapter, but an important concept about oral medication adherence derived from the schizophrenia literature is worth remembering: **adherence is dynamic, it is not static** [118]. Patients may take lithium religiously for months or years, but adverse effects, mood states (depression or mania/hypomania) or other circumstances may cause them to stop therapy without notifying their clinician. There are a variety of adherence definitions, but for medications taken once daily an accepted threshold is taking the full daily dose 70% or 80% of the time [119–121]. Among schizophrenia outpatients, adherence rates with oral antipsychotics using the 70% threshold range from 50% to 78.3% [122]. A consensus paper on medication adherence found that the majority of experts believe the average patient with schizophrenia or BD in their practice takes only 51–70% of their prescribed medication [119]. Importantly, nonadherence and discontinuation occur very quickly among new starts, highlighting the need for vigilance when patients start treatment. It is worth recalling that the 2007 Danish study of new lithium prescriptions for adults from 1995 to 2000 (n = 14,277) found the median time to discontinuation was 181.0 days (95% CI 135.7–181.0), and that 25% stopped lithium within 45.2 days [75].

For BD-1 and SAD-BT patients, nonadherence may not be identified until the patient is hospitalized for a mood episode, usually mania, so measures to monitor adherence must be employed to forestall decompensation. Pill count remains one of the most evidence based methods [119, 123]. While decidedly low tech, it is inexpensive, easily replicated, and can be performed when a patient is seen via telemedicine interface. As patients may forget to bring medications for an office visit, the telemedicine session offers an opportunity to have the patient retrieve their lithium prescription, count the pills together with the clinician and discuss issues with nonadherence that might prompt a referral for CAE or other interventions to promote adherence [83]. Serum levels offer another objective adherence measure based on the idea that over short periods of time (e.g. 12 months) there are limited changes in eGFR, so 12 h trough levels should also exhibit limited variation. A small 1984 study in 13 inpatients who had sequential 12 h trough levels obtained as part of a kinetic study found that the intraindividual coefficient of variation (CV) was only 9% [124]. One expects a greater degree of variability among outpatients followed for longer periods of time. For schizophrenia outpatients, a CV of 30% is acceptable among antipsychotic adherent individuals, meaning that trough antipsychotic levels which deviate by 30% or more from the established mean baseline are likely to be the product of medication nonadherence [4]. This conclusion for lithium is bolstered by data from a 12 month adherence study published in 2021 which noted that the subgroup on an extended release lithium preparation (n = 30) had very high rates of adherence – ≥ 85% at months 3, 6 and 12 – and thus could be used to examine serum level variability [125]. The CV for this subgroup at these three time points averaged 29%, suggesting that 12 h trough serum level deviations of 30% or more from the mean baseline value is a useful metric of lithium nonadherence. As always, one must note the time at which the sample was drawn, and also rule out dosing errors or new kinetic factors before concluding that a change in serum lithium level ≥ 30% from the baseline mean level represents nonadherence [4].

G **Target Level Ranges for Acute Mania, Bipolar Maintenance or Bipolar Depression, Unipolar Major Depression Adjunctive Use**

WHAT TO KNOW: TARGET SERUM LITHIUM LEVELS

- Acute mania: 1.00–1.20 mEq/l. Levels > 1.20 mEq/l are associated with increased risk of renal insufficiency.
- BD-1 maintenance: 0.60–0.80 mEq/l, with consideration of levels up to 1.00 mEq/l or as low as 0.40 mEq/l in select patients.
- BD-2 disorder or unipolar MDD adjunctive use: 0.40–0.60 mEq/l.

After 70 years, the psychiatric community has generally come to a consensus about target lithium levels for acute mania and mania prophylaxis and when used adjunctively to antidepressants in unipolar MDD patients [29, 30, 61]. In particular, the optimal range for BD-1 and SAD-BT maintenance is 0.60–0.80 mEq/l, with a higher level (0.80–1.00 mEq/l) reserved for those in whom symptom breakthrough dictates that this range must be used to maintain stability. Imaging studies find that the mean brain-to-serum (BTS) ratio averages 0.50, meaning that brain levels are 50% lower than serum levels [126]. However, this research also found marked interindividual differences in central nervous system lithium penetration, and older age in particular was associated with higher BTS ratios in some but not all studies [127–129]. As certain individuals may therefore experience comparatively higher brain lithium exposure for any peripheral level, it makes sense that a lower maintenance range of 0.40–0.60 mEq/l be considered for reasons of tolerability or historical stability with that level [61, 130]. Conceptually, SAD-BT patients are treated in the same manner as BD-1 since both groups share the history of mania; however, there is a paucity of data for BD-2 individuals, so the comments in Table 4.4 are not evidence based, but a recommendation that incorporates the idea that the demands for mood stabilization in BD-2 patients might initially permit use of the lower end of the BD maintenance range (0.40–0.60 mEq/l) [130]. For all lithium related uses, clinical course will determine the optimal place within the therapeutic range for a specific patient, acknowledging that risks for renal dysfunction increase when trough levels exceed 1.00 mEq/l, and especially if the level ever exceeds 1.20 mEq/l [61, 62].

The most difficult question to answer is not the recommended lithium level for a specific mood disorder, but the target level when a clinician wants to use lithium for its anti-suicide, anti-aggression or neuroprotective effects in a patient who does not have a bipolar spectrum disorder or unipolar MDD. While animal models and studies correlating suicide, homicide and dementia rates with lithium levels in the municipal water supply suggest that low levels of exposure might be sufficient for these effects, there are limited data to suggest a target level specifically for anti-aggression or anti-suicide purposes in a patient who does not require lithium's mood properties. In some instances the level of exposure might be sufficiently modest that the trough value will be below the laboratory limit of detection [131–138]. As discussed in Chapter 1, a small double-blind, placebo-controlled study of lithium's neurocognitive effects in 61 older adults with mild cognitive impairment (but not BD) found positive results over 2 years using a target serum lithium level range of 0.25–0.50 mEq/l [139]; however, whether this is the ideal range to realize lithium's neuroprotective effects will require replication.

Table 4.4 Target serum level ranges and rationale

Indication	Level range*	Rationale
Acute mania	1.00–1.20 mEq/l	Single levels > 1.20 mEq/l are associated with increased risk of renal insufficiency (odds ratio 1.74, 95% CI 1.33–2.25) [62]. Patients with inadequate mania control with a level of 1.20 mEq/l despite concurrent use of an antipsychotic will often need divalproex added to obtain optimal mood control.
BD-1 or SAD-BT maintenance	0.60–0.80 mEq/l (response, history and tolerability concerns may dictate a lower range of 0.40–0.60 mEq/l, or a higher range of 0.80–1.00 mEq/l).	Compelling evidence that many individuals remain stable in this range and with improved short-term and long-term tolerability compared with higher levels [61]. Clinical course will drive decisions to use the lower or higher ranges, but maintenance levels should not exceed 1.00 mEq/l, primarily to avert long-term renal adverse effects [62]. Individuals over age 50 often have higher brain-to-serum lithium levels than younger patients, and thus may respond to and better tolerate lithium when peripheral levels are in the lower range [128].
BD-2	Same as BD-1, but consider the lower end of the range	Limited data in this patient population, but the decreased severity of hypomania/mixed episodes compared with BD-1 may permit use of the lower end of the serum level range for those BD-2 patients who need mood stabilization.
Unipolar MDD adjunctive use	0.40–0.60 mEq/l	It's the level range best studied, and is included in many consensus recommendations. Levels < 0.4 mEq/l appear less effective [29].

* Based on 12 h levels with medication taken at bedtime as a single daily dose.

Comment: As noted in Chapter 3, Table 3.2, despite the long-term renal impact of multiple daily dosing [62], some patients may be wedded to twice daily (BID) dosing for a variety of reasons (e.g. historical stability and reluctance to change, prior episodes of gastrointestinal adverse effects on single QHS doses). The morning trough level would be 28% higher were the total BID dose converted to a QHS schedule, so the morning trough maintenance level on BID dosing for most patients should be no higher than 0.62 mEq/l, equivalent to 0.80 mEq/l from single QHS dosing. The maximum maintenance level on BID dosing is therefore 0.78 mEq/l, which would equate to 1.00 mEq/l if the entire dose were given QHS only. For acute mania, the BID maximal level is 0.94 mEq/l (comparable to 1.20 mEq/l for QHS dosing).

Summary Points

a. Engaging in an open dialog with a patient about their illness, the perceived need for any pharmacotherapy, and their thoughts about lithium is key to identifying issues that might induce nonadherence. CAE therapy should be considered in all patients who struggle with lithium adherence.

b. In modern usage, there is no need to search for an "ideal lithium monotherapy candidate" to commence treatment as many bipolar spectrum patients require additional medications for mania prophylaxis or for treatment of bipolar depression. Any patient with an evidence based indication and an eGFR ≥ 60 ml/min is a lithium candidate. For those patients with a *compelling indication for lithium* (e.g. prior failure of non-lithium therapies), a baseline eGFR in the range of 45–59 ml/min can be considered, albeit with vigilant eGFR monitoring.

c. The number of absolutely necessary items (laboratory measures, vital signs) to be obtained at baseline before commencing lithium is modest, although local protocols might require certain tests (e.g. ECG) despite the patient's age or lack of cardiac history.

d. There are evidence based methods to load or initiate lithium more rapidly for the management of inpatients with acute mania. Avoid extended titrations in acutely manic individuals that prolong patient morbidity and possibly disrupt the inpatient milieu or endanger others.

e. For bipolar spectrum patients, modern treatment guidelines suggest a maintenance lithium level in the range of 0.60–0.80 mEq/l, with select patients using a higher (0.80–1.00 mEq/l) or lower (0.40–0.60 mEq/l) range, depending on response and tolerability.

f. Routine laboratory monitoring is not very complicated for most patients: lithium level, eGFR, serum calcium and TSH every 6 months, with certain patients also needing an EMUO and/or urine ACR. The frequency of renal monitoring depends on changes in eGFR, or whether the eGFR falls below certain thresholds. The use of EMUO and the 24 h FIR is important to detect urine concentration problems at the earliest stage and forestall patient demands to discontinue lithium.

References

1. Öhlund, L., Ott, M., Oja, S., et al. (2018). Reasons for lithium discontinuation in men and women with bipolar disorder: A retrospective cohort study. *BMC Psychiatry*, 18, 37–46.

2. Jawad, I., Watson, S., Haddad, P. M., et al. (2018). Medication nonadherence in bipolar disorder: A narrative review. *Ther Adv Psychopharmacol*, 8, 349–363.

3. Abegaz, T. M., Shehab, A., Gebreyohannes, E. A., et al. (2017). Nonadherence to antihypertensive drugs: A systematic review and meta-analysis. *Medicine (Baltimore)*, 96, e5641.

4. Meyer, J. M. and Stahl, S. M. (2021). *The Clinical Use of Antipsychotic Plasma Levels* (Stahl's Handbooks). New York: Cambridge University Press.

5. Van Putten, T. (1975). Why do patients with manic-depressive illness stop their lithium? *Compr Psychiatry*, 16, 179–183.

6. Jamison, K. R., Gerner, R. H. and Goodwin, F. K. (1979). Patient and physician attitudes toward lithium: Relationship to compliance. *Arch Gen Psychiatry*, 36, 866–869.

7. Vestergaard, P. and Amdisen, A. (1983). Patient attitudes towards lithium. *Acta Psychiatr Scand*, 67, 8–12.

8. Pope, M. and Scott, J. (2003). Do clinicians understand why individuals stop taking lithium? *J Affect Disord*, 74, 287–291.

9. Schou, M. (1999). The early European lithium studies. *Aust N Z J Psychiatry*, 33 Suppl., S39–47.

10. Cole, N. and Parker, G. (2012). Cade's identification of lithium for manic-depressive illness—the prospector who found a gold nugget. *J Nerv Ment Dis*, 200, 1101–1104.

11. Rybakowski, J. K. (2018). Challenging the negative perception of lithium and optimizing its long-term administration. *Front Mol Neurosci*, 11, 1–8.

12. Kerner, B., Crisanti, A. S., DeShaw, J. L., et al. (2019). Preferences of information dissemination on treatment for bipolar disorder: Patient-centered focus group study. *JMIR Ment Health*, 6, e12848.

13. Scott, J. and Tacchi, M. J. (2002). A pilot study of concordance therapy for individuals with bipolar disorders who are non-adherent with lithium prophylaxis. *Bipolar Disord*, 4, 386–392.

14. Sugawara, N., Adachi, N., Kubota, Y., et al. (2022). Determinants of three-year clinical outcomes in real-world outpatients with bipolar disorder: The multicenter treatment survey for bipolar disorder in psychiatric outpatient clinics (MUSUBI). *J Psychiatr Res*, 151, 683–692.

15. Kessing, L. V., Vradi, E. and Andersen, P. K. (2014). Starting lithium prophylaxis early v. late in bipolar disorder. *Br J Psychiatry*, 205, 214–220.

16. Yoshimura, B., Yada, Y., So, R., et al. (2017). The critical treatment window of clozapine in treatment-resistant schizophrenia: Secondary analysis of an observational study. *Psychiatry Res*, 250, 65–70.

17. Griffiths, K., Millgate, E., Egerton, A., et al. (2021). Demographic and clinical variables associated with response to clozapine in schizophrenia: A systematic review and meta-analysis. *Psychol Med*, 51, 376–386.

18. Franchini, L., Zanardi, R., Smeraldi, E., et al. (1999). Early onset of lithium prophylaxis as a predictor of good long-term outcome. *Eur Arch Psychiatry Clin Neurosci*, 249, 227–230.

19. Baldessarini, R. J., Tondo, L. and Hennen, J. (2003). Treatment-latency and previous episodes: Relationships to pretreatment morbidity and response to maintenance treatment in bipolar I and II disorders. *Bipolar Disord*, 5, 169–179.

20. Bratti, I. M., Baldessarini, R. J., Baethge, C., et al. (2003). Pretreatment episode count and response to lithium treatment in manic-depressive illness. *Harv Rev Psychiatry*, 11, 245–256.

21. Baldessarini, R. J., Tondo, L., Baethge, C. J., et al. (2007). Effects of treatment latency on response to maintenance treatment in manic-depressive disorders. *Bipolar Disord*, 9, 386–393.

22. Burkhardt, E., Pfennig, A. and Leopold, K. (2021). Clinical risk constellations for the development of bipolar disorders. *Medicina (Kaunas)*, 57, 792–799.

23. Martini, J., Leopold, K., Pfeiffer, S., et al. (2021). Early detection of bipolar disorders and treatment recommendations for help-seeking adolescents and young adults: Findings of the Early Detection and Intervention Center Dresden. *Int J Bipolar Disord*, 9, 23.

24. Lim, M., Li, Z., Xie, H., et al. (2021). The effect of therapeutic alliance on attitudes toward psychiatric medications in schizophrenia. *J Clin Psychopharmacol*, 41, 551–560.

25. Nestsiarovich, A., Gaudiot, C. E. S., Baldessarini, R. J., et al. (2022). Preventing new episodes of bipolar disorder in adults: Systematic review and meta-analysis of randomized controlled trials. *Eur Neuropsychopharmacol*, 54, 75–89.

26. Öhlund, L., Ott, M., Bergqvist, M., et al. (2019). Clinical course and need for hospital admission after lithium discontinuation in patients with bipolar disorder type I or II: Mirror-image study based on the LiSIE retrospective cohort. *BJPsych Open*, 5, e101–112.

27. Lintunen, J., Taipale, H., Tanskanen, A., et al. (2021). Long-term real-world effectiveness of pharmacotherapies for schizoaffective disorder. *Schizophr Bull*, 47, 1099–1107.

28. Wingård, L., Brandt, L., Bodén, R., et al. (2019). Monotherapy vs. combination therapy for post mania maintenance treatment: A population based cohort study. *Eur Neuropsychopharmacol*, 29, 691–700.

29. Abou-Saleh, M. T., Muller-Oerlinghausen, B. and Coppen, A. J. (2017). Lithium in the episode and suicide prophylaxis and in augmenting strategies in patients with unipolar depression. *Int J Bipolar Disord*, 5, 11.

30. Undurraga, J., Sim, K., Tondo, L., et al. (2019). Lithium treatment for unipolar major depressive disorder: Systematic review. *J Psychopharmacol*, 33, 167–176.

31. Scott, F., Hampsey, E., Gnanapragasam, S., et al. (2023). Systematic review and meta-analysis of augmentation and combination treatments for early-stage treatment-resistant depression. *J Psychopharmacol*, 37, 268–278.

32. Sforzini, L., Worrell, C., Kose, M., et al. (2022). A Delphi-method-based consensus guideline for definition of treatment-resistant depression for clinical trials. *Mol Psychiatry*, 27, 1286–1299.

33. Malhi, G. S., Bell, E., Bassett, D., et al. (2021). The 2020 Royal Australian and New Zealand College of Psychiatrists clinical practice guidelines for mood disorders. *Aust N Z J Psychiatry*, 55, 7–117.

34. Henssler, J., Alexander, D., Schwarzer, G., et al. (2022). Combining antidepressants vs antidepressant monotherapy for treatment of patients with acute depression: A systematic review and meta-analysis. *JAMA Psychiatry*, 79, 300–312.

35. Vázquez, G. H., Bahji, A., Undurraga, J., et al. (2021). Efficacy and tolerability of combination treatments for major depression: Antidepressants plus second-generation antipsychotics vs. esketamine vs. lithium. *J Psychopharmacol*, 35, 890–900.

36. Heitzmann, E., Javelot, H., Weiner, L., et al. (2016). A case of aripiprazole-induced tardive dyskinesia with dramatic evolution. *Case Rep Psychiatry*, 2016, 7031245.

37. Gomaa, H., Mahgoub, Y. and Francis, A. (2021). Covert dyskinesia with aripiprazole: Tip of the iceberg? A case report and literature review. *J Clin Psychopharmacol*, 41, 67–70.

38. Preskorn, S., Flynn, A. and Macaluso, M. (2015). Determining whether a definitive causal relationship exists between aripiprazole and tardive dyskinesia and/or dystonia in patients with major depressive disorder: Part 1. *J Psychiatr Pract*, 21, 359–369.

39. Macaluso, M., Flynn, A. and Preskorn, S. (2016). Determining whether a definitive causal relationship exists between aripiprazole and tardive dyskinesia and/or dystonia in patients with major depressive disorder, part 2: Preclinical and early phase human proof of concept studies. *J Psychiatr Pract*, 22, 42–49.

40. Preskorn, S. H. and Macaluso, M. (2016). Determining whether a definitive causal relationship exists between aripiprazole and tardive dyskinesia and/or dystonia in patients with major depressive disorder, part 3: Clinical trial data. *J Psychiatr Pract*, 22, 117–123.

41. Macaluso, M., Flynn, A. and Preskorn, S. (2016). Determining whether a definitive causal relationship exists between aripiprazole and tardive dyskinesia and/or dystonia in patients with major depressive disorder, part 4: Case report data. *J Psychiatr Pract*, 22, 203–220.

42. Schneider, L. S., Dagerman, K. S. and Insel, P. (2005). Risk of death with atypical antipsychotic drug treatment for dementia: Meta-analysis of randomized placebo-controlled trials. *JAMA*, 294, 1934–1943.

43. Maust, D. T., Kim, H. M., Seyfried, L. S., et al. (2015). Antipsychotics, other psychotropics, and the risk of death in patients with dementia: Number needed to harm. *JAMA Psychiatry*, 72, 438–445.

44. Gerhard, T., Stroup, T. S., Correll, C. U., et al. (2020). Mortality risk of antipsychotic augmentation for adult depression. *PLoS One*, 15, e0239206.

45. Thomas, L., Li, F. and Pencina, M. (2020). Using propensity score methods to create target populations in observational clinical research. *JAMA*, 323, 466–467.

46. Davies, P., Ijaz, S., Williams, C. J., et al. (2019). Pharmacological interventions for treatment-resistant depression in adults. *Cochrane Database Syst Rev*, 12, Cd010557.

47. Lorentzen, R., Kjær, J. N., Østergaard, S. D., et al. (2020). Thyroid hormone treatment in the management of treatment-resistant unipolar depression: A systematic review and meta-analysis. *Acta Psychiatr Scand*, 141, 316–326.

48. Kessing, L. V., Gerds, T. A., Feldt-Rasmussen, B., et al. (2015). Use of lithium and anticonvulsants and the rate of chronic kidney disease: A nationwide population-based study. *JAMA Psychiatry*, 72, 1182–1191.

49. Sinha, A., Shariq, A., Said, K., et al. (2018). Medical comorbidities in bipolar disorder. *Curr Psychiatry Rep*, 20, 36.

50. Scott, J., Etain, B. and Bellivier, F. (2018). Can an integrated science approach to precision medicine research improve lithium treatment in bipolar disorders? *Front Psychiatry*, 9, 360.

51. Grillault Laroche, D., Etain, B., Severus, E., et al. (2020). Socio-demographic and clinical predictors of outcome to long-term treatment with lithium in bipolar disorders: A systematic review of the contemporary literature and recommendations from the ISBD/IGSLI Task Force on treatment with lithium. *Int J Bipolar Disord*, 8, 1–13.

52. Nunes, A., Ardau, R., Berghofer, A., et al. (2020). Prediction of lithium response using clinical data. *Acta Psychiatr Scand*, 141, 131–141.

53. Hui, T. P., Kandola, A., Shen, L., et al. (2019). A systematic review and meta-analysis of clinical predictors of lithium response in bipolar disorder. *Acta Psychiatr Scand*, 140, 94–115.

54. Baldessarini, R. J., Tondo, L., Floris, G., et al. (2000). Effects of rapid cycling on response to lithium maintenance treatment in 360 bipolar I and II disorder patients. *J Affect Disord*, 61, 13–22.

55. Strawbridge, R., Kurana, S., Kerr-Gaffney, J., et al. (2022). A systematic review and meta-analysis of treatments for rapid cycling bipolar disorder. *Acta Psychiatr Scand*, 146, 290–311.

56. Fountoulakis, K. N., Tohen, M. and Zarate, C. A. (2022). Lithium treatment of bipolar disorder in adults: A systematic review of randomized trials and meta-analyses. *Eur Neuropsychopharmacol*, 54, 100–115.

57. Lin, Y., Maihofer, A. X., Stapp, E., et al. (2021). Clinical predictors of non-response to lithium treatment in the Pharmacogenomics of Bipolar Disorder (PGBD) study. *Bipolar Disord*, 23, 821–831.

58. Sekula, N. M., Yocum, A. K., Anderau, S., et al. (2022). Lithium use associated with symptom severity in comorbid bipolar disorder I and migraine. *Brain Behav*, 12, e32585.

59. Jacobsen, K. K., Nievergelt, C. M., Zayats, T., et al. (2015). Genome wide association study identifies variants in NBEA associated with migraine in bipolar disorder. *J Affect Disord*, 172, 453–461.

60. Clos, S., Rauchhaus, P., Severn, A., et al. (2015). Long-term effect of lithium maintenance therapy on estimated glomerular filtration rate in patients with affective disorders: A population-based cohort study. *Lancet Psychiatry*, 2, 1075–1083.

61. Nolen, W. A., Licht, R. W., Young, A. H., et al. (2019). What is the optimal serum level for lithium in the maintenance treatment of bipolar disorder? A systematic review and recommendations from the ISBD/IGSLI Task Force on treatment with lithium. *Bipolar Disord*, 21, 394–409.

62. Castro, V. M., Roberson, A. M., McCoy, T. H., et al. (2016). Stratifying risk for renal insufficiency among lithium-treated patients: An electronic health record study. *Neuropsychopharmacol*, 41, 1138–1143.

63. Bisogni, V., Rossitto, G., Reghin, F., et al. (2016). Antihypertensive therapy in patients on chronic lithium treatment for bipolar disorders. *J Hypertens*, 34, 20–28.

64. Finley, P. R. (2016). Drug interactions with lithium: An update. *Clin Pharmacokinet*, 55, 925–941.

65. Oedegaard, K. J., Alda, M., Anand, A., et al. (2016). The Pharmacogenomics of Bipolar Disorder study (PGBD): Identification of genes for lithium response in a prospective sample. *BMC Psychiatry*, 16, 129.

66. Amare, A. T., Schubert, K. O., Hou, L., et al. (2018). Association of polygenic score for schizophrenia and HLA antigen and inflammation genes with response to lithium in bipolar affective disorder: A genome-wide association study. *JAMA Psychiatry*, 75, 65–74.

67. McCarthy, M. J., Wei, H., Nievergelt, C. M., et al. (2019). Chronotype and cellular circadian rhythms predict the clinical response to lithium maintenance treatment in patients with bipolar disorder. *Neuropsychopharmacol*, 44, 620–628.

68. Mishra, H. K., Ying, N. M., Luis, A., et al. (2021). Circadian rhythms in bipolar disorder patient-derived neurons predict lithium response: Preliminary studies. *Mol Psychiatry*, 26, 3383–3394.

69. Post, R. M., Leverich, G. S., Kupka, R., et al. (2016). Clinical correlates of sustained response to individual drugs used in naturalistic treatment of patients with bipolar disorder. *Compr Psychiatry*, 66, 146–156.

70. Calabrese, J. R., Shelton, M. D., Rapport, D. J., et al. (2005). A 20-month, double-blind, maintenance trial of lithium versus divalproex in rapid-cycling bipolar disorder. *Am J Psychiatry*, 162, 2152–2161.

71. Hou, L., Heilbronner, U., Degenhardt, F., et al. (2016). Genetic variants associated with response to lithium treatment in bipolar disorder: A genome-wide association study. *Lancet*, 387, 1085–1093.

72. McIntyre, R. S., Berk, M., Brietzke, E., et al. (2020). Bipolar disorders. *Lancet*, 396, 1841–1856.

73. Schumann, C., Lenz, G., Berghofer, A., et al. (1999). Non-adherence with long-term prophylaxis: A 6-year naturalistic follow-up study of affectively ill patients. *Psychiatry Res*, 89, 247–257.

74. Inoue, T., Sano, H., Kojima, Y., et al. (2021). Real-world treatment patterns and adherence to oral medication among patients with bipolar disorders: A retrospective, observational study using a healthcare claims database. *Neuropsychiatr Dis Treat*, 17, 821–833.

75. Kessing, L. V., Søndergård, L., Kvist, K., et al. (2007). Adherence to lithium in naturalistic settings: Results from a nationwide pharmacoepidemiological study. *Bipolar Disord*, 9, 730–736.

76. Harvey, N. S. (1991). The development and descriptive use of the Lithium Attitudes Questionnaire. *J Affect Disord*, 22, 211–219.

77. Singh, S., Kumar, S., Mahal, P., et al. (2019). Self-reported medication adherence and its correlates in a lithium-maintained cohort with bipolar disorder at a tertiary care centre in India. *Asian J Psychiatr*, 46, 34–40.

78. Rosa, A. R., Marco, M., Fachel, J. M., et al. (2007). Correlation between drug treatment adherence and lithium treatment attitudes and knowledge by bipolar patients. *Prog Neuropsychopharmacol Biol Psychiatry*, 31, 217–224.

79. Thompson, K., Kulkarni, J. and Sergejew, A. A. (2000). Reliability and validity of a new Medication Adherence Rating Scale (MARS) for the psychoses. *Schizophr Res*, 42, 241–247.

80. Even, C., Thuile, J., Kalck-Stern, M., et al. (2010). Psychoeducation for patients with bipolar disorder receiving lithium: Short and long term impact on locus of control and knowledge about lithium. *J Affect Disord*, 123, 299–302.

81. Colom, F. (2014). The evolution of psychoeducation for bipolar disorder: From lithium clinics to integrative psychoeducation. *World Psychiatry*, 13, 90–92.

82. Soo, S. A., Zhang, Z. W., Khong, S. J., et al. (2018). Randomized controlled trials of psychoeducation modalities in the management of bipolar disorder: A systematic review. *J Clin Psychiatry*, 79, 17r11750.

83. Sajatovic, M., Tatsuoka, C., Cassidy, K. A., et al. (2018). A 6-month, prospective, randomized controlled trial of Customized Adherence Enhancement versus bipolar-specific educational control in poorly adherent individuals with bipolar disorder. *J Clin Psychiatry*, 79, 17m12036.

84. Sajatovic, M., Levin, J. B., Ramirez, L. F., et al. (2021). Long-acting injectable antipsychotic medication plus customized adherence enhancement in poor adherence patients with bipolar disorder. *Prim Care Companion CNS Disord*, 23, 20m02888.

85. Canales, T., Rodman, S., Conklin, D., et al. (2022). Combining medication adherence support plus long-acting injectable antipsychotic medication: A post-hoc analysis of 3 pilot studies. *Psychopharmacol Bull*, 52, 41–57.

86. Baldessarini, R. J., Bolzani, L., Cruz, N., et al. (2010). Onset-age of bipolar disorders at six international sites. *J Affect Disord*, 121, 143–146.

87. Solmi, M., Radua, J., Olivola, M., et al. (2022). Age at onset of mental disorders worldwide: Large-scale meta-analysis of 192 epidemiological studies. *Mol Psychiatry*, 27, 281–295.

88. Smilowitz, S., Aftab, A., Aebi, M., et al. (2020). Age-related differences in medication adherence, symptoms, and stigma in poorly adherent adults with bipolar disorder. *J Geriatr Psychiatry Neurol*, 33, 250–255.

89. McVoy, M., Delbello, M., Levin, J., et al. (2022). A customized adherence enhancement program for adolescents and young adults with suboptimal adherence and bipolar disorder: Trial design and methodological report. *Contemp Clin Trials*, 115, 106729.

90. Sajatovic, M., Tatsuoka, C., Dines, P., et al. (2014). Patient choice as a driver of medication-switching in non-adherent individuals with bipolar disorder. *Patient Prefer Adherence*, 8, 487–491.

91. Judd, L. L., Akiskal, H. S., Schettler, P. J., et al. (2003). A prospective investigation of the natural history of the long-term weekly symptomatic status of bipolar II disorder. *Arch Gen Psychiatry*, 60, 261–269.

92. Kerckhoffs, A. P. M., Hartong, E. and Grootens, K. P. (2018). The perspectives of patients with lithium-induced end-stage renal disease. *Int J Bipolar Disord*, 6, 1–7.

93. Methaneethorn, J., Mannie, Z., Bell, E., et al. (2022). Lithium replacement dose recommendations using Monte Carlo simulations. *Bipolar Disord*, 24, 739–748.

94. Merwick, A., Cooke, J., Neligan, A., et al. (2011). Acute neuropathy in setting of diarrhoeal illness and hyponatraemia due to lithium toxicity. *Clin Neurol Neurosurg*, 113, 923–924.

95. Malhi, G. S., Gessler, D. and Outhred, T. (2017). The use of lithium for the treatment of bipolar disorder: Recommendations from clinical practice guidelines. *J Affect Disord*, 217, 266–280.

96. Meyer, J. M., Dollarhide, A. and Tuan, I.-L. (2005). Lithium toxicity after switch from fosinopril to lisinopril. *Int Clin Psychopharmacol*, 20, 115–118.

97. Sebo, P., Herrmann, F. R. and Haller, D. M. (2017). Accuracy of anthropometric measurements by general practitioners in overweight and obese patients. *BMC Obes*, 4, 23–29.

98. Chen, T. K., Knicely, D. H. and Grams, M. E. (2019). Chronic kidney disease diagnosis and management: A review. *JAMA*, 322, 1294–1304.

99. **Łukawska, E., Frankiewicz, D., Izak, M., et al. (2021).** Lithium toxicity and the kidney with special focus on nephrotic syndrome associated with the acute kidney injury: A case-based systematic analysis. *J Appl Toxicol*, 41, 1896–1909.

100. **Stookey, J. D. (2019).** Analysis of 2009–2012 Nutrition Health and Examination Survey (NHANES) data to estimate the median water intake associated with meeting hydration criteria for individuals aged 12–80 in the US population. *Nutrients*, 11, 657–700.

101. **Golic, M., Aiff, H., Attman, P. O., et al. (2021).** Starting lithium in patients with compromised renal function – is it wise? *J Psychopharmacol*, 35, 190–197.

102. **Presne, C., Fakhouri, F., Noel, L. H., et al. (2003).** Lithium-induced nephropathy: Rate of progression and prognostic factors. *Kidney Int*, 64, 585–592.

103. **Rej, S., Li, B. W., Looper, K., et al. (2014).** Renal function in geriatric psychiatry patients compared to non-psychiatric older adults: Effects of lithium use and other factors. *Aging Ment Health*, 18, 847–853.

104. **Lepkifker, E., Sverdlik, A., Iancu, I., et al. (2004).** Renal insufficiency in long-term lithium treatment. *J Clin Psychiatry*, 63, 850–856.

105. **Aiff, H., Attman, P.-O., Aurell, M., et al. (2014).** The impact of modern treatment principles may have eliminated lithium-induced renal failure. *J Psychopharmacol*, 28, 151–154.

106. **Nederlof, M., Heerdink, E. R., Egberts, A. C. G., et al. (2018).** Monitoring of patients treated with lithium for bipolar disorder: An international survey. *Int J Bipolar Disord*, 6, 12–20.

107. **Werneke, U., Ott, M., Renberg, E. S., et al. (2012).** A decision analysis of long-term lithium treatment and the risk of renal failure. *Acta Psychiatr Scand*, 126, 186–197.

108. **Bauer, M. and Gitlin, M. (2016).** *The Essential Guide to Lithium Treatment.* Basel: Springer International Publishing AG.

109. **Du, J., Quiroz, J., Yuan, P., et al. (2004).** Bipolar disorder: Involvement of signaling cascades and AMPA receptor trafficking at synapses. *Neuron Glia Biol*, 1, 231–243.

110. **Meyer, J. M. (2022).** Pharmacotherapy of psychosis and mania. In L. L. Brunton and B. C. Knollmann, eds., *Goodman & Gilman's The Pharmacological Basis of Therapeutics*, 14th Edition. Chicago: McGraw-Hill, pp. 357–384.

111. **Meyer, J. M. (2021).** Approach to bipolar diathesis in schizophrenia spectrum patients. In M. A. Cummings and S. M. Stahl, eds., *Management of Complex Treatment-Resistant Psychotic Disorders*. Cambridge: Cambridge University Press, pp. 42–50.

112. **Schou, M. (2004).** *Lithium Treatment of Mood Disorders* (6th edn.). Basel: S. Karger AG.

113. **Cooper, T. B., Bergner, P. E. and Simpson, G. M. (1973).** The 24-hour serum lithium level as a prognosticator of dosage requirements. *Am J Psychiatry*, 130, 601–603.

114. **Amdisen, A. (1977).** Serum level monitoring and clinical pharmacokinetics of lithium. *Clin Pharmacokinet*, 2, 73–92.

115. **Kook, K. A., Stimmel, G. L., Wilkins, J. N., et al. (1985).** Accuracy and safety of a priori lithium loading. *J Clin Psychiatry*, 46, 49–51.

116. **Heald, A. H., Holland, D., Stedman, M., et al. (2021).** Can we check serum lithium levels less often without compromising patient safety? *BJPsych Open*, 8, e18.

117. **Kirkham, E., Skinner, J., Anderson, T., et al. (2014).** One lithium level > 1.0 mmol/L causes an acute decline in eGFR: Findings from a retrospective analysis of a monitoring database. *BMJ Open*, 4, e006020.

118. **MacEwan, J. P., Forma, F. M., Shafrin, J., et al. (2016).** Patterns of adherence to oral atypical antipsychotics among patients diagnosed with schizophrenia. *J Manag Care Spec Pharm*, 22, 1349–1361.

119. **Velligan, D. I., Weiden, P. J., Sajatovic, M., et al. (2009).** The expert consensus guideline series: Adherence problems in patients with serious and persistent mental illness. *J Clin Psychiatry*, 70, 1–46.

120. Sylvia, L. G., Reilly-Harrington, N. A., Leon, A. C., et al. (2014). Medication adherence in a comparative effectiveness trial for bipolar disorder. *Acta Psychiatr Scand*, 129, 359–365.

121. Velligan, D. I., Maples, N. J., Pokorny, J. J., et al. (2020). Assessment of adherence to oral antipsychotic medications: What has changed over the past decade? *Schizophr Res*, 215, 17–24.

122. Yaegashi, H., Kirino, S., Remington, G., et al. (2020). Adherence to oral antipsychotics measured by electronic adherence monitoring in schizophrenia: A systematic review and meta-analysis. *CNS Drugs*, 34, 579–598.

123. Velligan, D. I., Wang, M., Diamond, P., et al. (2007). Relationships among subjective and objective measures of adherence to oral antipsychotic medications. *Psychiatr Serv*, 58, 1187–1192.

124. Swartz, C. M. and Wilcox, J. (1984). Characterization and prediction of lithium blood levels and clearances. *Arch Gen Psychiatry*, 41, 1154–1158.

125. Barbuti, M., Colombini, P., Ricciardulli, S., et al. (2021). Treatment adherence and tolerability of immediate- and prolonged-release lithium formulations in a sample of bipolar patients: A prospective naturalistic study. *Int Clin Psychopharmacol*, 36, 230–237.

126. Soares, J. C., Boada, F. and Keshavan, M. S. (2000). Brain lithium measurements with (7) Li magnetic resonance spectroscopy (MRS): A literature review. *Eur Neuropsychopharmacol*, 10, 151–158.

127. Moore, C. M., Demopulos, C. M., Henry, M. E., et al. (2002). Brain-to-serum lithium ratio and age: An in vivo magnetic resonance spectroscopy study. *Am J Psychiatry*, 159, 1240–1242.

128. Forester, B. P., Streeter, C. C., Berlow, Y. A., et al. (2009). Brain lithium levels and effects on cognition and mood in geriatric bipolar disorder: A lithium-7 magnetic resonance spectroscopy study. *Am J Geriatr Psychiatry*, 17, 13–23.

129. Machado-Vieira, R., Otaduy, M. C., Zanetti, M. V., et al. (2016). A selective association between central and peripheral lithium levels in remitters in bipolar depression: A 3 T-(7) Li magnetic resonance spectroscopy study. *Acta Psychiatr Scand*, 133, 214–220.

130. Hsu, C. W., Carvalho, A. F., Tsai, S. Y., et al. (2021). Lithium concentration and recurrence risk during maintenance treatment of bipolar disorder: Multicenter cohort and meta-analysis. *Acta Psychiatr Scand*, 144, 368–378.

131. Oliver, S. L., Comstock, G. W. and Helsing, K. J. (1976). Mood and lithium in drinking water. *Arch Environ Health*, 31, 92–95.

132. Helbich, M., Leitner, M. and Kapusta, N. D. (2012). Geospatial examination of lithium in drinking water and suicide mortality. *Int J Health Geogr*, 11, 19.

133. Ishii, N., Terao, T., Araki, Y., et al. (2015). Low risk of male suicide and lithium in drinking water. *J Clin Psychiatry*, 76, 319–326.

134. Nunes, M. A., Schowe, N. M., Monteiro-Silva, K. C., et al. (2015). Chronic microdose lithium treatment prevented memory loss and neurohistopathological changes in a transgenic mouse model of Alzheimer's disease. *PLoS One*, 10, e0142267.

135. Vita, A., De Peri, L. and Sacchetti, E. (2015). Lithium in drinking water and suicide prevention: A review of the evidence. *Int Clin Psychopharmacol*, 30, 1–5.

136. Kessing, L. V., Gerds, T. A., Knudsen, N. N., et al. (2017). Association of lithium in drinking water with the incidence of dementia. *JAMA Psychiatry*, 74, 1005–1010.

137. Barjasteh-Askari, F., Davoudi, M., Amini, H., et al. (2020). Relationship between suicide mortality and lithium in drinking water: A systematic review and meta-analysis. *J Affect Disord*, 264, 234–241.

138. Eyre-Watt, B., Mahendran, E., Suetani, S., et al. (2022). The association between lithium in drinking water and neuropsychiatric outcomes: A systematic review and meta-analysis from across 2678 regions containing 113 million. *Aust N Z J Psychiatry*, 55, 139–152.

139. Forlenza, O. V., Radanovic, M., Talib, L. L., et al. (2019). Clinical and biological effects of long-term lithium treatment in older adults with amnestic mild cognitive impairment: Randomised clinical trial. *Br J Psychiatry*, 215, 668–674.

5

Management of Routine Lithium Related Adverse Effects

Polyuria, Gastrointestinal Complaints; Altered Taste; Weight Gain; Thyroid and Parathyroid Dysfunction; ECG Changes; Hair Loss; Acneiform Eruptions and Other Skin Disorders; Neutrophilia; CNS Complaints (Tremor, Fatigue, Cognitive and Emotional Dulling, Nystagmus, Myoclonus and Idiopathic Intracranial Hypertension); Peripheral Edema

QUICK CHECK

PRINCIPLES

- Management of adverse effects is crucial to keeping patients on lithium. Aside from laboratory measures, the best screening tool is routine inquiry. By the time a spontaneous complaint emerges, a patient may already be at the point of stopping lithium.

- Amiloride is the gold standard for managing lithium-induced nephrogenic diabetic insipidus (NDI), and is started once polyuria/polydipsia complaints emerge, and early morning urine osmolality provides evidence of partial NDI. The carbonic anhydrase inhibitor acetazolamide is used adjunctively when maximal doses of amiloride are insufficient.

- As eGFR approaches stage G3b CKD (eGFR 30–44 ml/min), one must re-evaluate the compelling need to remain on lithium. Considerations include whether the patient has the support to obtain frequent laboratory monitoring, prior failure of non-lithium therapies, and patient preference for remaining on lithium.

- Common ECG changes are benign and not a reason to discontinue lithium. Rare patients with sinus node dysfunction may require treatment interruption until pacemaker placement. Brugada syndrome is an uncommon disorder easily diagnosed from characteristic ECG findings. It is suspected based on patient history of recurrent syncope, a history of sudden death in 1st degree family members under the age of 45, or a familial diagnosis of Brugada syndrome.

- Ask at every visit about skin changes (e.g. acneiform eruptions) and hair loss to detect these problems early and before the patient decides to stop lithium. Treatments for these conditions are effective but may require weeks to be visible to the patient.

- Lithium is associated with weight gain, so use of antipsychotics with weight gain liability must be avoided unless necessary. Metformin can be used to minimize weight gain, and injectable glucagon-like peptide 1 (GLP-1) agonists are indicated for obesity management in nondiabetics.

- Thyroid and parathyroid dysfunction can occur but are not reasons to stop lithium. Use of cinacalcet for hyperparathyroidism is an option in lieu of surgery for some patients. Lithium does not adversely impact bone density or sexual function.

- Management of diarrhea and nausea involves use of sustained release lithium preparations or ingestion with food. Altered taste and dry mouth due to lithium alone are rare, but may be related to high therapeutic lithium levels.

- Lithium induced tremor can occur and is managed by propranolol, primidone or level reduction. Other central nervous system complaints (e.g. cognitive slowing, fatigue, emotional blunting) require consideration of multiple causes (e.g. depressed mood, other medication effects) before deciding on a course of action. Nystagmus and myoclonus are rare but should be recognized as potential lithium related adverse effects. Idiopathic intracranial hypertension is often due to other causes (e.g. hypertension), with lithium possibly playing a role. Lithium discontinuation may not be necessary.

INTRODUCTION

WHAT TO KNOW: INTRODUCTION

- Adverse effects are a leading cause of lithium discontinuation. Routine inquiry remains the only practical method to identify the majority of lithium related adverse effects.
- A patient's sense of trust and confidence in their provider's ability to manage adverse effects is an important factor in maintaining individuals on long-term treatment.

Despite recent downward trends in lithium use for bipolar disorder (BD) [1], nearly every treatment guideline, meta-analysis or review published in the last decade has reinforced the notion that lithium remains the mood stabilizer of choice for acute or maintenance therapy in those with a history of mania (BD-1, schizoaffective disorder, bipolar type [SAD-BT]), and an important treatment option for other mood disorder spectrum patients (BD-2, unipolar major depressive disorder [MDD]) [2–4]. Moreover, compared with non-lithium medications, lithium confers unique benefits on suicidal behavior and neurocognition, thus presenting a constellation of activities not seen with any other biological therapy [5–8]. It is worth noting the difficulty in establishing the extent of lithium's anti-suicide properties in prospective studies, as discussed in Chapter 1. Analyses of pooled results from clinical trials and observational studies indicate that mean exposures of 18 months may be necessary to establish between-treatment differences on suicidal behavior [9]. The daunting impact of subject attrition and poor adherence over the course of long-term clinical trials can erode the statistical power of any study, thus leaving open the question surrounding lithium's anti-suicide effect size, and whether this benefit devolves more to BD spectrum than to unipolar MDD patients [8]. Nonetheless, the balance of the evidence weighs heavily toward lithium being superior to other treatments in this regard [10]; however, any therapeutic benefit from lithium for any indication only accrues to those who remain on it [4, 11]. It has been estimated that 40–50% of patients stop lithium during the first 6 months of treatment [12, 13], with certain factors such as substance use, recent stressors, personality disorder, lack of social support, inefficacy and illness severity emerging as significant contributors to lithium nonadherence [14–16]. While many of those factors lie beyond the clinician's short-term control, there are two issues leading to discontinuation that are eminently addressable: the patient's attitude toward the psychiatric disorder itself, and adverse effects [12, 17]. As discussed in Chapter 4, one motivation for discontinuing lithium relates to a patient's health beliefs and discomfort with use of any medication to control mood states, or the wish to avoid the daily reminder of a chronic illness that they may not fully accept [15, 18, 19]. For patients harboring those feelings, a referral for Customized Adherence Enhancement (CAE) therapy can be enormously productive, and the content is delivered over just 1–4 weekly visits [20]. While CAE requires a referral source and the personnel to administer the sessions, clinicians can immediately address most adverse effects and thereby avert discontinuation due to a manageable problem.

In spite of modern practice guidelines on lithium dosing and monitoring, adverse effects remain the leading cause of lithium discontinuation. A 2018 paper examined reasons for discontinuation among 873 lithium treated patients in Norrbotten, Sweden, from 1997–2013 [21]. Dispensing records indicated that 54% stopped lithium, comprising 561 episodes of lithium discontinuation (certain patients resumed and then stopped lithium more than once). In 62% of treatment episodes, lithium was stopped due to adverse effects, with the five most common reasons being diarrhea (13%), tremor (11%), polyuria/polydipsia (9%), creatinine increase (9%) and weight gain (7%). The top three on this list represent issues that should be manageable, while weight gain is not unique to lithium and is a problem shared with divalproex/valproate (VPA) and many second generation antipsychotics (SGAs) [17, 22]. As will be discussed later in this chapter, whether any patient with diminishing renal function should discontinue lithium is a decision that incorporates a number of inputs, including the patient's preference, the current estimated glomerular filtration rate (eGFR), the recent trajectory of eGFR declines, the burden and severity of medical comorbidities contributing to chronic kidney disease (CKD), and the clinical course of the mood disorder. Regardless of the reason for discontinuation, the fate of a patient who stops lithium presents a realistic concern over future psychiatric stability, especially as data on BD outcomes following lithium discontinuation emphasize that other treatments may not be equally effective (Figure 5.1) [23].

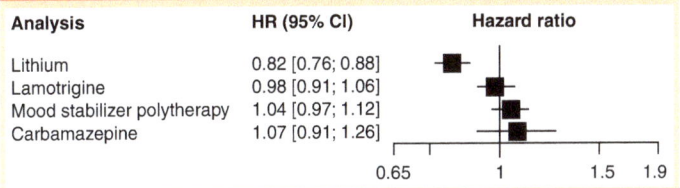

Figure 5.1 Using valproate as the reference, a within-individual Cox regression analysis of treatment failure with mood stabilizer monotherapy following lithium discontinuation shows that resumption of lithium is superior to trying other options [23]

(Adapted from: M. Holm, A. Tanskanen, M. Lahteenvuo, et al. [2022]. Comparative effectiveness of mood stabilizers and antipsychotics in the prevention of hospitalization after lithium discontinuation in bipolar disorder. *Eur Neuropsychopharmacol*, 61, 36–42.)

Laboratory or office monitoring is necessary to detect certain lithium related sequelae (e.g. declining eGFR, hypercalcemia, hypothyroidism, weight gain), but routine inquiry remains the only practical method to identify the majority of adverse effects that can lead to discontinuation (e.g. cognitive complaints, hair loss). The use of biomarkers to predict liability for certain adverse effects is not yet at the stage of clinical application, but a 2022 study suggests that this may be a reality in the near future [24]. While we await further research to identify biomarkers and demonstrate the impact of their use on patient outcomes, the one tool available to all clinicians is the ability to convey a willingness to hear about adverse effects as soon as they arise, and the ability to relate one's experience in managing these issues. As discussed in Chapter 4, patient rapport remains central to promoting medication adherence. Having agreed to a lithium trial, a patient's sense of trust and confidence in their provider's ability to manage adverse effects is an important factor in maintaining individuals on long-term treatment.

In-Depth 5.1 Identifying Biomarkers to Predict Risk for Lithium Related Adverse Effects

Using a sample of 66 lithium treated patients (81.8% BD), investigators examined associations between changes in expression of lithium related genes, and how this differential expression related to the serum lithium level and to common adverse effects. The lithium specific changes in gene expression were assessed using a non-lithium treated reference group that included 528 healthy controls and 856 individuals with a variety of psychiatric diagnoses on antipsychotics, antidepressants and anticonvulsants [24]. Lithium significantly altered the expression of 52 genes in a serum level-dependent manner, with 32 upregulated genes and 20 downregulated genes compared with lithium non-users. Tremor and dry mouth were significantly associated (p ≤ 0.01) with specific sets of 3 or more lithium-associated genes, and the adverse effect with the largest association was between nausea/vomiting and increased expression of calcium/calmodulin-dependent protein kinase 1 (p ≤ 0.01) [24].

A Renal Effects: Polyuria and Decreasing eGFR

WHAT TO KNOW: MANAGING POLYURIA AND DECREASING eGFR

- Polyuria arises from lithium's entry into collecting duct principal cells via the epithelial sodium channel (ENaC). Development of polyuria reflects the beginnings of a process that can lead to downstream long-term effects on renal function if left untreated, or to patient refusal.

- Polyuria is diagnosed by routine inquiry, use of early morning urine osmolality (EMUO) and the 24 h fluid intake record (FIR). It can be treated using amiloride, a potassium sparing diuretic that specifically inhibits ENaC. For inadequate response to amiloride there is recent evidence for adjunctive use of the carbonic anhydrase inhibitor acetazolamide.

- When lithium is dosed using modern precepts (single QHS dosing; maintenance levels ideally 0.60–0.80 mEq/l, but not exceeding 1.00 mEq/l), medical comorbidities such as hypertension and diabetes mellitus are the main contributors to accelerated eGFR declines, and are also the primary cause of proteinuria (as noted by an elevated albumin-to-creatinine ratio [ACR]).

- Appropriate monitoring of eGFR, EMUO and ACR can help determine when nephrology consultation is necessary.

- There are several important considerations in deciding whether a patient with an eGFR nearing CKD stage G3b should have lithium discontinued, including the presence of viable options, preferential reasons to remain on lithium (e.g. suicidality), and whether the patient has the resources to meet the demands of more intensive monitoring.

Clinician anxiety about lithium often revolves around uncertainties about lithium's renal effects, but over the past 20 years there is an increased appreciation of several core concepts:

i.   The earliest signal of lithium related renal dysfunction is polyuria [25], and this is seen as patient complaints of polydipsia or urinary frequency [26].

ii. Medical comorbidities such as hypertension and diabetes mellitus are significant contributors to accelerated eGFR declines, and the primary cause of proteinuria [27].

iii. Administering lithium once daily and keeping maintenance levels from exceeding 1.00 mEq/l minimizes long-term lithium related renal dysfunction [28, 29].

From an understanding of the literature covering the first concept, it becomes evident that early recognition and treatment of urinary concentration deficits might serve two goals: prevention of lithium discontinuation, and minimization of the long-term nephropathy risk related to unchecked lithium entry into collecting duct principal cells [30].

1   Managing Polyuria and Nephrogenic Diabetes Insipidus (NDI)

There are several evidence based tools for tracking lithium related changes in urine concentrating ability that herald the development of nephrogenic diabetes insipidus (NDI) [26]. As outlined in Chapter 4, Info Box 4.4, routine inquiry at each visit about polyuria/polydipsia should be supplemented with periodic use of the 24 h FIR and EMUO. In general, any patient complaint in this area must prompt further investigation to forestall lithium refusal. The data in Figures 5.2a and 5.2b come from an Irish study in which multiple measures were obtained in 79 lithium treated patients, including a 24 h urine collection to diagnose polyuria using the standard definition of 24 h output > 3 liters (Figure 5.2a, 5.2b) [26]. For patients with a 24 h FIR < 2000 ml, another cause must be sought for their complaint as this level of fluid intake is generally incompatible with a urine concentration problem (likelihood ratio for polyuria = 0.18) [26]. As the 24 h FIR reaches 3000 ml, the majority of patients will have polyuria and will merit treatment. Some individuals may not complain, hence the need to use EMUO, especially when the patient has difficulty performing the 24 h FIR [31]. An EMUO < 300 mOsm/kg represents full NDI – these patients deserve treatment regardless of the severity of their complaint as they are showing obvious signs of lithium's accumulation in collecting duct principal cells. While a normal EMUO is > 850 mOsm/kg, the question is which combination of data points (EMUO, 24 h FIR) best identifies those patients who must be treated in the absence of polyuria complaints. An EMUO < 600 mOsm/kg had 100% sensitivity for detecting lithium related polyuria in the Irish study, but low specificity [26]; however, the use of EMUO < 600 mOsm/kg and an FIR > 2500 ml improves the specificity significantly, as only a small fraction of patients without polyuria had 24 h FIR intake exceeding 2500 ml/day.

Figures 5.2a, 5.2b The relationship of lithium related polyuria and early morning urine osmolality (EMUO) or the 24 h fluid intake record (FIR) [26]

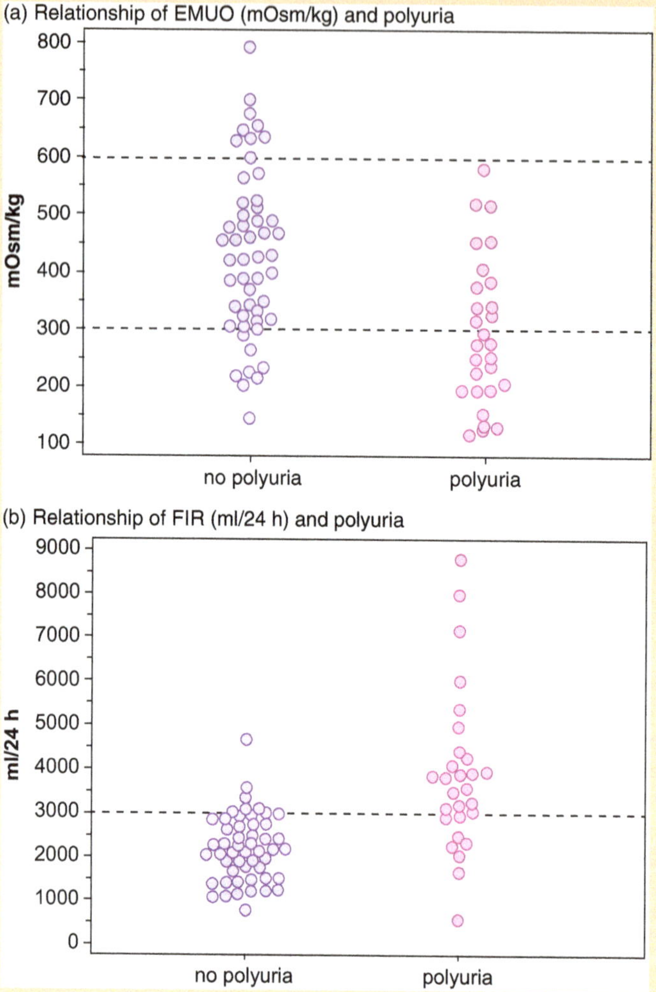

(a) Relationship of EMUO (mOsm/kg) and polyuria

(b) Relationship of FIR (ml/24 h) and polyuria

(Adapted from: J. C. Kinahan, A. NiChorcorain, S. Cunningham, et al. [2015]. Diagnostic accuracy of tests for polyuria in lithium-treated patients. *J Clin Psychopharmacol*, 35, 434–441.)

The approach to polyuria treatment rests on the principle that lithium induces polyuria through numerous effects on 2nd messenger systems in collecting duct principal cells, and it does so by entering these cells via the epithelial sodium channel (ENaC) on the apical surface [32]. The form of ENaC in these cells is often referred to as the amiloride-sensitive ENaC, since amiloride blocks the entry of sodium through this channel. ENaC is expressed in many areas of the body including the kidney, colon, lung and certain taste cells on the tongue, and its trimeric structure combines 3 of the 4 possible subunits (α, β, γ or β, γ, δ) to form the functioning channel [33]. As described in Chapter 2, the form of ENaC expressed on the apical surface of collecting duct principal cells is composed of an α, β and γ subunit, and this isoform is referred to as the amiloride-sensitive ENaC to differentiate it from variants in other tissues, and to reflect that the α subunit is required for amiloride sensitivity [34]. All ENaC isoforms that contain an α subunit exhibit 1.6-fold higher permeability for lithium than for sodium [34]. Unfortunately, lithium is a poor substrate for the Na^+/K^+-ATPase pump on the basolateral membrane and must rely exclusively on the Na^+/H^+ exchanger type 1 (NHE1) for transport out of the principal cell. In many patients, this NHE1 transport mechanism is insufficient, resulting in high intracellular lithium levels. The initial sequelae are downregulation of water absorbing aquaporin channels and vasopressin insensitivity; however, when this process is left unchecked over months and years, microcyst formation and interstitial fibrosis can result [35, 36]. Amiloride thus presents an elegant solution as it specifically prevents lithium from entering principal cells via the amiloride-sensitive ENaC (Figure 5.3) [36]. The initial reports of amiloride for this purpose are roughly 40 years old [37], and over time amiloride has emerged as the gold standard treatment for this problem (Info Box 5.1) [38]. Not only does amiloride improve urine osmolality and increase aquaporin 2 channel density after 6 weeks at modest doses (10 mg/d) [39], animal models of lithium induced renal injury note that amiloride ameliorates interstitial fibrosis. This finding suggests that use in patients with polyuria left untreated for years may still be beneficial [30]. Given its highly specific mechanism of action, the intriguing question is whether amiloride should be started prophylactically in all lithium treated patients, as early use might greatly reduce future risk of lithium related renal dysfunction. Recent papers have raised this question, but there are insufficient data to recommend starting amiloride routinely in all newly treated patients [38]; however, this view may change based on research and prevailing opinion.

Figure 5.3 Detailed view of collecting duct principal cells and the site of action for amiloride at the epithelial sodium channel (ENaC) [40]

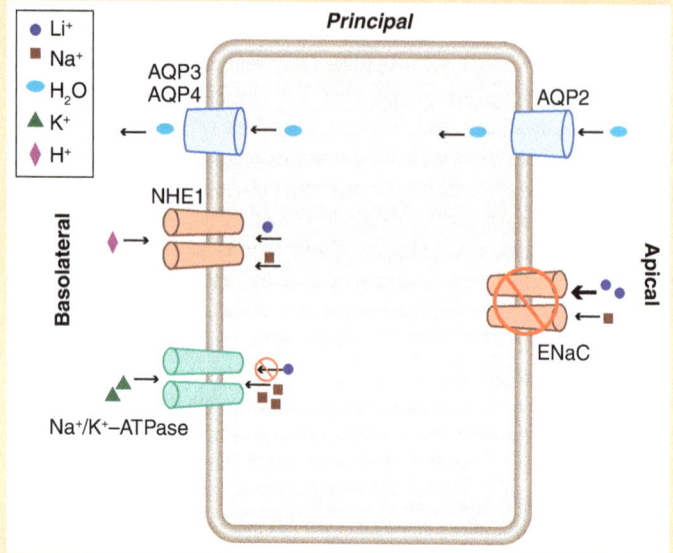

Legend AQP: aquaporin channel; ENaC: epithelial sodium channel; NHE1: sodium-hydrogen exchanger type 1; (Adapted from: J.-P. Grünfeld and B. C. Rossier [2009]. Lithium nephrotoxicity revisited. *Nat Rev Nephrol*, 5, 270–276.)

Info Box 5.1 When to Initiate Treatment for Polyuria and How to Use Amiloride

a. When to treat polyuria

  i. Patient complaints

    1. Treat for polyuria all patients with 24 h FIR > 2500 ml.

    2. Rationale: While not all patients complain about polyuria even when symptomatic [31], as 24 h FIR exceeds 2500 ml the majority of patients will have polyuria and will want clinical intervention. In these patients, the EMUO will typically be below 600 mOsm/kg, but should not be normal (> 850 mOsm/kg).

    3. Comment: If a patient complains of urinary frequency with a 24 h FIR < 2000 ml, another cause must be sought as this is less than the daily urine output for most adults (likelihood ratio for polyuria = 0.180) [26]. If no other cause is found, repeat the FIR and EMUO as one or both are likely to become abnormal if the etiology is lithium related.

ii. No patient complaints

1. Treat all patients with an EMUO < 600 mOsm/kg and 24 h FIR > 2500 ml.

2. Rationale: Based on the data from Figures 5.2a and 5.2b, an EMUO < 600 mOsm/kg appears to have 100% sensitivity for detecting lithium related polyuria, but low specificity; however, the use of EMUO < 600 mOsm/kg and an FIR > 2500 ml improves the specificity significantly as only a small fraction of patients without polyuria had a 24 h FIR intake exceeding 2500 ml [26].

b. Step 1: If on divided daily lithium dosing, consolidate lithium to bedtime (QHS)

i. Rationale: Divided doses increase risk of long-term renal insufficiency and short-term urine concentration deficits [41, 42].

ii. Adjust dose based on new level: After consolidation, the 12 h level will be 28% higher on average, and the new level may exceed the recommended range [43, 44].

iii. Expected result: A study of 51 BD patients found that switching from divided to QHS dosing for 12–18 months decreased urinary volume by 14%, but only in those on lithium < 5 years [45].

c. Step 2: Use amiloride

i. Avoiding interactions with other antihypertensives: Amiloride should be avoided with angiotensin converting enzyme inhibitors (ACEIs), angiotensin II receptor blockers (ARBs), spironolactone or triamterene due to hyperkalemia risk [46]. If these medications cannot be avoided, monitor serum Na^+ and K^+ every 3 months initially, and then every 6 months if normal after 1 year. An amiloride-hydrochlorothiazide (HCTZ) combination pill exists in some countries. Electrolyte monitoring should also be performed for this product [47, 48].

ii. Dosing

1. 5 mg QAM for 7 days, then increase to 5 mg BID. Repeat EMUO and 24 h FIR after 6 weeks to allow lithium to be cleared from principal duct cells and for its biological effects to dissipate [39].

2. May increase in 5 mg increments every 6 weeks, with FIR and EMUO prior to each dosage change. Maximum dosage is 10 mg BID. In some patients EMUO may never normalize, but the goal is limited patient complaints and a 24 h FIR < 2500 ml.

iii. Monitoring: Monitoring sodium and potassium is not necessary but may be considered every 6 months in patients with multiple medical problems or baseline poor renal function (eGFR < 60 ml/min).

d. Step 3: Use of adjunctive acetazolamide

i. **Rationale:** Persistent patient complaints may result in lithium discontinuation, so further treatment should be pursued when amiloride 10 mg BID for ≥ 6 weeks is insufficient.

ii. **Evidence:** Multiple studies indicate that acetazolamide decreases urinary volume in a lithium-induced NDI mouse model, although it may not increase urine concentration as much as amiloride [49–51]. There are also multiple case reports of successful use in patients including combination therapy with amiloride [52, 53].

iii. **Practical issues, allergies and drug interactions:** Avoid in those with sulfonamide allergy, and in patients with baseline low sodium or potassium values. Acetazolamide can increase cyclosporine and phenytoin exposure, but decreases primidone and lithium levels [54].

iv. **Dosing and monitoring:** 250 mg PO BID initially. Results may be seen within 7 days, but allow 2 weeks before rechecking EMUO and increasing to 750 mg/d. Maximum dose is 500 mg BID.

Amiloride is the preferred medication for lithium related NDI due to its specific action on ENaC, but there is literature on use of hydrochlorothiazide (HCTZ) for this same purpose dating back 50 years [55–57]. The explanation for the thiazide effect was unclear until research with mouse knockout models lacking the thiazide-sensitive Na^+-Cl^- cotransporter (NCC) found that HCTZ similarly reduced lithium induced polyuria in these animals [57]. As NCC is the primary target for thiazides, it was postulated that a secondary property, carbonic anhydrase inhibition, mediated thiazide effects on lithium induced NDI in NCC knockouts [57, 58]. This hypothesis was based on the knowledge that thiazides were originally derived from carbonic anhydrase inhibitors, and subsequent studies with the carbonic anhydrase inhibitor acetazolamide confirmed that this as an effective agent for lithium induced NDI, comparable to the effects of an amiloride/thiazide combination but without the thiazide related risks for hyperkalemia, hyponatremia and lithium toxicity [49, 51, 58]. The effect of acetazolamide on urinary volume is partially induced via a tubular-glomerular feedback response and/or a direct effect on collecting duct principal cells that reduces intracellular prostaglandin E2 levels [49, 51]. In mouse models, acetazolamide monotherapy decreases urinary volume but not urine concentrating ability [51]. If is for this reason, combined with amiloride's specific ENaC blocking properties, that acetazolamide is considered a useful medication for lithium related NDI, but is reserved for adjunctive use when maximal doses of amiloride are not sufficiently effective [53].

2   *Decreasing eGFR and When to Refer for Nephrology Consultation*

Age-related declines in eGFR typically do not exceed 1 ml/min per year independent of lithium exposure [59]. It is for this reason that age has been a core variable in eGFR estimation formulas in the past two decades, including the 2021 version of the Chronic Kidney Disease Epidemiology Collaboration equation (CKD-EPI 2021) eGFR$_{cr-cys}$ that removed the problematic race coefficient, and in doing so also improved performance across diverse populations [60]. When lithium is prescribed using modern principles, including administering lithium once daily and keeping maintenance levels from exceeding 1.00 mEq/l, the independent impact of lithium on long-term renal function may be modest [27–29]. The purpose of monitoring eGFR every 6 months is to detect accelerated declines in eGFR (> 2 ml/min over 6 months or > 4 ml/min over 12 months, as verified by a repeat specimen) and facilitate two important interventions: increasing the eGFR monitoring frequency, and making sensible adjustments to the lithium regimen (e.g. consolidating divided daily doses to QHS, or lowering doses slightly if recent maintenance levels have exceeded 1.00 mEq/l). Lamentably, it is medical comorbidities such as hypertension and diabetes mellitus that emerge as the main contributors to accelerated eGFR declines when lithium is dosed according to modern precepts, and these comorbidities are also the primary cause of proteinuria [27]. BD and schizophrenia spectrum patients are a group of individuals with high rates of cardiometabolic disorders, but the management of those problems is largely out of the control of the lithium prescriber [61–63]. Nonetheless, as mental health providers routinely track blood pressure, serum lipids and fasting glucose (or A1C) as part of antipsychotic monitoring, undertreated hypertension, dyslipidemia or prediabetes/diabetes should be brought to the attention of the primary care provider to prevent long-term morbidity, and especially the impact on eGFR. While many nonpsychiatric clinicians are quick to blame all forms of renal dysfunction on lithium, this is also an opportune moment to inform those clinicians about measures used to minimize lithium related risks (low maintenance serum level, once nightly dosing) so that energies can be focused on the medical comorbidities.

When eGFR declines exceed 2 ml/min over 6 months, or 4 ml/min over 12 months, as verified by a repeat specimen, nephrology consultation can be helpful to see whether an undetected problem is present, especially where there are limited CKD risk factors. Referral is also necessary for hematuria and severe forms of albuminuria. There are no agreed upon criteria in published guidelines on when such a referral should occur, so the list in Info Box 5.2 represents a synthesis of available recommendations [38]. The nephrology consultant may also blame the renal dysfunction on lithium, despite measures being taken to minimize lithium related risks, but this is not true for all renal specialists, and some very much recognize the unique clinical value of lithium and that management of medical comorbidity is often the proper course of action, not lithium discontinuation [38]. In that sense, the nephrology consultant may be your ally in working with other medical providers to better manage the obvious problem of poorly controlled hypertension or diabetes.

Info Box 5.2 When to Consult a Nephrologist

a. eGFR: Second decline in eGFR > 2 ml/min over 6 months or > 4 ml/min over 12 months as verified by a repeat specimen

b. eGFR < 45 ml/min as verified by a repeat specimen

c. Urine albumin-to-creatinine ratio (ACR): Stage A3 (> 300 mg/g)

d. Nephrogenic diabetes insipidus (EMUO values < 300 mOsm/kg) unresponsive to maximal doses of amiloride (10 mg BID) plus adjunctive use of acetazolamide (up to 500 mg BID) for 6 weeks

e. Hematuria

3 *Stopping Lithium for Low eGFR: Considerations*

As discussed in Chapter 4, for patients who present a *compelling indication* for lithium, initiation with eGFR as low as 45 ml/min is not unreasonable provided there is diligent and frequent eGFR monitoring. The converse situation involves deciding when the risk–benefit calculus leans toward discontinuation, especially when eGFR declines are significant, and underlying medical comorbidities associated with CKD (e.g. hypertension, diabetes mellitus) are poorly controlled. As outlined in Info Box 5.3, there is no absolute eGFR threshold at which lithium must be stopped, but the literature indicates that as eGFR dips below 45 ml/min and enters stage G3b CKD the risk of progression even after lithium is stopped is appreciable [64]. For example, in one analysis of long-term lithium exposure (n = 74, mean exposure 19.8 years), the outcomes among those who underwent lithium discontinuation depended greatly on renal function at the time lithium was stopped (using an older metric, creatinine clearance [CL_{Cr}]): 5 of 7 improved when CL_{Cr} exceeded 40 ml/min, while 12 of 18 experienced further declines when CL_{Cr} was ≤ 40 ml/min. Moreover, all patients experienced further declines when CL_{Cr} was less than 25 ml/min at the time lithium was stopped [65].

Another important factor is whether the patient has viable alternatives to lithium and is willing to consider them. If not willing to look at other options, one must investigate whether the patient understands the morbidity and mortality risk of advanced CKD [66, 67], and has the cognitive, physical and support resources needed to withstand the demands of dialysis if needed. Given the potential objections from other medical providers or family/caregivers to continuing lithium in someone with advanced CKD (stages G4–G5), it may be necessary to convene a panel that includes an ethicist to reach a shared decision. When there is a compelling reason to continue lithium, a 2022 systematic review covering the treatment course in 18 patients receiving dialysis noted that lithium was typically dosed 3 times per week, with each dose administered following dialysis (see Chapter 7) [68]. However, the review stated that a flexible approach to dosing is necessary for two reasons: (a) the pharmacokinetic properties of lithium in dialysis are not well characterized and can be complicated in some patients by a rebound in serum levels postdialysis due to a two-compartment volume of distribution; and (b) postdialysis diuresis in other patients may hasten lithium clearance and necessitate administering lithium more frequently than 3 times per week following each dialysis treatment. The review commented that lithium was clearly effective in all 18 patients, with some demonstrating rapid improvement after initiation, and only one patient required lithium discontinuation [68]. The overriding principle is that those patients with no other options, and for whom lithium has demonstrated unique efficacy, have earned the right to continue lithium assuming measures are in place to assure success with whatever care is needed for their declining renal function (Info Box 5.3). The goal is to avert, if possible, poor psychiatric outcomes of the type described in the older literature, where suicides occurred after lithium was withdrawn in the face of significant renal dysfunction [69]. These are difficult, complicated and individualized decisions that incorporate a number of considerations to arrive at a course of action.

Info Box 5.3 Unique Considerations Concerning Discontinuing Lithium for Low eGFR

a. **Is the eGFR close to stage G3b (30–44 ml/min)?** While the contribution of lithium to eGFR declines may be modest overall [27], this may not be true for specific individuals, especially those with concurrent medical comorbidities contributing to CKD [70]. The issues include:

   i. Literature indicates that stopping lithium when eGFR is in this range may help stabilize renal function despite the presence of medical comorbidities, while waiting until stage G4 may increase risk of further accelerated progression, reduced quality of life and increased risk of mortality [64, 65, 67, 70].

    ii. The presence of a low eGFR poses a greater risk for lithium toxicity. An episode of toxicity might cause non-renal medical morbidity (e.g. bradycardia, central nervous system effects) and possibly induce further renal injury.

b. Does the patient have a support structure to ensure that frequent, necessary laboratory monitoring is obtained? Maintaining a patient with low renal function on lithium requires vigilant monitoring, with eGFR values and lithium levels every 6 weeks. If physical limitations, cognitive issues, lack of insight or transportation preclude the ability to perform necessary monitoring, this may make persistence with lithium untenable.

c. Does the patient have a compelling reason to remain on lithium? Assuming a patient has the support to meet the challenges of aggressive monitoring or renal replacement therapy (e.g. dialysis or transplantation), inadequate response to non-lithium therapies – particularly suicide attempts on other treatments or when the patient was nonadherent with lithium – presents a compelling reason why stakeholders involved in the case (e.g. patients, family, clinicians) might meet together with an ethicist, and together decide that remaining on lithium is the prudent course of action, even if CKD progresses to the need for renal replacement therapy.

    i. Does the patient appreciate the demands of dialysis? Where there is concern that the patient does not fully appreciate the demands of dialysis, consultation with a nephrologist may be helpful, along with a tour of a dialysis center, and perhaps a demand that the patient report to the dialysis center 3 times per week for 4 hours (the average dialysis session is 3–5 hours) for a full month to assess the impact on their life.

    ii. Using lithium in dialyzed patients: The kinetics and safety of lithium with dialysis is documented in the literature, so this may be a feasible option where no other medication choices exist (see Chapter 7) [68]. While cause and effect is not easily established, the literature also documents instances where lithium is discontinued due to advanced CKD and the patient later commits suicide [69].

B | **Cardiovascular Effects: Sinus Node Dysfunction, ECG Changes, Brugada Syndrome**

WHAT TO KNOW: ECG EFFECTS

- A baseline ECG is suggested in those above age 40 to find undetected cardiac issues related to age or medical comorbidity. An ECG is suggested for any patient/family history of syncope or sudden cardiac death (SCD) to screen for ion channelopathies such as Brugada syndrome.

- The impact of lithium on inward sodium currents only starts at concentrations > 1.00 mEq/l. Any impact of lithium on the ECG is unlikely to be seen in most patients at therapeutic serum levels.

- Bradycardia or sick sinus syndrome usually (but not always) appears in the context of supratherapeutic levels. Much of the literature noting serious ECG changes is based on case reports or series, often associated with episodes of toxicity (levels > 1.50 mEq/l) not seen in routine practice.

- There is no need to discontinue therapy due to a novel ECG finding, as very few lithium related ECG manifestations present a medical emergency.

- Benign ECG findings seen with long-term treatment include PR interval prolongation, T-wave changes and development of U-waves. These ECG changes reflect the chronicity of lithium exposure and accumulation in myocytes, and do not represent a source of SCD risk.

The impact of psychotropics on cardiac function is a broad area of concern for many clinicians, in part due to the association between SCD and use of certain antipsychotics, and possibly lamotrigine [71, 72]. The reassuring finding from 70 years of clinical use is that lithium is not associated with SCD, and that ECG changes are typically benign or represent easily diagnosed issues such as bradycardia or sick sinus syndrome that usually (but not always) appear in the context of supratherapeutic levels (Table 5.1) [73–76]. Unlike antipsychotics, tricyclic antidepressants, citalopram, escitalopram and lamotrigine, lithium carries no package insert warning about QT prolongation, and, outside of overdose situations, no language about routine ECG monitoring [77]. However, comments added to lithium labeling in 2011 about Brugada syndrome, combined with the fact that long-term lithium treatment can be associated with ECG changes (albeit benign in most circumstances), can cause some clinicians to conclude incorrectly that lithium is inherently cardiotoxic when the evidence suggests otherwise [75].

Lithium is a monovalent cation, but the extent to which it interacts with any ion channel or ion pump is quite variable, a property now appreciated with respect to lithium's renal trafficking, as reviewed in Chapter 2. Any concern for cardiac effects relates to lithium action at the voltage-dependent sodium channel (I_{Na}) and impact on the velocity of the inward current. *In vitro* studies using cultured cells expressing various isoforms of I_{Na} find that the impact of lithium on sodium currents only starts to become evident at concentrations of 1.00 mmol/l (equivalent to 1.00 mEq/l), a result in keeping with evidence dating back 40 years that any acute impact of lithium on the ECG is unlikely to be seen in most patients at therapeutic serum levels [78–80]. Researchers using other techniques have been able to demonstrate an effect on peak I_{Na} kinetics, but they acknowledge the results of any ion current experiment depend on the animal species, cardiac cell type and region, and the *in vitro* and *in vivo* conditions, and thus cannot hope to reproduce the net effects in an intact human heart [79, 81]. Detailed analyses of lithium treated patients confirm impressions from older literature that bradycardia or T-wave inversions are more pronounced with supratherapeutic levels > 1.20 mEq/l [82].

A 2017 meta-analysis and review provided the most comprehensive assessment of the evidence for lithium related ECG changes, and commented that much of the literature is based on case reports or series, often associated with episodes of toxicity (levels > 1.50 mEq/l) not seen in routine practice (Table 5.1) [75]. The reasons to obtain a baseline ECG are thus largely directed at discovering previously undetected cardiac issues related to age or medical comorbidity, especially given the high prevalence of cardiometabolic disorders in patients with serious mental disorders. The other reason is to screen those with a patient/family history of syncope or SCD for ECG findings suggestive of ion channelopathies such as Brugada syndrome (Chapter 4, Table 4.3). Certain ECG findings can emerge with long-term treatment, such as prolongation of the PR interval (reflecting a slowing of atrial conduction), T-wave changes, and development of U-waves that resemble those seen with hypokalemia. These ECG changes are more evident over time due to the chronicity of lithium exposure and accumulation in myocytes, and do not represent a source of SCD risk [75].

Table 5.1 Summary of evidence regarding impact of lithium on the ECG from a 2017 meta-analysis [75]

ECG component	Findings	Level of evidence*	Human or animal evidence	Number of supporting literature references
Rate and rhythm	– Sinus node dysfunction and bradycardia	2a	Human/animal	4
	– Increased atrial conduction time	2b	Human	1
	– Atrial flutter	5	Human	1
	– Sick sinus syndrome	5	Human	1
	– Cardiac asystole	4	Human	1

ECG component	Findings	Level of evidence*	Human or animal evidence	Number of supporting literature references
P wave and PR interval	– Sinoatrial blocks	4	Human	3
	– PR prolongation and atrioventricular blocks	3b	Human	4
QRS complex	– Incomplete bundle branch block	4	Human	1
	– Right bundle branch block	5	Human	1
	– Nonspecific intraventricular conduction delay	5	Human	1
	– Left bundle branch block	5	Human	1
ST segment	– Depression	4	Human	1
	– Elevation	4	Human	3
	– Brugada pattern	5	Human	2
T wave and QTc interval	– T wave flattening or inversion	2a	Human	4
	– QTc prolongation	5	Human	1
	– Higher QT dispersion ratio	2a	Human	2
	– Ventricular tachyarrhythmias	4	Human	1

* Level of evidence descriptors:

1a: multiple/homogeneous randomized clinical trials

1b: individual randomized clinical trial

2a: multiple/homogeneous prospective cohort studies

2b: individual prospective cohort study

3a: multiple/homogeneous retrospective studies

3b: individual retrospective study

4: case series or more than 3 case reports

5: isolated case reports or expert opinion

(Adapted from: N. Mehta and R. Vannozzi [2017]. Lithium-induced electrocardiographic changes: A complete review. *Clin Cardiol*, 40, 1363–1367.)

There is no need to discontinue therapy due to a novel ECG finding, as nearly every lithium related ECG manifestation is not a medical emergency but one that can be addressed with consultation to rule out the need for intervention.

For example, certain common age-related ECG changes, such as right bundle branch block, are markers for other cardiovascular pathology due to hypertension and do not relate to the chronicity of lithium use [83]. The one exception where lithium might need to be discontinued is the rare patient who develops bradycardia with therapeutic lithium levels, as this likely represents unmasking of sick sinus syndrome [75]. This syndrome is most commonly due to age-related degenerative fibrosis of the sinus node and is often asymptomatic during the early course, but eventually may present with bradycardia and near syncope. Lithium itself does not induce the pathology but hastens its identification in these rare patients. Lithium use may have to be temporarily interrupted in symptomatic patients until pacemaker implantation is arranged.

For those nervous about lithium's electrical effects, the language added to product labeling in 2011 about Brugada syndrome may have generated an unnecessary level of clinician concern simply due to unfamiliarity with this disorder. In 1989 it was recognized that certain ECG patterns were associated with likelihood of future SCD. For decades there was awareness of the heritability of SCD, but it was not until 1996 that two cardiologist brothers from Spain, Josep and Ramon Brugada, linked the association of a specific ECG pattern and SCD risk in a manner that set investigators on a search for the cause and for reliable diagnostic criteria [84]. As we now understand it, Brugada syndrome is an uncommon heritable disorder, with a prevalence estimate between 1 in 2000 and 1 in 5000, whose genetic basis is chiefly due to polymorphisms in the alpha subunit of a sodium channel protein (SCN5A) found primarily in cardiac muscle cells [84]. SCN5A polymorphisms account for 30% of all cases where a genetic basis can be found, and 2–5% of cases have polymorphisms in other genes that relate to sodium, potassium or calcium related channels or cellular processes. Nonetheless, 70% of families have no implicated genetic variant, and the diagnosis is established based on specific ECG findings agreed upon in 2012, with type 1 morphology recognized as the pattern associated with SCD risk. (Modern ECG machines are programmed to distinguish this pattern: coved ST elevation ≥ 2 mm in at least 1 right precordial lead ending with a negative T wave.) As this ECG pattern is now widely recognized, it has become apparent that up to 2/3 of patients with a type 1 ECG pattern are asymptomatic, that the rate of SCD as first presentation of Brugada syndrome is low (< 5%), and that future arrhythmia risk also remains low (5%) [84]. Since many remain symptom free, the true SCD risk and prevalence will be refined over time as surveillance data provide more insight. Asymptomatic patients are usually identified due to an abnormal ECG pattern when being screened for other purposes, or when provocative drug testing is performed due to clinical suspicion (i.e. from family or patient history), using intravenous administration of sodium channel blockers (e.g. ajmaline, flecainide) under highly controlled conditions that elicit ST changes (Info Box 5.4) [85].

Info Box 5.4 Brugada Syndrome and Lithium Use

a. **What is it and how is it diagnosed?** A rare heritable disorder associated with risk for sudden cardiac death (SCD), typically involving genetic polymorphisms of voltage gated sodium channels, but with 70% of patients having no identifiable genetic basis [84]. As many remain asymptomatic, the true prevalence is unknown but estimated to be 1 in 2000 to 1 in 5000, with less than 5% having their first presentation as SCD, and only 5% having a future risk for arrhythmia. Diagnosis of those with SCD risk is based on a classic type 1 pattern that involves a coved ST elevation ≥ 2 mm in at least 1 right precordial lead ending with a negative T wave.

b. **How commonly does lithium unmask this syndrome?** Only 13 cases of Brugada syndrome being unmasked by lithium have ever been reported, with 12/13 having the type 1 ECG pattern, and 1 patient having a variant (type 2 pattern) but a history of recurrent syncope [86]. 10/13 cases were > age 40 and would normally be picked up by a routine pre-lithium ECG recommended for that age group, or by surveillance ECG monitoring after starting lithium. One of the cases (age 42) had the type 2 pattern, but also a history of syncope. Of the three cases under age 40, two had strongly suggestive histories (recurrent near syncope, cardiac arrest), while one patient aged 39 had a type 1 ECG pattern on admission for mania. This patient is the only known death, and that occurred after all psychotropics were stopped and his ECG had normalized.

c. **What is the level of risk?** A nonprofit initiative was developed by physicians from the University of Amsterdam Academic Medical Center Department of Cardiology, in collaboration with a panel of world experts on Brugada syndrome, to assist clinicians in clinical decision-making. Their level of risk assessment for lithium is **Class IIb**, implying conflicting evidence/opinions (see www.brugadadrugs.org/avoid/Brugada for their risk assessment).

d. **What should I ask a patient?** Ask whether there is a history of recurrent syncope, sudden death in 1st degree family members under the age of 45, or a familial diagnosis of Brugada syndrome. An answer of "yes" should prompt a baseline ECG (see ECG screening recommendations in Chapter 4, Table 4.3). This approach is largely consistent with the package insert language, such as that below from 2020 [77]:

Cardiologist consultation is recommended if: (1) treatment with lithium is under consideration for patients suspected of having Brugada Syndrome or patients with risk factors for Brugada Syndrome, e.g., unexplained syncope, a family history of Brugada Syndrome, or a family history of sudden unexplained death before the age of 45 years, (2) patients who develop unexplained syncope or palpitations after starting lithium therapy.

Since the recognition of Brugada syndrome nearly 30 years ago, only 13 cases associated with lithium use have been reported as of 2020. Among these 13 cases, 12 had the type 1 ECG pattern (92.3%), while 1 had a variant (type 2 pattern) but also had a history of recurrent syncope [86]. 77% of these patients were over the age of 40 and thus would have been detected by routine ECG surveillance prior to or while on lithium (Chapter 4, Table 4.3). Among the 3 subjects under the age of 40, 2 of 3 had symptoms prior to starting lithium that would prompt a clinician to obtain a baseline ECG: history of recurrent near syncope (age 26), prior episode of sudden cardiac arrest (age 38) [86]. A manic patient with unknown family history (he was adopted) was found to have a type 1 pattern and QTc prolongation (540 msec) when an ECG was obtained during medical screening for psychiatric admission. At the time, he was on the combination of a tricyclic antidepressant (amitriptyline 200 mg qhs), high dose haloperidol (10 mg TID) and lithium 400 mg/d [87]. The QTc prolongation was deemed related to high tricyclic antidepressant levels, but the decision was made to discontinue all psychiatric medications nonetheless. The resulting ECG normalized and the patient was transferred to a psychiatric inpatient unit. Unfortunately, before he could return for follow-up and provocative flecainide testing, the patient died suddenly [87]. Based on the available case data, the approach to risk management in Info Box 5.4 relies on obtaining a baseline history suggestive of Brugada risk before starting lithium. It is a rare patient who will have a family history of SCD or have heard the term Brugada syndrome, but some may endorse recurrent syncope and yet never have had an ECG. The other point of emphasis is to ask patients, including those who don't require a baseline ECG, to report immediately palpitations or syncope upon starting lithium [85]. The management of Brugada patients is individualized as many are and will remain asymptomatic, and the placement of an implantable cardiac defibrillator (ICD) can be associated with complications [85]. For patients with an ICD, there is no further risk from lithium. For those in whom an ICD is not indicated, close consultation with the cardiologist is necessary to determine the best clinical strategy when there is a compelling reason to use lithium (e.g. failure of non-lithium therapies).

C Dermatological Effects on Skin and Hair

WHAT TO KNOW: SKIN AND HAIR EFFECTS

- Routine inquiry *at every visit* is the best method for detecting dermatological problems. Early detection is particularly crucial as treatment may require many weeks to resolve certain adverse effects (e.g. acne, alopecia).

- The true incidence is unknown but includes new onset problems (e.g. alopecia, acneiform eruptions, folliculitis, maculopapular rash), or an exacerbation of existing issues (e.g. acne, psoriasis).
- Lithium discontinuation is not always necessary for many dermatological adverse effects. Clinicians should become adept at using topical 5% minoxidil for men or women as soon as an alopecia complaint appears. A 2% strength is also available if scalp irritation occurs, but men and women typically remain on and tolerate the 5% solution.

The literature in this area is comprised predominantly of case reports or case series, leaving unresolved the extent to which lithium increases the risk for a variety of skin and hair related conditions. The wide disparity in reported rates (3–45%) is also of little help to clinicians [88–90]. Moreover, a 2012 meta-analysis looking at a range of adverse effects identified little high-quality evidence supporting the association between lithium and cutaneous reactions. Of 77 publications that met inclusion criteria, 68 were case reports, and only two randomized clinical trials (RCTs) reported skin disorder outcomes [91]. Unfortunately, due to the limited data available, the meta-analysis found no significant difference in the prevalence of skin disorders between patients on lithium and those on placebo (OR 1.28, 95% CI 0.49–3.36, $p = 0.62$) [91]. A 2017 review found only one additional RCT, and also concluded that the incidence of cutaneous adverse reactions was not significantly different from placebo (OR 1.14, 95% CI 0.44–2.94, $p = 0.78$), or between lithium and other treatments (OR 0.61, 95% CI 0.34–1.11, $p = 0.11$) [92].

The absence of systematic data should not lead anyone to assume the absence of an association, as there are sufficient examples of patients experiencing exacerbations of existing problems (e.g. psoriasis), or new problems (e.g. acneiform eruptions, folliculitis, maculopapular rash, alopecia), that clinicians must pay attention to these issues, discuss them proactively with patients when starting lithium, and routinely ask about these adverse effects at every visit (Info Box 5.5) [88]. In 2022, an Australian group explored to what extent this type of screening was performed at a clinic in Ipswich, Queensland, and found that less than half of new lithium users were asked about pre-existing skin conditions, and no patient chart showed documentation that any dermatological side effects were discussed [90]. Among patients who were asked about cutaneous disorders, 45% endorsed some prior or current issue, a fact of crucial importance given the probable association between lithium use and psoriasis or acne exacerbation in some patients. While psoriasis and acne were not among the top 10 causes of lithium discontinuation in a large retrospective study (n = 873, Norrbotten, Sweden, 1997–2013), these two specific disorders were responsible for 1.8% and 1.4% of discontinuations, respectively [21]. The importance of early detection relates in part to the cosmetic nature of cutaneous disorders, and the reality that interventions for hair loss, acne or psoriasis can require weeks for effects to be seen. The treatment strategies are straightforward: a new problem that appears related to lithium with an obvious treatment option should allow the patient to remain on lithium. In instances without an obvious option other than discontinuation (e.g. maculopapular rash), tapering lithium might be prudent in the short term, with dermatology consultation if one wishes to rechallenge the patient. (See Ch 8 for rationale behind tapering lithium slowly over 15-30 days when it must be stopped.)

Info Box 5.5 Management of Skin and Hair Disorders on Lithium

General approach for all patients: Ask about skin eruptions and hair loss on every visit. For specific issues:

a. **New onset maculopapular rash upon starting lithium:** Onset with starting lithium is usually clear, so the course of action for maculopapular rash is to taper off lithium over 15-30 days while using another mood stabilizer until the rash clears [93]. If there is a compelling need to rechallenge with lithium, consider dermatology consultation to help rule out other causes if the rash recurs.

b. **Acneiform eruptions, folliculitis (new, or exacerbation):** Both of these are treatable with topical medications, and thus should not necessitate lithium discontinuation [94]. The treatment of folliculitis may require antibacterial, antifungal or steroid medication, the choice of which is best left to the dermatologist. An initial treatment for acne is over-the-counter benzoyl peroxide 2%–10% twice daily, and this will allow some time to arrange for dermatology follow-up should this prove insufficiently effective. Some patients may require the addition of topical retinoids, and for more severe cases oral antibiotics or hormonal therapy, all of which are best prescribed by a dermatologist based on the severity, type and distribution of the acne [94].

c. **Dry skin:** The association with lithium may be tenuous, but this is a treatable problem using moisturizing lotions and bath products containing colloidal oats as initial strategies. Difficult-to-manage cases should be referred to a dermatologist, as should cases where eczema is suspected.

d. **Psoriasis (new, or exacerbation):** For a patient with known psoriasis, there should be an honest discussion about the prospect of lithium exacerbating the condition, while also expressing the particular advantages of lithium for the patient and your willingness to work with their dermatologist to manage the problem. Treatment reviews in dermatology journals cite discontinuation of the offending agent as the initial strategy, but recent advances in psoriasis treatment, including new biological agents, may allow some patients to remain on lithium [95]. In certain cases, however, management of the psoriasis may be too difficult while the patient remains on lithium.

e. **Hair loss:** There has been a longstanding recommendation to consider a daily multivitamin with at least 100 mcg of selenium and 15 mg of zinc, but evidence for this is virtually nonexistent. Topical minoxidil is one of three United States FDA-approved treatments for male and female pattern hair loss, and should be tried since the problem may not relate to lithium (although lithium is blamed), and it may yet be effective even if lithium is the culprit. As soon as the complaint appears, topical 5% minoxidil should be started for men or women, and is over-the-counter in most countries. A 2% strength is available if scalp irritation occurs, but men and women typically remain on and tolerate the 5% strength, available in foam and liquid solutions [96]. Effects are most pronounced in the frontal regions of the scalp and at the vertex. Oral finasteride and other options can be considered, but must be initiated by a dermatologist.

The mechanisms by which lithium induces any cutaneous adverse effect are largely unknown, but hair loss has been studied in experimental models. As noted in Chapters 1 and 2, lithium is a potent inhibitor of GSK3-β activity, an aspect of its therapeutic mechanism, but one which causes problems leading to polyuria when lithium accumulates in collecting duct principal cells [35, 97, 98]. One consequence of GSK3-β inhibition is intracellular accumulation of β-catenin, a widely expressed protein involved in cellular adhesion and gene transcription [30]. In theory, lithium's effects should mitigate the impact of androgen-induced downregulation of intracellular β-catenin levels and promote hair growth [99, 100], so the fact that lithium is associated with alopecia is somewhat perplexing, and the mechanism unknown. The literature in this area is even more sparse than for other cutaneous problems, with the few trials recording this adverse effect describing small but nonsignificant differences from placebo [91, 93]. The prevalence of alopecia is also unclear since all of the literature is based on patient self-report. Nonetheless, older reviews cite alopecia rates of 10% for lithium, compared with 12% for VPA, and less than 6% for carbamazepine [101]. There are no systematic treatment trials, so management is the same as for other causes of alopecia (e.g. androgen-induced). Hair regrowth is a slow process – early detection by vigorous and repeated inquiry is the best method for attacking the problem before it gets to the point at which a patient wants to stop lithium.

Endocrine Effects (Hypothyroidism, Hyperparathyroidism, Hypercalcemia, Weight Gain), and Lack of Impact on Bone Density or Sexual Function

WHAT TO KNOW: ENDOCRINE ADVERSE EFFECTS

- The annual incidence of new onset hypothyroidism during lithium treatment is 1.5%, but may be 3-fold higher in women. L-thyroxine is the treatment of choice for hypothyroidism – lithium discontinuation is never necessary. Lithium is not associated with increased risk for Hashimoto's thyroiditis, Graves' disease or thyroid tumors. Cases of hyperthyroidism are likely to be incidental to lithium use and not due to a direct lithium effect.

- Lithium can alter the calcium sensing mechanism resulting in hyperparathyroidism. Routine serum calcium monitoring will identify this adverse effect, with ionized calcium and parathyroid hormone levels used for confirmation. Calcimimetic agents offer a nonsurgical treatment option. Lithium does not cause osteoporosis.

- Weight gain is primarily related to use of other psychotropics (e.g. valproate, antipsychotics) that carry weight gain liabilities, but can be due to lithium. GLP-1 agonists are the preferred agents for managing weight gain.

- Sexual dysfunction is common in stable BD patients related to multiple factors (mood, antipsychotics, medical comorbidity), all of which must be investigated. Lithium is not typically the cause. Erectile dysfunction may have central or peripheral causes but often responds to phosphodiesterase 5 (PDE_5) inhibitors (e.g. sildenafil, tadalafil, vardenafil).

The spectrum of endocrine and metabolic issues includes specific effects on thyroid or parathyroid function, along with weight gain and sexual dysfunction. The last item on this list, sexual dysfunction, is the most difficult of these adverse effects to assess, as numerous factors can contribute to patient complaints of sexual dissatisfaction, including depressed mood, the absence of hypomania, use of other psychiatric and nonpsychiatric medications that induce sexual dysfunction, and the impact of age-related medical comorbidities and lifestyle habits (e.g. smoking) [102, 103]. Moreover, the complaint is often addressed in the absence of objective findings. On the other hand, weight gain is easily tracked using a scale, and laboratory monitoring of thyroid stimulating hormone (TSH) and serum calcium readily permit identification of hypothyroidism, hyperparathyroidism and, occasionally, hyperthyroidism during long-term lithium treatment [2, 104, 105].

Lithium related sexual dysfunction is the least studied, but all of these issues have evidence based management strategies that can obviate the need for lithium discontinuation and ideally improve patient retention when implemented early.

1 Hypothyroidism and Hyperthyroidism

The association between lithium exposure and increased rates of hypothyroidism has been documented for over 50 years, but in that time frame important conclusions have become evident: (a) the presence of hypothyroidism is not a reason to avoid lithium or to discontinue it [106]; (b) lithium treatment is not associated with development of antithyroid antibodies consistent with Hashimoto's thyroiditis or Graves' disease, or higher rates of thyroid tumors [106, 107]; (c) TSH is a sufficient screening tool (Info Box 5.6) [108]. Lithium is associated with a 1.5% annual incidence of hypothyroidism in longer-term studies, but hyperthyroidism is relatively rare and more likely to be incidental to lithium use and not the product of lithium exposure. Using the Oxford University Hospitals National Health Service (NHS) Trust laboratory database, a group investigated the incidence of hyperthyroidism (defined as TSH < 0.2 mIU/l) in adult patients who had at least 2 TSH or lithium measurements between October 1, 1982, and March 31, 2014 (n = 1916), compared with controls without lithium exposure (n = 234,034) [109]. After adjustment for age, sex and a diagnosis of diabetes, use of lithium was not associated with hyperthyroidism (OR 1.22, 95% CI 0.96–1.55; p = 0.1010) or a raised adjusted calcium concentration (OR 1.08, 95% CI 0.88–1.34; p = 0.46) [109]. There is also one propensity score adjusted longitudinal cohort study published in 2016 that used UK electronic health records from 1995–2013 to examine a broad range of adverse effect outcomes in BD patients on olanzapine, quetiapine, valproate or lithium monotherapy [110]. The primary outcome measure was rate per 100 person-years at risk (PYAR) of the adverse effect. There were 41 cases of hyperthyroidism among the 2148 lithium treated patients (median duration of exposure 1.48 years), with a PYAR value of 0.78, a result that was not significantly different than for quetiapine (n = 1376), but was higher than olanzapine (n = 1477) or VPA (n = 1670) [110]. The authors of this paper note the inconsistent associations between lithium and hyperthyroidism in the literature, and suggest that the most prudent course of action given the rarity of these events is routine TSH monitoring. The scarcity of hyperthyroidism cases is reinforced by a 2019 review which found only 39 individual case reports, 3 case series and 10 cross-sectional, case–control or cohort studies. After excluding the 41 cases identified in the 2016 paper, the total number of cases from the reports/series was 46, and only 8 cases from the remaining 9 out of 10 cohort studies, although some reports mentioned additional numbers of subclinical hyperthyroidism patients with low TSH but normal free thyroxine levels (n = 7). When measured, antibodies were positive in less than 50% of patients, and the time course from starting lithium was highly variable, suggesting that many of the cases were due to other problems such as Hashimoto's disease or Graves' disease, which have prevalence rates of 5% and 0.5% respectively in the population. This is especially relevant given the absence of an association with hyperthyroidism in the Oxford University Trust database study, and the lack of association between lithium exposure and the development of antithyroid antibodies in other studies [107]. In all instances where a low TSH is detected, one should continue lithium, consult with a primary care provider about obtaining other measures (e.g. thyroxine [T_4], triiodothyronine [T_3]), discuss when one should repeat the TSH, and, if low, any necessary laboratory work-up for Hashimoto's disease (e.g. antithyroid peroxidase antibodies) or for Graves' disease (e.g. thyroid-stimulating antibodies) [111]. Depending on the etiology of hyperthyroidism, appropriate treatment may proceed and is not influenced by the presence of lithium.

Info Box 5.6 **Essential Facts about Lithium and Hypothyroidism**

a. **Can lithium be used in a patient with a prior history of hypothyroidism?** A history of hypothyroidism is not a reason to deprive a patient of lithium therapy [17].

b. **Can lithium be continued in a patient with new onset hypothyroidism?** The development of hypothyroidism is not a reason to discontinue lithium therapy [17].

c. **What is the annual incidence of hypothyroidism during lithium therapy?** In long-term follow-up studies, the annual incidence of newly diagnosed hypothyroidism is approximately 1.5%, with females having 3 times higher rates than males [112].

d. **Is lithium associated with higher rates of anti-thyroid antibodies or thyroid tumors?** Long-term lithium treatment is not associated with increased prevalence of autoantibodies to thyroid peroxidase, thyroglobulin or the TSH receptor, compared with age- and gender-matched peers [107, 112, 113]. There is also no association with increased risk of developing thyroid tumors [106].

e. **What are the mechanisms by which lithium induces hypothyroidism?** The Na^+/I^- symporter (NIS) transports iodide into the thyroid cell where it is oxidized by thyroid peroxidase (TPO), and TPO then iodinates select tyrosine residues on thyroglobulin (Tg) [114]. Tg is the intracellular repository of inactive forms of iodine and thyroid hormones (T_4 and T_3) in the lumen of the thyroid follicle. T_4 and T_3 are attached to Tg after synthesis, and this aggregate forms the colloid within the follicle.

Stimulation by TSH causes portions of the colloid to move from the follicular lumen into the surrounding thyroid follicular epithelial cell by endocytosis where it is cleaved by proteases to separate Tg from T_4 and T_3, thus allowing T_4 and T_3 to be secreted. Lithium does not alter iodide uptake or efflux [115], but lithium is an NIS substrate, leading to accumulation in the thyroid gland at levels 3–4 times higher than in plasma [116]. There are multiple reversible effects, although occasional patients may have persistent hypothyroidism after lithium is stopped due to other causes [117]. The most prominent effects of lithium are:

i. inhibition of T_4 and T_3 release from the thyroid gland [116]

ii. altered conformation of Tg, with inhibited coupling of its iodinated tyrosine residues to form T_4 and T_3 [114]

iii. altered binding of T_4 and T_3 to hypothalamic receptors thereby downregulating expression of genes for certain receptor isoforms [114].

f. **What is the management strategy for hypothyroidism?**

i. L-thyroxine is the treatment of choice, not lithium discontinuation, and is started based on the TSH [108]. The normal TSH range is 0.35 to 4.5 mIU/l, with 4.5–9.9 mIU/l designated as subclinical hypothyroidism [108]. There is debate about these ranges, and the upper limit of normal for younger females might be lower (2.5 mIU/l) [118]. The debate about "normal" ranges for subgroups argues for a flexible treatment approach. For example, a patient with TSH 4.0 mIU/l and significant symptoms of hypothyroidism might do better with a TSH closer to 1.00 mIU/l.

ii. Subclinical hypothyroidism is sometimes not treated, but middle-aged patients with subclinical hypothyroidism may have measurable cognitive dysfunction and nonspecific symptoms such as fatigue and altered mood [108]. While the association between hypothyroidism and depression is not robust in the general population, BD patients are unique in this regard [119]. A 1999 study noted that BD patients with lower mean serum free T_4 levels experienced more affective episodes and greater depression severity, and a follow-up study by the same investigators noted that lithium treated BD patients who required depression treatment had a significantly higher adjusted mean TSH level (4.4 mIU/l) compared with those not requiring depression intervention (2.4 mIU/l) [120, 121]. Other data indicate that elevated pre-treatment TSH values in depressed BD patients may slow treatment response [122].

iii. There is no indication for routine thyroid ultrasound or autoantibody testing, and the need for laboratory measures beyond TSH should be dictated by the clinician prescribing L-thyroxine and clinical course. The use of T_3 levels or the T_4:T_3 ratio is a subject of debate, but there is recognition that the normal T_4:T_3 ratio of 3 is often not achieved with L-thyroxine, with one large surveillance study (n = 1800) noting a mean ratio of 4 among patients who underwent thyroidectomy and were receiving L-thyroxine monotherapy [123]. The American Thyroid Association, British Thyroid Association and European Thyroid Association held a joint conference on November 3, 2019, and published a consensus document that discussed methods to characterize the need for T_4/T_3 combination therapy with clinical trials [124].

2 *Hypercalcemia, Hyperparathyroidism and Protective Effects on Bone Health*

Hypothyroidism is not challenging to treat in most instances, and is never a reason to discontinue lithium or a reason to avoid lithium since it represents one of the more manageable issues during lithium therapy [17]. Although the association between lithium exposure and hypothyroidism is clear, studies on lithium's impact on calcium metabolism and rates of hyperparathyroidism are proportionately fewer. In 2012, a systematic review and meta-analysis concerning a range of lithium related adverse effects found a number of relevant published studies (4 cohort, 14 case-control, 36 case reports, 6 cross-sectional), but the total sample size from these publications was modest (n = 699) [91]. The meta-analysis found that total calcium was increased by 0.09 mmol/l (95% CI 0.02–0.17 mmol/l, p = 0.009), and parathyroid hormone (PTH) by 7.32 pg/ml (95% CI 3.42–11.23 pg/ml, p < 0.0001) [91]. This result was at odds with the larger Oxford University Hospitals NHS Trust laboratory database study (n = 1916) which found no increased lithium related risk for raised albumin-adjusted calcium concentration (OR 1.08, 95% CI 0.88–1.34; p = 0.46) after adjustment for age, sex and a diagnosis of diabetes [109]. Despite the apparent discrepancy, there are sufficient human and animal data to indicate that lithium exposure can induce hypercalcemia through a number of mechanisms, including increased gastrointestinal and renal calcium reabsorption, a direct impact on calcium sensing, and secondary or independent effects on parathyroid gland function [125]. A case-control study of 112 adults with BD found that the lithium treated cohort (n = 56, mean 60.8 ± 74.8 months exposure) had higher ionized calcium but not PTH levels [126]. The prevalence of hypercalcemia and primary hyperparathyroidism is 2.5-fold greater among women and is also age dependent, with a 3-fold higher prevalence in patients > 80 years of age compared with those ages 20–29 [125]. Hypercalcemia prevalence in the general population is approximately 1–2%, with 90% of the cases due to primary hyperparathyroidism and malignancy-associated hypercalcemia. The prevalence of primary hyperparathyroidism in the general population ranges from 0.2% to 0.8%, although it may be as high as 2.1% in postmenopausal women [127]. For lithium treated patients there are limited prevalence estimates, but the 2012 meta-analysis found an absolute risk for hypercalcemia and hyperparathyroidism of 10% [91], although the case-control study cited above reported a hyperparathyroidism prevalence of 8.6%, and 24.1% for hypercalcemia [126].

In-Depth 5.2 Lithium's Impact on Parathyroid Function

In a manner that mirrors lithium related issues in collecting duct principal cells, lithium can enter the parathyroid gland and inhibit GSK3-β activity, but in this instance GSK3-β inhibition leads to disruption of the calcium-sensing receptor pathway in parathyroid chief cells. The result is a shifting of the PTH set point to the right so that a higher serum calcium level is required to suppress PTH secretion [128]. This effect is measurable with brief exposures, although not clinically relevant at that stage, and is reversible upon discontinuation [125, 128]. Chronic lithium therapy in a subset of patients appears to induce more durable changes in parathyroid gland function due to unmasking of latent hyperparathyroidism in those with a subclinical parathyroid adenoma, or some direct process leading to multiglandular hyperparathyroidism (i.e. hyperplasia). Duration of lithium therapy has been correlated with increasing parathyroid gland mass, but when parathyroid hyperplasia or adenomas become evident the problem often persists even in the absence of lithium use. The clinical picture is thus identical to that of primary hyperparathyroidism, and the approach is the same: lithium discontinuation is not the initial strategy, and in some instances of no value [125].

On the basis of the available data, the earliest impact of lithium will be seen on serum calcium levels, hence the logic for routine monitoring outlined in Chapter 4. Traditionally, the management of hyperparathyroidism relied on surgery as the gold standard approach, and in the hands of experienced parathyroid surgeons the outcomes are excellent (Info Box 5.7) [125, 129]. As most patients are diagnosed when asymptomatic, the indications for surgery in this group are based on studies which show that a third of these individuals have disease progression and complications (e.g. renal stones, osteoporosis). The consensus surgical criteria for asymptomatic patients include: age < 50 years; serum calcium more than 1 mg/dl above the upper limit of normal; bone density T-score less than −2.5 at the lumbar spine, femoral neck, total hip, or distal one-third radius in peri- or postmenopausal women, and Z-score less than −2.5 in premenopausal women and men younger than 50 years [129]. Patients who do not meet these criteria are candidates for surveillance, but there is increasing evidence that calcimimetic agents developed for CKD-related secondary hyperparathyroidism (e.g. cinacalcet) are effective for lithium-induced hyperparathyroidism, and can be used in those who do not meet surgery criteria, are poor surgical candidates, or who are wary of surgery [125]. Calcimimetics allosterically activate the calcium-sensing receptor, thereby counteracting lithium's action, with multiple case reports documenting the use of cinacalcet as a nonsurgical option in lieu of parathyroidectomy for lithium treated patients [125, 128, 130]. Prior to the development of calcimimetics, there were limited nonsurgical options to manage primary hyperparathyroidism, so lithium discontinuation may have been considered necessary when surgery wasn't feasible despite evidence that stopping lithium may not reverse parathyroid hyperplasia or adenoma formation. Hypercalcemia and hyperparathyroidism are no longer considered reasons to stop lithium, and ongoing serial monitoring of serum calcium will detect these problems at a stage that allows for early treatment.

Info Box 5.7 The Approach to Elevated Serum Calcium and Hyperparathyroidism

a. **Initial elevated serum calcium:** Sporadic elevated total calcium values can be seen, so obtaining a repeat measure in 3–6 months is reasonable to look for persistence. When the total calcium remains elevated, a more specific test must be obtained. Calcium is highly bound to serum proteins such as albumin and in prior years formulas were used to adjust for albumin levels, but an ionized calcium assay is the confirmatory test to order as it measures free calcium levels [126]. The normal ranges for total calcium and ionized calcium are below:

	Lower limit of normal	Upper limit of normal
Total calcium	8.5 mg/dl (2.2 mmol/l)	10.5 mg/dl (2.8 mmol/l)
Ionized calcium	4.4 mg/dl (1.1 mmol/l)	5.2 mg/dl (1.3 mmol/l)

b. **Elevated ionized calcium**: The follow-up test to order when ionized calcium is high is a parathyroid hormone (PTH) level, with subsequent referral to an endocrinologist for assessment. A preliminary discussion with the consultant about the benefit of lithium for that patient and need to remain on lithium might avert a reflexive recommendation to discontinue lithium. The normal range for PTH is 10–65 pg/ml, with some variation between laboratories. It is worth noting that patients with CKD can have elevated PTH (secondary hyperparathyroidism), but this will occur in the context of hyperphosphatemia; hypocalcemia, not hypercalcemia; and low levels of calcitriol (1,25-(OH)$_2$ Vitamin D$_3$) [131].

c. **Work-up:** Further testing to assess the extent of the problem and rule out other causes (e.g. genetic, malignancy, etc.) will be determined by the endocrinologist [125, 128].

d. **Treatment:**

   i. Lithium discontinuation is not necessary, and may be of no benefit in instances of glandular hyperplasia or parathyroid adenoma [128].

   ii. Surgery is recommended for all symptomatic patients [129], but routine serum calcium monitoring during lithium therapy will mostly diagnose patients who are asymptomatic. The consensus surgical criteria for asymptomatic patients include: age < 50 years; serum calcium more than 1 mg/dl above the upper limit of normal; bone density T-score less than −2.5 at the lumbar spine, femoral neck, \total hip, or distal one-third radius in peri- or postmenopausal women, and Z-score less than −2.5 in premenopausal women and men younger than 50 years [129]. With modern intraoperative imaging and surgical techniques, outcomes in experienced hands are excellent.

   iii. Calcimimetic treatment is considered in those who do not meet surgery criteria, are poor surgical candidates, or who refuse surgery. Multiple reports document the value of calcimimetics such as cinacalcet for lithium-associated hyperparathyroidism [125, 128, 130].

Patients with BD have a number of medical comorbidities, especially cardiometabolic and renal (independent of lithium use) [62, 132], but concerns were raised about bone health over the past 20 years by studies associating psychotropic exposure and increased fracture risk among older BD patients [133], and by literature noting that depression is a risk factor for poor bone health and osteoporosis, mediated by lifestyle factors such as poor diet and lack of physical activity [134]. Among psychotropic medications, sedating agents (e.g. benzodiazepines, quetiapine, mirtazapine) increase fracture risk due to falls; however, potent serotonin reuptake inhibitors block serotonin transporters on osteoblasts and osteocytes resulting in osteopenia [135], and prolactin elevation by D_2 antagonist antipsychotics induces hypogonadism in males and females that can result in demineralization [136]. To examine diagnosis related risk, investigators used Taiwanese National Health Insurance medical claims data from 1997–2013 to look at rates of bone fracture in 3705 BD patients and 10 demographically matched controls without BD [137]. After adjusting for covariates, BD patients had a 32% higher fracture risk than controls (17.6% vs 11.7%; HR 1.32, 95% CI 1.20–1.45, $p < 0.001$). Interestingly the HR was greater among BD patients with a history of psychiatric hospitalization (n = 847, 22.9%), with a 76% increased risk of fracture

(HR = 1.76, 95% CI 1.50–2.06) compared with controls, while BD patients without history of psychiatric hospitalization had only a 20% increased risk (HR = 1.20, 95% CI 1.08–1.34). Other established risk factors such as female gender, older age, previous exposure to benzodiazepines or GABA-agonist hypnotics (e.g. zolpidem), substance abuse and a diagnosis of osteoporosis were also associated with greater risk for bone fracture, but higher cumulative exposure to antipsychotics or mood stabilizers did not increase risk [137].

Although the Taiwanese study did not find an association between increased mood stabilizer use and fracture risk, there is a significant body of preclinical animal studies documenting that lithium directly improves bone mineral density and stimulates bone formation as a consequence of GSK3-β inhibition. As mentioned in the context of hair loss, GSK3-β inhibition by lithium increases the intracellular accumulation of β-catenin, a widely expressed protein involved in cellular adhesion and gene transcription [30]. For osteoblasts, the higher level of β-catenin activity during lithium treatment has the potential to improve fracture healing in later phases of repair once mesenchymal cells are committed to the osteoblast lineage [138]. Moreover, in a genetic knockout mouse model of osteoporosis related to inadequate osteoblast renewal, lithium exposure restored bone metabolism and bone mass to levels close to that of wild type mice [139]. Other 2nd messenger pathways are also implicated, with a 2020 review concluding that preclinical data indicating lithium's skeletal protective effects are exciting, but validation from human trials is needed to assess any effect in clinical use [140].

In an attempt to isolate drug related effects, a group used the Danish Psychiatric Central Research Register to identify 22,912 adults (median age 50.4 years) with an initial BD diagnosis from January 1, 1996 to January 1, 2019, and matched them with 5 age- and sex-matched individuals randomly selected from the general population [134]. Those with a schizophrenia spectrum disorder diagnosis prior to receiving a BD diagnosis and those with osteoporosis prior to the index date were excluded. For the BD cohort, treatment periods with lithium, antipsychotics, VPA, and lamotrigine were examined, and the primary outcome was a new diagnosis of osteoporosis for those age ≥ 40 as identified by hospital diagnosis codes and prescribed medications. After a median follow-up of 7.68 years, the incidence of osteoporosis per 1000 person-years was 14% higher in the BD cohort (hazard rate ratio (HRR) 1.14, 95% CI 1.08–1.20), with rates of 8.70 (95% CI 8.28–9.14) for the BD patients vs. 7.90 (95% CI 7.73–8.07) among matched controls. Patients in the BD cohort were often on polytherapy, and during the period of observation 38.2% received lithium, 73.6% received an antipsychotic, 16.8% received VPA, and

33.1% received lamotrigine. Based on periods of exposure, BD patients on lithium had 38% decreased risk of osteoporosis (HRR, 0.62; 95% CI 0.53–0.72) compared with patients not receiving lithium, while treatment with antipsychotics, VPA and lamotrigine was not associated with reduced risk [134]. Though numerous temporal factors can contribute to fracture risk (e.g. sedating medications, mood states), the Danish study is the first to link lithium use with improved bone health as noted by the 14% lower osteoporosis rate in lithium exposed BD patients, thus providing the first human evidence of the effect seen in animal models. This finding from a well-designed case-control trial, combined with lithium's neuroprotective effects [7], provides further support for lithium's preferential use in older BD patients.

3   *Weight Gain*

A 2020 review on interventions for weight loss in BD noted that 68% of treatment-seeking BD patients are overweight or obese, but clinical trials in this area are woefully inadequate, with significant methodological issues [141]. Cardiovascular disease is the leading cause of premature death in BD, with BD patients expiring at least 10 years earlier than demographically matched peers. Contributors to increased mortality include illness-related factors (i.e. mania or depression), treatment-related factors (weight implications and other side effects of medications) [142] and lifestyle factors (physical inactivity, poor diet, smoking, substance use) [141]. The approaches to weight management in BD patients are very similar to those for patients with schizophrenia spectrum disorders and include nonpharmacological strategies (i.e. dietary, lifestyle), pharmacological interventions (i.e. weight loss medications, medication switching) and bariatric surgery (Info Box 5.8). Unfortunately, the literature for BD individuals is not sufficiently robust to suggest one particular option, but clinical action must be taken. Obesity not only contributes to medical comorbidity, it was also the 5th leading cause of adverse effect related lithium discontinuation in the Norrbotten study [21]. Beyond the effect on lithium adherence, weight gain may have direct neuropsychiatric consequences. The literature is clear that a significant association exists between obesity and depressive episodes and impaired cognitive function in BD patients, an effect likely mediated by higher levels of systemic inflammation [62, 143].

That lithium treatment may be associated with weight gain has been known for 50 years, but an important point to consider is that weight gain is greater during exposure to VPA or certain SGAs, especially olanzapine and quetiapine [91, 144]. A 2012 meta-analysis examining lithium related adverse effects located 14 studies with sufficient weight data to estimate the impact of treatment, and concluded that lithium did increase the risk of > 7% weight gain compared with placebo (OR = 1.89; 95% CI 1.27–2.82; p = 0.002); however, it should be noted that this risk *was 3 times lower than that for olanzapine* (n = 285; OR 0.32, 95% CI 0.21–0.49, p < 0.0001) [91]. The 2016 UK electronic health records study of adverse effects among BD patients on monotherapy with olanzapine, quetiapine, VPA or lithium found that the rates of weight gain exceeding 15% on valproate, olanzapine and quetiapine were 62–84% higher than for lithium: VPA HR 1.62; 95% CI 1.31–2.01, p < 0.001; olanzapine HR 1.84; 95% CI 1.47–2.30, p < 0.001; quetiapine HR 1.67; 95% CI 1.24–2.20, p < 0.001 [110].

Although weight gain can occur with lithium, it lacks the association with other forms of metabolic dysfunction seen with many SGAs. A cross-sectional study of 129 BD patients aged 18–85 years followed at tertiary care clinics in Montreal compared mean BMI and metabolic syndrome prevalence between lithium treated patients and those not on lithium [145]. The mean age of the sample was 47.9 years, 39.12% were obese and 40.4% met metabolic syndrome criteria. Mean BMI was not significantly different between lithium and non-lithium using cohorts (29.10 ± 6.70 kg/m^2 vs. 30.2 ± 8.57 kg/m^2, p = 0.184), and the lithium and non-lithium groups were also not significantly different in the prevalence of obesity or metabolic syndrome. However, compared with the non-lithium group, lithium users had lower hemoglobin A1C (5.24 ± 0.53 vs. 6.01 ± 1.83, p = 0.006) and lower serum triglycerides (129.2 ± 77.9 mg/dl vs. 177.8 ± 110.6 mg/dl, p = 0.020), although it should be noted that lithium non-users comprised a greater proportion of antipsychotic-treated individuals. The important conclusion is that there is a high prevalence of obesity and metabolic syndrome among BD patients, but this did not appear to be specifically associated with lithium use when compared with those not on lithium due to the weight gain liability often encountered with non-lithium therapies (e.g. SGAs, valproate) [145].

Info Box 5.8 Approach to Weight Gain

a. **Concomitant medications:** If possible, avoid antipsychotics with high weight gain liability unless clinically necessary (e.g. need for clozapine to manage treatment resistant mania). For bipolar depression, lurasidone, cariprazine and lumateperone are preferable to quetiapine or the olanzapine/fluoxetine combination [146, 147]. Lamotrigine has low risk for weight gain but cannot be used for acute bipolar depression due to the prolonged titration required to minimize risk of Stevens–Johnson Syndrome. Divalproex is also associated with weight gain, so clinical assessment of the need for combined therapy should be considered; however, there are many patients who require lithium and VPA concurrently for adequate mood control [11, 148].

b. Diet and lifestyle modification: Educational initiatives in these areas have been designed for patients with schizophrenia, but a 2020 Cochrane review of interventions for the management of obesity in people with bipolar disorder lamented that no study met review criteria due to quality issues [141]. Nonetheless, patients should be offered whatever options are available for nutritional counseling, exercise and other lifestyle modifications to promote weight management.

c. Metformin: Metformin has been studied for antipsychotic-induced weight gain in adolescents and adults, primarily in those on olanzapine or clozapine, with greatest benefit when started at the onset of therapy [149]. There is one case report of metformin for weight gain in a patient on lithium monotherapy in which the patient lost 8 kg after 6 months on metformin 500 mg BID [150]. As many BD-1 and all SAD-BT patients will be on lithium plus an antipsychotic, start metformin as early as possible. The slow early titration is to minimize gastrointestinal adverse effects (e.g. diarrhea). If these develop, use an extended release formulation. Vitamin B12 levels should be checked yearly. Metformin has no risk of lactic acidosis with eGFR $\geq$ 30 ml/min, but use caution as eGFR drops below 45 ml/min [151]. **Suggested adult metformin titration:**

   i. 500 mg PO QAM with food x 3 weeks

   ii. 500 mg BID with meals x 1 week

   iii. 500 mg QAM (with food) / 1000 mg qpm (with dinner) x 1 week

   iv. 1000 mg BID with meals

d. GLP-1 agonist: Originally developed for type 2 DM but approved as subcutaneous injections for weight loss in *nondiabetics* (semaglutide) [152, 153]. There is no contraindication to use in patients on lithium, and there are studies of GLP-1 agonists used in patients on clozapine noting significant weight loss [154]. Tirzepatide is an agonist at GLP-1 and glucose-dependent insulinotropic polypeptide (GIP) receptors with pending approval for weight loss.

   i. Indications: Obesity (BMI $\geq$ 30 kg/m^2) or overweight (BMI $\geq$ 27 kg/m^2) with at least one weight-related comorbid condition (e.g. hypertension, type 2 diabetes mellitus or dyslipidemia).

   ii. Adverse effects concerns: Pancreatitis, rapid weight loss inducing cholelithiasis, cholecystitis. Association with thyroid C-cell tumors including medullary thyroid carcinoma (MTC) was seen in rodent models but the relevance is unknown. Cases of MTC with liraglutide were reported in the postmarketing period, but the data are insufficient to establish or exclude a causal relationship. There are reports of new or worsening depression or suicidality - patients should report any mood changes immediately.

e. Bariatric surgery: For many individuals, this is a life-saving procedure, and having a mental illness such as BD or even schizophrenia does not automatically preclude one from consideration [155]. Obese patients who have failed the above strategies should be referred for consideration, preferably to a group who has previously worked with BD or schizophrenia spectrum patients and will consider each case individually.

i. **Considerations:** The primary concern in lithium treated patients is the multiple changes to diet prior to and after surgery (e.g. low sodium diet), along with alterations in body weight and composition that impact lithium clearance [155]. Postoperative lithium levels can increase 2-fold to 5-fold regardless of the type of bariatric procedure, a situation that can result in lithium toxicity (see Chapter 3) [76, 155–161].

ii. **Lithium dosing:** Once the bariatric surgery is performed, immediately lower postoperative doses by 50%, and obtain a level 1 week after the surgery. Future lithium dosing can then be adjusted to mirror the baseline level. Even after the initial postoperative period of dosage adjustment, recent papers recommend rechecking the eGFR and lithium level weekly for the first 6 weeks, and extending the interval to every 2 weeks for the next 6 months as ongoing weight loss may further alter lithium clearance [155].

The biological mechanism by which lithium causes weight gain is unknown, but increased appetite is the net result, and impaired satiety will be exacerbated by use of other medications that induce weight gain. The reported range of weight gain after 1 year is highly variable, but values of 4–10 kg are cited in papers dating back 20 years, although significant outliers may skew these findings [144]. As discussed in Info Box 5.8, the clinician should exercise discretion in the use of SGAs, eschewing those with significant weight gain liability as much as possible [142, 147]. Diet and lifestyle modification should be offered in whatever form is available to the patient based on local expertise. At the onset of lithium therapy, strong consideration should be given to starting metformin, a medication extensively studied for moderating SGA-related weight gain, especially as many BD-1 and SAD-BT patients will be on combination treatment with an SGA [150]. For obese patients, GLP-1 agonists (e.g. subcutaneous semaglutide) are approved for weight loss in nondiabetics with a BMI ≥ 30 kg/m^2, or for persons who are overweight (BMI ≥ 27 kg/m^2) who have at least one weight-related comorbid condition (e.g. hypertension, type 2 diabetes mellitus, or dyslipidemia) [152, 153]. This represents an option open to anyone, even those with severe mental illnesses such as treatment resistant schizophrenia or mania patients on clozapine [149, 162, 163]. (Tirzepatide is an agonist at GLP-1 and glucose-dependent insulinotropic polypeptide (GIP) receptors with pending approval for weight loss.) Lastly, having a psychiatric disorder does not preclude referral for bariatric surgery. Once surgery is performed, clinicians must decrease the lithium dose postoperatively to prevent postoperative lithium toxicity (see Info Box 5.8, and also Chapter 3, Section E **"Other Factors Affecting Lithium Levels"** for details).

4   *Sexual Dysfunction*

Sexual function is an important part of human experience, and many factors (medical comorbidity, smoking, medication, mood state) contribute to dysfunction among patients with BD or SAD-BT [102, 164]. A 2015 review covering sexual dysfunction in stable BD patients lamented that this is an under-researched area and deserves greater attention [103]. One of the few systematic studies in this area was an assessment of sexual functioning in 100 clinically stable BD adults with minimal depressive or manic symptoms receiving treatment at an academic psychiatric clinic in Chandigarh, India [102]. The mean sample age was 44.3 years, and 18% of the subjects had at least one medical comorbidity (hypertension, diabetes mellitus, hypothyroidism). The mean duration of lithium use was 9.97 ± 8.3 years, and mean lithium dose 799.5 ± 251.4 mg/d [102]. The sample was 85% male and 98% married, with 52% self-identifying as smokers, and 85% were on lithium monotherapy. Using the Arizona Sexual Experience scale (ASEX), sexual dysfunction was defined as an ASEX total score ≥ 19, or a score ≥ 5 on any 1 item or a score of ≥ 4 on any 3 items. In this study, 37% had some form of sexual dysfunction; the rates did not differ between males and females and were nearly identical when analyzed separately for the 85 subjects on lithium monotherapy. Compared with those without sexual dysfunction, those with sexual dysfunction were older ($p = 0.003$), had a higher number of other lithium related adverse effects (2.9 vs. 1.4; $p < 0.001$), and poorer medication adherence. This study mirrors those from the older literature indicating that sexual dysfunction is a prevalent problem in stable BD patients, and that it must be addressed by routine patient inquiry and treated [165]. A comprehensive 2022 review of the epidemiological and biological association between lithium exposure and sexual dysfunction noted that lithium may decrease desire and arousal for all genders, that concurrent benzodiazepine use exacerbates this problem, and that reversible erectile dysfunction (ED) has been described [165]. Preclinical studies associate lithium's impact on erectile function to both central and peripheral mechanisms, with the latter related to effects on 2nd messenger systems, especially prostaglandin physiology [165]. Supporting the hypothesis that lithium may cause an imbalance in prostaglandin production resulting in impaired endothelial relaxation response, exposure to indomethacin, a cyclooxygenase (COX) inhibitor, reversed these effects in an animal model. Moreover, the one double-blind, placebo-controlled clinical trial for lithium related ED in 32 stable male BD patients found that 6 weeks of aspirin 80 mg TID significantly improved lithium related ED compared with placebo as measured by the International Index for Erectile Function [166].

289

In-Depth 5.3 Erectile Dysfunction Is Prevalent in Bipolar Disorder

A Taiwanese study of 5150 adult males newly diagnosed with BD from 2000 to 2010 compared new onset ED rates and the associations with psychotropic exposure with demographically matched peers without BD [164]. The mean sample age was 36.71 ± 12.74 years, and the BD group had higher rates of a number of medical comorbidities compared with the healthy controls, including hypertension (15.88% vs. 12.37%) and dyslipidemia (13.13% vs. 11.87%). After adjusting for obesity, medical comorbidities and alcohol use disorders, BD patients were two times more likely to develop ED than controls (HR 1.95, 95% CI 1.47–2.58, p < 0.0001) (Figure 5.4) [164]. Independent risk factors included hypertension (HR 2.23) and dyslipidemia (HR 1.57); however, not being treated with a mood stabilizer (HR 2.22) or an antipsychotic (HR 2.26) did not moderate the relationship between ED and the BD diagnosis, stressing the concept that issues inherent to the BD patient population contribute to any form of sexual dysfunction, including ED. Importantly, exposure to VPA increased ED risk almost 6-fold (HR 5.73), and carbamazepine 3-fold (HR 3.41), but lithium exposure did not increase ED risk [164].

Figure 5.4 Proportion of individuals without new onset erectile dysfunction following a new bipolar disorder diagnosis among a cohort of 5150 Taiwanese males aged 15–64, and compared with 10,300 matched general population controls [164]

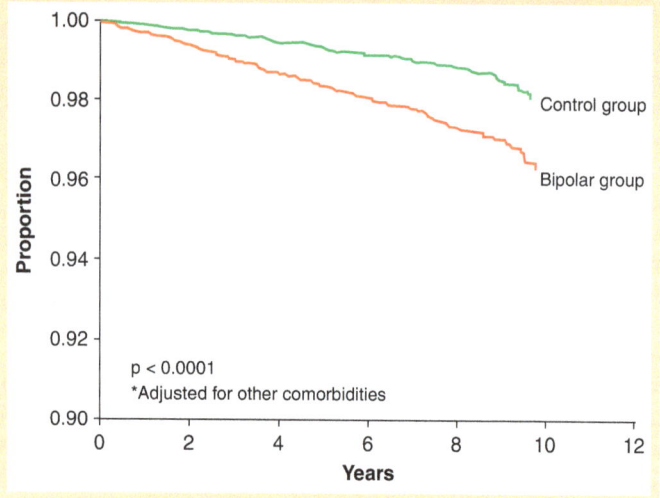

(Adapted from: P. H. Hou, F. C. Mao, G. R. Chang, et al. [2018]. Newly diagnosed bipolar disorder and the subsequent risk of erectile dysfunction: A nationwide cohort study. *J Sex Med*, 15, 183–191.)

The conclusion from Taiwanese data and other studies is that ED and other forms of sexual dysfunction are common in BD patients, and that ongoing discussion is needed to pinpoint treatment approaches, especially when there is a temporal association between sexual dysfunction and mood states or certain medications. COX inhibitors may treat ED specifically attributable to lithium, but ongoing use of aspirin presents concerns about bleeding risk due to antiplatelet activity. Fortunately, erectile dysfunction from psychotropics responds to the use of phosphodiesterase 5 (PDE$_5$) inhibitors widely prescribed for this purpose since 1998 (e.g. sildenafil, tadalafil, vardenafil) [167]. Although these agents are generally well tolerated, all PDE$_5$ inhibitors contain contraindications to use with nitrates or related vasodilating medications or with guanylate cyclase inhibitors used for pulmonary hypertension, due to the risk of significant hypotension. PDE$_5$ inhibitors are typically prescribed by the primary care provider to permit screening for important drug–drug interactions or medical conditions. As sexual dysfunction is prevalent in BD patients, clinicians must talk about this important area to identify causes, reframe medication related concerns that clearly appear to be driven by mood states (e.g. depression, or absence of hypomania), and offer suggested treatment options including removal of potential offending medications (e.g. benzodiazepines). Lithium is but one factor that may underlie ED complaints, but one should reinforce the benefits of lithium, educate that ED can be caused by other mood stabilizing medications (e.g. VPA), smoking or medical comorbidities (e.g. hypertension, dyslipidemia) and that there is treatment in the form of PDE$_5$ inhibitors. Again, the goal is to maintain patients on lithium and avert the potential for decompensation related to refusal or medication switching (Info Box 5.9) [168].

Info Box 5.9 **Lithium, Sexual Dysfunction and Bipolar Disorder**

a. **Establish a pre-lithium baseline:** It is important to appreciate that ED and other forms of sexual dysfunction are common in BD patients. In clinical practice it may be difficult to determine the exact cause of a sexual complaint for a patient, given the large number of factors that impact sexual functioning; however, establishing a pretreatment baseline greatly assists with future assessment.

b. **Complaints arising during lithium treatment:** When complaints are elicited, attempt to explore to what extent any issue pre-dated lithium use, with the aim of averting patient insistence that lithium is the sole cause, and explore any temporal relationship with use of other medications or with mood states.

c. **Approach to complaints of low arousal:** This is usually due to other factors than lithium, especially mood state (depression or the absence of hypomania), other psychotropics (due to sedation or endocrine effects) or medical comorbidity. The course of action depends greatly on the suspected etiology.

d. Approach to complaints of erectile dysfunction: Medical conditions with vascular consequences (e.g. hypertension, dyslipidemia, diabetes mellitus), smoking, psychotropics, nonpsychiatric medications (antihypertensives) and lithium are all possibilities. Lithium's impact on erectile function appears related to effects on second messenger systems, especially prostaglandin physiology. Fortunately, regardless of etiology, the class of phosphodiesterase 5 (PDE$_5$) inhibitors (e.g. sildenafil, tadalafil, vardenafil) are generally effective [167]. Clinicians should consult with the patient's primary care provider to rule out any medical contraindications before prescribing such medications.

E | Gastrointestinal and Oral Adverse Effects (Diarrhea, Nausea, Altered Taste and Dry Mouth)

WHAT TO KNOW: GASTROINTESTINAL AND ORAL ADVERSE EFFECTS

- Diarrhea and nausea can be dose related, but there are other strategies to manage these issues.
- Nausea is related to lithium ion absorption in the proximal jejunum. Switching from standard lithium to an extended release preparation or taking lithium with dinner helps mitigate nausea.
- Diarrhea is related to ion absorption in the lower gastrointestinal tract. Switching from an extended release preparation (which delivers lithium distally) to standard lithium or taking lithium with dinner helps resolve this problem.
- Taste abnormalities are very uncommon (< 1%), and may relate to variations in expression of amiloride-sensitive forms of ENaC in taste buds that signal salty taste. Whether amiloride can remedy this in the rare patient with this complaint is not known.
- Dry mouth is an uncommon complaint (< 5%), and the majority of patients who have dry mouth are relating a problem due to thirst (from polyuria) or direct effects of other medications. Both of these possibilities should be investigated.

1 *Diarrhea and Nausea*

Diarrhea during lithium use has been described for decades, and 13% of those who stopped lithium for a somatic adverse effect in the 2018 Norrbotten study did so for this reason [21]. That diarrhea was the leading somatic cause of lithium discontinuation either speaks to a lack of clinical attention to this problem, or lack of expertise in managing this complaint. The primary hypothesis for the induction of loose stools or diarrhea relates to lithium ion delivery to the large intestine, an issue that was problematic with older sustained release preparations with extremely long T_{Max} values (e.g. 12 h), but is seen less with current sustained release formulations that have T_{Max} values of 3–6 h. Changes in drug preparations over the years may be one reason that the literature presents a broad range of estimates for diarrhea incidence, but papers do consistently note an association with higher lithium levels (6–28%) [169–171]. The relevance of the serum level to diarrhea complaints was documented in a 1988 study which described a correlation between diarrhea and lithium levels > 0.80 mEq/l (Figure 5.5) [170]. A 2012 40 week double-blind extension of a 12 week lithium vs. aripiprazole BD-1 maintenance trial reported a 13.2% incidence of diarrhea, although 35% of lithium treated subjects had mean serum levels during the last 4 weeks of the extension phase that exceeded

Figure 5.5 Association between complaints of diarrhea and serum lithium level [170]

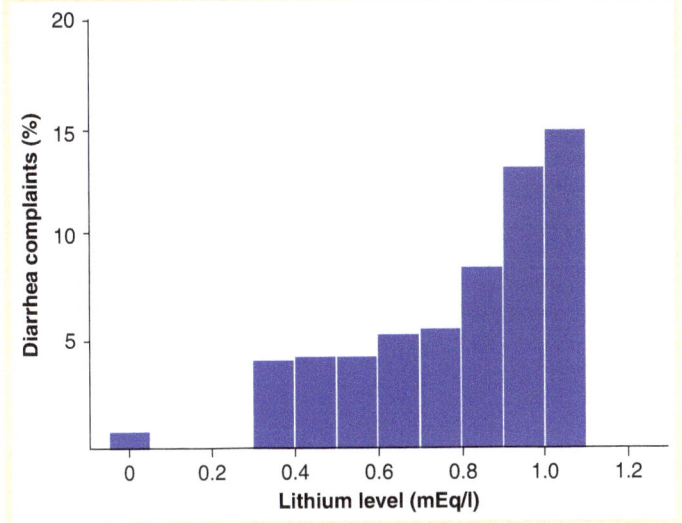

(Adapted from: P. Vestergaard, I. Poulstrup and M. Schou [1988]. Prospective studies on a lithium cohort. 3. Tremor, weight gain, diarrhea, psychological complaints. *Acta Psychiatr Scand*, 78, 434–441.)

0.80 mEq/l [172]. Nonetheless, some patients are clearly more sensitive to this problem than others, with a long-term trial of lithium (n = 77) vs. lamotrigine (n = 78) monotherapy as maintenance treatment for BD-1 reporting a 28% incidence of diarrhea in the lithium cohort despite a mean endpoint serum lithium level of 0.69 ± 0.20 mEq/l and a study design aimed at keeping levels within the range of 0.50–1.00 mEq/l [171]. There is limited literature on management strategies, but the options outlined in Info Box 5.10 include taking lithium with food to delay gastrointestinal (GI) transit, trying standard lithium in lieu of a sustained release formulation and lowering the lithium level, especially if it exceeds 0.80 mEq/l (Info Box 5.10).

Approximately 5–20% of patients experience nausea from upper GI tract lithium ion delivery to the small intestine, but this problem does improve with use of sustained release preparations or food intake [171, 173]. The value of sustained release products lies in their lower C_{Max}, and delayed T_{Max}, and modern sustained release products do not delay absorption so excessively (e.g. T_{Max} 12 h) that they induce diarrhea [17]. Administering lithium with food won't significantly alter bioavailability. Although the C_{Max} is measurably higher with food intake of any composition (e.g. standard meal, high fat, high fat and high protein) [174], it has been known since 1975 that ingestion after a meal minimizes GI adverse effects. The impact of food on GI complaints is especially effective for diarrhea related to rapid passage into the lower GI tract, but sometimes for nausea as well [175]. If use of a sustained release formulation does not resolve nausea, ingestion of lithium after a meal should be tried. The important principle is to identify these GI complaints early, recognize how distressing they can be, and act quickly, especially when diarrhea is the problem. While diarrhea tends to occur more often with lithium than with other mood stabilizers, VPA may also induce nausea, even the sustained released formulation. The 2021 product information for extended release divalproex notes the following rates of GI adverse effects compared with placebo in adult acute mania trials: nausea – VPA 19% vs. PBO 13%; vomiting – VPA 13% vs. PBO 5%; diarrhea – VPA 12% vs. PBO 8% [176].

Info Box 5.10 Approach to Lithium Related Gastrointestinal Adverse Effects

a. **Monitoring:** Ask about gastrointestinal (GI) adverse effects at every office visit during the first 6 months of treatment. Most patients will complain of diarrhea and nausea, but some might not. Early detection is important as diarrhea is a leading somatic cause of lithium discontinuation [21].

b. Treatment options:

i. Administering lithium with dinner: It has been known since 1975 that ingestion after a meal minimizes GI adverse effects, especially diarrhea related to rapid passage into the lower GI tract [175]. Ingesting lithium with dinner is preferable to eating more food at bedtime given the high prevalence of obesity among BD and schizophrenia spectrum patients [141, 145]. Patients should be advised to eat dinner somewhat late on the evening before a 12 h trough level is to be obtained so that they can go the laboratory at an hour that is feasible the next morning.

ii. Lowering the serum level: One study noted an association between levels > 0.80 mEq/l and increased rates of diarrhea [170]. This is a consideration, especially during the early phase of treatment when the optimal serum level for maintenance has not yet been established. Many patients may do equally well with a level in the lower end of the maintenance range (0.60–0.80 mEq/l) [177].

iii. Changing to a sustained release preparation: Delaying lithium ion delivery and lowering the C_{Max} might lessen patient complaints of nausea without necessarily inducing diarrhea. Older sustained released formulations with very long T_{Max} values (e.g. 12 h) often caused diarrhea by dumping most of the lithium ion into the lower GI tract, but modern formulations have T_{Max} values in the range of 3–6 h and generally should not make diarrhea worse, and can improve nausea by slowing upper GI tract absorption [173].

2 *Altered Taste and Dry Mouth*

Taste problems are uncommon, but have been reported in the literature for over 40 years and variably described as metallic taste, dysgeusia, taste distortion or salty taste [178, 179]. One conjecture was that this might be related to the lithium containing tablet touching the tongue, with some authors suggesting use of a capsule form to mitigate this issue, but when reports emerged among patients on capsule-based preparations it cast doubt on this explanation [178]. A more likely hypothesis relates to the fact that salty taste in mammalian species is mediated via amiloride-sensitive and insensitive forms of ENaC [180, 181]. It is the amiloride-sensitive isoform containing the α subunit which exhibits 1.6-fold higher affinity for lithium than for sodium, and thus might be sensitive to lithium related effects on 2nd messenger systems in a manner akin to that in collecting duct principal cells [34].

Although salty taste in mammals is mediated by ENaC, one issue in developing a link between lithium use and abnormal taste relates to the fact that human taste buds were thought not to express the amiloride-sensitive ENaC isoform containing the α subunit, but only express an ENaC composed of β, γ and δ subunits [33]. The absence of the α subunit means that lithium would not readily enter ENaC isoforms on human taste buds [34], with some studies indicating that application of amiloride solutions to the tongue had little impact on salt taste in humans [181]. However, there are discrepant results in the literature that may relate to the site of application (anterior tongue vs. whole mouth), and amiloride concentration, with many studies finding that humans do have a population of amiloride-sensitive channels mediating salty taste on the anterior tongue [180]. Using human volunteers, investigators measured the transepithelial voltage drop following application of a salt solution to tongue mucosa to see if this current can be blocked by amiloride in the same manner as in mouse models. Electrophysiological recordings in response to focal salt stimulation provided evidence that, in some individuals, amiloride was able to reduce the voltage drop caused by salt application, but the effect was highly variable between individuals, ranging from 0% to 42% inhibition [180]. The fact that not all subjects were sensitive to amiloride's electrophysiological effects on salt stimulation suggests that population differences in ENaC expression among tongue taste cells may underlie taste changes described by a subset of patients during lithium treatment.

Fortunately, complaints of lithium induced taste changes appear relatively uncommon, with a 1988 long-term follow-up study of 471 lithium treated BD patients noting that only 5 individuals (1%) described alterations in taste sensation [170]. There are also very few reports in recent years, with many of the cases relating the onset of the complaint to supratherapeutic lithium levels [182, 183]. The connection between taste changes and higher lithium levels is supported by a BD maintenance study which found this complaint in 17% of those randomized to a lithium serum level range of 0.80–1.00 mEq/l, but in none of the patients assigned to the 0.40–0.60 mEq/l range [184]. These findings suggest that the optimal approach to the rare complaint of unusual taste phenomena is to recheck the serum lithium level and consider very modest reductions in the level, especially if the level is at the higher end of the therapeutic range (0.80–1.00 mEq/l). As the complaint is unusual, an occasional inquiry might be helpful as patients might not have known what to make of the changes in taste sensation or that there might be a possible remedy. Whether amiloride might be useful for altered taste has not been studied, nor are there case reports as of this writing.

Many patients on lithium complain of thirst due to uncontrolled polyuria, but this is not the same as xerostomia or dry mouth. In this regard, the literature is difficult to interpret as older studies either fail to distinguish these two phenomena, or report rates in patients on other medications (antipsychotics, antiparkinsonian medications, tricyclic antidepressants) that clearly possess anticholinergic properties which interfere with salivary flow [185]. For example, a 2021 genome-wide association study and review of lithium related dry mouth stated that the rate may be as high as 70%, citing a 1980 paper as one source [186]; however, that 1980 paper never uses the terms "dry mouth" or "xerostomia" although it lists other complaints (e.g. salty taste, diminished taste) [169]. What is reported in that paper is a 70% rate of patients complaining of increased thirst in the context of excessive urine output [169]. A 2020 review of mood stabilizer adverse effects is more circumspect in their reading of the literature and does not mention dry mouth among lithium related adverse effects, although it is described for carbamazepine and other anticonvulsants [187]. Lithium prescribing information in Japan notes the rate of dry mouth as 2.4%, although the source of the data is unknown [188]. Perhaps the best modern estimate is from the 2012 40-week double-blind extension of a 12-week lithium vs. aripiprazole BD-1 maintenance monotherapy trial which reported a 4.4% incidence of dry mouth [172]. The Norrbotten study listed xerostomia as the cause of lithium discontinuation in only 0.9% of patients. Given the low prevalence, these data indicate it is a problem patients may not tolerate for long when it does occur [21].

For this reason, it is incumbent on the clinician to investigate complaints of dry mouth, and determine whether other medications are contributing to the problem (e.g. psychostimulants, anticholinergics, norepinephrine reuptake inhibitors, anticonvulsants), or if this is an expression of thirst due to increased urine output. Assessment of polyuria related complaints is discussed in detail in this chapter, and the approach to that problem is clear once one has the 24 h FIR and EMUO data to provide evidence for impaired urine concentration. There is a big push to minimize anticholinergic burden in older individuals and those with severe mental illnesses to avert the cognitive impact, but tapering off these agents slowly might also remove a problem incorrectly ascribed to lithium [189, 190]. The same is true for other medications also associated with dry mouth – consider tapering them off slowly if possible and finding other options if necessary. For those rare patients on lithium monotherapy with no evidence of polyuria, there is no obvious management strategy as the mechanism for inducing dry mouth is unknown, but the plausible treatment choices are artificial saliva mouth rinses or sprays, or very modest reductions in the lithium level, especially if at the higher end of the therapeutic range (0.80–1.00 mEq/l). Fortunately, it is likely that the majority of patients who have dry mouth are relating a problem due to thirst or direct effects from other medications.

F | Hematological Effects – Neutrophilia

WHAT TO KNOW: NEUTROPHILIA

- Lithium enhances the production of granulocyte colony stimulating factor (G-CSF) and this stimulates bone marrow to create more neutrophils.

- This property has been exploited by hematologists to boost neutrophil counts following chemotherapy or prior to bone marrow transplantation. It is also used in the context of clozapine prescribing.

- The phenomenon of lithium related neutrophilia is known to many, but not all, clinicians. A brief communication about this effect to the patient and to their primary care provider can obviate unnecessary worry and a needless work-up for occult infection.

The association between lithium and granulocytosis (i.e. elevated neutrophil counts) has been recognized for decades, but it was not proven until 1978 that lithium-induced neutrophilia is not merely a redistribution of neutrophils that are marginated or are in bone marrow reserves (see Chapter 1) [191]. Lithium enhances the production of granulocyte colony stimulating factor (G-CSF), and directly stimulates the proliferation of pluripotential stem cells [191]. During lithium exposure, there are significant increases in bone marrow colony-forming units and bone marrow organ cellularity. This effect occurs reproducibly in animal and human studies, and exhibits a dose dependency within the serum range of 0.30–1.00 mEq/l (0.30–1.00 mmol/l) [191]. At therapeutic doses of 900–1200 mg/d, the mean increase in absolute neutrophil count (ANC) averaged 88% in one small trial, and the effect was seen in the first week after lithium was initiated, though peak absolute neutrophil counts may not occur until week 2 or 3 [192]. While not an adverse effect per se, clinicians not familiar with lithium's impact on ANC might incorrectly assume an infectious or inflammatory process and subject the patient to unnecessary work-up. In some instances, neutrophilia is used to the clinician's benefit, especially for clozapine treated patients whose ANC might dip below certain thresholds that necessitate increased frequency of ANC monitoring or clozapine interruption [193]. In general, no action need be taken to monitor for neutrophilia, but one should educate the patient and other medical providers about the association with lithium to avert inappropriate concerns about an elevated ANC in an otherwise asymptomatic patient.

 Central Nervous System Effects: Tremor, Cognitive Dysfunction, Fatigue, Muscle Weakness, Parkinsonism, Nystagmus, Myoclonus, Idiopathic Intracranial Hypertension (IIH), and Limited Impact on EEG

 WHAT TO KNOW: CNS EFFECTS

- Lithium related tremor is typically level dependent, and modest dose reduction remains an option, but other contributing causes (e.g. medications) should also be ruled out.

- Lithium tremor is typically a fine postural tremor of 8–12 Hz that closely resembles essential tremor and whose medication management is similar (once other causes have been addressed): propranolol initially, other anticonvulsants (e.g. primidone, topiramate) if absolutely necessary.

- Cognitive dysfunction or emotional dulling is frustrating to both patients and prescribers. Lithium can be a cause of these complaints, but numerous other medication, mood and medical issues (e.g. hypothyroidism) must be examined. When other etiologies have been addressed or ruled out, modest serum level reduction should be entertained under the hypothesis that this patient may be experiencing higher CNS levels than other individuals for a given serum level.

- Lithium uncommonly can impact dopamine neurotransmission, with cases of parkinsonism reported in older patients, or exacerbation of Parkinson's disease. The decision to stop lithium should be balanced against lithium's neuroprotective effects in this population.

- Nystagmus is a very rare complication of long-term lithium use, and nearly always reversible upon discontinuation. Myoclonus is also exceedingly rare, and only seen after long-term use. It appears related to lithium's effects on serotonergic neurotransmission. Unlike with nystagmus, patients with mild symptoms may choose to remain on lithium and use adjunctive medications to manage their movement symptoms.

- Lithium is not associated with pathological EEG changes aside from overdose situations.

- As of 2020, only 17 cases of IIH associated with lithium have been reported despite the high prevalence of obesity (the most common IIH risk factor) in BD spectrum patients. In some instances, use of other offending medications (e.g. minocycline) make the connection with lithium difficult to establish.

A number of central nervous system (CNS) complaints may surface during routine treatment, with some having clear associations to lithium exposure (e.g. postural tremor); however, for many CNS adverse effects the association with lithium therapy is circumstantial and more likely due to confounding issues, such as medical comorbidity, depressed mood or concurrent medications. The clinical challenge is to reframe the complaint as one with multiple possible etiologies, whose solution may not be lithium discontinuation but adjustments to the serum level, removal of or the addition of medications, or more detailed work-up. By understanding the prevalence of and differential diagnosis of these heterogeneous CNS adverse effect issues, one can take initial steps that, in most instances, will resolve the problem, and thereby avoid delegating the work-up to a provider who may be less knowledgeable about these issues and whose reflexive response might be lithium discontinuation.

1 *Tremor*

Tremor is one of the cardinal signs of lithium toxicity due to supratherapeutic levels, but it remains a common enough occurrence during maintenance treatment for it to be the second leading somatic cause of lithium cessation in the Norrbotten study, accounting for 11% of discontinuations [21]. A broad range of prevalence estimates are reported in the literature (4–65%), many of which date to the early years of lithium therapy when maintenance levels > 1.00 mEq/l were commonly employed [194]. Other complicating issues in establishing the true prevalence is the failure to exclude a prior history of tremor, and the nonsystematic nature of data collection in this area, with some studies relying on patient self-report after a prompting question about hand tremor, but others counting observed tremor that may not be bothersome to the patient [194]. Nonetheless, the association between lithium tremor and serum level is well established, with approximately 36% of those in a maintenance trial randomized to a lithium serum level range of 0.80–1.00 mEq/l experiencing tremor vs. 18% of the patients assigned to the 0.40–0.60 mEq/l range [184]. Lithium tremor is typically a fine postural tremor, meaning that it is usually seen during voluntary maintenance of a particular posture held against gravity, primarily in the hands. The characteristic frequency is 8–12 Hz, and it appears as an exaggerated physiologic tremor that closely resembles essential tremor, with the difference being reversibility upon lithium discontinuation, except for rare instances when it is the sequela of significant lithium toxicity (e.g. prior episodes of serum levels ≫ 1.5 mEq/l, especially in older patients) [194]. Tremor typically appears during early treatment, but in some cases the onset may be delayed by months, or rarely years. In a 40-week double-blind extension of a 12-week lithium vs. aripiprazole BD-1 maintenance monotherapy trial, 13.8% noted tremor during the first 12 weeks of lithium treatment, but only 7.9% experienced new onset tremor during the extension phase [172].

The first step in addressing this issue is to assess what other factors are contributing to the tremor and are exaggerating the central 8–12 Hz component or the peripheral mechanical component. The CNS component will be worsened by use of VPA or lamotrigine, or a prior history of idiopathic familial tremor. The peripheral component is enhanced by sympathomimetics such as oral decongestants, inhaled β_2 agonists, psychostimulants, norepinephrine reuptake inhibitors and caffeine, or when the patient is experiencing hyperthyroidism, anxiety or alcohol/benzodiazepine withdrawal [194]. Lastly, patients may have a parkinsonian tremor due to the concurrent use of D_2 antagonists, or a complex tremor with contributions from both lithium and the antipsychotic. The approach to tremor involves assessment of risk factors, modification of other medications or lithium dosing as seems appropriate, and then use of adjunctive strategies (see Info Box 5.11) [187, 194]. Given the visible nature of lithium related tremor and the functional impact, this is an adverse effect that should be inquired about during each visit, and responded to with alacrity to prevent the patient refusing to continue with lithium. Patients should also be counseled that VPA and lamotrigine both have tremor risk, but lack lithium's spectrum of benefits for those with a history of mania or whose past behavior suggests a risk for completed suicide.

Info Box 5.11 **Approach to the Assessment and Management of Tremor [187, 194]**

a. Assessment

　i. **Patient factors:** Personal or 1st degree family history of essential tremor, hyperthyroidism, alcohol or benzodiazepine withdrawal, anxiety.

　ii. **Medications – sympathomimetics:** Use of decongestants, inhaled β-2 agonists, psychostimulants, norepinephrine reuptake inhibitors (NRIs) and caffeine.

　iii. **Medications – other:** VPA (and note serum level), lamotrigine, dopamine D_2 antagonist/partial agonists.

　　• If dopamine D_2 modulators are present, is there evidence for parkinsonism (e.g. coarse 3–7 Hz pill rolling tremor at rest, masked facies, rigidity, bradykinesia, or festination)?

　iv. **Lithium:** Latest level, changes in severity with higher levels.

b. Management

　i. **Treat other modifiable patient risk factors:** Address hyperthyroidism. Manage alcohol or benzodiazepine withdrawal and anxiety, but avoid long-term benzodiazepine use due to dependence and cognitive effects.

ii. Modify other medication exposures:

- **Sympathomimetics:** NRIs, decongestants, psychostimulants can often be avoided. Use of inhaled β-2 agonists may be unavoidable, and many patients are reluctant to moderate caffeine intake (unless there is evidence it is excessive).

- **Other medications:** Reassess need for VPA and whether the VPA level can be lowered if necessary. Reassess need for lamotrigine. If evidence of parkinsonism, consider modest (e.g. 10% per month) antipsychotic dose reduction, or use of amantadine as it lacks the cognitive and peripheral adverse effects of anticholinergics. The usual amantadine starting dose is 100 mg QAM, increasing to 100 mg BID; maximal dose is 200 mg BID. There are rare reports of symptom exacerbation in psychosis/mania patients, but this is very uncommon at doses ≤ 400 mg/d. Amantadine is renally cleared, so for those with eGFR 30–50 ml/min, the recommended dose is 200 mg x 1, then 100 mg Q24 H.

- **Lithium:** For all patients with evidence of level-dependent effects, especially those with levels > 0.80 mEq/l, consider modest dose reduction, assuming the prior history indicates that this approach will not result in decompensation. As the CNS $T_{1/2}$ of lithium may be as long as 48 hours, allow at least 1–2 weeks to recheck the serum level at the new steady state and ascertain the impact on tremor severity. A discussion should be held with the patient about the need to balance the risk for mood relapse with the need to manage the tremor. In some instances, the preferred option will be use of an adjunctive medication.

iii. Adjunctive medications

- **β-adrenergic antagonists (beta blockers):** Propranolol is the best studied, but has been evaluated more systematically for essential tremor where the effect size is 50% [195]. It has a short half-life (4–5 hours), is started at 10 mg BID and the dose advanced every 2 days as tolerated until the tremor is not bothersome, or the patient experiences dose-limiting adverse effects (tiredness, fatigue, orthostasis). Once a dose of 60 mg/d is reached, there are extended release forms that should be used and are dosed QAM. If tolerated, doses as high as 320 mg/d have been used for hypertension, although tremor often responds to doses < 100 mg/d. Absolute contraindications are sick sinus syndrome, sinus bradycardia, 1st degree heart block or congestive heart failure. A history of asthma, chronic obstructive pulmonary disease or diabetes mellitus are not contraindications in most patients, but the primary care provider should be consulted. Peripherally acting beta blockers (e.g. atenolol) can be considered if CNS side effects (e.g.

fatigue) become limiting, and have shown efficacy in some studies [194]. Atenolol is a once daily medication, and can be advanced in 12.5 mg increments every 2 days as tolerated until the tremor is not bothersome, or the patient experiences dose-limiting adverse effects (orthostasis). Beta blockers must be tapered off and not stopped abruptly due to rebound effects.

- **Primidone:** Effective for lithium and essential tremor with an effective size of 50% for the latter [195]. The active metabolite phenylethylmalonamide (PEMA) does not appear to mediate effects on tremor. Approximately 15% is converted to phenobarbital, a potent hepatic inducer which can lower levels of many antipsychotics and anticonvulsants [194]. Primidone has a $T_{1/2}$ of 29–36 h. The starting dose is 100 mg QHS, advancing by 50 mg QHS every 3 days as tolerated, with most patients responding to doses ≤ 250 mg/d [194]. Major limiting side effects are fatigue or sedation, but rapid titration can cause ataxia, vertigo and nausea. Primidone must be tapered off to avoid withdrawal symptoms.

- **Other anticonvulsants:** Topiramate (200–400 mg/d) and gabapentin (1200–3600 mg/d) have been studied for essential tremor, but topiramate has more robust supporting evidence [195]. Topiramate is titrated slowly, starting at 25 mg BID, increasing by 25 mg BID every week as tolerated. Topiramate can induce sedation, marked cognitive impairment and metabolic acidosis necessitating periodic monitoring of bicarbonate levels. Topiramate has a fairly extensive list of precautions in the product label that should be reviewed prior to initiation.

2   *Cognitive and Emotional Blunting*

Bipolar I disorder and SAD-BT clearly have cognitive components, and the high prevalence of cardiometabolic comorbidity and lifestyle factors (e.g. smoking) further add to the risk of cognitive dysfunction due to macroscopic or microscopic vascular insults [7]. The other complicating issue when assessing cognitive complaints is the role of mood related cognitive dysfunction from depressive symptoms (or the absence of hypomania), the effects of sedating medications, and the role that depressed mood plays in the rates of CNS adverse effect complaints independent of serum lithium level [196, 197]. The complaint of emotional blunting in particular may be a product of similar factors, with perhaps a greater focus on assessing the psychological impact of the absence of hypomania, or the loss of the highs and emotional range that some patients enjoyed. Emotional blunting may be a proxy for other cognitive complaints, but it was not rare in the Norrbotten study, and ranked as the 7th leading somatic cause of lithium stoppage, accounting for 6.5% of all discontinuations [21]. On the other hand, other specific cognitive complaints were not among the top 10 reasons for lithium discontinuation. While there is limited literature to quantify lithium's impact on emotional experience, a 2009 meta-analysis found 12 studies with cognitive outcomes involving 276 lithium treated patients and 263 control subjects or the same subjects during a lithium-free period. Lithium was taken for a mean duration of 3.9 years by the mood disorder patients with mean level 0.80 mEq/l. Lithium use was associated with small impairments in immediate verbal learning and memory (effect size [ES] = 0.24; 95% CI 0.05–0.43) and creativity (ES = 0.33; 95% CI 0.02–0.64), whereas delayed verbal memory, visual memory, attention, executive function, processing speed and psychomotor performance were not significantly affected. Longer-term lithium treatment also was associated with an impact on psychomotor performance (ES = 0.62; 95% CI 0.27–0.97) [197]. A subsequent 2016 review also commented that mood recurrence may adversely affect cognitive performance, as noted in studies where excellent lithium responders with few affective recurrences performed comparably on cognitive functions testing to age-matched, healthy control subjects [6]. The most persuasive data come from a detailed neurocognitive battery performed on 262 BD patients on lithium monotherapy enrolled in a multicenter clinical trial [198]. There were no differences in baseline neurocognitive performance between those taking lithium and those who were not. However, at follow-up, significant neurocognitive improvement in the global cognitive index score (F = 31.69; p < 0.001) was detected among the lithium treated subjects. The longitudinal effects of lithium were specifically examined in the subset of 88 BD-1 patients who achieved mood stabilization with lithium monotherapy. This subgroup had mean age 40.9 years, with mean premorbid IQ of 103.1 [198]. The follow-up cognitive assessment was performed after a mean of 132.1 ± 90.3 days from the 1st assessment, at which time the mean serum lithium level was 0.65 ± 0.22 mEq/l. The follow-up testing suggested that lithium may be beneficial to neurocognitive functioning in BD-1 patients, and that at the very least it did not seem to impair cognition significantly [198]. Nonetheless, there are studies which show an impact on psychomotor speed, a finding that might be due to age-related differences in brain lithium levels and an impact on dopamine neurotransmission in sensitive patients (see section below on parkinsonism) [199].

Lithium may certainly induce complaints of cognitive dysfunction or emotional blunting in new users, and these complaints must be taken seriously to prevent discontinuation; however, the effects of other factors such as medical illnesses (e.g. hypothyroidism), co-medication and depressed mood must be assessed, with a careful plan devised to taper off sedating and anticholinergic medications, treat depressed symptoms with nonsedating agents effective for bipolar depression (e.g. lurasidone, lumateperone, cariprazine), and then consider reduction in the serum lithium level (Info Box 5.12) [196]. The imaging literature shows clearly that some patients achieve higher brain levels for any given peripheral level, so it is not unreasonable to surmise that excessive brain levels in certain patients might underlie cognitive complaints. Steady state brain levels generally correlate with serum levels [200–202], but there are marked interindividual differences in brain lithium penetration, with older age emerging as one factor in some but not all studies [201, 203, 204]. In one study, elevations in brain (but not serum) lithium levels in those over age 50 were associated with frontal lobe dysfunction and higher depression rating scores, suggesting that a cognitive effect may be related to supratherapeutic CNS exposure [201]. It is for this reason that one should consider dose reduction in select individuals when other causes of cognitive dysfunction have been ruled out, especially medical comorbidity, mood and other medications. This is particularly true when serum levels are at the higher end of the therapeutic range or there appears to be a direct correlation between titration to a higher serum lithium level and emergence of the cognitive complaint.

 Info Box 5.12 **Considerations When Addressing Cognitive Dysfunction and Emotional Dulling**

a. **Other medications:** The concurrent use of sedating and anticholinergic medications significantly adds to the risk of these complaints. Before concluding that lithium is the primary cause, other offending medications should be tapered off, and less sedating replacements found (e.g. amantadine in lieu of anticholinergic antiparkinsonian medication, cariprazine/lurasidone/lumateperone in lieu of quetiapine for bipolar depression, etc.)

b. **Comorbid medical conditions and medications:** Changes in the severity of certain conditions (e.g. heart failure), inadequately treated hypothyroidism, and nonpsychiatric medications may also play a role. A temporal relationship to the onset of the CNS complaints can help quickly rule out to what extent these issues are relevant.

c. **The role of mood state:** The CNS complaints may be related to residual symptoms of depressed mood, or to the patient missing the emotional range of hypomania/mania. Bipolar depression should be managed aggressively, and psychotherapeutic options offered to help patients who are struggling with the absence of those "highs" associated with periods of hypomania/mania.

d. **The role of lithium:** Certain patients may be more sensitive to lithium's CNS effects, possibly due to greater relative brain penetration that results in higher central levels. Careful downward dose titration can be considered when other causes have been excluded.

The absence of hypomania is also a concept that must be processed with certain patients who may be wedded to the idea that they cannot perform adequately unless in a hyperthymic state, or that they feel "blunted" when unable to experience elevated mood states after starting lithium. As with all adverse effect complaints, one should listen empathically, educate the patient, and explain your rationale for making certain recommendations with the aim of reaching a shared decision that furthers the patient's goals. In most instances, lithium discontinuation is not necessary, but careful reductions in the serum lithium level might allow for resolution of the complaint when other factors have been ruled out. In the absence of clinically available neuroimaging to track brain lithium levels, it is not unreasonable to hypothesize that complaints of cognitive or emotional blunting, especially in newly treated patients, reflect supratherapeutic brain lithium levels *for that patient.*

3   *Fatigue, Muscle Weakness, Motor Speed, Parkinsonism*

The assessment of fatigue mirrors the approach to cognitive complaints since numerous underlying causes must be considered, including depressed mood (or the absence of hypomania), effects of other medications (D_2 blockade, histamine H_1 antagonism, antimuscarinic effects, benzodiazepines), hypothyroidism, hypercalcemia, and medical issues unrelated to the psychiatric disorder or its treatment (e.g. congestive heart failure) [17, 196]. Fatigue was the 6th most common cause of lithium discontinuation in the Norrbotten study, at 5.9%, just outranking nausea (5.7%), so clinicians must become adept at reasoning through the possible etiologies [21]. Among this list of potential etiologies, depressed mood, other medication effects and hypothyroidism (or TSH levels at the upper end of the therapeutic range) represent the most likely targets, especially considering the association between depression in BD patients and increased complaints of lithium related adverse effects of all types [108, 121, 196]. The need for any medical work-up will be guided by other signs and symptoms suggestive of a specific problem (e.g. new onset edema raising suspicion for congestive heart failure [CHF] or nephrotic syndrome) [205]. As with cognitive dysfunction, consider dose reduction in select individuals when other causes of fatigue have been ruled out, when lithium levels are at the higher end of the therapeutic range, or there appears to be a direct correlation between the titration to higher serum levels and emergence of fatigue. Complaints of muscular weakness are a separate issue. Weakness is an uncommon complaint, but it can be an early symptom of lithium toxicity or hypercalcemia [17]. In that instance, a lithium level and serum calcium should be checked before considering other etiologies and requesting a neurology consultation. Complaints of slowing motor speed in the absence of D_2 blockade should be approached in the same manner as fatigue.

Most clinicians may never encounter this effect, but there is evidence of lithium's reversible impact on D_2 neurotransmission that in rare cases presents as drug-induced parkinsonism (DIP) [206]. Not surprisingly, the common demographic feature among all of these reports is older age [207–209]. Dopamine transporter (DaT) SPECT scanning was performed in 9 cases to diagnose primary Parkinson's disease, and in 8 of 9 patients the scans were normal, effectively ruling out an underlying neurodegenerative disorder [209]. This imaging finding, and the reversibility upon lithium dose reduction or discontinuation [210], indicates that any effect of lithium is transient, that lithium is not causing loss of dopaminergic neurons or some other degenerative process, and that the incidence is extremely low, even among older patients [209]. Animal studies indicate that lithium does not increase the sensitivity to haloperidol-induced D_2 related adverse effects [211], and a 2022 Japanese study of 3521 lithium treated BD patients found no association with increased risk of Parkinson-like events [212]. It is worth noting that imaging studies of BD patients with parkinsonism suggest that a subset of this patient population (20%) may have a dopaminergic deficit, a finding that might explain the rare cases of lithium related parkinsonism [213]. Medium spiny neurons in the striatum receive serotonergic input, and medications that act as serotonin agonists directly or indirectly (e.g. selective serotonin reuptake inhibitors [SSRIs]) can induce DIP, akathisia and other movement disorders [209, 214]. Lithium facilitates serotonin release in part by actions at the $5HT_{1B}$ autoreceptor [215], so any effect on dopamine neurotransmission likely occurs via serotonergic agonism in vulnerable patients, a mechanism also postulated to underlie the rare cases of lithium related myoclonus [209, 213, 216, 217]. Interestingly, one hypothesis for the lower rates of Parkinson's disease and brain α-synuclein deposition in smokers relates to lithium levels in tobacco leaf. Over time, sufficient CNS lithium exposure may occur, resulting in inhibition of GSK3-β and enhancement of β-catenin mediated activity (e.g. gene transcription) [217]. Whether lithium offers any neuroprotective benefit in patients with primary Parkinson's disease is unknown, but its advantages (e.g. reduction in risk of suicide related death, mood stability, decreased dementia risk) outweigh the motor effects in most Parkinson's disease patients, especially since VPA is also associated with reports of DIP or exacerbation of motor symptoms in Parkinson's disease [209]. For patients with lithium related DIP, a normal DaT scan and no use of D_2 modulating antipsychotics, lowering lithium exposure may improve the problem. A VPA trial can be considered if DIP persists despite low therapeutic levels (e.g. 0.40 mEq/l), but with the understanding that VPA may induce DIP; moreover, rare reports also exist for DIP in patients treated with carbamazepine or lamotrigine [218].

4   *Nystagmus, Myoclonus, EEG Changes, and Idiopathic Intracranial Hypertension*

Nystagmus is an adverse effect seen with supratherapeutic anticonvulsant levels, excessive exposure to other medications (e.g. benzodiazepines, amphetamines, SSRIs, psychedelics), alcohol intoxication or thiamine deficiency [187], but there are rare reports of nystagmus and other oculomotor abnormalities (smooth pursuit abnormalities, horizontal gaze palsy) during routine lithium treatment not related to episodes of toxicity [210–228]. Fortunately, there are fewer than 40 cases in the literature, and nearly all occurred in patients aged 60 and over. Work-up reveals normal MRI findings, absence of other causes and nontoxic lithium levels (e.g. < 1.5 mEq/l), but those experiencing new onset nystagmus have usually been on lithium for years, suggesting a cumulative effect in certain individuals, especially a subset with greater age-related brain penetration of lithium [201, 203, 204]. Removal of lithium is necessary due to the marked visual impairment, and VPA represents an acceptable alternative not associated with worsening of the oculomotor symptoms [219]. In almost all instances, nystagmus resolves upon lithium discontinuation, but with two caveats: the time course to resolution may be slow in some patients (i.e. weeks, months); there are several cases in which nystagmus did not resolve after lithium discontinuation. Baclofen is the medication of choice in patients with persistent nystagmus, and one case report documents complete response after gradual titration to 20 mg TID in a patient whose nystagmus did not remit 3 months after lithium discontinuation [222]. Pathological nystagmus is the result of drug effects to the vestibular system, but the exact mechanism by which any individual medication induces this problem is often unclear. While a rare adverse effect, it is one that should be evaluated immediately by a neurologist or ophthalmologist to confirm the diagnosis, and a plan subsequently created to find another mood stabilizing medication for the patient. (Options for the patient who discontinues lithium are presented in Chapter 8.)

Myoclonus is often not pathological, with many experiencing it as a hypnic jerk while falling asleep. The definition of myoclonus is a brief, involuntary, nonrhythmic twitching of a muscle or muscle group. While not necessarily pathological, in some instances it is the marker of a disease state (e.g. multiple sclerosis, Parkinson's disease, Alzheimer's disease, myoclonic epilepsy, Creutzfeldt–Jakob disease) or a drug induced issue (e.g. serotonin syndrome, anticonvulsant or clozapine related) [193, 216, 218, 220]. A broad array of medications can induce myoclonus, but the association with serotonergic agonism has emerged as the best explanatory hypothesis for lithium related cases [209, 216, 230, 231]. While lithium facilitates serotonin release by actions at the $5HT_{1B}$ autoreceptor, this agonist effect is clearly not as potent as with SSRI antidepressants; however, in select sensitive patients, it is sufficient to induce myoclonus and the effect may be additive with concurrent SSRI exposure [215, 231]. The number of reported cases is fewer than 25, but two features emerge: many of the patients are older and have been exposed to lithium for years; and the myoclonic movements may be fine enough and sufficiently rhythmic in their presentation to be deemed "a tremor," although the underlying diagnosis is cortical myoclonus [231]. When myoclonic movements present as a sudden and brief twitch, the diagnosis is obvious, but some forms of myoclonus may fit into a broader definition of tremor. From the clinician's perspective, the presence of myoclonus should be considered when a tremor complaint emerges after years, and when level reduction, propranolol or primidone do not adequately address the problem. The distinction between tremor and myoclonus can be difficult in the clinical setting, so specialized testing that includes electrophysiological studies may be needed to accurately confirm the diagnosis.

In-Depth 5.5 A Detailed Study of Lithium Related Myoclonus Cases

A 2019 paper performed an exhaustive work-up on eight cases, including magnetic resonance imaging (MRI) with magnetic resonance spectroscopy (MRS), EEG and electrophysiology studies [231]. 75% of the patients were 55 and above, and 75% were female. One patient was eventually diagnosed with a central tremor, leaving seven cases of cortical myoclonus for analysis. Based on medical history and concurrent medication use, the authors reached some important conclusions about lithium related myoclonus: (1) All cases were associated with prolonged exposure to lithium (7–40 years); (2) Use of serotonin agonist antidepressants may exacerbate the problem (86% of the sample); (3) Among the five cases who underwent MRI/MRS imaging, all exhibited abnormalities in cerebellar vermis function based on the N-acetyl-aspartate/creatine ratio; (4) 57% of the myoclonus cases had gluten sensitivity compared with the population prevalence of 11%, and this comorbidity is linked in the literature to cerebellar ataxia or cortical myoclonus [231]. There were no characteristic EEG findings.

In a manner akin to nystagmus, there is a small subset of patients who may develop lithium related CNS issues after years of exposure to therapeutic levels, but the approach to myoclonus is not identical. Some patients may have mild disability and either choose no treatment or use of propranolol to dampen the amplitude of the movements [231]. Removal of other offending agents (e.g. SSRIs, SNRIs) should be considered, lowering the lithium level is an option, as is switching to a gluten free diet for 6 months [231]. In some instances, myoclonus may not remit upon lithium discontinuation. Depending on the severity, propranolol or anticonvulsants (e.g. levetiracetam) may be helpful to manage the problem. Armed with the knowledge that myoclonus can occur, and that in some patients the presentation may be subtle, one can help point a patient toward obtaining the correct diagnosis and the optimal treatment.

The absence of EEG findings in the myoclonus study parallels the literature amassed over the past 50 years showing that lithium monotherapy is not associated with characteristic pathological EEG changes [232]. The best evidence of this is a study of 15 lithium treated patients who had serum lithium levels, electrolytes, thyroid function, urine creatinine and an EEG obtained every 6 months for 2 years [232]. During follow-up, the mean serum lithium level was 0.64 mEq/l and did not change over the 2 years. Compared with the pretreatment EEG, endpoint EEG did not reveal any specific potentials, focal signs or asymmetric phenomena [232]. There has been little evidence to the contrary except in conditions of lithium neurotoxicity and supratherapeutic serum levels [233]. A number of findings may be seen in that context, including focal sharp epileptiform waves, paroxysmal bursts of slowing without full seizure activity, and generalized slowing [234, 235]. Somewhat interestingly, lithium appears to have a protective effect on pentylenetetrazole induced seizures in animal models, but the combination of lithium and the muscarinic agonist pilocarpine is used as a model for temporal lobe seizures in other studies [236, 237]. Although anecdotal reports exist [238], concerns that lithium may alter seizure threshold have virtually disappeared from the literature, and a history of seizure disorder is not a consideration in starting lithium. Except in overdose situations, new onset seizure activity is unlikely to be lithium related, and other etiologies should be sought and treated.

Last on the list of rare CNS adverse effects associated with lithium treatment is the development of idiopathic intracranial hypertension (IIH), a condition resulting in high intracranial pressure (ICP) without a known cause. (The old name for this condition is pseudotumor cerebri, but this is not commonly used except as a historical reference.) Modified Dandy criteria are used to establish the diagnosis of IIH and include the following six elements: (1) symptoms of raised ICP (headache, nausea, vomiting, transient visual obscurations, or papilledema); (2) no localizing signs, with the exception of abducens (6th ocular nerve) palsy; (3) the patient is awake and alert; (4) normal CT/MRI findings without evidence of thrombosis; (5) lumbar puncture (LP) opening pressure > 25 cm H_2O and normal biochemical and cytological composition of cerebrospinal fluid; (6) no other explanation for the raised ICP [239]. The country specific adult incidence of IIH varies from 0.03 to 4.7 per 100,000 inhabitants [240]. Although the etiology of IIH is unclear, several potential risks associated with the disorder have been described, with female gender and obesity having the most robust link [240]. However, other factors are associated with IIH, including CKD, systemic lupus erythematosus, Addison's disease and iron deficiency anemia, along with exposure to a number of medications such as tetracycline related antibiotics, hormonal contraceptives, vitamin A and lithium [240]. Paralleling the increasing rates of obesity in Western countries, the rate of IIH has also increased, but a 2020 review of drug-induced IIH noted only 17 cases associated with lithium, despite the high prevalence of obesity in BD and SAD-BT patients [239]. In some instances, the patient was also on other offending medications (e.g. minocycline), making the connection with lithium difficult to establish [241, 242]. Serum lithium levels were reported to be within the therapeutic range, but unfortunately the review did not analyze demographic or IIH other risk factors.

In-Depth 5.6 Findings Related to Lithium and IIH from a Population Based Study

In 2021 a group used the Swedish national database to investigate the incidence and factors associated with IIH in adults. Cases were identified with the ICD diagnosis code G93.2 during 2000–2016, and the IIH diagnosis validated by having the code G93.2 recorded three times [240]. Each IIH case was demographically matched to five randomly selected individuals from the general population and also to five obese individuals. Overall, the mean age at IIH diagnosis in Sweden was 32.2 years, and during the last 4 years of the study the female:male ratio was almost exactly 9:1. The highest associations (OR > 10.0) vs. general population controls were for hypertension (OR 17.53), systemic lupus erythematosus (OR 13.81) and renal dysfunction (OR 13.16), with the latter category represented by the ICD-10 codes N17, N18 and N19. N18 in particular subsumed all gradations of CKD from stage G1 to stage G5, and end-stage renal disease. Given the known effect of obesity on IIH rates, the paper calculated the OR for IIH vs. general population and also vs. the obese controls. For lithium, the OR vs. general population controls was: OR 7.70 (95% CI 2.76–21.99), while the OR vs. obese controls was 50% lower: OR 4.75 (95% CI 1.97–11.47) [240]. This finding would be of greater concern except for a major methodological issue of particular relevance to lithium treated patients: the failure to account for confounding bias (aside from obesity) in a patient population prescribed lithium that has high rates of hypertension and CKD [243].

It is difficult to know what the rate of lithium induced IIH might be after adjustment for hypertension and CKD, but the small number of cases speaks to an extremely uncommon condition during lithium treatment, regardless of etiology [243]. No routine monitoring is necessary, but clinicians should maintain an index of suspicion for raised ICP if a patient complains of persistent headache (as opposed to episodic migraine-like phenomena), particularly if this evolves over time into a syndrome with nausea, vomiting or transient visual changes. Referral to a clinician who can examine the patient for papilledema and perform a lumbar puncture (LP) is necessary to establish or rule out the diagnosis. Given the tenuous association with lithium, lithium discontinuation should not be the first consideration, especially when risk factors (e.g. obesity, hypertension, CKD) are present [243]. The patient and the consulting neurologist should be included in a discussion concerning whether other medications or comorbidities are inducing IIH, and whether the patient has other viable mood stabilizer options. In some cases, a protracted period off lithium might be necessary to satisfy the concerns of all stakeholders regarding the extent of its contribution to the development of IIH [243].

H Miscellaneous Effects: Peripheral Edema, Reduced Cancer Risk

WHAT TO KNOW: EDEMA AND REDUCED CANCER RISK

- Peripheral edema is an uncommon cause of lithium discontinuation (< 4%) and not unique to lithium: the rate of edema during VPA exposure is 8%.

- Assuming medical conditions have been ruled out (nephrotic syndrome, heart failure, venous insufficiency), treatment options for edema include furosemide or acetazolamide. As furosemide can increase lithium levels in older patients, acetazolamide is preferable as it will not cause lithium toxicity since it lowers lithium levels by 31%. Dose adjustment based on serum levels is necessary regardless of which diuretic is chosen.

- Long-term lithium use does not increase risk for any malignancy, and is associated with risk reductions in certain data sets. Whether the latter is a direct biological effect of lithium or the result of lifestyle modifications (e.g. less smoking), or improved attention to nonpsychiatric medical issues in clinically stable patients, is not known.

Although complaints of peripheral edema are listed in the lithium product labeling, the prevalence and correlates are poorly described in the literature, as is the preferred treatment strategy. In the Norrbotten study, edema was responsible for 3.4% of lithium discontinuations, with the authors noting that women outnumbered men in this regard, and hypothesizing whether hormonal factors might possibly underlie this difference [21, 244]. A comprehensive review of lithium's pharmacology, safety and efficacy published by Grandjean and Aubry in 2009 described extremity edema as a rare adverse effect, but without commenting on the differential diagnosis or its management [245]. This problem is not unique to lithium, as edema represents a well-known adverse effect of VPA with a rate of 8% (vs. 3% on placebo) [176]. Edema arising during VPA treatment is secondary to diminished albumin production [246]; however, except in rare instances, lithium is not a cause of significant proteinuria and does not impact albumin production, so the mechanism by which lithium might cause edema is unknown [247].

Before concluding that edema is simply a bothersome drug related adverse effect from lithium or VPA, it is important to consider medical comorbidities as a potential cause. Although the differential diagnosis of edema is quite broad, the work-up will be guided by signs and symptoms suggestive of a more general problem (e.g. nephrotic syndrome, CHF) or a local issue (e.g. venous insufficiency and dependent lower extremity edema). CHF can be associated with CKD, and its management may require use of agents that have significant kinetic interactions with lithium, so close monitoring of lithium levels and eGFR will be paramount. Glomerular pathology from lithium is exceedingly rare, with only 36 reported cases of lithium induced nephrotic syndrome (i.e. proteinuria > 3.5 g/24 h) reported as of 2021 [247]. Proteinuria can develop insidiously due to relatively common systemic disorders (e.g. hypertension, diabetes mellitus) [248], so regular monitoring of the ACR in patients with these comorbidities will pick up albuminuria that pre-dates lithium, or which may have worsened during the course of lithium treatment (see Chapter 4, Info Box 4.4) [248]. In the extremely rare instances of lithium related nephrotic syndrome, the presentation will be dramatic, with marked generalized edema and systemic complaints (e.g. fatigue) suggestive of a serious medical issue [247].

Once other causes of edema have been ruled out or addressed, the question of treatment is important. Diuretics such as furosemide are commonly employed, but one must be mindful of the risk for lithium toxicity that loop diuretics pose in older patients [249]. An alternative to consider is the carbonic anhydrase inhibitor acetazolamide. Unlike other diuretics that can cause lithium toxicity, acetazolamide lowers lithium levels by 31%, an interaction easily compensated for by lithium dose adjustment [250, 251]. As with other adverse effects, offering a treatment option for the problem may prevent patient demands to stop lithium despite its therapeutic advantages for them.

Until recently, there had been no association between lithium use and increased cancer risk, with older literature generally suggesting no impact or a small protective effect, although the quality of these studies is suspect [252]. However, in February 2015, the European Medicines Agency advised lithium manufacturers to add a product label warning indicating that long-term lithium exposure (> 10 years) may increase risk for benign renal lesions (microcysts), but also for malignancies such as oncocytomas and collecting duct renal carcinomas [253]. This warning was surprising in light of earlier studies [252], so Professor Lars Kessing (Psychiatric Center Copenhagen, Rigshospitalet, University of Copenhagen) and colleagues performed a nationwide, population based longitudinal study of cancer incidence for the years 1995–2012 that included all lithium exposed patients (n = 24,272), all individuals with a diagnosis of BD (n = 9651), those exposed to anticonvulsants for any reason (n = 386,255), and a randomly selected sample of 1,500,000 adults from the Danish population [254]. The outcomes were hazard rate ratios (HR) for malignant or benign renal upper tract tumors, adjusted for numerous covariates including concurrent medications, medical comorbidities, age, gender, calendar year and a BD diagnosis. This detailed, methodologically rigorous analysis found that continued treatment with lithium was not associated with increased rates of malignant or benign renal upper tract tumors: HR for malignant or benign tumors: 0.67–1.18, $p = 0.70$; HR malignant tumors only: 0.61–1.34, $p = 0.90$; HR benign tumors only: 0.74–1.18, $p = 0.70$ [254]. This lack of association with increased risk for renal tract tumors was subsequently confirmed in multiple other studies [253, 255].

These findings conclusively dispelled the notion that lithium induces renal malignancy, but other investigators subsequently strove to examine the association between lithium exposure and cancer risk of all types. A Swedish group performed a nationwide register study of incidence rate ratios (IRRs) for any cancer and specific cancers among adults with BD aged 50–84 years, diagnosed from July 2005 to December 2009 (n = 5442), compared with rates in the general population, stratified by lithium exposure [256]. The study found that there was no difference in overall cancer risk compared with the general population for BD patients receiving lithium treatment [IRR = 1.04, 95% CI 0.89–1.23], nor for BD patients without lithium treatment (IRR = 1.03, 95% CI 0.89–1.19). Interestingly, site specific cancer risk was significantly increased in BD patients without lithium treatment in the digestive organs (IRR = 1.47, 95% CI 1.12–1.93), in the respiratory system and intrathoracic organs (IRR = 1.72, 95% CI 1.11–2.66), and in the endocrine glands and related structures (IRR = 2.60, 95% CI 1.24–5.47), but not in lithium treated BD patients [256]. A Taiwanese group used their nationwide database to compare cancer incidence in adults with BD exposed to lithium only, anticonvulsants only, or both agents during the years 1998–2009 after excluding those with < 1 year of drug exposure or pre-existing cancer diagnoses [257]. The median duration of medication exposure was 7.1 years for the lithium only group, 5.2 years for the anticonvulsant only group, and 7.5 years for the combined group. Compared with anticonvulsant-only exposure, lithium exposure was associated with significantly lower cancer risk (HR = 0.74, 95% CI 0.55–0.97), and this risk decreased in a dose dependent manner: the HR for those with the highest tertile of lithium exposure (> 810 mg/d) was 0.55 (95% CI 0.37–0.83) [257]. In 2021, an international collaborative team performed a systematic review and meta-analysis of the literature, with analyses based on outcomes of 2,606,187 individuals from five studies [258]. This comprehensive examination of the literature did not show an increased risk of cancer in BD patients using lithium, and even suggested a small but nonsignificant protective effect for any malignancy (RR = 0.94, 95% CI 0.72–1.22; p = 0.66] and urinary cancer (RR = 0.93; 95% CI 0.75–1.14; p = 0.48] [258]. While one would not prescribe lithium under the presumption that it reduces cancer risk, one can be confident that it does not increase risk.

 Summary Points

a. Laboratory or office monitoring is needed to detect certain lithium related issues (e.g. declining eGFR, hypercalcemia, hypothyroidism, weight gain), but routine inquiry is the best method to identify the majority of adverse effects, especially CNS, skin/hair and sexual complaints.

b. Lithium discontinuation is necessary for only a small subset of adverse effects (e.g. sick sinus syndrome, nystagmus) with many common adverse effects having evidence based management strategies (e.g. polyuria, tremor, hypothyroidism, hyperparathyroidism).

c. Weight gain is best managed by minimizing the contributions from other medications (e.g. SGAs).

d. The decision regarding when or whether to stop lithium for low eGFR is a nuanced one based on a number of considerations for each individual case.

References

1. Zivanovic, O. (2017). Lithium: A classic drug frequently discussed, but, sadly, seldom prescribed! *Aust N Z J Psychiatry*, 51, 886–896.

2. Malhi, G. S., Gessler, D. and Outhred, T. (2017). The use of lithium for the treatment of bipolar disorder: Recommendations from clinical practice guidelines. *J Affect Disord*, 217, 266–280.

3. Fountoulakis, K. N., Tohen, M. and Zarate, C. A. (2022). Lithium treatment of bipolar disorder in adults: A systematic review of randomized trials and meta-analyses. *Eur Neuropsychopharmacol*, 54, 100–115.

4. Kishi, T., Ikuta, T., Matsuda, Y., et al. (2022). Pharmacological treatment for bipolar mania: A systematic review and network meta-analysis of double-blind randomized controlled trials. *Mol Psychiatry*, 27, 1136–1144.

5. Benard, V., Vaiva, G., Masson, M., et al. (2016). Lithium and suicide prevention in bipolar disorder. *Encephale*, 42, 234–241.

6. Rybakowski, J. K. (2016). Effect of lithium on neurocognitive functioning. *Curr Alzheimer Res*, 13, 887–893.

7. Velosa, J., Delgado, A., Finger, E., et al. (2020). Risk of dementia in bipolar disorder and the interplay of lithium: A systematic review and meta-analyses. *Acta Psychiatr Scand*, 141, 510–521.

8. Baldessarini, R. J. and Tondo, L. (2021). Testing for antisuicidal effects of lithium treatment. *JAMA Psychiatry*, 79, 9–10.

9. Baldessarini, R. J., Tondo, L., Davis, P., et al. (2006). Decreased risk of suicides and attempts during long-term lithium treatment: A meta-analytic review. *Bipolar Disord*, 8, 625–639.

10. Del Matto, L., Muscas, M., Murru, A., et al. (2020). Lithium and suicide prevention in mood disorders and in the general population: A systematic review. *Neurosci Biobehav Rev*, 116, 142–153.

11. Kishi, T., Ikuta, T., Matsuda, Y., et al. (2021). Mood stabilizers and/or antipsychotics for bipolar disorder in the maintenance phase: A systematic review and network meta-analysis of randomized controlled trials. *Mol Psychiatry*, 26, 4146–4157.

12. Schumann, C., Lenz, G., Berghofer, A., et al. (1999). Non-adherence with long-term prophylaxis: A 6-year naturalistic follow-up study of affectively ill patients. *Psychiatry Res*, 89, 247–257.

13. Kessing, L. V., Søndergård, L., Kvist, K., et al. (2007). Adherence to lithium in naturalistic settings: Results from a nationwide pharmacoepidemiological study. *Bipolar Disord*, 9, 730–736.

14. Aagaard, J., Vestergaard, P. and Maarbjerg, K. (1988). Adherence to lithium prophylaxis: II. Multivariate analysis of clinical, social, and psychosocial predictors of nonadherence. *Pharmacopsychiatry*, 21, 166–170.

15. Maarbjerg, K., Aagaard, J. and Vestergaard, P. (1988). Adherence to lithium prophylaxis: I. Clinical predictors and patient's reasons for nonadherence. *Pharmacopsychiatry*, 21, 121–125.

16. Jawad, I., Watson, S., Haddad, P. M., et al. (2018). Medication nonadherence in bipolar disorder: A narrative review. *Ther Adv Psychopharmacol*, 8, 349–363.

17. Gitlin, M. (2016). Lithium side effects and toxicity: Prevalence and management strategies. *Int J Bipolar Disord*, 4, 27–36.

18. Pope, M. and Scott, J. (2003). Do clinicians understand why individuals stop taking lithium? *J Affect Disord*, 74, 287–291.

19. McVoy, M., Delbello, M., Levin, J., et al. (2022). A customized adherence enhancement program for adolescents and young adults with suboptimal adherence and bipolar disorder: Trial design and methodological report. *Contemp Clin Trials*, 115, 106729.

20. Sajatovic, M., Tatsuoka, C., Cassidy, K. A., et al. (2018). A 6-month, prospective, randomized controlled trial of Customized Adherence Enhancement versus bipolar-specific educational control in poorly adherent individuals with bipolar disorder. *J Clin Psychiatry*, 79, 17m12036 e12031–e12010.

21. Öhlund, L., Ott, M., Oja, S., et al. (2018). Reasons for lithium discontinuation in men and women with bipolar disorder: A retrospective cohort study. *BMC Psychiatry*, 18, 37–46.

22. Bai, Y., Yang, H., Chen, G., et al. (2020). Acceptability of acute and maintenance pharmacotherapy of bipolar disorder: A systematic review of randomized, double-blind, placebo-controlled clinical trials. *J Clin Psychopharmacol*, 40, 167–179.

23. Holm, M., Tanskanen, A., Lahteenvuo, M., et al. (2022). Comparative effectiveness of mood stabilizers and antipsychotics in the prevention of hospitalization after lithium discontinuation in bipolar disorder. *Eur Neuropsychopharmacol*, 61, 36–42.

24. Krull, F., Akkouh, I., Hughes, T., et al. (2022). Dose-dependent transcriptional effects of lithium and adverse effect burden in a psychiatric cohort. *Prog Neuropsychopharmacol Biol Psychiatry*, 112, 110408.

25. Davis, J., Desmond, M. and Berk, M. (2018). Lithium and nephrotoxicity: A literature review of approaches to clinical management and risk stratification. *BMC Nephrol*, 19, 305.

26. Kinahan, J. C., NiChorcorain, A., Cunningham, S., et al. (2015). Diagnostic accuracy of tests for polyuria in lithium-treated patients. *J Clin Psychopharmacol*, 35, 434–441.

27. Clos, S., Rauchhaus, P., Severn, A., et al. (2015). Long-term effect of lithium maintenance therapy on estimated glomerular filtration rate in patients with affective disorders: A population-based cohort study. *Lancet Psychiatry*, 2, 1075–1083.

28. Kirkham, E., Skinner, J., Anderson, T., et al. (2014). One lithium level > 1.0 mmol/L causes an acute decline in eGFR: Findings from a retrospective analysis of a monitoring database. *BMJ Open*, 4, e006020.

29. Castro, V. M., Roberson, A. M., McCoy, T. H., et al. (2016). Stratifying risk for renal insufficiency among lithium-treated patients: An electronic health record study. *Neuropsychopharmacology*, 41, 1138–1143.

30. Kalita-De Croft, P., Bedford, J. J., Leader, J. P., et al. (2018). Amiloride modifies the progression of lithium-induced renal interstitial fibrosis. *Nephrology (Carlton)*, 23, 20–30.

31. Pradhan, B. K., Chakrabarti, S., Irpati, A. S., et al. (2011). Distress due to lithium-induced polyuria: Exploratory study. *Psychiatry Clin Neurosci*, 65, 386–388.

32. Kortenoeven, M. L., Li, Y., Shaw, S., et al. (2009). Amiloride blocks lithium entry through the sodium channel thereby attenuating the resultant nephrogenic diabetes insipidus. *Kidney Int*, 76, 44–53.

33. Vandenbeuch, A. and Kinnamon, S. C. (2020). Is the amiloride-sensitive Na+ channel in taste cells really ENaC? *Chem Senses*, 45, 233–234.

34. Vallée, C., Howlin, B. and Lewis, R. (2021). Ion selectivity in the ENaC/DEG family: A systematic review with supporting analysis. *Int J Mol Sci*, 22, 10998, 10991–10922.

35. Trepiccione, F. and Christensen, B. M. (2010). Lithium-induced nephrogenic diabetes insipidus: New clinical and experimental findings. *J Nephrol*, 23 Suppl. 16, S43–48.

36. Davis, J., Desmond, M. and Berk, M. (2018). Lithium and nephrotoxicity: Unravelling the complex pathophysiological threads of the lightest metal. *Nephrology (Carlton)*, 23, 897–903.

37. Batle, D. C., von Riotte, A. B., Gaviria, M., et al. (1985). Amelioration of polyuria by amiloride in patients receiving long-term lithium therapy. *NEJM*, 312, 408–414.

38. Schoot, T. S., Molmans, T. H. J., Grootens, K. P., et al. (2020). Systematic review and practical guideline for the prevention and management of the renal side effects of lithium therapy. *Eur Neuropsychopharmacol*, 31, 16–32.

39. Bedford, J. J., Weggery, S., Ellis, G., et al. (2008). Lithium-induced nephrogenic diabetes insipidus: Renal effects of amiloride. *Clin J Am Soc Nephrol*, 3, 1324–1331.

40. Grünfeld, J.-P. and Rossier, B. C. (2009). Lithium nephrotoxicity revisited. *Nat Rev Nephrol*, 5, 270–276.

41. Schou, M., Amdisen, A., Thomsen, K., et al. (1982). Lithium treatment regimen and renal water handling: The significance of dosage pattern and tablet type examined through comparison of results from two clinics with different treatment regimens. *Psychopharmacology*, 77, 387–390.

42. Song, J., Bergen, S. E., Di Florio, A., et al. (2016). Genome-wide association study identifies SESTD1 as a novel risk gene for lithium-responsive bipolar disorder. [Erratum appears in *Mol Psychiatry* (2017). Aug. 22(8): 1223; PMID: 28194006.] *Mol Psychiatry*, 21, 1290–1297.

43. Amdisen, A. (1977). Serum level monitoring and clinical pharmacokinetics of lithium. *Clin Pharmacokinet*, 2, 73–92.

44. Swartz, C. M. (1987). Correction of lithium levels for dose and blood sampling times. *J Clin Psychiatry*, 48, 60–64.

45. Kusalic, M. and Engelsmann, F. (1996). Renal reactions to changes of lithium dosage. *Neuropsychobiology*, 34, 113–116.

46. Roush, G. C. and Sica, D. A. (2016). Diuretics for hypertension: A review and update. *Am J Hypertens*, 29, 1130–1137.

47. Mehta, B. R. and Robinson, B. H. (1980). Lithium toxicity induced by triamterene-hydrochlorothiazide. *Postgrad Med J*, 56, 783–784.

48. Dorevitch, A. and Baruch, E. (1986). Lithium toxicity induced by combined amiloride HCl-hydrochlorothiazide administration. *Am J Psychiatry*, 143, 257–258.

49. de Groot, T., Sinke, A. P., Kortenoeven, M. L., et al. (2016). Acetazolamide attenuates lithium-induced nephrogenic diabetes insipidus. *J Am Soc Nephrol*, 27, 2082–2091.

50. Gordon, C. E., Vantzelfde, S. and Francis, J. M. (2016). Acetazolamide in lithium-induced nephrogenic diabetes insipidus. *N Engl J Med*, 375, 2008–2009.

51. de Groot, T., Doornebal, J., Christensen, B. M., et al. (2017). Lithium-induced NDI: Acetazolamide reduces polyuria but does not improve urine concentrating ability. *Am J Physiol Renal Physiol*, 313, F669–676.

52. Sands, J. M. and Bichet, D. G. (2006). Nephrogenic diabetes insipidus. *Ann Intern Med*, 144, 186–194.

53. Macau, R. A., da Silva, T. N., Silva, J. R., et al. (2018). Use of acetazolamide in lithium-induced nephrogenic diabetes insipidus: A case report. *Endocrinol Diabetes Metab Case Rep*, 2018, 17-0154.

54. Alembic Pharmaceuticals Inc. (2022). *Acetazolamide capsule, extended release package insert*. Bedminster, NJ.

55. Thomsen, K. and Schou, M. (1973). The effect of prolonged administration of hydrochlorothiazide on the renal lithium clearance and the urine flow of ordinary rats and rats with diabetes insipidus. *Pharmakopsychiatr Neuropsychopharmakol*, 6, 264–269.

56. Kim, G.-H., Lee, J. W., Oh, Y. K., et al. (2004). Antidiuretic effect of hydrochlorothiazide in lithium-induced nephrogenic diabetes insipidus is associated with upregulation of aquaporin-2, Na-Cl co-transporter, and epithelial sodium channel. *J Am Soc Nephrol*, 15, 2836–2843.

57. Sinke, A. P., Kortenoeven, M. L., de Groot, T., et al. (2014). Hydrochlorothiazide attenuates lithium-induced nephrogenic diabetes insipidus independently of the sodium–chloride cotransporter. *Am J Physiol Renal Physiol*, 306, F525–F533.

58. Sands, J. M. (2016). Water, water everywhere: A new cause and a new treatment for nephrogenic diabetes insipidus. *J Am Soc Nephrol*, 27, 1872–1874.

59. Chen, T. K., Knicely, D. H. and Grams, M. E. (2019). Chronic kidney disease diagnosis and management: A review. *JAMA*, 322, 1294–1304.

60. **Delgado, C., Baweja, M., Crews, D. C., et al. (2021).** A unifying approach for GFR estimation: Recommendations of the NKF–ASN Task Force on Reassessing the Inclusion of Race in Diagnosing Kidney Disease. *Am J Kidney Dis*, 79, 268–288.e261.

61. **Fagiolini, A., Chengappa, K. N., Soreca, I., et al. (2008).** Bipolar disorder and the metabolic syndrome: Causal factors, psychiatric outcomes and economic burden. *CNS Drugs*, 22, 655–669.

62. **McElroy, S. L. and Keck, P. E., Jr. (2014).** Metabolic syndrome in bipolar disorder: A review with a focus on bipolar depression. *J Clin Psychiatry*, 75, 46–61.

63. **Godin, O., Leboyer, M., Belzeaux, R., et al. (2021).** Non-alcoholic fatty liver disease in a sample of individuals with bipolar disorders: Results from the FACE-BD cohort. *Acta Psychiatr Scand*, 143, 82–91.

64. **Lepkifker, E., Sverdlik, A., Iancu, I., et al. (2004).** Renal insufficiency in long-term lithium treatment. *J Clin Psychiatry*, 63, 850–856.

65. **Presne, C., Fakhouri, F., Noel, L. H., et al. (2003).** Lithium-induced nephropathy: Rate of progression and prognostic factors. *Kidney Int*, 64, 585–592.

66. **Fotso Soh, J., Kiil-Drori, S. and Rej, S. (2019).** Using lithium in older age bipolar disorder: Special considerations. *Drugs Aging*, 36, 147–154.

67. **Golic, M., Aiff, H., Attman, P. O., et al. (2021).** Starting lithium in patients with compromised renal function – is it wise? *J Psychopharmacol*, 35, 190–197.

68. **McGrane, I. R., Omar, F. A., Morgan, N. F., et al. (2022).** Lithium therapy in patients on dialysis: A systematic review. *Int J Psychiatry Med*, 57, 187–201.

69. **Markowitz, G. S., Radhakrishnan, J., Kambham, N., et al. (2000).** Lithium nephrotoxicity: A progressive combined glomerular and tubulointerstitial nephropathy. *J Am Soc Nephrol*, 11, 1439–1448.

70. **Rej, S., Abitbol, R., Looper, K., et al. (2013).** Chronic renal failure in lithium-using geriatric patients: Effects of lithium continuation versus discontinuation – a 60-month retrospective study. *Int J Geriatr Psychiatry*, 28, 450–453.

71. **Amaro-Hosey, K., Castells, X., Blanco-Silvente, L., et al. (2022).** Drug-induced sudden death: A scoping review. *Curr Drug Saf*, https://doi.org/10.2174/1574886317666220525115232 (online ahead of print).

72. **Bunschoten, J. W., Husein, N., Devinsky, O., et al. (2022).** Sudden death and cardiac arrythmia with lamotrigine: A rapid systematic review. *Neurology*, 98, e1748–e1760.

73. **Meyer, J. M., Dollarhide, A. and Tuan, I.-L. (2005).** Lithium toxicity after switch from fosinopril to lisinopril. *Int Clin Psychopharmacol*, 20, 115–118.

74. **Sabharwal, M. S., Annapureddy, N., Agarwal, S. K., et al. (2013).** Severe bradycardia caused by a single dose of lithium. *Int Med*, 52, 767–769.

75. **Mehta, N. and Vannozzi, R. (2017).** Lithium-induced electrocardiographic changes: A complete review. *Clin Cardiol*, 40, 1363–1367.

76. **Dahan, A., Porat, D., Azran, C., et al. (2019).** Lithium toxicity with severe bradycardia post sleeve gastrectomy: A case report and review of the literature. *Obes Surg*, 29, 735–738.

77. **ANI Pharmaceuticals Inc. (2020).** *LithoBID package insert*. Baudette, MN.

78. **Bucht, G., Smigan, L., Wahlin, A., et al. (1984).** ECG changes during lithium therapy: A prospective study. *Acta Med Scand*, 216, 101–104.

79. **Josephson, I. R., Lederer, W. J. and Hartmann, H. A. (2006).** Letter regarding article by Darbar et al, "unmasking of Brugada syndrome by lithium." *Circulation*, 113, e408; author reply e408.

80. **Yanagita, T., Maruta, T., Uezono, Y., et al. (2007).** Lithium inhibits function of voltage-dependent sodium channels and catecholamine secretion independent of glycogen synthase kinase-3 in adrenal chromaffin cells. *Neuropharmacology*, 53, 881–889.

81. Darbar, D., Yang, T., Churchwell, K., et al. (2005). Unmasking of brugada syndrome by lithium. *Circulation*, 112, 1527–1531.

82. Hsu, C. H., Liu, P. Y., Chen, J. H., et al. (2005). Electrocardiographic abnormalities as predictors for over-range lithium levels. *Cardiology*, 103, 101–106.

83. Bussink, B. E., Holst, A. G., Jespersen, L., et al. (2013). Right bundle branch block: Prevalence, risk factors, and outcome in the general population. Results from the Copenhagen City Heart Study. *Eur Heart J*, 34, 138–146.

84. Brugada, J., Campuzano, O., Arbelo, E., et al. (2018). Present status of Brugada Syndrome: JACC state-of-the-art review. *J Am Coll Cardiol*, 72, 1046–1059.

85. Gourraud, J. B., Barc, J., Thollet, A., et al. (2017). Brugada syndrome: Diagnosis, risk stratification and management. *Arch Cardiovasc Dis*, 110, 188–195.

86. Ravi, V., Serafini, N. J., Pulipati, P., et al. (2020). Lithium-induced Brugada pattern: A case report and review of literature. *Cureus*, 12, e9351–e9537.

87. Roberts-Thomson, K. C., Teo, K. S. and Young, G. D. (2007). Drug-induced Brugada syndrome with ST-T wave alternans and long QT. *Intern Med J*, 37, 199–200.

88. Jafferany, M. (2008). Lithium and skin: Dermatologic manifestations of lithium therapy. *Int J Dermatol*, 47, 1101–1111.

89. Suganya Priyadharshini, B. S. and Ummar, I. S. (2017). Prevalence and sociodemographic profile of lithium-induced cutaneous side effects in bipolar affective disorder patients: A 1-year prospective observational study in South India. *Indian J Psychol Med*, 39, 648–652.

90. Cox, C. and George, M. (2022). Monitoring of cutaneous manifestations of lithium treatment in mental health inpatients. *Aust N Z J Psychiatry*, 56, 863.

91. McKnight, R. F., Adida, M., Budge, K., et al. (2012). Lithium toxicity profile: A systematic review and meta-analysis. *Lancet*, 379, 721–728.

92. Pinna, M., Manchia, M., Puddu, S., et al. (2017). Cutaneous adverse reaction during lithium treatment: A case report and updated systematic review with meta-analysis. *Int J Bipolar Disord*, 5, 20.

93. McKnight, R. F., Geddes, J. R. and Goodwin, G. M. (2017). Short- and midterm side effects of lithium therapy. In G. S. Malhi, M. Masson and F. Bellivier, eds., *The Science and Practice of Lithium Therapy*. Basel: Springer International Publishing AG, pp. 249–264.

94. Eichenfield, D. Z., Sprague, J. and Eichenfield, L. F. (2021). Management of acne vulgaris: A review. *JAMA*, 326, 2055–2067.

95. Balak, D. M. and Hajdarbegovic, E. (2017). Drug-induced psoriasis: Clinical perspectives. *Psoriasis (Auckl)*, 7, 87–94.

96. Nestor, M. S., Ablon, G., Gade, A., et al. (2021). Treatment options for androgenetic alopecia: Efficacy, side effects, compliance, financial considerations, and ethics. *J Cosmet Dermatol*, 20, 3759–3781.

97. Kozikowski, A. P., Gaisina, I. N., Yuan, H., et al. (2007). Structure-based design leads to the identification of lithium mimetics that block mania-like effects in rodents – possible new GSK-3beta therapies for bipolar disorders. *J Am Chem Soc*, 129, 8328–8332.

98. Freland, L. and Beaulieu, J. M. (2012). Inhibition of GSK3 by lithium, from single molecules to signaling networks. *Front Mol Neurosci*, 5, 14.

99. Kang, J. I., Kim, S. C., Kim, M. K., et al. (2015). Effects of dihydrotestosterone on rat dermal papilla cells in vitro. *Eur J Pharmacol*, 757, 74–83.

100. Xiao, S., Wang, J., Chen, Q., et al. (2019). The mechanism of activated platelet-rich plasma supernatant promotion of hair growth by cultured dermal papilla cells. *J Cosmet Dermatol*, 18, 1711–1716.

101. McKinney, P. A., Finkenbine, R. D. and DeVane, C. L. (1996). Alopecia and mood stabilizer therapy. *Ann Clin Psychiatry*, 8, 183–185.

102. Grover, S., Ghosh, A., Sarkar, S., et al. (2014). Sexual dysfunction in clinically stable patients with bipolar disorder receiving lithium. *J Clin Psychopharmacol*, 34, 475–482.

103. Elnazer, H. Y., Sampson, A. and Baldwin, D. (2015). Lithium and sexual dysfunction: An under-researched area. *Hum Psychopharmacol*, 30, 66–69.

104. Wiggers, S. (1968). [Effects of lithium on the thyroid gland]. *Ugeskr Laeger*, 130, 1523–1525.

105. Garfinkel, P. E., Ezrin, C. and Stancer, H. C. (1973). Hypothyroidism and hyperparathyroidism associated with lithium. *Lancet*, 2, 331–332.

106. Ambrosiani, L., Pisanu, C., Deidda, A., et al. (2018). Thyroid and renal tumors in patients treated with long-term lithium: Case series from a lithium clinic, review of the literature and international pharmacovigilance reports. *Int J Bipolar Disord*, 6, 17.

107. Kraszewska, A., Ziemnicka, K., Sowinski, J., et al. (2019). No connection between long-term lithium treatment and antithyroid antibodies. *Pharmacopsychiatry*, 52, 232–236.

108. Biondi, B., Cappola, A. R. and Cooper, D. S. (2019). Subclinical hypothyroidism: A review. *JAMA*, 322, 153–160.

109. Shine, B., McKnight, R. F., Leaver, L., et al. (2015). Long-term effects of lithium on renal, thyroid, and parathyroid function: A retrospective analysis of laboratory data. *Lancet*, 386, 461–468.

110. Hayes, J. F., Marston, L., Walters, K., et al. (2016). Adverse renal, endocrine, hepatic, and metabolic events during maintenance mood stabilizer treatment for bipolar disorder: A population-based cohort study. *PLoS Med*, 13, e1002058.

111. Fairbrother, F., Petzl, N., Scott, J. G., et al. (2019). Lithium can cause hyperthyroidism as well as hypothyroidism: A systematic review of an under-recognised association. *Aust N Z J Psychiatry*, 53, 384–402.

112. Kibirige, D., Luzinda, K. and Ssekitoleko, R. (2013). Spectrum of lithium induced thyroid abnormalities: A current perspective. *Thyroid Res*, 6, 3–7.

113. Kupka, R. W., Nolen, W. A., Post, R. M., et al. (2002). High rate of autoimmune thyroiditis in bipolar disorder: Lack of association with lithium exposure. *Biol Psychiatry*, 51, 305–311.

114. Czarnywojtek, A., Zgorzalewicz-Stachowiak, M., Czarnocka, B., et al. (2020). Effect of lithium carbonate on the function of the thyroid gland: Mechanism of action and clinical implications. *J Physiol Pharmacol*, 71, 191–199.

115. Liu, Y. Y., van der Pluijm, G., Karperien, M., et al. (2006). Lithium as adjuvant to radioiodine therapy in differentiated thyroid carcinoma: Clinical and in vitro studies. *Clin Endocrinol (Oxf)*, 64, 617–624.

116. Lerena, V. S., León, N. S., Sosa, S., et al. (2022). Lithium and endocrine dysfunction. *Medicina (B Aires)*, 82, 130–137.

117. Lieber, I., Ott, M., Öhlund, L., et al. (2020). Lithium-associated hypothyroidism and potential for reversibility after lithium discontinuation: Findings from the LiSIE retrospective cohort study. *J Psychopharmacol*, 34, 293–303.

118. Biondi, B. (2013). The normal TSH reference range: What has changed in the last decade? *J Clin Endocrinol Metab*, 98, 3584–3587.

119. Bode, H., Ivens, B., Bschor, T., et al. (2021). Association of hypothyroidism and clinical depression: A systematic review and meta-analysis. *JAMA Psychiatry*, 78, 1375–1383.

120. Frye, M. A., Denicoff, K. D., Bryan, A. L., et al. (1999). Association between lower serum free T4 and greater mood instability and depression in lithium-maintained bipolar patients. *Am J Psychiatry*, 156, 1909–1914.

121. Frye, M. A., Yatham, L., Ketter, T. A., et al. (2009). Depressive relapse during lithium treatment associated with increased serum thyroid-stimulating hormone: Results from two placebo-controlled bipolar I maintenance studies. *Acta Psychiatr Scand*, 120, 10–13.

122. Cole, D. P., Thase, M. E., Mallinger, A. G., et al. (2002). Slower treatment response in bipolar depression predicted by lower pretreatment thyroid function. *Am J Psychiatry*, 159, 116–121.

123. McAninch, E. A. and Bianco, A. C. (2016). The history and future of treatment of hypothyroidism. *Ann Intern Med*, 164, 50–56.

124. Jonklaas, J., Bianco, A. C., Cappola, A. R., et al. (2021). Evidence-based use of levothyroxine/liothyronine combinations in treating hypothyroidism: A consensus document. *Thyroid*, 31, 156–182.

125. Shapiro, H. I. and Davis, K. A. (2015). Hypercalcemia and "primary" hyperparathyroidism during lithium therapy. *Am J Psychiatry*, 172, 12–15.

126. Albert, U., De Cori, D., Aguglia, A., et al. (2013). Lithium-associated hyperparathyroidism and hypercalcaemia: A case-control cross-sectional study. *J Affect Disord*, 151, 786–790.

127. Catalano, A., Chilà, D., Bellone, F., et al. (2018). Incidence of hypocalcemia and hypercalcemia in hospitalized patients: Is it changing? *J Clin Transl Endocrinol*, 13, 9–13.

128. Mifsud, S., Cilia, K., Mifsud, E. L., et al. (2020). Lithium-associated hyperparathyroidism. *Br J Hosp Med (Lond)*, 81, 1–9.

129. Islam, A. K. (2021). Advances in the diagnosis and the management of primary hyperparathyroidism. *Ther Adv Chronic Dis*, 12, 20406223211015965.

130. Pattan, V., Singh, B., Abdelmoneim, S. S., et al. (2021). Lithium-induced hyperparathyroidism: An ill-defined territory. *Psychopharmacol Bull*, 51, 65–71.

131. Ketteler, M., Bover, J. and Mazzaferro, S. (2022). Treatment of secondary hyperparathyroidism in non-dialysis CKD: An appraisal 2022s. *Nephrol Dial Transplant*, DOI: 10.1093/ndt/gfac236.

132. Kessing, L. V., Gerds, T. A., Feldt-Rasmussen, B., et al. (2015). Use of lithium and anticonvulsants and the rate of chronic kidney disease: A nationwide population-based study. *JAMA Psychiatry*, 72, 1182–1191.

133. Takkouche, B., Montes-Martínez, A., Gill, S. S., et al. (2007). Psychotropic medications and the risk of fracture: A meta-analysis. *Drug Saf*, 30, 171–184.

134. Köhler-Forsberg, O., Rohde, C., Nierenberg, A. A., et al. (2022). Association of lithium treatment with the risk of osteoporosis in patients with bipolar disorder. *JAMA Psychiatry*, 79, 454–463.

135. Zhou, C., Fang, L., Chen, Y., et al. (2018). Effect of selective serotonin reuptake inhibitors on bone mineral density: A systematic review and meta-analysis. *Osteoporos Int*, 29, 1243–1251.

136. De Hert, M., Detraux, J. and Stubbs, B. (2016). Relationship between antipsychotic medication, serum prolactin levels and osteoporosis/osteoporotic fractures in patients with schizophrenia: A critical literature review. *Expert Opin Drug Saf*, 15, 809–823.

137. Su, J. A., Cheng, B. H., Huang, Y. C., et al. (2017). Bipolar disorder and the risk of fracture: A nationwide population-based cohort study. *J Affect Disord*, 218, 246–252.

138. Chen, Y., Whetstone, H. C., Lin, A. C., et al. (2007). Beta-catenin signaling plays a disparate role in different phases of fracture repair: Implications for therapy to improve bone healing. *PLoS Med*, 4, e249.

139. Clément-Lacroix, P., Ai, M., Morvan, F., et al. (2005). Lrp5-independent activation of Wnt signaling by lithium chloride increases bone formation and bone mass in mice. *Proc Natl Acad Sci USA*, 102, 17406–17411.

140. Wong, S. K., Chin, K. Y. and Ima-Nirwana, S. (2020). The skeletal-protecting action and mechanisms of action for mood-stabilizing drug lithium chloride: Current evidence and future potential research areas. *Front Pharmacol*, 11, 1–17.

141. Tully, A., Smyth, S., Conway, Y., et al. (2020). Interventions for the management of obesity in people with bipolar disorder. *Cochrane Database Syst Rev*, 7, Cd013006.

142. Doane, M. J., Bessonova, L., Friedler, H. S., et al. (2022). Weight gain and comorbidities associated with oral second-generation antipsychotics: Analysis of real-world data for patients with schizophrenia or bipolar I disorder. *BMC Psychiatry*, 22, 114–125.

143. Dalkner, N., Bengesser, S. A., Birner, A., et al. (2021). Metabolic syndrome impairs executive function in bipolar disorder. *Front Neurosci*, 15, 717824.

144. Vanina, Y., Podolskaya, A., Sedky, K., et al. (2002). Body weight changes associated with psychopharmacology. *Psychiatr Serv*, 53, 842–847.

145. Prillo, J., Soh, J. F., Park, H., et al. (2021). Obesity and metabolic comorbidity in bipolar disorder: Do patients on lithium comprise a subgroup? A naturalistic study. *BMC Psychiatry*, 21, 558–565.

146. Vieta, E., Locklear, J., Gunther, O., et al. (2010). Treatment options for bipolar depression: A systematic review of randomized, controlled trials. *J Clin Psychopharmacol*, 30, 579–590.

147. Huhn, M., Nikolakopoulou, A., Schneider-Thoma, J., et al. (2019). Comparative efficacy and tolerability of 32 oral antipsychotics for the acute treatment of adults with multi-episode schizophrenia: A systematic review and network meta-analysis. *The Lancet*, 394, 939–951.

148. Wingård, L., Brandt, L., Bodén, R., et al. (2019). Monotherapy vs. combination therapy for post mania maintenance treatment: A population based cohort study. *Eur Neuropsychopharmacol*, 29, 691–700.

149. Wang, Y., Wang, D., Cheng, J., et al. (2021). Efficacy and tolerability of pharmacological interventions on metabolic disturbance induced by atypical antipsychotics in adults: A systematic review and network meta-analysis. *J Psychopharmacol*, 35, 1111–1119.

150. Praharaj, S. K. (2016). Metformin for lithium-induced weight gain: A case report. *Clin Psychopharmacol Neurosci*, 14, 101–103.

151. Lipska, K. J., Bailey, C. J. and Inzucchi, S. E. (2011). Use of metformin in the setting of mild-to-moderate renal insufficiency. *Diabetes Care*, 34, 1431–1437.

152. Novo Nordisk Inc. (2021). *Wegovy package insert*. Plainsboro, NJ.

153. Novo Nordisk Inc. (2022). *Saxenda package insert*. Plainsboro, NJ.

154. Larsen, J. R., Vedtofte, L., Jakobsen, M. S. L., et al. (2017). Effect of liraglutide treatment on prediabetes and overweight or obesity in clozapine- or olanzapine-treated patients with schizophrenia spectrum disorder: A randomized clinical trial. *JAMA Psychiatry*, 74, 719–728.

155. Ayub, S., Saboor, S., Usmani, S., et al. (2022). Lithium toxicity following Roux-en-Y gastric bypass: Mini review and illustrative case. *Ment Health Clin*, 12, 214–218.

156. Bingham, K. S., Thoma, J., Hawa, R., et al. (2016). Perioperative lithium use in bariatric surgery: A case series and literature review. *Psychosomatics*, 57, 638–644.

157. Musfeldt, D., Levinson, A., Nykiel, J., et al. (2016). Lithium toxicity after Roux-en-Y bariatric surgery. *BMJ Case Rep*, 2016.

158. Niessen, R., Sottiaux, T., Schillaci, A., et al. (2018). [Lithium toxicity after bariatric surgery]. *Rev Med Liege*, 73, 82–87.

159. Jamison, S. C. and Aheron, K. (2020). Lithium toxicity following bariatric surgery. *SAGE Open Med Case Rep*, 8, 2050313x20953000.

160. Lin, Y. H., Liu, S. W., Wu, H. L., et al. (2020). Lithium toxicity with prolonged neurologic sequelae following sleeve gastrectomy: A case report and review of literature. *Medicine (Baltimore)*, 99, e21122.

161. Marques, A. R., Alho, A., Martins, J. M., et al. (2021). Lithium intoxication after bariatric surgery: A case report. *Acta Med Port*, 34, 382–386.

162. Pratley, R., Amod, A., Hoff, S. T., et al. (2019). Oral semaglutide versus subcutaneous liraglutide and placebo in type 2 diabetes (PIONEER 4): A randomised, double-blind, phase 3a trial. *Lancet*, 394, 39–50.

163. Alsugair, H. A., Alshugair, I. F., Alharbi, T. J., et al. (2021). Weekly semaglutide vs. liraglutide efficacy profile: A network meta-analysis. *Healthcare (Basel)*, 9, 1125.

164. Hou, P. H., Mao, F. C., Chang, G. R., et al. (2018). Newly diagnosed bipolar disorder and the subsequent risk of erectile dysfunction: A nationwide cohort study. *J Sex Med*, 15, 183–191.

165. Sheibani, M., Ghasemi, M. and Dehpour, A. R. (2022). Lithium and erectile dysfunction: An overview. *Cells*, 11, 171.

166. Saroukhani, S., Emami-Parsa, M., Modabbernia, A., et al. (2013). Aspirin for treatment of lithium-associated sexual dysfunction in men: Randomized double-blind placebo-controlled study. *Bipolar Disord*, 15, 650–656.

167. Gopalakrishnan, R., Jacob, K. S., Kuruvilla, A., et al. (2006). Sildenafil in the treatment of antipsychotic-induced erectile dysfunction: A randomized, double-blind, placebo-controlled, flexible-dose, two-way crossover trial. *Am J Psychiatry*, 163, 494–499.

168. Öhlund, L., Ott, M., Bergqvist, M., et al. (2019). Clinical course and need for hospital admission after lithium discontinuation in patients with bipolar disorder type I or II: Mirror-image study based on the LiSIE retrospective cohort. *BJPsych Open*, 5, e101–112.

169. Vestergaard, P., Amdisen, A. and Schou, M. (1980). Clinically significant side effects of lithium treatment: A survey of 237 patients in long-term treatment. *Acta Psychiatr Scand*, 62, 193–200.

170. Vestergaard, P., Poulstrup, I. and Schou, M. (1988). Prospective studies on a lithium cohort. 3. Tremor, weight gain, diarrhea, psychological complaints. *Acta Psychiatr Scand*, 78, 434–441.

171. Licht, R. W., Nielsen, J. N., Gram, L. F., et al. (2010). Lamotrigine versus lithium as maintenance treatment in bipolar I disorder: An open, randomized effectiveness study mimicking clinical practice. The 6th trial of the Danish University Antidepressant Group (DUAG-6). *Bipolar Disord*, 12, 483–493.

172. El-Mallakh, R. S., Marcus, R., Baudelet, C., et al. (2012). A 40-week double-blind aripiprazole versus lithium follow-up of a 12-week acute phase study (total 52 weeks) in bipolar I disorder. *J Affect Disord*, 136, 258–266.

173. Barbuti, M., Colombini, P., Ricciardulli, S., et al. (2021). Treatment adherence and tolerability of immediate- and prolonged-release lithium formulations in a sample of bipolar patients: A prospective naturalistic study. *Int Clin Psychopharmacol*, 36, 230–237.

174. Gai, M. N., Thielemann, A. M. and Arancibia, A. (2000). Effect of three different diets on the bioavailability of a sustained release lithium carbonate matrix tablet. *Int J Clin Pharmacol Ther*, 38, 320–326.

175. Jeppsson, J. and Sjögren, J. (1975). The influence of food on side effects and absorption of lithium. *Acta Psychiatr Scand*, 51, 285–288.

176. AbbVie Inc. (2021). *Depakote ER package insert*. North Chicago, IL.

177. Nolen, W. A., Licht, R. W., Young, A. H., et al. (2019). What is the optimal serum level for lithium in the maintenance treatment of bipolar disorder? A systematic review and recommendations from the ISBD/IGSLI Task Force on treatment with lithium. *Bipolar Disord*, 21, 394–409.

178. Rogers, G. A. (1981). Flavors altered by lithium. *Am J Psychiatry*, 138, 261.

179. Glenmark Pharmaceuticals Inc. (2020). *Lithium Carbonate capsule package insert*. Mahwah, NJ.

180. Bigiani, A. (2020). Does ENaC work as sodium taste receptor in humans? *Nutrients*, 12, 1195.

181. Lossow, K., Hermans-Borgmeyer, I., Meyerhof, W., et al. (2020). Segregated expression of ENaC subunits in taste cells. *Chem Senses*, 45, 235–248.

182. Terao, T., Watanabe, S., Hoaki, N., et al. (2011). Strange taste and mild lithium intoxication. *BMJ Case Rep*, 2011.

183. Hanyu, S., Sugita, N., Matsuda, M., et al. (2020). Lithium intoxication-induced dysgeusia accompanied by glossalgia in a patient receiving lithium carbonate: A case report. *J Med Case Rep*, 14, 149.

184. Gelenberg, A. J., Kane, J. M., Keller, M. B., et al. (1989). Comparison of standard and low serum levels of lithium for maintenance treatment of bipolar disorder. *N Engl J Med*, 321, 1489–1493.

185. Proctor, G. B. and Carpenter, G. H. (2014). Salivary secretion: Mechanism and neural regulation. *Monogr Oral Sci*, 24, 14–29.

186. Wu, L. S., Huang, M. C., Chen, C. K., et al. (2021). Genome-wide association study of lithium-induced dry mouth in bipolar I disorder. *J Pers Med*, 11, 1265.

187. Orsolini, L., Pompili, S. and Volpe, U. (2020). The "collateral side" of mood stabilizers: Safety and evidence-based strategies for managing side effects. *Expert Opin Drug Saf*, 19, 1461–1495.

188. Seki, T., Aki, M., Kawashima, H., et al. (2019). Electronic health record nested pragmatic randomized controlled trial of a reminder system for serum lithium level monitoring in patients with mood disorder: KONOTORI study protocol. *Trials*, 20, 706.

189. Joshi, Y. B., Thomas, M. L., Braff, D. L., et al. (2021). Anticholinergic medication burden-associated cognitive impairment in schizophrenia. *Am J Psychiatry*, 178, 838–847.

190. Lupu, A. M., MacCamy, K. L., Gannon, J. M., et al. (2021). Less is more: Deprescribing anticholinergic medications in persons with severe mental illness. *Ann Clin Psychiatry*, 33, 80–92.

191. Focosi, D., Azzara, A., Kast, R. E., et al. (2009). Lithium and hematology: Established and proposed uses. *J Leukoc Biol*, 85, 20–28.

192. Ballin, A., Lehman, D., Sirota, P., et al. (1998). Increased number of peripheral blood CD34+ cells in lithium-treated patients. *Br J Haematol*, 100, 219–221.

193. Meyer, J. M. and Stahl, S. M. (2019). *The Clozapine Handbook* (Stahl's Handbooks). Cambridge: Cambridge University Press.

194. Baek, J. H., Kinrys, G. and Nierenberg, A. A. (2014). Lithium tremor revisited: Pathophysiology and treatment. *Acta Psychiatr Scand*, 129, 17–23.

195. Schneider, S. A. and Deuschl, G. (2014). The treatment of tremor. *Neurotherapeutics*, 11, 128–138.

196. Wilting, I., Heerdink, E. R., Mersch, P. P., et al. (2009). Association between lithium serum level, mood state, and patient-reported adverse drug reactions during long-term lithium treatment: A naturalistic follow-up study. *Bipolar Disord*, 11, 434–440.

197. Wingo, A. P., Wingo, T. S., Harvey, P. D., et al. (2009). Effects of lithium on cognitive performance: A meta-analysis. *J Clin Psychiatry*, 70, 1588–1597.

198. Burdick, K. E., Millett, C. E., Russo, M., et al. (2020). The association between lithium use and neurocognitive performance in patients with bipolar disorder. *Neuropsychopharmacology*, 45, 1743–1749.

199. Paterson, A. and Parker, G. (2017). Lithium and cognition in those with bipolar disorder. *Int Clin Psychopharmacol*, 32, 57–62.

200. Soares, J. C., Boada, F. and Keshavan, M. S. (2000). Brain lithium measurements with (7) Li magnetic resonance spectroscopy (MRS): A literature review. *Eur Neuropsychopharmacol*, 10, 151–158.

201. Forester, B. P., Streeter, C. C., Berlow, Y. A., et al. (2009). Brain lithium levels and effects on cognition and mood in geriatric bipolar disorder: A lithium-7 magnetic resonance spectroscopy study. *Am J Geriatr Psychiatry*, 17, 13–23.

202. Lee, J. H., Adler, C., Norris, M., et al. (2012). 4-T 7Li 3D MR spectroscopy imaging in the brains of bipolar disorder subjects. *Magn Reson Med*, 68, 363–368.

203. Moore, C. M., Demopulos, C. M., Henry, M. E., et al. (2002). Brain-to-serum lithium ratio and age: An in vivo magnetic resonance spectroscopy study. *Am J Psychiatry*, 159, 1240–1242.

204. Machado-Vieira, R., Otaduy, M. C., Zanetti, M. V., et al. (2016). A selective association between central and peripheral lithium levels in remitters in bipolar depression: A 3 T-(7)Li magnetic resonance spectroscopy study. *Acta Psychiatr Scand*, 133, 214–220.

205. Tandon, P., Wong, N. and Zaltzman, J. S. (2015). Lithium-induced minimal change disease and acute kidney injury. *N Am J Med Sci*, 7, 328–331.

206. Basile, G., Epifanio, A., Mandraffino, R., et al. (2014). Parkinsonism and severe hypothyroidism in an elderly patient: A case of lithium toxicity due to pharmacological interactions. *J Clin Pharm Ther*, 39, 452–454.

207. Hermida, A. P., Janjua, A. U., Glass, O. M., et al. (2016). A case of lithium-induced parkinsonism presenting with typical motor symptoms of Parkinson's disease in a bipolar patient. *Int Psychogeriatr*, 28, 2101–2104.

208. Marras, C., Herrmann, N., Fischer, H. D., et al. (2016). Lithium use in older adults is associated with increased prescribing of Parkinson medications. *Am J Geriatr Psychiatry*, 24, 301–309.

209. Friedman, J. H. (2020). Movement disorders induced by psychiatric drugs that do not block dopamine receptors. *Parkinsonism Relat Disord*, 79, 60–64.

210. Hsieh, H. T. and Yeh, Y. W. (2020). Dose-dependent effects of lithium treatment on the aggravation of antipsychotic-induced Pisa syndrome. *Clin Neuropharmacol*, 43, 90–91.

211. Tatara, A., Shimizu, S., Shin, N., et al. (2012). Modulation of antipsychotic-induced extrapyramidal side effects by medications for mood disorders. *Prog Neuropsychopharmacol Biol Psychiatry*, 38, 252–259.

212. Uwai, Y. and Nabekura, T. (2022). Relationship between lithium carbonate and the risk of Parkinson-like events in patients with bipolar disorders: A multivariate analysis using the Japanese adverse drug event report database. *Psychiatry Res*, 314, 114687.

213. Erro, R., Landolfi, A., D'Agostino, G., et al. (2021). Bipolar disorder and Parkinson's Disease: A (123)I-Ioflupane dopamine transporter SPECT study. *Front Neurol*, 12, 652375.

214. Revet, A., Montastruc, F., Roussin, A., et al. (2020). Antidepressants and movement disorders: A postmarketing study in the world pharmacovigilance database. *BMC Psychiatry*, 20, 308.

215. Chenu, F. and Bourin, M. (2006). Potentiation of antidepressant-like activity with lithium: Mechanism involved. *Curr Drug Targets*, 7, 159–163.

216. Janssen, S., Bloem, B. R. and van de Warrenburg, B. P. (2017). The clinical heterogeneity of drug-induced myoclonus: An illustrated review. *J Neurol*, 264, 1559–1566.

217. Guttuso, T., Jr. (2019). High lithium levels in tobacco may account for reduced incidences of both Parkinson's disease and melanoma in smokers through enhanced β-catenin-mediated activity. *Med Hypotheses*, 131, 109302.

218. Sáenz-Farret, M., Tijssen, M. A. J., Eliashiv, D., et al. (2022). Antiseizure drugs and movement disorders. *CNS Drugs*, 36, 859–876.

219. Williams, D. P., Troost, B. T. and Rogers, J. (1988). Lithium-induced downbeat nystagmus. *Arch Neurol*, 45, 1022–1023.

220. Halmagyi, G. M., Lessell, I., Curthoys, I. S., et al. (1989). Lithium-induced downbeat nystagmus. *Am J Ophthalmol*, 107, 664–670.

221. Rosenberg, M. L. (1989). Permanent lithium-induced downbeating nystagmus. *Arch Neurol*, 46, 839.

222. Lee, M. S. and Lessell, S. (2003). Lithium-induced periodic alternating nystagmus. *Neurology*, 60, 344.

223. Monden, M. A., Nederkoorn, P. J. and Tijsma, M. (2015). [Downbeat nystagmus – a rare side-effect of lithium carbonate]. *Tijdschr Psychiatr*, 57, 49–53.

224. Jørgensen, J. S., Landschoff Lassen, L. and Wegener, M. (2016). Lithium-induced downbeat nystagmus and horizontal gaze palsy. *Open Ophthalmol J*, 10, 126–128.

225. Rust, H., Lutz, N., Honegger, F., et al. (2016). Periodic alternating nystagmus in a patient on long-term lithium medication. *J Neurol Sci*, 369, 252–253.

226. Schein, F., Manoli, P. and Cathébras, P. (2017). Lithium-induced downbeat nystagmus. *Am J Ophthalmol Case Rep*, 7, 74–75.

227. Hong, H. and Lyu, I. J. (2019). A case of skew deviation and downbeat nystagmus induced by lithium. *BMC Ophthalmol*, 19, 257.

228. Peng, Y. Y. (2019). Reversible hand tremors, downbeat nystagmus, and an unsteady gait with nontoxic lithium level. *Clin Case Rep*, 7, 599–600.

229. Boyer, E. W. and Shannon, M. (2005). The serotonin syndrome. *N Engl J Med*, 352, 1112–1120.

230. Caviness, J. N. and Evidente, V. G. (2003). Cortical myoclonus during lithium exposure. *Arch Neurol*, 60, 401–404.

231. Sarrigiannis, P. G., Zis, P., Unwin, Z. C., et al. (2019). Tremor after long term lithium treatment; is it cortical myoclonus? *Cerebellum Ataxias*, 6, 5.

232. Kocher, R. and Richter, R. (1978). Routine EEG examinations accompanying lithium therapy over two years. *Arzneimittelforschung*, 28, 1524–1525.

233. Hanak, A. S., Malissin, I., Poupon, J., et al. (2017). Electroencephalographic patterns of lithium poisoning: A study of the effect/concentration relationships in the rat. *Bipolar Disord*, 19, 135–145.

234. Swartz, C. M. and Dolinar, L. J. (1995). Encephalopathy associated with rapid decrease of high levels of lithium. *Ann Clin Psychiatry*, 7, 207–209.

235. Señga, M. M., Sarapuddin, G. and Saniel, E. (2020). A case report on an atypical presentation of the Syndrome of Irreversible Lithium-Effectuated Neurotoxicity (SILENT) in a war veteran with bipolar disorder and PTSD. *Case Rep Psychiatry*, 2020, 5369297.

236. Brandt, C., Töllner, K., Klee, R., et al. (2015). Effective termination of status epilepticus by rational polypharmacy in the lithium–pilocarpine model in rats: Window of opportunity to prevent epilepsy and prediction of epilepsy by biomarkers. *Neurobiol Dis*, 75, 78–90.

237. Payandemehr, B., Bahremand, A., Ebrahimi, A., et al. (2015). Protective effects of lithium chloride on seizure susceptibility: Involvement of α2-adrenoceptor. *Pharmacol Biochem Behav*, 133, 37–42.

238. Garcia, G., Crismon, M. L. and Dorson, P. G. (1994). Seizures in two patients after the addition of lithium to a clozapine regimen. *J Clin Psychopharmacol*, 14, 426–428.

239. Tan, M. G., Worley, B., Kim, W. B., et al. (2020). Drug-induced intracranial hypertension: A systematic review and critical assessment of drug-induced causes. *Am J Clin Dermatol*, 21, 163–172.

240. Sundholm, A., Burkill, S., Waldenlind, E., et al. (2021). A national Swedish case-control study investigating incidence and factors associated with idiopathic intracranial hypertension. *Cephalalgia*, 41, 1427–1436.

241. Hexom, B. and Barthel, R. P. (2004). Lithium and pseudotumor cerebri. *J Am Acad Child Adolesc Psychiatry*, 43, 247–248.

242. Jonnalagadda, J., Saito, E. and Kafantaris, V. (2005). Lithium, minocycline, and pseudotumor cerebri. *J Am Acad Child Adolesc Psychiatry*, 44, 209.

243. Callens, P., Sienaert, P., Demyttenaere, K., et al. (2012). [Is there a causal link between idiopathic intracranial hypertension and the use of lithium? A case-study and a review of the literature]. *Tijdschr Psychiatr*, 54, 453–462.

244. Stachenfeld, N. S., Taylor, H. S., Leone, C. A., et al. (2003). Estrogen effects on urine concentrating response in young women. *J Physiol (Lond).* 552, 869–880.

245. Grandjean, E. M. and Aubry, J.-M. (2009). Lithium: Updated human knowledge using an evidence-based approach: Part III: Clinical safety. *CNS Drugs,* 23, 397–418.

246. Rugino, T. A., Janvier, Y. M., Baunach, J. M., et al. (2003). Hypoalbuminemia with valproic acid administration. *Pediatr Neurol,* 29, 440–444.

247. Łukawska, E., Frankiewicz, D., Izak, M., et al. (2021). Lithium toxicity and the kidney with special focus on nephrotic syndrome associated with the acute kidney injury: A case-based systematic analysis. *J Appl Toxicol,* 41, 1896–1909.

248. Levey, A. S., Grams, M. E. and Inker, L. A. (2022). Uses of GFR and albuminuria level in acute and chronic kidney disease. *N Engl J Med,* 386, 2120–2128.

249. Juurlink, D. N., Mamdani, M. M., Kopp, A., et al. (2004). Drug-induced lithium toxicity in the elderly: A population-based study. *J Am Geriatr Soc,* 52, 794–798.

250. Thomsen, K. and Schou, M. (1968). Renal lithium excretion in man. *Am J Physiol,* 215, 823–827.

251. Atherton, J. C., Doyle, A., Gee, A., et al. (1991). Lithium clearance: Modification by the loop of Henle in man. *J Physiol,* 437, 377–391.

252. Cohen, Y., Chetrit, A., Cohen, Y., et al. (1998). Cancer morbidity in psychiatric patients: Influence of lithium carbonate treatment. *Med Oncol,* 15, 32–36.

253. Gahr, M., Wezel, F., Bolenz, C., et al. (2019). Lithium therapy associated with renal and upper and lower urinary tract tumors: Results from a retrospective single-center analysis. *J Clin Psychopharmacol,* 39, 530–532.

254. Kessing, L. V., Gerds, T. A., Feldt-Rasmussen, B., et al. (2015). Lithium and renal and upper urinary tract tumors – results from a nationwide population-based study. *Bipolar Disord,* 17, 805–813.

255. Pottegård, A., Hallas, J., Jensen, B. L., et al. (2016). Long-term lithium use and risk of renal and upper urinary tract cancers. *J Am Soc Nephrol,* 27, 249–255.

256. Martinsson, L., Westman, J., Hallgren, J., et al. (2016). Lithium treatment and cancer incidence in bipolar disorder. *Bipolar Disord,* 18, 33–40.

257. Huang, R. Y., Hsieh, K. P., Huang, W. W., et al. (2016). Use of lithium and cancer risk in patients with bipolar disorder: Population-based cohort study. *Br J Psychiatry,* 209, 393–399.

258. Anmella, G., Fico, G., Lotfaliany, M., et al. (2021). Risk of cancer in bipolar disorder and the potential role of lithium: International collaborative systematic review and meta-analyses. *Neurosci Biobehav Rev,* 126, 529–541.

6

Lithium Toxicity

Manifestations and Management of Lithium Toxicity and Overdose; Debate About Hemodialysis Implementation; Safe Use of Lithium During ECT; Clinical Situations When Lithium Should Be Temporarily Discontinued

QUICK CHECK

PRINCIPLES

- Many of the risks for lithium toxicity can be managed by a combination of routine monitoring, patient education, and collaboration with other health-care providers. Collaboration with colleagues is crucial to minimizing the risk related to new medications that interact with lithium, and for managing lithium dosing and fluid requirements around the time of surgery. Patients are at risk for lithium toxicity following bariatric surgery, so lithium dose reduction and level monitoring must be part of the postoperative plan.

- The symptoms of lithium toxicity depend greatly on the pattern of overdose: acute, acute on chronic, or chronic. Acute on chronic overdose and chronic toxicity represent more serious situations due to the presence of a pre-existing brain lithium level. Toxicity symptoms are predominantly gastrointestinal (nausea, vomiting, diarrhea) or neurological (new or worse fine tremor, ataxia, dysarthria, choreiform movements, coarse tremors, fasciculations, myoclonus, nystagmus, hyperreflexia, delirium, seizure, coma). Lithium does not have significant ECG effects but it may induce bradycardia, QTc prolongation, and Brugada-like or pseudoinfarction patterns.

- Patients with lithium levels ≥ 2.00 mEq/l are referred for emergency room evaluation. For levels under 2.00 mEq/l, the presentation, clinical context, and history of intentional overdose are factors in determining who requires emergency room evaluation. Lab error resulting in a high level can occur if the sample was placed in a heparinated tube.

- Recent literature challenges the concept that the combination of lithium and ECT is unsafe or is associated with increased risk for cognitive dysfunction. Lithium is often held the night before ECT, but this decision should be based on whether ECT being used to manage mania or depression, patient age and baseline lithium level.

- Dialysis criteria following lithium overdose were established in 2015, but are a subject of debate. Nonetheless, the use of hemodialysis and modern critical care has resulted in fatality rates for lithium overdose that are comparable to that for other mood stabilizers. In rare instances, patients may suffer from persistent neurological sequelae of overdose, with fever increasing this risk.

INTRODUCTION

WHAT TO KNOW: INTRODUCTION

- Lithium toxicity is preventable, and prevention relies on three core principles: ongoing lithium related monitoring, patient education, and collaboration with other prescribers. Collaboration allows appropriate monitoring when kinetically interacting medications are added or withdrawn or when surgery is planned.

- The early symptoms of lithium intoxication have been described since Cade's 1949 case series [1], and include gastrointestinal and neurological manifestations, and an impact on sinus node function presenting initially as bradycardia.

- The use of dialysis over the past 50 years has made fatality a rare occurrence following lithium overdose or intoxication. There is ongoing debate about the 2015 EXtracorporeal TReatments In Poisoning (EXTRIP) working group recommendations due to the recognition that overly aggressive mobilization of CNS lithium stores might induce neurological consequences in overdose patients who had been on chronic lithium treatment. Newer and more easily implemented criteria have been suggested in recent years.

- Permanent neurological sequela of severe overdose go by the acronym SILENT (syndrome of irreversible lithium-effectuated neurotoxicity). With modern critical care methods including dialysis, only 123 cases have been reported over the past half-century.

Medical journals from the late nineteenth and early twentieth centuries contained descriptions of lithium toxicity derived from animal experiments, some of which resulted in fatal outcomes; however, a 1903 paper reviewed this animal and human literature extensively and noted that, when lithium carbonate was used in daily doses of 975 mg – 1300 mg as a putative gout treatment, the adverse effects were quite modest and gastrointestinal in nature [2]. Perhaps emboldened by this finding, a Michigan physician, Dr. Clarence Cleaveland, decided in 1913 to experiment on himself by ingesting 14 grams (g) of lithium chloride (equivalent to 12,380 mg of lithium carbonate) in divided doses over a period of 28 h (2 g at 1 pm, 9 pm and 7 am, then 8 g at 7 pm) and document the outcome [3]. While he experienced minimal adverse effects following the first two doses, after the third dose Cleaveland developed dizziness, weakness, tremors and tinnitus, and, following the fourth and largest dose, developed vertigo, tremors, dizziness, blurred vision and ataxia of such severity that he remained bed bound. The tinnitus and ocular symptoms persisted for 36 hours, but the tremors and weakness lasted for 5 days. Nonetheless, Cleaveland commented on the absence of diarrhea or abdominal pain, side effects that he had anticipated. Having completely recovered, Cleaveland repeated the experiment several months later and noted that, after the second 2 gm dose he again experienced weakness, dizziness, tinnitus and blurred vision, but this time the weakness lasted only 1 day and was less severe than experienced from the prior larger ingestion. Cleaveland did not succumb from his experiment, but when John Cade undertook the decision to test lithium carbonate on himself in 1949 after completing his animal experiments, he did so with full knowledge that use of lithium chloride as a salt substitute had been associated with numerous deaths, including those reported in medical journals that same year [1, 4–9].

Having satisfied himself that lithium ingestion within certain limits was not fatal, Cade's initial case series of 10 patients confirmed Cleaveland's finding that lithium toxicity was dose dependent, and that this was manageable by dose reduction [1]. Cade used a lithium carbonate dose of 650 mg TID for acute mania, but recommended this be decreased "once emotional tone is attained," noting that a high proportion of patients exhibited toxicity after 1–3 weeks on that dosage [1]. Cade warned that if the appearance of such symptoms is not immediately followed by cessation of intake, "there is little doubt that they can progress to a fatal issue," based on examples from uncontrolled lithium chloride ingestion [1]. The common toxicity symptoms seen in Cade's initial case series were broadly divided into gastrointestinal (GI) complaints (e.g. abdominal pain, anorexia, nausea, vomiting, occasional mild diarrhea), and central nervous system (CNS) related symptoms (e.g. giddiness, tremor, ataxia, slurred speech, myoclonic twitching, depression). At that time, lithium assays were technically difficult and somewhat unreliable, so Cade did not employ any method to track systemic exposure. Sadly, a 1950 Australian case series of similarly unmonitored patients described serious instances of toxicity and the first reported fatality; moreover, Cade himself later treated two patients who died during a lithium trial [10, 11].

In-Depth 6.1 Early Insights from 1950–1951 on Lithium's Maximum Maintenance Serum Level

The modern era of lithium treatment for neuropsychiatric purposes is the result of two publications in 1950 and 1951 documenting that lithium appears safe and well tolerated at serum levels ≤ 1.00 mEq/l. The January 1950 paper by US physician John Talbott was the direct result of the 1949 US Food and Drug Administration decision to withdraw lithium chloride-containing salt substitutes from the US market due to multiple deaths [12]. Talbott does not specify the assay method, but his paper provides the first detailed exploration of the association between adverse effects, lithium carbonate dose and serum levels across a variety of clinical conditions: in a "normal" individual given 1560 mg/d for 21 days; in 11 hospitalized patients with a variety of medical conditions; and in 9 cases of alleged lithium intoxication. While not denying that excessive exposure to lithium could prove fatal, Talbott's paper found that 10 of 11 supposed lithium intoxication cases he investigated had serum levels ≤ 1.50 mEq/l and had other causes for their physical complaints. Importantly, he noted that the majority of lithium related adverse effects, including gastrointestinal (GI) issues, were not seen with serum levels < 1.00 mEq/l [12]. This paper did not go unnoticed in Australia, and was cited by two Melbourne physicians, Noack and Trautner, in their 1951 article which recorded the first use of serum levels to manage lithium treatment for psychiatric disorders [11].

This routine use of serum levels outside of a research setting became possible because Professor Victor Wynn, also of Melbourne, developed a flame spectrophotometry assay for serum sodium and potassium levels in 1950, a method that could also be used for lithium [13]. A historical review commented that the Noack and Trautner 1951 study was influential in promoting lithium therapy by demonstrating that lithium toxicity could be avoided through level monitoring, and by endorsing the concept that, following high dose use for acute mania, clinicians should heed Talbott's suggestion that lithium's tolerability is significantly improved when levels are kept under 1.00 mEq/l [11, 14].

The need to monitor maintenance levels to minimize routine adverse effects became accepted practice, but experience with overdose cases over the years illustrated that massive lithium ingestions could prove fatal, that dialysis can be extremely helpful in managing severe lithium toxicity, and that a prior history of lithium exposure is an important factor in the clinical outcome. The relationship to lithium exposure is based on the concept that a significant sequela of overdose is persistent CNS dysfunction. Patients chronically treated with lithium have sufficiently high brain levels that the insult from acute ingestion or from prolonged exposure to toxic levels (e.g. typically ≥ 2.0 mEq/l) will be associated with poorer outcomes than comparable exposures in lithium naïve patients [15]. The three overdose patterns are thus termed acute, acute on chronic, or chronic, with the latter two being more serious in nature and comprising more than 90% of overdose or toxicity cases. In 2010, toxicologists affiliated with the California Poison Control System (CPCS) examined the outcomes of 502 lithium exposure cases reported to CPCS from 2003 to 2007 in which lithium was the sole ingestion and the patient hospitalized [15]. The pattern of overdose was evident in 450 cases, and the breakdown was as follows: 9.8% – acute lithium exposure; 27.6% – acute on chronic overdose; 62.6% – chronic overdose. Among the total sample of 502 cases, 69 patients received hemodialysis, but there were only 4 total deaths [15]. The rarity of fatal outcomes following lithium overdose/ intoxication is reflected in a large data set on single ingestion cases, amassed from regional poison centers serving all 50 US states, Puerto Rico and the District of Columbia, for 2000–2014 [16]. Among the 46,286 lithium exposures, there were only 61 deaths reported; moreover, as a point of comparison, during this same time frame there were 35 deaths from 48,286 serotonin norepinephrine reuptake inhibitor (SNRI) ingestions (venlafaxine, desvenlafaxine, duloxetine, milnacipran, levomilnacipran). The mortality ratio per 10,000 single overdose exposures was 13.2 (95% CI 10.1–16.9) for lithium, with the 95% confidence interval almost overlapping that for the SNRI class (MR 7.2, 95% CI 5.0–10.0).

Advances in critical care have dramatically reduced fatalities from lithium intoxication, but a small fraction of overdose/intoxication patients suffer from permanent neurological sequelae, with cerebellar symptoms being the most common feature [17]. In the late 1980s, the acronym SILENT was coined (**s**yndrome of **i**rreversible **l**ithium-**e**ffectuated **n**euro**t**oxicity), to reflect that some have persistent CNS consequences of excessive lithium exposure due to a single overdose, or, more commonly, acute on chronic or chronic overdose [18]. Despite decades of use, the first large case series describing persistent lithium neurotoxicity was not published until 1984 by the Danish psychiatrist Mogens Schou (n = 40) [17], and the first comprehensive review of the world's literature from 1948 to 1984 appeared in 1986, penned by Professor Rif El-Mallakh (n = 213 cases) [19]. Schou reported ongoing cerebellar symptoms, ataxia and scanning speech in his cases, and El-Mallakh provided the following breakdown: ataxia (50.0%), tremor (45.8%), dysarthria (37.5%), "organic brain syndrome" (25.0%) and dysmetria (16.7%). The rate of persistent symptoms in El-Mallakh's review was 32.5%, but this is difficult to interpret as hemodialysis was not commonly employed in this era, leading to prolonged periods of supratherapeutic lithium levels that lasted for weeks in certain instances [20]. As practices surrounding lithium dosing, level monitoring and use of hemodialysis have changed dramatically in the last 40 years, the true incidence of SILENT is unknown, but a 2020 review was able to find only 123 cases published from 1965 to 2019, suggesting that measures which limit fatalities may also have the same effect on the risk for permanent neurological sequelae from acute or chronic lithium toxicity [18].

In contemporary usage, lithium toxicity is often defined as a serum level ≥ 1.5 mEq/l. The use of modern monitoring schemes and serum level ranges has significantly lowered rates of lithium toxicity, with an incidence of 0.01 per patient-year reported in longitudinal studies [21–23]. One example of such research is an analysis of 1340 lithium treated patients in Norrbotten, Sweden, for the years 1997–2013, that quantified rates of lithium intoxication using the above definition (i.e. any lithium level ≥ 1.5 mEq/l). An average of 667 patients per year were treated with lithium (equal to > 10,000 patient-years), yet only 96 experienced at least 1 episode of lithium intoxication [22]. Practice patterns have changed over time, but recent analyses confirm that the risk factors for lithium toxicity incorporated into the monitoring guidelines outlined in Chapter 4 remain relevant. The Kaiser network is a large US based health maintenance organization whose vertically integrated system permits data mining often not possible in fragmented care settings. The Kaiser Colorado system analyzed data from 3115 individuals treated with lithium to identify contributors to lithium toxicity in the 70 individuals who experienced this complication and required acute care service utilization [24]. After matching patients with an episode of lithium toxicity 1:5 with other lithium treated patients, the following risk factors were noted: a newly initiated potentially interacting medication (odds ratio [OR] 30.30, 95% CI 2.32–394.95), a higher number of treated chronic diseases (OR 1.28, 95% CI 1.12–1.45), older age (OR 1.05, 95% CI 1.02–1.09), and higher total daily lithium dose (OR 1.00, 95% CI 1.00–1.00) [24]. These findings are not surprising, but illustrate that even in a system where all providers (e.g. pharmacists, prescribers) have access to a patient's medication records, episodes of lithium toxicity from kinetic interactions can occur. Iatrogenic issues account for a substantial portion of the more chronic toxicity cases [25], so all lithium prescribers must be aware that lithium related drug interactions can escape oversight of the health-care system or the dispensing pharmacy.

 Info Box 6.1 Methods to Mitigate Lithium Toxicity

a. **Monitor:** Monitor serum levels and eGFR more frequently in those with low eGFR (< 60 ml/min), especially in the presence of chronic kidney disease (CKD) risks (e.g. hypertension, diabetes mellitus, peripheral vascular disease) or higher levels (0.80–1.00 mEq/l) (Chapter 4, Info Box 4.4).

b. **Educate:** Remind patients of procedures to follow with illnesses that induce vomiting or diarrhea, or during periods of excessive sweating, how to use nonsteroidal anti-inflammatory medications safely, and to notify you immediately of new medications that may interact with lithium. A summary sheet of such medications is helpful [26].

c. **Collaborate:** For all individuals, especially older patients (≥ 60 years of age), those with CKD risks, or eGFR ≤ 60 ml/min, develop a relationship with the primary care provider to obviate the use of medications that kinetically interact with lithium, and to establish a means for the provider to contact you when such medications are necessary [27]. When surgery is scheduled, collaborate with the surgeon and anesthesiologist on management of lithium during the preoperative and postoperative period, especially when bariatric surgery is planned, oral intake will be limited for many days, or when persistent polyuria will drastically alter intraoperative and postoperative fluid requirements (see Info Box 6.6) [28, 29].

d. **Suspect:** Be suspicious of **lab error** with extremely high levels in an asymptomatic patient. The sample may have been placed in a heparinated (**green top**) tube that contains lithium heparin. A repeat level will clarify the issue.

Diminishing renal function due to age or medical comorbidities contributes to toxicity risk, but often the precipitant relates to the combined effects of multiple issues or temporal factors in the form of sodium depletion related to GI or other major illness (e.g. COVID), or excessive sweating [30, 31]. As discussed in Chapters 2 and 3, the common element in those scenarios is excessive volume and electrolyte loss due to fever, sweating, vomiting or diarrhea, compounded by the use of free water as volume replacement, thereby inducing a state of sodium depletion. Given that a confluence of factors often underlies episodes of nonintentional lithium toxicity, a small number of measures can be implemented to help manage this risk (Info Box 6.1). Among these measures is more frequent monitoring of lithium levels and eGFR for patients with eGFR < 60 ml/min (Chapter 4, Info Box 4.4) [32], patient education about drug interactions and management of GI illnesses, and collaboration with other providers (e.g. the primary care clinician) to facilitate communication when medications must be used that interact kinetically with lithium so appropriate dosage adjustment and lithium level monitoring can be implemented (Chapter 3, Table 3.6). Despite these measures, and despite lithium's anti-suicide properties, overdose and toxicity situations can happen due to intentional or accidental events. An important aspect of collaborative care is having familiarity with modern dialysis recommendations and the evolving nature of these guidelines based on the increasing appreciation that rapid mobilization of lithium ion in chronic users may itself induce neurological sequelae [33–35]. Another area where clinicians must collaborate is when patients have surgical procedures that may limit oral intake or drastically alter lithium kinetics (e.g. bariatric surgery) [28], or when lithium treated patients require electroconvulsive therapy (ECT). The recent ECT literature indicates that the combination of lower maintenance lithium levels (especially compared with prior decades), unilateral electrode placement and ultrabrief pulse width stimulation is not associated with cognitive dysfunction or other safety concerns (e.g. postictal delirium, prolonged seizure duration) in lithium treated patients [36–38]. The important conclusion from the past 70 years of lithium usage is that the risks are generally foreseeable and manageable, and that the risk:benefit equation for lithium strongly favors net benefit when clinicians attend to a small number of core principles, many of which derive from contemporary use of lower maintenance levels, improved understanding of the need for diligent monitoring of serum levels and renal function, and a prompt response when new medications are added that reduce lithium clearance.

A Signs and Symptoms of Toxicity, and Clinical Predictors of Toxicity

WHAT TO KNOW: SIGNS AND SYMPTOMS OF TOXICITY, AND CLINICAL PREDICTORS OF TOXICITY

- Early GI symptoms of lithium intoxication include nausea, vomiting, diarrhea and, rarely, ileus. Neurological signs initially appear as tremor, but progress in more serious situations to ataxia, dysarthria, choreiform movements, coarse tremors, fasciculations, myoclonus, nystagmus, hyperreflexia, and eventually stupor or coma.

- ECG changes may be nonspecific, but, at levels ≫ 1.50 mEq/l, bradycardia, QT prolongation and Brugada-like patterns may be seen.

- The need for admission depends on multiple factors but is often not indicated with levels < 2.00 mEq/l.

- The single-ingestion fatality rate for lithium is not significantly different than for valproate, carbamazepine or lamotrigine.

- Hemodialysis has markedly reduced rates of fatality and neurological sequelae. The new *Paris* criteria are an attempt to obviate issues with the EXTRIP 2015 recommendations. Use of intravenous saline is not helpful in improving outcomes but may be useful in volume depleted patients needing fluid resuscitation to optimize renal perfusion.

- The biggest predictor of lithium toxicity is the addition of a new medication that kinetically interacts with lithium (30-fold increased risk) while medical comorbidity by itself only increases risk by 28%.

1 *Signs and Symptoms of Lithium Toxicity*

By the 1970s, it was recognized that the clinical manifestations of lithium toxicity may not always correlate with the ingested dose or the serum level, so the alacrity in response should be in proportion to the patient's presentation. In 1978, Danish psychiatrists Hansen and Amdisen proposed three categories of adverse effects to help clinicians rate clinical severity, graded on a I–III scale [39]:

Grade I (mild intoxication): nausea, vomiting, tremor, hyperreflexia, agitation, muscle weakness, ataxia

Grade II (moderate intoxication): stupor, rigidity, hypertonia, hypotension

Grade III (severe intoxication): coma, convulsions, myoclonus, collapse

Although certain items found in contemporary lists are missing from the 1978 scheme (e.g. bradycardia, Brugada-like ECG changes), this picture of lithium toxicity remains largely accurate almost 50 years later (Info Box 6.2). What changed in the ensuing decades is an emphasis on the pattern of lithium exposure prior to the episode of lithium toxicity, with more favorable outcomes for acute ingestions in lithium naïve patients [40]. By 1993, the terminology of acute, acute on chronic, and chronic lithium intoxication was well established in the literature, and this terminology reified the concept that a pre-existing CNS lithium level alters the relationship between the peripheral serum level and intracellular brain concentration during overdose or chronic toxicity situations. Earlier papers attempted to assign specific serum level thresholds to the emergence of certain signs or symptoms, but in practice there are too many variables to make these correlations clinically useful. The lithium naïve patient who presents just 6 hours after an ingestion with a serum level of 4.0 mEq/l may be much less symptomatic than a patient exposed chronically to a level of 2.0 mEq/l [19, 40]. Laboratories typically alert clinicians when lithium levels exceed a certain threshold (e.g. 1.2 mEq/l) [41], but the initial question to address when levels are modestly elevated (< 2.00 mEq/l) is whether this reflects an easily remedied situation that can be managed as an outpatient (e.g. one-time dosing error, diarrhea with inadequate electrolyte replacement), or whether it demands emergency room evaluation for hospitalization.

 Info Box 6.2 Signs and Symptoms and Patterns of Lithium Toxicity, and the Need for Hospitalization

a. Patterns of toxicity in relationship to prior treatment
Comment:
   i. Acute: overdose in a lithium naïve individual
   ii. Acute on chronic: overdose in a lithium treated individual
   iii. Chronic: persistently high lithium levels in a lithium treated individual

b. The spectrum of symptoms
   i. **Gastrointestinal:** nausea, vomiting, diarrhea, rarely ileus
   ii. **Neurological:**
      1. Early neuromuscular manifestation: fine intention tremor that is new or worse than the patient's baseline
      2. Later neuromuscular manifestations: ataxia, dysarthria, choreiform movements, coarse tremors, fasciculations, myoclonus (ocular and axial), nystagmus, hyperreflexia
      3. Generalized: delirium, seizure, nonconvulsive status epilepticus, coma
   iii. **Cardiovascular:** lithium does not have significant ECG effects but it may induce bradycardia (reduced sinus node automaticity), QTc prolongation, Brugada-like and pseudoinfarction patterns
   iv. **Systemic:** hyperthermia (rare)

c. **The need for emergency room evaluation and potential hospitalization**

   i. **Serum level 1.50–1.99 mEq/l is due to acute but not persistent circumstances:** Asymptomatic or minimally symptomatic patients (e.g. mild tremor) whose levels are elevated due to transient events that are expected to resolve or be easily corrected can be managed as outpatients (e.g. one-time dosing error, addition of a kinetically interfering medication, GI illness with poor oral salt and water intake in a patient with eGFR ≥ 60 ml/min). The typical approach is to hold lithium for 24 to 36 h, recheck the morning level, and adjust lithium dosing if necessary (e.g. to compensate for the impact of a new medication which is altering lithium kinetics). New onset sinus bradycardia will require admission or an emergency room stay for ECG monitoring even among asymptomatic patients, especially older individuals with medical comorbidity.

   ii. **Serum level 1.50–1.99 mEq/l is due to intentional overdose or chronic toxicity:** Asymptomatic patients with acute or acute on chronic intentional overdoses are admitted for psychiatric safety (i.e. due to the intentional overdose). When the high level is the product of transient factors as noted above (e.g. dosing error, new medication added that delays lithium clearance), patients are typically admitted for observation even if asymptomatic, especially when the time since ingestion is short and the clinical picture is expected to evolve. Some patients with acute on chronic ingestions, or chronic toxicity involving prolonged exposure (e.g. weeks) to serum levels close to 2.00 mEq/l may be quite ill and require extensive supportive care.

   iii. **Serum level ≥ 2.00 mEq/l:** All patients with levels in this range should present to a hospital for evaluation. In some instances, the stay may be very brief as the patient is asymptomatic, the underlying problem easily correctable (e.g. dosing error, dehydration) and there is no need for ECG monitoring. The need for prolonged stay, intensive support and hemodialysis will depend on the patient's clinical status, the level, and the pattern of intoxication (e.g. acute vs. acute on chronic vs. chronic toxicity).

2 Predictors of Lithium Toxicity

The 2018 Kaiser study identified a short list of lithium toxicity risk factors, two of which (older age, presence of medical comorbidities) can be easily managed by more frequent monitoring of eGFR and lithium levels as dictated by declining renal function, proteinuria or CKD comorbidities (Chapter 4, Info Box 4.4) [24]. Unfortunately, the largest effect involved initiation of a kinetically interacting medication, and this alone increased the odds of lithium toxicity 30-fold [24].

To a large extent, drug interaction risk is also a product of age and lower baseline renal function, in part because older individuals are more likely to require antihypertensives and diuretics, and because having a lower eGFR reduces the safety margin when lithium clearance is reduced [32]. The method for mitigating risk imposed by new medications is not laboratory based, but rests on maintaining open lines of communication with the patient and the primary care provider about the potential impact of certain medications on lithium clearance, and the need to alter lithium dosing immediately upon starting such agents (Info Box 6.1). One should not assume that the other provider is knowledgeable in this area, as they may have limited experience with lithium treated patients, nor should one assume that a pharmacy will flag the interaction or prevent the new prescription from being filled. Kinetic drug interactions with lithium are usually manageable (Chapter 3, Table 3.6) provided a clinician is given sufficient warning to anticipate the extent of the interaction, adjust the lithium dose and order a follow-up level.

Death from lithium intoxication is exceedingly rare, but clinicians are often presented with the conundrum of wanting to use lithium in a mood disorder patient with a history of suicide attempts specifically for its anti-suicide effects, while simultaneously worrying that the patient may overdose on lithium before realizing that benefit. There is no evidence based method that perfectly addresses this clinical bind, but there are data that can inform the care of such patients. The first consideration is that mortality from self-poisoning is no greater for lithium than for other mood stabilizers, and may be lower than for carbamazepine when mixed with other medications [42]. This assertion is based on analyses of large data sets, such as that published in 2018 by a UK group that used the British Office for National Statistics cases of fatal self-poisoning, and also examined the Multicentre Study of Self-Harm in England for instances of nonfatal self-poisoning, both for the years 2005–2012 [42]. From this combined massive data set, they calculated the case fatality rate (the ratio between rates of fatal and nonfatal self-poisoning) among individuals aged ≥ 15 years for the mood stabilizers lithium, valproate (VPA), carbamazepine and lamotrigine [42]. As seen in Table 6.1, the rates of self-poisoning per 100,000 patient-years was numerically lower for lithium than for other mood stabilizers. Moreover, the case fatality index relative to lithium was not significantly different for any of the other agents studied, as evidenced by the fact that the 95% confidence intervals for each of the other medications overlapped 1.0 [42]. Additionally, among multiple ingestions where carbamazepine was listed as the primary drug, its case fatality index was 2-fold higher than for lithium: OR 2.37 (95% CI 1.16–4.85). Using other mood stabilizers in lieu of lithium to reduce the rate and risk of self-poisoning or suicide related death is not supported by these and other data [43].

Table 6.1 Number and rates of suicides involving single drugs in England among individuals aged 15 years and over (2005–2012) [42]

	Single drug deaths	Average number of prescriptions per year	Prescription rate (per 100,000 person-yrs)	Self-poisoning rate (per 100,000 person-yrs)	Single drug case fatality index relative to lithium (95% CI)
Lithium	6	4956	107.24	1.64	–
Valproate	15	15,433	333.97	4.45	0.92 (0.35–2.45)
Carbamazepine	33	18,836	407.62	3.87	2.33 (0.94–5.74)
Lamotrigine	5	7635	165.22	2.02	0.68 (0.20–2.28)

The approach to this difficult situation will always be individualized, but it is not unreasonable to engage in a frank discussion with the patient regarding why lithium is being chosen (especially if a history of self-harm is part of that decision), the dangers of overdose with lithium or any mood stabilizer, and initial measures one may wish to implement until the patient is established on lithium, such as limiting drug dispensing to a 1-week supply. There are limited data on the onset of lithium's anti-suicide properties, but some information was provided in a 2006 meta-analysis that examined 85,229 person-years of lithium risk-exposure from 31 papers providing data on attempted and completed suicides in lithium and non-lithium treated mood spectrum patients [44]. One important finding was that the reduction in risk of completed suicide or serious attempts appeared consistent across diagnostic categories, with 5-fold higher risk in the non-lithium groups (see Chapter 1, Info Box 1.1). Another finding was that studies of shorter duration, with mean length 1.41 years (primarily randomized clinical trials), saw lesser effects from lithium than those of longer duration (mean 7.77 years). Balancing out the effect of longer treatment duration is the fact that any recent use of lithium decreases suicide related risk. The conclusion comes from an analysis of hazard ratios (HRs) for suicide related events, completed suicide, and all-cause mortality among Taiwanese adults with BD for the years 2000–2005, which indicated that use of any mood stabilizer in the prior month decreased risk for these outcomes [43]. While this study lacked the statistical power to find differences between the mood stabilizers, the investigators did note that no suicide deaths occurred when lithium was prescribed during the final exposure period, and that the risk of all-cause mortality was significantly higher in the group not exposed to mood stabilizers compared with the lithium only cohort (HR 29.34, 95% CI 21.22–40.57; p < 0.0001) [43]. There are many factors that contribute to intentional overdose, including active substance use, clinician rapport and psychiatric stability, but the Taiwanese findings suggest that lithium's anti-impulsive effects might be seen after a month of treatment, although the greatest anti-suicide impact may take longer, as noted in the meta-analysis. Limiting early prescription amounts among patients with multiple risk factors seems prudent, but gradual extension of prescription quantities is not unreasonable once other factors contributing to self-poisoning risk are quiescent, and especially as patients remain on lithium for extended periods (e.g. 18 months or more) without incidents.

Managing Overdose and Severe Toxicity (Levels ≥ 2.00 mEq/l), and the Debate over When to Use Dialysis

WHAT TO KNOW: MANAGING OVERDOSE AND SEVERE TOXICITY (LEVELS ≥ 2.00 mEQ/l), AND THE DEBATE OVER WHEN TO USE DIALYSIS

- Clinical assessment (especially CNS manifestations), ingestion of other medications, the pattern of overdose (e.g. acute vs. acute on chronic), baseline renal function, laboratory abnormalities and the trajectory of serum lithium levels determine the level of supportive care required.

- Lithium is an ion and is not removed by activated charcoal. Intravenous saline is not a treatment for overdose and is not a replacement for hemodialysis. However, in volume depleted patients, fluid resuscitation with normal saline optimizes renal perfusion and facilitates lithium excretion by reducing proximal lithium reabsorption.

- Hemodialysis vastly improves outcomes, but there is ongoing debate about the 2015 EXTRIP algorithm. In 2021, a French group published the *Paris* criteria based on extensive analyses of outcomes from a tertiary care hospital. These simpler *Paris* criteria recommend initiating dialysis for a lithium level ≥ 5.2 mEq/l and/or a serum creatinine ≥ 2.26 mg/dl.

1 *Patient Assessment, Frequency of Lithium Level Monitoring and Other Considerations*

The correlation between serum level and clinical signs or symptoms is often poor, and depends greatly on both the amount of ingestion (if intentional), the time since ingestion, and, importantly, whether this is an acute overdose in a lithium naïve patient or an acute on chronic or chronic intoxication [40]. Lithium naïve patients may not have significant symptoms in the early hours because the primary manifestation of serious lithium poisoning is the CNS lithium level. The CNS T_{Max} is delayed at least 3 h from the peripheral T_{Max}, and lithium naïve patients are starting from a baseline of no prior brain intracellular lithium exposure, so there may be an insufficient CNS level for many hours before neurological symptoms are present [45, 46]. Nonetheless, patient assessment is crucial to determining the speed at which interventions should proceed, as some patients are obtunded enough to require ventilatory support and urgent considerations for dialysis, while others may require much less intensive care [35, 47]. The patient's report of ingested dosages and use of other substances is helpful, but should not be relied upon, and toxicology testing is always a part of overdose management regardless of the agent involved. Lithium clearance varies dramatically between individuals, based upon renal function, prior history of lithium use and exposure to medications that impair lithium clearance, so lithium levels are typically checked every 2–4 hours until a peak is established, especially as the peak may be delayed if the overdose involved a sustained release preparation [47]. Despite advances in critical care, fatalities can and do occur from lithium overdose; however, these are such rare occurrences that hospitalists may have cared for multiple lithium toxicity patients during their career yet never seen a death.

2 Decontamination and Dialysis

Like many acids, bases, and metals, lithium is not removed by activated charcoal, and this should not be administered unless indicated for other co-occurring ingestions. The most effective method for hastening lithium clearance is hemodialysis, with the first reports of its use for lithium intoxication emerging in the late 1960s [48]. Previously, the standard treatment for lithium toxicity involved administration of large doses of sodium chloride, often intravenously, in an attempt to compete with lithium and improve the clinical symptoms [4]. This seemed helpful in cases where lithium was used as a salt substitute, particularly when patients had been on a sodium restricted diet [4]. However, it became evident that sodium chloride or potassium chloride by themselves were largely ineffective, with a 1968 paper by Mogens Schou, covering eight cases of lithium poisoning, stating: "Most of the patients were given sodium chloride, 10–12 gm per day, or potassium chloride, 2–4 gm per day, or both. Neither of these treatments produced any clearcut change in the patient's clinical condition; nor could increase of the fall rate of serum lithium during the administration of these compounds be noted" [49]. Sadly, even papers as late as 1987 still endorsed the use of saline diuresis as the primary treatment

Info Box 6.3 Patient Assessment, Level Monitoring and Other Considerations in Overdose and Severe Toxicity Situations

a. Patient assessment: History is obtained about other co-ingested medications or substances, and an attempt made to quantify the lithium ingestion. As this information may be unreliable or unobtainable, initial treatment relies on lithium levels, toxicology screens, chemistry panel (for electrolyte disturbances and renal function), and clinical examination (especially presence of neurological signs and symptoms).

b. Frequency of lithium level determinations: Kinetics following toxic exposures depend on a number of variables, especially renal function, whether the patient is lithium naïve or has significant tissue lithium stores, and if the ingestion involved standard or delayed release lithium. The trajectory of lithium excretion and determination of whether levels have peaked requires frequent lithium levels obtained every 2–4 hours until a maximum is seen. A nomogram was developed by one group to help clinicians predict which patients might have a lithium level at 36 h that exceeds 1.0 mEq/l, and thus possibly be dialysis candidates per the 2015 EXTRIP criteria (see Info Box 6.4 for further discussion) [34].

c. Intravenous saline: This is not a replacement for hemodialysis, but in volume depleted patients the use of fluid resuscitation with normal saline (0.9% NaCl) optimizes renal perfusion and facilitates lithium excretion by reducing proximal reabsorption of lithium [47].

d. Other measures: The need for ventilatory support, dialysis, arrhythmia management, seizure control and other care depends on the clinical picture. As discussed in Info Box 6.4 and illustrated below, in patients with acute on chronic or chronic intoxication, lithium will be mobilized from tissue stores following dialysis and the level can rise several hours later. Further dialysis may be necessary to lessen the time spent above the initial target level of 1.0 mEq/l (see Figure 6.1) [33].

modality, with dialysis only reserved for instances of renal failure [50]. The kinetic differences in these approaches are readily apparent: in a case series of 22 toxicity patients, the lithium half-life ($T_{1/2}$) decreased to 3.5 ± 0.8 h following the first session of hemodialysis, compared with 29 ± 14 h and 29 ± 6 h during therapy with diuretics or supportive treatment, respectively [51]. While saline infusion will not replace dialysis, many lithium intoxication patients present in a hypovolemic state, especially those with chronic lithium exposure and polyuria, and these individuals need fluid resuscitation. In those instances, the use of normal saline (0.9% NaCl) not only restores a euvolemic state and improves renal perfusion, the added sodium load facilitates lithium excretion by reducing proximal reabsorption of lithium [47].

There is no debate that any form of dialysis improves lithium clearance (Figure 6.1), and that hemodialysis is more effective than other forms of renal replacement therapy (e.g. peritoneal dialysis), yet the criteria for employing dialysis have been the subject of intense debate since publication of the EXtracorporeal TReatments In Poisoning (EXTRIP) lithium workgroup paper in 2015 (Info Box 6.4) [33]. While this paper was the product of an extensive review of the literature, the workgroup acknowledged that most of this literature comprised case reports, and for this reason there was very low-quality evidence for all recommendations [35]. Nonetheless, critical care specialists applauded this effort to arrive at an evidence based algorithm and thus bring a sense of order to an area with multiple and conflicting recommendations.

Figure 6.1 Serum and cerebrospinal fluid (CSF) lithium levels following a single session of dialysis [48]

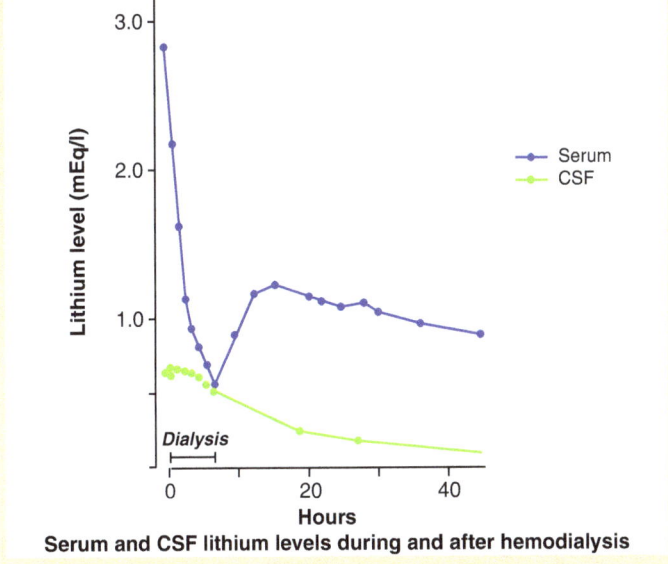

Serum and CSF lithium levels during and after hemodialysis

(Adapted from: A. Amdisen and H. Skjoldborg [1969]. Haemodialysis for lithium poisoning. *Lancet*, 2, 213.)

As clinicians started to operationalize the EXTRIP algorithm, a practical issue was that one of the suggested criteria was based on whether the expected lithium level "with optimal management" would be ≥ 1.0 mEq/l at 36 h (i.e. ≥ 2.5 mEq/l 24 h after hospital admission) [33]. The kinetics in lithium naïve overdose patients or those with chronic toxicity are relatively predictable using serial lithium levels and eGFR, but lithium clearance in cases of acute on chronic toxicity are not so easily predicted. An Australian group analyzed 111 acute on chronic cases and 250 chronic lithium toxicity cases with lithium levels ≥ 1.3 mEq/l in an attempt to find a method that facilitated implementation of this EXTRIP criterion [34]. Lithium levels among chronic toxicity patients generally fell steadily, but those in the acute on chronic overdoses were unpredictable, with some experiencing rising concentrations for up to 24 h. Despite these issues, the authors developed a nomogram based on initial eGFR and lithium level that performed best in chronic cases but could be used for acute on chronic overdose situations. In their concluding remarks, the authors commented that, overall, the EXTRIP criteria were overly broad. If the 2015 EXTRIP *suggested* criteria were followed, dialysis would have been instituted for 211 of the chronic toxicity patients, yet only 51 of this cohort fulfilled both the serum level and a clinical criterion that would have demanded dialysis [34].

Aside from the complex kinetics with acute on chronic overdose, another source of concern was the impact of significant ion shifts in patients with chronic lithium exposure, and specifically whether overly aggressive use of dialysis may induce more CNS problems than it prevents (Info Box 6.4) [35]. As reviewed in Info Box 6.4, a comprehensive analysis of 128 lithium toxicity cases from a tertiary care hospital in Paris found those who did not get dialyzed despite meeting EXTRIP criteria had shorter ICU stays ($p < 0.05$). Importantly, forgoing dialysis in those cases did not result in greater neurological impairment on discharge compared with patients who received hemodialysis, and with no increase in the fatality rate [35]. From this large data set, the authors proposed a parsimonious set of dialysis criteria that obviated the need for kinetic modeling, and also removed any confusion engendered by the EXTRIP terms *recommended* and *suggested*. These simpler *Paris* criteria recommend initiating dialysis for a lithium level ≥ 5.2 mEq/l and/or a serum creatinine ≥ 2.26 mg/dl [35]. Replication and refinement of these criteria will be necessary (e.g. use of eGFR in lieu of serum creatinine), but outcomes analyses from contemporary data sets, as were produced by the Australian and Parisian groups, will help drive the field to a set of consensus criteria that incorporate new understandings in this area and might be easier to implement than the 2015 EXTRIP recommendations.

Info Box 6.4 The Debate about When to Use Dialysis

Background: Dialysis will rapidly remove lithium from the vascular compartment, and in many instances can be life-saving and potentially lessen the chances of permanent central nervous system (CNS) sequelae, but for decades there was no consensus on when to use hemodialysis or other renal replacement therapy (e.g. peritoneal dialysis) [33, 34]. In 2015, the Extracorporeal Treatments in Poisoning (EXTRIP) lithium intoxication workgroup proposed criteria based on their review of 166 articles [33]. The workgroup acknowledged in their report a very low quality of evidence for all recommendations as most publications were case reports (n = 228 with patient-level data) [33]. Despite this, they concluded decisively that hemodialysis was the preferred extracorporeal treatment when such treatment was indicated, but other methods could be used, although they are less efficient. They noted that clinical decisions on when to use extracorporeal treatment should take into account the lithium level, renal function, pattern of lithium toxicity, clinical status and availability of extracorporeal treatments, but with those caveats in mind the following were recommended:

The EXTRIP workgroup *recommended* extracorporeal treatment if:

a. The lithium level is > 4.0 mEq/l **and at least one of the following:** eGFR < 45 ml/min; acute kidney injury stage 2–3; serum creatinine ≥ 2.00 mg/dl if < age 65 or ≥ 1.50 mg/dl if age ≥ 65; presence of oliguria/anuria *OR*

b. There is a decreased level of consciousness (i.e. Glasgow coma scale < 12), seizures, or life-threatening dysrhythmias, irrespective of the lithium level

The EXTRIP workgroup *suggested* extracorporeal treatment if:

a. The lithium level is > 5.0 mEq/l *OR*

b. Significant confusion is present (i.e. Glasgow coma scale 12–13) *OR*

c. If the expected lithium level with optimal management will be ≥ 1.0 mEq/l at 36 h (i.e. ≥ 2.5 mEq/l 24 h after hospital admission)

Extracorporeal treatment should be continued until clinical improvement is apparent, the serum level is < 1.0 mEq/l, or for a minimum of 6 hours if the lithium level cannot be readily measured.

Issues: By 2020, authors had called for some refinements to the EXTRIP recommendations. This was based in part on difficulty in implementing the third suggested criterion since it demanded complex kinetic calculations related to the serum level and eGFR [34]. As the vast majority of episodes occur in situations of acute on chronic or chronic lithium intoxication, there was also significant concern about complications arising from rapid CNS ion shifts related to the movement of lithium from its intracellular locations in patients on chronic therapy [34, 35].

2020 *Paris criteria*: In 2020, a French group performed an outcomes analysis of 128 cases and found those who did not get dialyzed despite meeting EXTRIP criteria had shorter ICU stays ($p < 0.05$) without a significant increase in fatalities or neurological impairment on discharge, compared with those who received hemodialysis [35]. From these cases, the authors proposed a set of simpler *Paris* criteria:

- Initiate dialysis for lithium levels ≥ 5.2 mEq/l and/or serum creatinine ≥ 2.26 mg/dl

Comment: These criteria are much easier to implement, represent a detailed analysis of a large number of cases from a tertiary care facility, and incorporate the concept that nearly all overdose/toxicity situations occur in patients chronically treated with lithium (i.e. acute on chronic or chronic toxicity). Replication and further refinement of these criteria (e.g. use of eGFR in lieu of serum creatinine) will provide clinicians with an easily implemented tool to help decide upon the use of hemodialysis. Importantly, these criteria acknowledge the possible neurological consequences of overly aggressive dialysis in chronically lithium treated patients.

 C Sequelae of Toxicity, SILENT, and Lithium Dosing in Patients Undergoing ECT

 WHAT TO KNOW: NEUROTOXICITY (SILENT) FOLLOWING OVERDOSE, AND LITHIUM USE DURING ECT

- Use of hemodialysis has lowered the rates of adverse neurological outcomes, but some patients have persistent sequelae which go by the acronym SILENT (**s**yndrome of **i**rreversible **l**ithium-**e**ffectuated **n**euro**t**oxicity), and are typically manifested as cerebellar signs (truncal or central ataxia, dysmetria, intention tremor, dysdiadochokinesia).

- Fever or infection increases the risk for developing persistent cerebellar sequelae 14-fold in those with peak serum levels < 2.5 mEq/l. Aggressive treatment of fever and its underlying cause is crucial to minimizing neurological consequences.

- The use of unilateral ECT electrode placement and ultrabrief pulse widths has lessened the cognitive impact of ECT. For patients > 50 years of age and those with 12 h trough levels ≥ 0.80 mEq/l, holding lithium the night before ECT treatment is a reasonable approach.

1   *Sequelae of Lithium Toxicity (SILENT)*

Acute neurological symptoms following lithium overdose were described in Cleaveland's 1913 self-experiment [3], but many US physicians received first-hand experience of these manifestations in 1949 as the result of numerous hospitalizations and deaths from use of Westsal®, a lithium containing salt substitute developed by the Foster-Milburn Co. of Buffalo, New York, in spring of 1948 [4]. While neurological symptoms appeared to resolve among those who survived their unsupervised use of Westsal® [4, 5, 7], case reports emerged in the literature recording persistent neurological sequelae of lithium overdose, with Schou describing in his 1984 case series (n = 40) cerebellar symptoms including ataxia and scanning speech [17]. El-Mallakh's 1986 comprehensive review of 213 lithium neurotoxicity cases published from 1948–1984 reported that 32.5% developed persistent neurological symptoms: ataxia (50.0%), tremor (45.8%), dysarthria (37.5%), "organic brain syndrome" (25.0%) and dysmetria (16.7%) [19]. The reported rate of persistent neurological symptoms is difficult to interpret since hemodialysis was not commonly used even through the mid-1980s [20]. Nonetheless, subsequent reviews of persistent neurological sequelae from severe overdose confirmed that cerebellar symptoms predominate, including truncal or central ataxia, dysmetria, intention tremor and dysdiadochokinesia (decreased ability to perform rapid alternating movements) [52]. Among those with evidence of cerebellar dysfunction, 50% also had some form of dysarthria (e.g. scanning or slurred speech), and this can be present without ataxia [52]. The acronym SILENT was created in the late 1980s (**s**yndrome of **i**rreversible **l**ithium-**e**ffectuated **n**eurotoxicity) to reflect that patients can suffer from persistent CNS consequences of excessive lithium exposure, and to serve as a reminder that routine monitoring of lithium levels is crucial, as is the need to keep maintenance levels below 1.00 mEq/l [18]. Routine eGFR and lithium level monitoring combined with use of hemodialysis has dramatically reduced rates of lithium related fatality [42], but the true incidence of SILENT in modern practice remains unknown. A 2021 review only found 123 published cases from 1965 to 2019, suggesting that measures which limit fatalities may also have the same effect on risk for permanent neurological sequelae from acute on chronic or from chronic overdose [18]. The 2021 paper did point out a finding which Schou had mentioned in his 1984 paper, but which was given limited emphasis in subsequent literature: fever plays a pivotal role in the development of persistent neurological symptoms [17, 18]. Among the 123 SILENT cases reviewed, 48% had fever or infection; moreover, among the subset of 51 cases with persistent cerebellar symptoms whose peak lithium levels were under 2.5 mEq/l, neither age ≥ 50 years, female gender nor antipsychotic use were significantly associated with the outcome, but the presence of fever or infection increased the risk almost 14-fold (OR 13.9, 95% CI 3.21– 60.05). Fever was not a significant predictor of cerebellar sequelae in the 34 cases with peak lithium levels ≥ 2.5 mEq/l, suggesting that the toxic effects of lithium are sufficient to produce cerebellar symptoms with sufficiently high exposure. That SILENT can rarely occur with lower serum levels strongly suggests that fever and the underlying infectious cause should be aggressively managed in any lithium treated individual, especially with levels ≥ 1.00 mEq/l [18].

2 *Lithium and Electroconvulsive Therapy (ECT) – the Modern Perspective*

The ECT literature has also evolved greatly over the last 20 years with recognition that exposure to lithium itself is not associated with cognitive dysfunction or other safety concerns (e.g. postictal delirium, prolonged apnea, prolonged seizure duration) [36–38]. Although older case reports raised many of these safety issues, by 2005 larger case series emerged reporting no unusual response when ECT is administered to patients on lithium, and which questioned the assumption that this combination should be avoided except in extreme circumstances [36]. A comprehensive 2021 review on the use of ECT to treat mania also commented that adverse events related to the concurrent use of lithium were the product of higher serum levels commonly employed in past decades, and that recent literature fails to suggest an increased risk for delirium, other cognitive complaints or prolonged anesthesia recovery (see Info Box 6.5) [37]. While ECT is used for short periods to manage manic episodes, long-term use for depression treatment allows the opportunity to examine to what extent the combination of ECT and lithium generates any unexpected neurocognitive adverse effects. The most rigorous study to address this was a multicenter 6-month trial that explicitly examined neurocognitive outcomes in older unipolar depressed patients (mean age 70.5 years) who were randomized to venlafaxine + lithium vs. venlafaxine + lithium + ECT [38]. The ECT method chosen employed right unilateral electrode placement and ultrabrief pulse width to minimize any cognitive impact from ECT itself. Both groups experienced neurocognitive improvements over the 6 months of the study on most measures, with no endpoint difference between those who did or did not receive ECT [38]. From the available modern literature, it can be concluded that use of lithium by itself does not pose a safety issue during ECT, but that there should be certain considerations around when to hold the lithium dose the night before ECT, especially when ECT is used to treat mania, or when the baseline serum level is ≥ 0.80 mEq/l.

Info Box 6.5 Lithium and Electroconvulsive Therapy (ECT)

a. **Treatment principles:** Much of the literature documenting adverse responses during the ECT procedure (prolonged seizure, postictal confusion, delayed recovery from anesthesia) relates to cases with higher serum levels than those recommended in contemporary guidelines [23, 37]. A common practice is to hold lithium for 24 h prior to ECT, but whether one does this depends on a few variables: is ECT being used for mania or for depression, is the baseline lithium level ≥ 0.80 mEq/l, and is the patient's age > 50 years [38]? Imaging research indicates that certain patients achieve higher brain levels for any given peripheral level [53–55], with age > 50 years emerging as one possible factor in some but not all studies [54, 56, 57].

b. **Anesthesia concerns:** Lithium is rarely reported to potentiate the action of neuromuscular blockers through a hypothesized presynaptic mechanism [58], but almost all cases were reported in the 1970s [59]. In 2020, one group from Japan published a case report which noted that the action of a modest rocuronium dose (50 mg) in a lithium treated 64-year-old female was greater than expected after 1 hour, although it was reversible with sugammadex [60]. The absence of recent cases is likely related to modern practices involving more careful titration of neuromuscular blockade, use of a nerve stimulation device to assess paralytic activity, and administration of reversal agents if the extent of neuromuscular blockade is more severe or persistent than expected [60]. Use of lithium is not a consideration in deciding to employ ECT or in the choice of muscle relaxants.

c. **Is there a greater risk for cognitive effects when ECT is used in lithium treated patients?** Most of the literature in this area comes from longitudinal studies of patients receiving ECT for major depression, but the answer appears to be "no" [38]. In part, this is due to recent emphasis on unilateral ECT treatment to mitigate the putatively greater cognitive impact from bilateral electrode placement. In 2022, results of a 6-month study (Phase 2 of the Prolonging Remission in Depressed Elderly [PRIDE] trial) were published that specifically compared neurocognitive outcomes in patients with mean age 70.5 years receiving symptom-titrated, algorithm based longitudinal ECT in combination with venlafaxine and lithium vs. those on pharmacotherapy alone (venlafaxine and lithium) [38]. The main hypothesis was that use of right unilateral and ultrabrief pulse width ECT will be effective with relatively benign cognitive adverse effects, and the results bore this out [38]. Most areas of neurocognitive functioning improved in both groups over 6 months, with no significant between-group differences at 6 months in psychomotor processing speed, autobiographical memory consistency, short-term and long-term verbal memory, phonemic fluency, inhibition, complex visual scanning and cognitive flexibility.

d. **To hold or not to hold lithium when ECT is used for mania:** Minimizing any safety issues from the use of higher lithium levels to manage mania is one concern, but another dilemma is whether lowering the lithium level will interfere with achieving mood stability. For patients > 50 years of age and those with 12 h trough levels ≥ 0.80 mEq/l, holding lithium the night before ECT treatment is a reasonable approach. Ideally, ECT is administered early in the morning, thereby allowing the held lithium dose from the night before to be given before noon. The usual evening dose should also be given that night to maintain the pre-ECT lithium level [37].

e. **To hold or not to hold lithium when ECT is used for depression:** In this situation, the primary concern is not whether lowering the lithium level will interfere with obtaining euthymia, but with minimizing adverse effects especially when ECT is administered in an older population. The protocol used in the PRIDE study (see above) was very straightforward: lithium levels were ideally kept in the range of 0.4–0.6 mEq/l since it was being used adjunctively for unipolar depression; lithium was held a minimum of 24 h before each ECT session; and additional time for lithium clearance was allotted when levels were above 0.8 mEq/l [38].

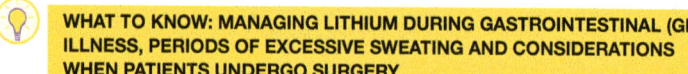

D **Managing Lithium during Episodes of Gastrointestinal (GI) Illness, Periods of Excessive Sweating and Considerations When Patients Undergo Surgery**

WHAT TO KNOW: MANAGING LITHIUM DURING GASTROINTESTINAL (GI) ILLNESS, PERIODS OF EXCESSIVE SWEATING AND CONSIDERATIONS WHEN PATIENTS UNDERGO SURGERY

- Patients must be educated that sodium and volume losses from heavy sweating or prolonged GI illness (diarrhea, vomiting) must be replaced with electrolyte solutions. Use of free water creates a scenario that may result in lithium toxicity. For GI illnesses that persist, communication with the prescriber is reasonable. With a CNS $T_{1/2}$ of 28–48 h, holding lithium for 24 h or 48 h until the patient has resumed oral intake is unlikely to induce any psychiatric sequelae.

- Lithium need not be held prior to surgery and can be resumed once the patient is able to drink fluids. For patients with untreated polyuria and fluid requirements ≥ 3 liters/24 h, the anesthesiologist and surgeon must be alerted so adequate fluid replacement can be provided in the intraoperative and postoperative period.

1 *Gastrointestinal (GI) Illness, Periods of Excessive Sweating*

Lithium competes with sodium for proximal renal reabsorption, so conditions associated with excessive sodium loss can result in lithium toxicity, *but only when patients replace volume losses with free water that lacks sodium.* The most common scenarios include GI disorders that induce persistent vomiting or diarrhea (e.g. ≥ 12 h), or environmental situations that promote excessive sweating [30, 61–63]. It is worth noting that studies exploring the effects of ambient temperature, the season, sweating or strenuous exercise do not show an independent effect on lithium levels [62, 64, 65]. High temperatures or vigorous exercise should only be associated with lithium toxicity when patients lose significant amounts of sodium and when free water without electrolytes is used for rehydration. The educational efforts outlined in Info Box 6.6 emphasize the role of sodium depletion in causing lithium toxicity, the use of electrolyte replacement solutions or packets under such circumstances, and the need to hold lithium and contact the prescriber when unable to tolerate oral intake for extended periods due to GI illness. Lithium's CNS $T_{1/2}$ is 28–48 h, and patients should be reminded that forgoing lithium for 1–2 days is unlikely to impact psychiatric stability and may be the best course of action when very ill, especially until such time as they can confer with the mental health professional prescribing the lithium.

 Info Box 6.6 Holding Lithium for Extended Periods When Gastrointestinal (GI) Illness Limits Oral Fluid Intake or following Surgery

GI Illness

a. **Principles:** The scenario leading to lithium toxicity involves a dehydrated patient repleting losses from GI illness (vomiting, diarrhea) with free water instead of a balanced electrolyte solution [66]. While free water will restore vascular volume, it does not restore depleted sodium stores, thereby resulting in hyponatremia. Any state that induces sodium depletion can potentially cause lithium toxicity as lithium will be preferentially reabsorbed proximally by the sodium hydrogen exchanger 3 (NHE3) due to the paucity of sodium [67, 68].

b. **Patient education:** Patients must be educated that free water is not ideal during situations of extreme water and sodium loss (e.g. vomiting, diarrhea, excessive sweating in high temperatures), and about the need to use electrolyte replacement packets or ready-made electrolyte solutions for rehydration (see Chapter 3 for more discussion). The availability of electrolyte solutions initially geared for pediatric use has broadened into a market with numerous products for adults. When persistent vomiting or diarrhea precludes acceptable oral intake for more than 12 h, patients should hold lithium for 24 h and contact their prescriber for guidance on resuming lithium or seeking medical attention if the GI illness does not improve. Once the patient is able to resume adequate oral intake, the usual lithium dose is restarted unless some other serious issue (e.g. acute kidney injury from severe dehydration) is detected, especially in situations where the patient needed medical help.

With a CNS $T_{1/2}$ of 28–48 h, holding lithium for 24 h or 48 h is unlikely to induce any psychiatric sequelae. After longer periods without lithium, the clinician may consider a modest loading procedure (e.g. two 10 mg/kg doses over 24 h) to hasten the time to steady state therapeutic levels, with a follow-up level after 5 days on the prior stable dose.

Surgery

a. **Fluid balance and polyuria:** This is a crucial area where collaboration is necessary to prevent patients from experiencing dehydration and hypernatremia related to inadequate fluid replacement during protracted periods without oral intake. For patients with known polyuria complaints, the fact that their fluid requirements may be 3 liters/24 h or more must be communicated to the anesthesiologist so that adequate fluid replacement can be provided in the intraoperative and postoperative period while the patient is not drinking. This is especially critical when procedures involve major fluid shifts, significant blood loss or extended periods (e.g. days) where the patient will be NPO.

b. **Lithium dosing:** There is no compelling reason to hold lithium prior to surgery. As noted in Info Box 6.5 (ECT), concerns about interactions with neuromuscular blockers are mostly a vestige of older practices. Except for the period following bariatric surgery (see Info Box 6.7), most patients can resume their usual lithium dose following the majority of surgeries once oral intake is permitted. The obvious exceptions relate to procedures involving major fluid shifts, major blood loss or other factors that significantly influence cardiac output, renal function or electrolyte balance (e.g. coronary artery bypass surgery, nephrectomy, major hemorrhage, trauma). Assessment of eGFR and electrolyte balance (especially serum sodium), review of current treatment to look for new medications that alter lithium clearance and consultation with the hospitalist are recommended before resuming lithium.

Interestingly, there is an effect of high altitude on renal hemodynamics that acutely decreases lithium clearance when individuals are exposed to elevations ≥ 3000 meters [69]. Patients need to be counseled that this effect can be seen within 48 h of ascending to altitude and instructed to be vigilant for signs of lithium toxicity appearing in the form of new or worsening adverse effects [70]. If lithium treated individuals planning on high-altitude exposure are concerned about this effect, one can discuss a possible modest dose reduction (e.g. 25–33%) starting 24 h prior to the trip. Since acetazolamide is used for acute mountain sickness, patients should also be educated that a carbonic anhydrase inhibitor will lower lithium levels approximately 30% if used persistently (e.g. when used for acute mountain sickness prophylaxis) [71]. In general, this effect is not sufficient to destabilize most individuals, but rare sensitive patients might notice the emergence of subthreshold symptoms if the lithium level drops low enough for an extended period of time.

2 *Considerations for Patients Undergoing Surgery*

Concerns about lithium interactions with neuromuscular blocking agents have abated in the past 30 years (see Chapter 3), so the primary focus in patients undergoing surgery is whether there will be an extended period without oral intake, and whether the surgery may result in electrolyte imbalance, or diminished cardiac or renal function. Patients with polyuria are vulnerable to dehydration and hypernatremia during periods without oral intake, especially if the extent of polyuria is significant and the duration of NPO status lasts $\geq$ 24 h. In those instances, anesthesiologists and critical care team members must be apprised that this particular patient's daily fluid requirements will be substantially greater than that of typical patients, and of the need to monitor serum sodium and renal function daily while the patient remains NPO. Resumption of lithium after most surgeries will be at the prior stable dose with two exceptions: following bariatric surgery (see Info Box 6.7), and following major surgeries that could impact cardiac or renal function or alter electrolyte levels (e.g. coronary artery bypass surgery). In the latter circumstance, collaboration with other medical providers combined with a review of the current eGFR, serum sodium level and medications will be necessary to ascertain how best to resume lithium.

E | **Managing Lithium Dosing in Patients Undergoing Bariatric Surgery**

WHAT TO KNOW: MANAGING LITHIUM DOSING IN PATIENTS UNDERGOING BARIATRIC SURGERY

- Bariatric surgery is a unique situation associated with 2–5-fold increases in postoperative lithium levels both acutely (i.e. the first week after surgery) and more chronically as the patient experiences weight loss in the first 12 months. This is true regardless of the type of procedure.

- The postoperative lithium dose must be decreased by 50% and the level checked within 1 week, with further downward dosing adjustments based on the level. Very frequent lithium level monitoring is necessary during the first 12 months until weight stabilizes.

Bariatric surgery can impact the kinetics of many oral medications by altering GI motility, absorptive surface area, and time spent in the acidic stomach environment

[72]; however, lithium clearance is more greatly influenced by all of the factors associated with such surgery, including dietary changes and significant alterations to body weight and composition [28]. The net effect is that postoperative lithium levels increase 2-fold to 5-fold regardless of the type of bariatric surgery, a situation that can result in lithium toxicity within weeks of the procedure [28, 73–79]. A 2022 literature review of 11 cases found that the onset of postoperative lithium toxicity ranged from 9 days to 6 months, with 8 of 11 cases having their onset within the first month after bariatric surgery [28]. Bariatric surgery requires careful planning, so clinicians can use this time to engage in discussions about postoperative lithium dosage adjustments, and to map out a strategy for regular postoperative eGFR and lithium level monitoring to minimize the risk of lithium toxicity (see Info Box 6.7).

 Info Box 6.7 **Management of Lithium Dosing for Patients Undergoing Bariatric Surgery**

a. **Principles:** Postoperative lithium levels may increase 2–5-fold following bariatric surgery, regardless of the type of procedure. A 2022 review of 11 cases found that 73% experienced postoperative lithium toxicity within the first month after the bariatric procedure when continuing the usual preoperative dose [28].

b. **Preoperative levels:** As some patients may alter their diet, lose weight or be on sodium-restricted diets, a 12 h trough level should be obtained several weeks before the planned surgery. For levels above 1.00 mEq/l, the lithium dose should be lowered and a repeat level checked 1 week later.

c. **Postoperative dosing and monitoring**

  i. **Immediate postoperative period:** Postoperative lithium doses should be reduced by 50% and a level obtained 1 week after resuming oral intake. The initial goal is a postoperative level at or slightly below the preoperative baseline level, anticipating that the lithium level will increase over subsequent weeks as the patient loses weight.

  ii. **Weeks 1–6 after surgery:** Recheck the eGFR and lithium level weekly for the first 6 weeks. Adjust lithium doses as necessary based on the preoperative level.

  iii. **Weeks 7–24 after surgery:** Recheck the eGFR and lithium level every 2 weeks through week 12, tapering down to monthly levels as the patient approaches 6 months from the date of surgery.

  iv. **Months 6–12 after surgery:** As it may take 6–12 months to recover from bariatric surgery, consider monthly lithium level and eGFR monitoring during months 6–9 as the patient's body adapts to the rapid changes induced by the surgery, and then an eGFR and lithium level every 2 months through the end of the first year.

Summary Points

a. Many of the risk factors for and scenarios leading to lithium toxicity (e.g. gastrointestinal illness, drug interactions) are well established, and manageable by a combination of routine eGFR and lithium level monitoring, patient education, and collaboration with other health-care providers.

b. The combination of lithium and ECT is not unsafe nor associated with evidence of increased cognitive dysfunction. Lithium is typically held the night before ECT, but this decision should be based on whether ECT is being used to manage mania or depression, whether the patient is over 50 years of age, or if 12 h trough levels are ≥ 0.80 mEq/l.

c. Use of lithium is rarely associated with fatal intentional overdose, and rates of such fatalities appear comparable to those of other mood stabilizers. Patients with an indication for lithium who have a history of self-harm should not be deprived of a lithium trial, especially given its anti-suicide benefits; however, certain measures may be implemented during the early course of treatment to manage this risk (e.g. limited prescription fills).

d. The symptoms of lithium toxicity may not always correlate with the dose, and often depend on whether the situation involves an acute ingestion in a lithium naïve patient, chronic toxicity, or an acute on chronic overdose. There is considerable debate about the 2015 EXTRIP dialysis criteria, especially related to concerns about implementation, and also consequences of rapid ion shifts in brain lithium stores when chronically treated patients are dialyzed.

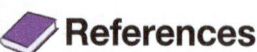
References

1. Cade, J. F. J. (1949). Lithium salts in the treatment of psychotic excitement. *Med J Aust*, 36, 349–351.

2. Good, C. A. (1903). An experimental study of lithium. *Am J Med Sci*, 125, 273–284.

3. Cleaveland, S. A. (1913). A case of poisoning by lithium presenting some new features. *JAMA*, 60, 722.

4. Corcoran, A. C., Taylor, R. D. and Page, I. H. (1949). Lithium poisoning from the use of salt substitutes. *JAMA*, 139, 685–688.

5. Hanlon, L. W., Romaine III, M., Gilroy, F. J., et al. (1949). Lithium chloride as a substitute for sodium chloride in the diet: Observations on its toxicity. *JAMA*, 139, 688–692.

6. Peters, H. A. (1949). Lithium intoxication producing chorea athetosis with recovery. *Wis Med J*, 48, 1075.

7. Stern, R. L. (1949). Severe lithium chloride poisoning with complete recovery; report of case. *JAMA*, 139, 710.

8. Waldron, A. M. (1949). Lithium intoxication occurring with the use of a table salt substitute in the low sodium dietary treatment of hypertension and congestive heart failure. *Univ Hosp Bull*, 15, 9.

9. Cade, J. F. (1999). John Frederick Joseph Cade: Family memories on the occasion of the 50th anniversary of his discovery of the use of lithium in mania. 1949. *Aust N Z J Psychiatry*, 33, 615–618.

10. Roberts, E. L. (1950). A case of chronic mania treated with lithium citrate and terminating fatally. *Med J Aust*, 2, 261–262.

11. Noack, C. H. and Trautner, E. M. (1951). The lithium treatment of maniacal psychosis. *Med J Aust*, 2, 219–222.

12. Talbott, J. H. (1950). Use of lithium salts as a substitute for sodium chloride. *Arch Int Med*, 85, 1–10.

13. Wynn, V., Simon, S., Morris, R. J., et al. (1950). The clinical significance of sodium and potassium analyses of biological fluids: Their estimation by flame spectrophotometry. *Med J Aust*, 1, 821–835.

14. Johnson, G. and Gershon, S. (1999). Early North American research on lithium. *Aust N Z J Psychiatry*, 33 Suppl., S48–53.

15. Offerman, S. R., Alsop, J. A., Lee, J., et al. (2010). Hospitalized lithium overdose cases reported to the California Poison Control System. *Clin Toxicol (Phila)*, 48, 443–448.

16. Nelson, J. C. and Spyker, D. A. (2017). Morbidity and mortality associated with medications used in the treatment of depression: An analysis of cases reported to U.S. poison control centers, 2000–2014. *Am J Psychiatry*, 174, 438–450.

17. Schou, M. (1984). Long-lasting neurological sequelae after lithium intoxication. *Acta Psychiatr Scand*, 70, 594–602.

18. Verdoux, H., Debruyne, A. L., Queuille, E., et al. (2021). A reappraisal of the role of fever in the occurrence of neurological sequelae following lithium intoxication: A systematic review. *Expert Opin Drug Saf*, 20, 827–838.

19. El-Mallakh, R. S. (1986). Acute lithium neurotoxicity. *Psychiatric Developments*, 4, 311–328.

20. El-Mallakh, R. S. (1984). Treatment of acute lithium toxicity. *Vet Hum Toxicol*, 26, 31–35.

21. Aiff, H., Attman, P.-O., Aurell, M., et al. (2014). The impact of modern treatment principles may have eliminated lithium-induced renal failure. *J Psychopharmacol*, 28, 151–154.

22. Ott, M., Stegmayr, B., Salander Renberg, E., et al. (2016). Lithium intoxication: Incidence, clinical course and renal function – a population-based retrospective cohort study. *J Psychopharmacol*, 30, 1008–1019.

23. Nolen, W. A., Licht, R. W., Young, A. H., et al. (2019). What is the optimal serum level for lithium in the maintenance treatment of bipolar disorder? A systematic review and recommendations from the ISBD/IGSLI Task Force on treatment with lithium. *Bipolar Disord*, 21, 394–409.

24. Heath, L. J., Billups, S. J., Gaughan, K. M., et al. (2018). Risk factors for utilization of acute care services for lithium toxicity. *Psychiatr Serv*, 69, 671–676.

25. Oakley, P. W., Whyte, I. M. and Carter, G. L. (2001). Lithium toxicity: An iatrogenic problem in susceptible individuals. *Aust N Z J Psychiatry*, 35, 833–840.

26. Bisogni, V., Rossitto, G., Reghin, F., et al. (2016). Antihypertensive therapy in patients on chronic lithium treatment for bipolar disorders. *J Hypertens*, 34, 20–28.

27. Juurlink, D. N., Mamdani, M. M., Kopp, A., et al. (2004). Drug-induced lithium toxicity in the elderly: A population-based study. *J Am Geriatr Soc*, 52, 794–798.

28. Ayub, S., Saboor, S., Usmani, S., et al. (2022). Lithium toxicity following Roux-en-Y gastric bypass: Mini review and illustrative case. *Ment Health Clin*, 12, 214–218.

29. Richards, E., Pankhania, M., Thomas, C., et al. (2022). Perioperative management of lithium in the patient undergoing pituitary surgery: A case report. *Br J Neurosurg*. https://doi.org/10.1080/02688697.2021.2010651.

30. Pi, H. T. and Surawicz, F. G. (1978). Severe neurotoxicity and lithium therapy. *Clin Toxicol*, 13, 479–486.

31. Pai, N. M., Malyam, V., Murugesan, M., et al. (2022). Lithium toxicity at therapeutic doses as a fallout of COVID-19 infection: A case series and possible mechanisms. *Int Clin Psychopharmacol*, 37, 25–28.

32. Tobita, S., Sogawa, R., Murakawa, T., et al. (2021). The importance of monitoring renal function and concomitant medication to avoid toxicity in patients taking lithium. *Int Clin Psychopharmacol*, 36, 34–37.

33. Decker, B. S., Goldfarb, D. S., Dargan, P. I., et al. (2015). Extracorporeal treatment for lithium poisoning: Systematic review and recommendations from the EXTRIP Workgroup. *Clin J Am Soc Nephrol*, 10, 875–887.

34. Buckley, N. A., Cheng, S., Isoardi, K., et al. (2020). Haemodialysis for lithium poisoning: Translating EXTRIP recommendations into practical guidelines. *Br J Clin Pharmacol*, 86, 999–1006.

35. Vodovar, D., Beaune, S., Langrand, J., et al. (2020). Assessment of Extracorporeal Treatments in Poisoning criteria for the decision of extracorporeal toxin removal in lithium poisoning. *Br J Clin Pharmacol*, 86, 560–568.

36. Dolenc, T. J. and Rasmussen, K. G. (2005). The safety of electroconvulsive therapy and lithium in combination: A case series and review of the literature. *J ECT*, 21, 165–170.

37. Elias, A., Thomas, N. and Sackeim, H. A. (2021). Electroconvulsive therapy in mania: A review of 80 years of clinical experience. *Am J Psychiatry*, 178, 229–239.

38. Lisanby, S. H., McClintock, S. M., McCall, W. V., et al. (2022). Longitudinal neurocognitive effects of combined electroconvulsive therapy (ECT) and pharmacotherapy in major depressive disorder in older adults: Phase 2 of the PRIDE study. *Am J Geriatr Psychiatry*, 30, 15–28.

39. Hansen, H. E. and Amdisen, A. (1978). Lithium intoxication. (Report of 23 cases and review of 100 cases from the literature.). *Q J Med*, 47, 123–144.

40. Jaeger, A., Sauder, P., Kopferschmitt, J., et al. (1993). When should dialysis be performed in lithium poisoning? A kinetic study in 14 cases of lithium poisoning. *J Toxicol Clin Toxicol*, 31, 429–447.

41. Hiemke, C., Bergemann, N., Clement, H. W., et al. (2018). Consensus guidelines for therapeutic drug monitoring in neuropsychopharmacology: Update 2017. *Pharmacopsychiatry*, 51, 9–62.

42. Ferrey, A. E., Geulayov, G., Casey, D., et al. (2018). Relative toxicity of mood stabilisers and antipsychotics: Case fatality and fatal toxicity associated with self-poisoning. *BMC Psychiatry*, 18, 399.

43. Tsai, C. J., Cheng, C., Chou, P. H., et al. (2016). The rapid suicide protection of mood stabilizers on patients with bipolar disorder: A nationwide observational cohort study in Taiwan. *J Affect Disord*, 196, 71–77.

44. Baldessarini, R. J., Tondo, L., Davis, P., et al. (2006). Decreased risk of suicides and attempts during long-term lithium treatment: A meta-analytic review. *Bipolar Disord*, 8, 625–639.

45. Komoroski, R. A., Newton, J. E., Sprigg, J. R., et al. (1993). In vivo 7Li nuclear magnetic resonance study of lithium pharmacokinetics and chemical shift imaging in psychiatric patients. *Psychiatry Res*, 50, 67–76.

46. Plenge, P., Stensgaard, A., Jensen, H. V., et al. (1994). 24-hour lithium concentration in human brain studied by Li-7 magnetic resonance spectroscopy. *Biol Psychiatry*, 36, 511–516.

47. Baird-Gunning, J., Lea-Henry, T., Hoegberg, L. C. G., et al. (2017). Lithium poisoning. *J Intensive Care Med*, 32, 249–263.

48. Amdisen, A. and Skjoldborg, H. (1969). Haemodialysis for lithium poisoning. *Lancet*, 2, 213.

49. Schou, M., Amdisen, A. and Trap-Jensen, J. (1968). Lithium poisoning. *Am J Psychiatry*, 125, 520–527.

50. Dyson, E. H., Simpson, D., Prescott, L. F., et al. (1987). Self-poisoning and therapeutic intoxication with lithium. *Hum Toxicol*, 6, 325–329.

51. Eyer, F., Pfab, R., Felgenhauer, N., et al. (2006). Lithium poisoning: Pharmacokinetics and clearance during different therapeutic measures. *J Clin Psychopharmacol*, 26, 325–330.

52. Kores, B. and Lader, M. H. (1997). Irreversible lithium neurotoxicity: An overview. *Clin Neuropharmacol*, 20, 283–299.

53. Soares, J. C., Boada, F. and Keshavan, M. S. (2000). Brain lithium measurements with (7) Li magnetic resonance spectroscopy (MRS): A literature review. *Eur Neuropsychopharmacol*, 10, 151–158.

54. Forester, B. P., Streeter, C. C., Berlow, Y. A., et al. (2009). Brain lithium levels and effects on cognition and mood in geriatric bipolar disorder: A lithium-7 magnetic resonance spectroscopy study. *Am J Geriatr Psychiatry*, 17, 13–23.

55. Lee, J. H., Adler, C., Norris, M., et al. (2012). 4-T 7Li 3D MR spectroscopy imaging in the brains of bipolar disorder subjects. *Magn Reson Med*, 68, 363–368.

56. Moore, C. M., Demopulos, C. M., Henry, M. E., et al. (2002). Brain-to-serum lithium ratio and age: An in vivo magnetic resonance spectroscopy study. *Am J Psychiatry*, 159, 1240–1242.

57. Machado-Vieira, R., Otaduy, M. C., Zanetti, M. V., et al. (2016). A selective association between central and peripheral lithium levels in remitters in bipolar depression: A 3 T-(7) Li magnetic resonance spectroscopy study. *Acta Psychiatr Scand*, 133, 214–220.

58. Abdel-Zaher, A. O. (2000). The myoneural effects of lithium chloride on the nerve–muscle preparations of rats: Role of adenosine triphosphate-sensitive potassium channels. *Pharmacol Res*, 41, 163–178.

59. Jefferson, J. W. (1978). Lithium–pancuronium interaction. *Ann Intern Med*, 88, 577.

60. Kishimoto, N., Yoshikawa, H. and Seo, K. (2020). Potentiation of rocuronium bromide by lithium carbonate: A case report. *Anesth Prog*, 67, 146–150.

61. Aref, M. A., El-Badramany, M., Hannora, N., et al. (1982). Lithium loss in sweat. *Psychosomatics*, 23, 407.

62. Jefferson, J. W., Greist, J. H., Clagnaz, P. J., et al. (1982). Effect of strenuous exercise on serum lithium level in man. *Am J Psychiatry*, 139, 1593–1595.

63. Grandjean, E. M. and Aubry, J.-M. (2009). Lithium: Updated human knowledge using an evidence-based approach. Part III: Clinical safety. *CNS Drugs*, 23, 397–418.

64. Wilting, I., Fase, S., Martens, E. P., et al. (2007). The impact of environmental temperature on lithium serum levels. *Bipolar Disord*, 9, 603–608.

65. Cheng, S., Buckley, N. A., Siu, W., et al. (2020). Seasonal and temperature effect on serum lithium concentrations. *Aust N Z J Psychiatry*, 54, 282–287.

66. Merwick, A., Cooke, J., Neligan, A., et al. (2011). Acute neuropathy in setting of diarrhoeal illness and hyponatraemia due to lithium toxicity. *Clin Neurol Neurosurg*, 113, 923–924.

67. Davis, J., Desmond, M. and Berk, M. (2018). Lithium and nephrotoxicity: A literature review of approaches to clinical management and risk stratification. *BMC Nephrol*, 19, 305.

68. Davis, J., Desmond, M. and Berk, M. (2018). Lithium and nephrotoxicity: Unravelling the complex pathophysiological threads of the lightest metal. *Nephrology (Carlton)*, 23, 897–903.

69. Arancibia, A., Paulos, C., Chavez, J., et al. (2003). Pharmacokinetics of lithium in healthy volunteers after exposure to high altitude. *Int J Clin Pharmacol Ther*, 41, 200–206.

70. Uber, A. and Twark, C. (2022). Symptom overlap of acute mountain sickness and lithium toxicity: A case report. *High Alt Med Biol*, 23, 291–293.

71. Thomsen, K. and Schou, M. (1968). Renal lithium excretion in man. *Am J Physiol*, 215, 823–827.

72. McGrane, I. R., Salyers, L. A., Molinaro, J. R., et al. (2021). Roux-en-Y gastric bypass and antipsychotic therapeutic drug monitoring: Two cases. 34, 3, 503–506.

73. Bingham, K. S., Thoma, J., Hawa, R., et al. (2016). Perioperative lithium use in bariatric surgery: A case series and literature review. *Psychosomatics*, 57, 638–644.

74. Musfeldt, D., Levinson, A., Nykiel, J., et al. (2016). Lithium toxicity after Roux-en-Y bariatric surgery. *BMJ Case Rep*, 2016.

75. Niessen, R., Sottiaux, T., Schillaci, A., et al. (2018). [Lithium toxicity after bariatric surgery]. *Rev Med Liege*, 73, 82–87.

76. Dahan, A., Porat, D., Azran, C., et al. (2019). Lithium toxicity with severe bradycardia post sleeve gastrectomy: A case report and review of the literature. *Obes Surg*, 29, 735–738.

77. Jamison, S. C. and Aheron, K. (2020). Lithium toxicity following bariatric surgery. *SAGE Open Med Case Rep*, 8, 2050313x20953000.

78. Lin, Y. H., Liu, S. W., Wu, H. L., et al. (2020). Lithium toxicity with prolonged neurologic sequelae following sleeve gastrectomy: A case report and review of literature. *Medicine (Baltimore)*, 99, e21122.

79. Marques, A. R., Alho, A., Martins, J. M., et al. (2021). Lithium intoxication after bariatric surgery: A case report. *Acta Med Port*, 34, 382–386.

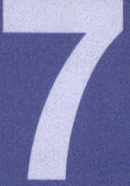

7

Special Populations and Circumstances

Older Bipolar Disorder Patients; Child and
Adolescent Bipolar Disorder Patients;
Pregnant and Breastfeeding Patients;
Lithium Use During Renal Dialysis

PRINCIPLES

- Lithium is effective in older bipolar disorder (BD) patients, and can be used safely by employing modern lithium prescribing and monitoring principles, and by being attentive to kinetic drug interactions. Lithium use in older BD-1 patients is not associated with greater risk for any measure of medical service use compared with divalproex. The frequency of lithium related laboratory monitoring is determined by estimated glomerular filtration rate (eGFR) and not by age.

- Mania in child/adolescent bipolar disorder (CA-BD) patients presents with mood symptomatology. It is diagnosed based not on irritability or severe aggression, but on episodic mood symptoms. CA-BD has significant diagnostic stability, especially the BD-1 subtype. Lithium is the most extensively studied mood stabilizer, is approved in the US for CA-BD in patients aged 7–17, and its use as monotherapy is not associated with significant weight gain. Kinetic studies recommend a daily dose of 25 mg/kg. Unlike in adults, more rapid lithium clearance in younger patients (e.g. those under age 13) often dictates twice daily dosing.

- The risk for any major congenital malformation from 1st trimester pregnancy exposure (including Ebstein's anomaly and other cardiovascular malformations) is much lower than previously thought, with a number needed to harm (NNH) of 37. Patients who need lithium to maintain 1st trimester psychiatric stability should not be dissuaded from its use. Lithium levels need to be monitored periodically during pregnancy due to 2nd trimester increases in eGFR. Lithium exposure may need to be reduced modestly in the week prior to delivery as newborn reactivity is greater when maternal levels are below 0.64 mEq/l at time of birth.

- Recent literature indicates that breastfeeding while taking lithium does not pose risks to the majority of infants, with infant lithium levels dropping significantly after the 2nd week of life as renal function matures. Lithium treated women should not be discouraged from breastfeeding; however, monitoring of infant growth and lithium related laboratory measures is important, especially during the early weeks and months after birth.

- There are lithium treated patients who must continue therapy during dialysis, based on a compelling reason to stay on lithium. The case literature suggests that lithium is tolerated in these patients, with dosing typically occurring three times per week following each dialysis session.

INTRODUCTION

WHAT TO KNOW: INTRODUCTION

- A 2022 meta-analysis on age of onset for major mental disorders noted that, among bipolar disorder (BD) spectrum patients, 5.1% have onset by age 14, and 13.7% by age 18. When child/adolescent patients are accurately diagnosed with BD by mental health specialists, 95% will retain a BD diagnosis after 4 years of follow-up, with BD-1 individuals most likely to retain their subtype.

- There is one important reason to keep older BD patients on lithium: long-term lithium use decreases rates of dementia nearly 50%. Decisions about starting or continuing lithium should be based on eGFR and not age alone. Laboratory monitoring frequency is also driven by eGFR and not by patient age.

- Collaboration with other medical providers is central to the management of older BD patients on lithium, and the same is true when managing lithium treated women through pregnancy and breastfeeding.

Recent findings have significantly altered the perception of lithium risk from 1st trimester exposure and during breastfeeding, while emphasizing that BD patients risk destabilization when not adequately treated during pregnancy.

- For the rare dialysis patient who requires lithium, there are evidence based methods for minimizing the risk of lithium toxicity.

The 2017 International Society for Bipolar Disorders (ISBD) Task Force report on pediatric bipolar disorder (BD) cemented the concept that BD can have onset before the age 18, and that establishing the diagnosis should be based on symptoms of mania or hypomania, while chronic irritability by itself is not sufficient to establish a BD diagnosis [1, 2]. A 2010 study of 1566 patients from six international sites documented that approximately 5% of BD-1 and 5% of BD-2 cases had onset before the age of 20 (Figure 7.1), although the authors noted that only 34.1% of patients were evaluated at onset of their BD, so investigators had to rely on patient

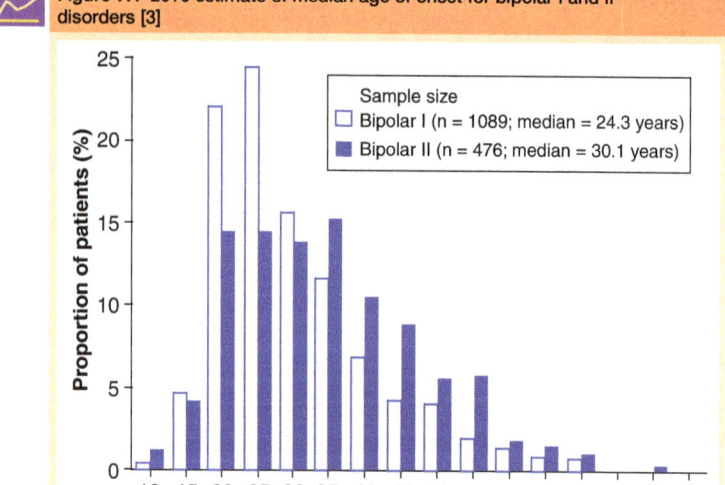

Figure 7.1 2010 estimate of median age of onset for bipolar I and II disorders [3]

(Adapted from: R. J. Baldessarini, L. Bolzani, N. Cruz, et al. [2010]. Onset-age of bipolar disorders at six international sites. *J Affect Disord*, 121, 143–146.)

recall for two-thirds of the sample. The largely retrospective nature of many studies means that the true prevalence of BD before age 18 is not clear, although a 2022 meta-analysis reported that 5.1% have onset by age 14, and 13.7% by age 18 (Figure 7.2) [3, 4].

Descriptive studies of child/adolescent onset BD (CA-BD) over the past decade provided clinicians and researchers with the ability to distinguish CA-BD from other diagnoses such as attention deficit hyperactivity disorder (ADHD) or disruptive mood dysregulation disorder, and this improved recognition should clarify the CA-BD prevalence [5–7]. What is clear is that CA-BD patients have significant diagnostic stability, indicating that this is indeed a persistent disorder and will require similar interventions to adult onset BD. In a sample of 72 Spanish

Figure 7.2 2022 meta-analysis of age of onset for any bipolar disorder diagnosis showing peak age of onset of initial symptoms at age 19.5 years, with a second peak at age 50.5 years [4]

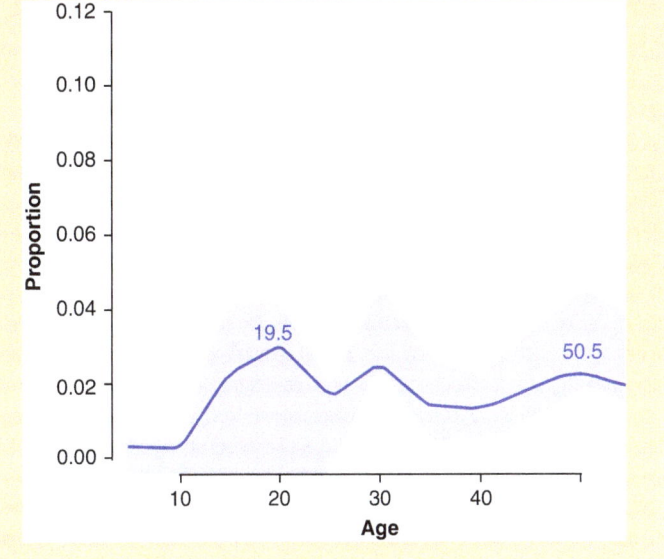

(Adapted from: M. Solmi, J. Radua, M. Olivolaet al. [2022]. Age at onset of mental disorders worldwide: Large-scale meta-analysis of 192 epidemiological studies. *Mol Psychiatry*, 27, 281–295.)

youth assessed in a specialty clinic, the median age of BD onset was 12.6 years, and 95.8% of the sample retained their BD diagnosis after a median follow-up of 3.86 years, with BD-1 individuals most likely to also retain their subtype [8]. Importantly, there was a median delay from symptom onset to BD diagnosis of 2.3 years, speaking to challenges that CA-BD patients may experience before they are accurately diagnosed [8]. A 2022 paper reported similar findings of syndromic persistence from a CA-BD sample recruited via a Harvard University affiliated clinic at Massachusetts General Hospital, and followed for an average of 5.8 ± 1.8 years [9]. Of the original cohort of 105 individuals, 84% (n = 88) returned for at least one follow-up assessment, with no significant demographic differences between those who remained in the study and those lost to follow-up, except for one: individuals who continued in the study had higher socioeconomic status. During the year prior to their last assessment, only 6% of these BD-1 youths were euthymic with normal functioning (i.e. functional remission) and 18% were euthymic but with impaired functioning (Figure 7.3). Among the remaining 76% of the sample, the majority continued to meet full diagnostic criteria for BD-1 (48%) (i.e. syndromic persistence), while 11% continued to have persistent subthreshold BD-1 disorder, or symptomatic persistence (17%) [9].

These findings are sobering and strongly indicate that clinicians treating patients with early onset BD should be diligent about informing all parties about the diagnosis, seeking expert consultation where doubt exists, and using the most evidence-based pharmacological strategies to achieve mood stability, including lithium for those with a history of mania [10, 11]. Multiple studies over the past 20 years have examined the use of lithium in children and adolescents, providing guidance on drug kinetics, dosing strategies, and comparative outcomes vs. divalproex and antipsychotics [11, 12]. Although the literature on maintenance lithium use is not as well developed as for adults, the same methods are available to monitor laboratory parameters (e.g. thyroid stimulating hormone, serum calcium, lithium levels, renal function) and track urine concentration problems (e.g. 24 h fluid intake record [FIR], early morning urine osmolality [EMUO]), to optimize and manage lithium therapy in younger BD patients [13]. Earlier onset often portends a form of the illness that is more difficult to treat, whether it is schizophrenia or BD. There is now sufficient published information to guide all forms of pharmacotherapy in CA-BD patients, with lithium being a core element in the medication toolbox for younger BD individuals [6, 12, 14].

With the increasing recognition that BD onset can occur at any time from childhood to age 70, and that older BD patients might preferentially benefit from

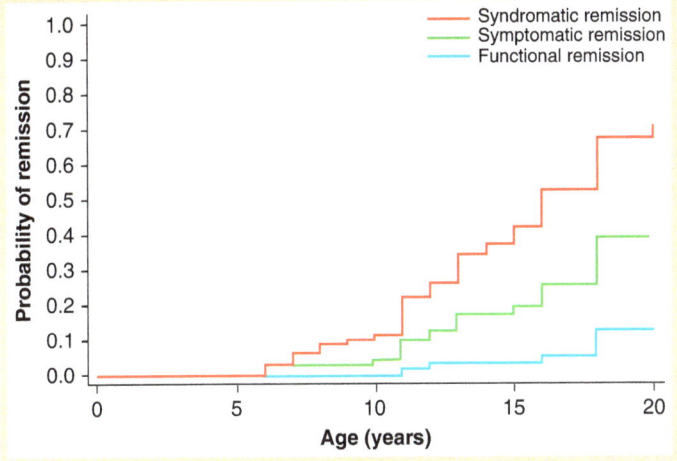

Figure 7.3 Probability of remission during long-term follow-up of child/adolescent onset bipolar I disorder [9]

(Adapted from: J. Wozniak, M. DiSalvo, A. Farrell, et al. [2022]. Long term outcomes of pediatric bipolar-I disorder: A prospective follow-up analysis attending to full syndromic, subsyndromal and functional types of remission. *J Psychiatr Res*, 151, 667–675.)

remaining on lithium due to its neuroprotective properties [15, 16], there is an ever expanding body of efficacy and safety literature to inform rational prescribing practices based on age-dependent differences in lithium kinetics, tolerability and the presence of medical comorbidities [11, 17]. Prospective, randomized studies have established that lithium is effective across the age spectrum for acute mania and for BD maintenance, and for adjunctive use to treat unipolar depression in adults [10, 18–21]. Unfortunately, addressing certain safety concerns cannot be done within the confines of controlled trials and requires a retrospective examination of large data sets [22]. For example, investigators in Ontario, Canada, examined medical outcomes (emergency room visits, nonpsychiatric hospitalizations) for the 1 year following a psychiatric admission in 1388 BD-1 patients with mean age 72.2 years to explore differences in medical service utilization between lithium and non-lithium therapies (e.g. divalproex, antipsychotics) [23]. This naturalistic analysis found that lithium (n = 279) was not associated with greater risk for any measure of medical service use in older BD-1 patients compared with divalproex (n = 452) or to antipsychotic exposure (n = 657) [23]. These findings, combined with the recent focus on using lower maintenance lithium levels led a 2021 review to conclude that with more frequent estimated glomerular filtration rate (eGFR) monitoring and vigilance in responding to the addition of kinetically interacting medications, lithium trials in older bipolar patients can be recommended [24]. As discussed in Chapter 4, starting lithium in individuals with baseline eGFR < 60 ml/min requires careful thought regardless of age (Info Box 7.1).

Info Box 7.1 What Is an Acceptable Baseline eGFR for Commencing Lithium?

a. For a patient with any evidence based indication for lithium:
minimum eGFR ≥ 60 ml/min

Rationale:

i. The Golic 2021 study illustrated that many patients with mean age 55 years who start lithium with an eGFR close to 60 ml/min (54 ml/min) do not exhibit significant annual eGFR declines over the next 6–8 years of treatment [25].

ii. The value of 60 ml/min represents the lower bound of stage G2 CKD, and is an easily remembered cutpoint, often referred to as the limit of "normal" in many papers and laboratory reports.

b. For any patient with a *compelling indication* for lithium:
minimum eGFR ≥ 45 ml/min

Rationale:

i. For patients who failed non-lithium therapies, especially where some of lithium's advantages are relevant (e.g. reduction in risk of completed suicide, 50% lower dementia risk in older BD patients), the risk–benefit equation now tilts toward accepting more baseline risk, since other therapies have not been sufficiently effective. Embedded in the acceptance of a lower baseline eGFR is the concern about depriving patients of lithium who lack options [26].

ii. Every patient newly started on lithium receives more frequent monitoring during the first 6 months of treatment regardless of eGFR (see Chapter 4, Info Box 4.4). To manage the risk in those starting with an eGFR 45–59 ml/min, especially in the presence of CKD risks due to advanced age and medical comorbidity, eGFR will be monitored every 6 weeks during the first 6 months, with future monitoring dictated by the eGFR. The goal is to identify quickly those who are rapidly progressing to stage G3b CKD after starting lithium (eGFR 30–44 ml/min).

iii. For patients continuing on lithium, monitoring frequency will also depend on the same clinical factors: eGFR, trends in eGFR, and the presence of renal and other medical comorbidities (see Info Box 7.2).

The frequency of lithium level monitoring is driven by eGFR values and trends, and by the presence of medical comorbidity, not age itself. While age is often a proxy for lower eGFR and medical comorbidity, there are varying trajectories of eGFR changes in patients of all ages, with some older patients experiencing limited changes in eGFR. Evidence for the latter comes from a retrospective study which found a lack of eGFR changes over 7.9 years of follow-up in a subgroup of patients aged 55.5 ± 16.8 years with mean eGFR 54 ± 15 ml/min when newly initiated on lithium [25]. To manage the risks in those commencing lithium with stage G3a chronic kidney disease (CKD) (45–59 ml/min), especially in the presence of CKD risks due to advanced age and medical comorbidity, eGFR and lithium levels should be monitored every 6 weeks during the first 6 months, with future monitoring dictated by the eGFR and the need to reassure the patient and all other interested parties that lithium is being safely prescribed (Info Box 7.2) [27–29].

Info Box 7.2 Considerations When Using Lithium in Older BD Patients

a. **Efficacy:** Lithium appears equally efficacious to divalproex in acutely manic/hypomanic older BD-1 patients [19]. Having a BD diagnosis increases dementia risk almost 3-fold (OR 2.96, 95% CI 2.09–4.18), but long-term lithium exposure is associated with a 50% reduction in dementia risk [15].

b. **Safety and tolerability:** During acute mania treatment, lithium is as well tolerated as divalproex [19]; moreover, with increased recognition of potential drug interactions in older patients [22, 30], longer-term use is not associated with higher rates of emergency room use, medical hospitalization or duration of inpatient medical stay compared with divalproex (see Table 7.1) [23]. Recent studies also suggest that lithium use may slow atherosclerosis progression during long-term use (using ultrasound measures of carotid intimal thickness), and may have certain cardioprotective effects [31, 32].

c. **Target levels:** Blood-brain barrier permeability can change as patients age, and this can result in greater central nervous system (CNS) lithium levels despite stable peripheral levels [33–35]. Consider using lower maintenance levels initially in new starts (e.g. the lower end of the range from 0.60–0.80 mEq/l), and modifying lithium doses in long-term users who develop new-onset complaints suggestive of increasing CNS lithium levels over time.

d. **Monitoring frequency:** All decisions about when to monitor serum lithium levels and eGFR more frequently are based on eGFR, with the understanding that age is one of the coefficients in the CKD-EPI 2021 eGFR equation [36, 37]. Large retrospective studies indicate that newly initiated, kinetically interacting medications are the major preventable cause of lithium toxicity, while age, medical comorbidity and daily lithium dose are less significant factors [30]. Nonetheless, in those with low eGFR (< 60 ml/min), the presence of medical comorbidities associated with CKD risk (e.g. hypertension, diabetes mellitus, peripheral vascular disease) may abruptly alter the eGFR, hence the rationale for more diligent monitoring. Info Box 7.3 contains the routine monitoring scheme also presented in Chapter 4, Info Box 4.4.

e. **Collaborate:** Patients ≥ 60 years of age represent a group with higher rates of medical comorbidities, higher rates of more advanced CKD (e.g. eGFR ≤ 60 ml/min) and greater use of medications with kinetic interactions. Develop a collaborative relationship with the primary care provider to obviate the use of medications that kinetically interact with lithium, and to establish a means for the provider to contact you when such medications are necessary [22].

f. **Educate:** Advise patients that more frequent monitoring is needed to prescribe lithium safely in certain circumstances, to report any new medications that might interact with lithium, and how to handle situations where dehydration, excessive sweating or gastrointestinal sodium losses might create a risk scenario for lithium toxicity (see Chapter 6, Info Box 6.1).

There are numerous reasons why older patients may need to commence or remain on lithium. For patients who have failed non-lithium therapies, especially where some of lithium's putative advantages are relevant (e.g. reduction in risk of completed suicide, antidepressant actions, improved cognitive performance, 50% lower dementia risk in older BD patients) [15, 38], the risk–benefit assessment leans toward accepting more baseline risk since non-lithium therapies have not been sufficiently effective. Embedded in the acceptance of a lower baseline eGFR for these individuals is the concern about depriving patients of lithium who lack therapeutic options (Info Box 7.3) [26]. No patient should be denied a lithium trial or have lithium discontinued due to age alone without consideration of all the clinical variables, including prior history of lithium response and stability. A 2022 publication used data from the Global Aging & Geriatric Experiments in Bipolar Disorder multicenter trial to perform a cross-sectional analysis of the differences and similarities between lithium users and non-users among 986 BD patients with mean age 63.5 years [38]. Bearing in mind the limitations of cross-sectional studies, this analysis found that older BD patients treated with lithium had lower mean depression ratings, were less likely to be categorized as having moderate or severe depression, had better performance on global cognitive state and functional assessments, required less antipsychotic use, and had fewer cardiovascular comorbidities than non-lithium treated peers [38].

Info Box 7.3 Routine Monitoring

a. **Vital signs:** Weight at every visit with BMI calculated, blood pressure every 6 months.

b. **ECG:** A follow-up should be obtained once lithium is at steady state after initial titration (e.g. week 12) *only in those who required an ECG upon lithium initiation (certain patients > 40 years old, younger patients with cardiac risk factors, or if required by institutional protocol).* In those patients an annual ECG may be required by local protocol or the presence of pre-existing abnormalities. An annual ECG is not recommended by most treatment guidelines for other patients [39].

c. **Serum calcium and TSH:** Every 6 months. As discussed in Chapter 5, an increase in the frequency or the need to add additional laboratory measures (e.g. ionized calcium, parathyroid hormone, T3, T4, free T4 index) will be dictated by the presence of abnormalities.

d. **Lithium level:**

   i. **New lithium starts:** A 12 h trough should be obtained approximately 1 week after any dosage change or introduction or removal of a medication having kinetic interactions with lithium. Through week 24 (6 months) the level should be obtained with the eGFR.

   ii. **Established therapy:** The 12 h trough level should be obtained with the eGFR, and the frequency dictated by the eGFR. For patients with low eGFR values, this may necessitate levels every 6 weeks. For those whose maintenance levels are in the range of 0.80–1.00 mEq/l, consider increasing the frequency of levels to every 3 months to minimize the occurrence of supratherapeutic levels that might incur risk for renal toxicity [27–29].

e. **Renal:**

   i. **Monitoring for the first 6 months of lithium treatment**

	6 weeks	3 months	18 weeks	6 months
eGFR (baseline eGFR ≥ 60 ml/min)	X	X		X
eGFR (baseline eGFR 45–59 ml/min)	X	X	X	X
24 h FIR	X	X		X
EMUO	X	X		X
ACR		X		X

Notes

• eGFR: After 6 months the monitoring frequency depends on CKD stage.

• 24 h FIR (Fluid intake record): Ask the patient to record fluid intake for two separate days and average the result

• EMUO: Should also be added following a new complaint of polyuria/polydipsia.

• ACR (Albumin-to-creatinine ratio): At 3 months and 6 months for those with baseline eGFR < 90 ml/min **or** risk factors for renal dysfunction. After 6 months monitoring frequency depends on the ACR stage.

ii. Routine 6-month monitoring during established lithium therapy

1. Review medical history for renal dysfunction risk factors and use of nephrotoxic medications.

2. eGFR

3. 24 h FIR: Ask the patient to record fluid intake for two separate days and average the result.

4. EMUO: For those with polyuria complaints, on stable amiloride treatment, or for patients whose most recent EMUO value is ≤ 850 mOsm/kg as verified by a repeat specimen.

5. ACR: For those with eGFR < 90 ml/min **or** risk factors for renal dysfunction as noted above.

iii. Increase frequency of labs to every 3 months during established lithium therapy when one of the following is present: (higher-risk patients)

1. eGFR value: When values are < 60 ml/min.

2. eGFR trends: Initial evidence of a decline in eGFR > 2 ml/min over 6 months or > 4 ml/min over 12 months as verified by a repeat specimen.

3. EMUO: For increased or new complaints of polyuria, when titrating amiloride (or adjunctive acetazolamide) to manage polyuria, or for urine osmolality values < 300 mOsm/kg.

4. ACR: If ACR has progressed from stage A1 to A2 as verified by a repeat specimen.

iv. When to consult a nephrologist

1. eGFR: Second decline in eGFR > 2 ml/min over 6 months or > 4 ml/min over 12 months as verified by a repeat specimen.

2. eGFR < 45 ml/min as verified by a repeat specimen.

3. ACR: Stage A3.

4. Nephrogenic diabetes insipidus (EMUO values < 300 mOsm/kg) unresponsive to maximal doses of amiloride (10 mg BID) plus adjunctive use of acetazolamide (up to 500 mg BID) for 6 weeks.

5. Hematuria

Collaboration with other medical providers is central to the management of older BD patients on lithium, and the same is true when managing lithium treated women through pregnancy and breastfeeding. There are randomized trial data on lithium use in older BD-1 patients, but one area of medical practice where drug related safety issues are not explored in prospective randomized trials involves medications employed during pregnancy and lactation [40–42]. Recent literature indicates that infant adverse effects from maternal lithium use during breastfeeding may be manageable with diligent monitoring [43], but the area of greatest concern for clinicians and patients relates to the impact of 1st trimester lithium exposure on risk for major congenital malformations (MCMs), specifically cardiovascular anomalies [44]. One of the greatest advances in the field of maternal health is not from a new understanding of how lithium may increase risk for Ebstein's anomaly, but in the development of sophisticated methods appropriate for the analysis of large data sets (e.g. 1.3 M pregnancies) to more accurately distinguish drug effect from what is termed *confounding bias* related to health habits, concomitant medications and comorbidities in the treated population [45, 46]. As discussed in Chapters 2 and 4, some of the presumed lithium related impact on CKD risk is due to high rates of cardiometabolic disorders among lithium treated patients [47], with lithium assuming a more modest influence on eGFR trends when dosed using modern principles (e.g. once daily dosing, maintenance levels < 1.00 mEq/l) [28, 48].

Similar considerations apply when attempting to examine lithium related MCM risk, as the patient pool is comprised predominantly of individuals with BD or schizoaffective disorder, bipolar type (SAD-BT), a group with higher rates of smoking, substance use, medical conditions, concurrent medication use, housing instability and health-care disparities than demographically matched women [40, 49]. By employing advanced statistical techniques, including propensity score matching and covariate balancing, investigators at the Harvard T. H. Chan School of Public Health published a rigorous analysis quantifying the risk of any cardiovascular malformation (CVM) (e.g. Ebstein's and other CV anomalies) following 1st trimester lithium exposure [44]. The novel finding of this study is that maternal lithium doses ≤ 900 mg/d did not significantly increase CVM risk; moreover, after accounting for potential differences in the probability of termination of malformed fetuses among lithium-exposed and unexposed women, the range of plausible adjusted relative risk (RR) values for any CVM among lithium-exposed infants across all doses was estimated to be 1.67–1.80. Since the base rate of CVM in unexposed infants is 1.15%, using the upper RR value of 1.80, one can calculate the number needed to harm (NNH) at 108. Even for patients on daily lithium doses > 900 mg, this translates to an NNH of 39 [44]. In women whose psychiatric stability necessitates continuation of lithium in the 1st trimester, this well-designed analysis indicates that lithium is not associated with an inordinately increased CVM risk, and provides a risk estimate to guide individualized decisions when patients require doses > 900 mg/d. Moreover, this study and another by this same group of Harvard researchers also noted no increased MCM risk with 1st trimester lamotrigine or antipsychotic exposure, thus providing women evidence-based choices to best manage their bipolar disorder during pregnancy [40, 44]. The conclusions from a

2020 review of lithium use during pregnancy confirm the findings of the Harvard paper, and reminded clinicians that maternal psychiatric stability provides the best chance for optimal infant outcomes during and after pregnancy [49]. A cooperative approach with obstetricians and pediatricians who understand this concept and are conversant in the latest data on lithium related risks can provide patients with the support needed to achieve this goal [49].

As alluded to above and in Chapter 4, there may be important reasons why patients remain on lithium even with extremely low eGFR values [50, 51]. In some instances, long-term patients may value the psychiatric response achieved with lithium, and others may have experienced significant instability or even attempted suicide during non-lithium treatment. Though rarely encountered by most psychiatric providers, the extreme example is a patient with end-stage renal disease who cannot be managed successfully without lithium, and where lithium must be continued during ongoing renal replacement therapy in the form of dialysis. Although the kinetics become more complicated due to the periodic impact of dialysis, a 2022 review noted that, of the 18 reported cases, 94% were able to remain on lithium, with most patients having lithium dosed three times per week following each dialysis session [51]. Management of such cases will require cooperation from all stakeholders (e.g. the patient, the nephrologist); however, with diligent and frequent pre- and postdialysis lithium level monitoring, and by correlating these levels with response and adverse effects, a clinician can quickly establish the dose and pattern of dosing which best suits that patient. The need to provide lithium's efficacy during dialysis mirrors the same considerations for patients with age-related renal and medical comorbidities, or for pregnant/ breastfeeding women: creative, evidence based strategies can be implemented to help patients who need to remain on lithium. Bipolar disorder can be a factor during any stage in an individual's life cycle. The sophisticated prescriber should be conversant in the issues involved in prescribing lithium across the age spectrum, thereby helping patients achieve their psychiatric and functional goals.

 A **Use of Lithium in Older Bipolar Disorder Patients**

 WHAT TO KNOW: USING LITHIUM IN OLDER BIPOLAR DISORDER PATIENTS

- Collaboration with other medical providers is central to the management of older BD patients. The most important risk factor for lithium toxicity in adults is adding a potentially interacting medication (odds ratio [OR] 30). Medical comorbidities and age have a markedly lower independent impact on this risk (OR 1.28 and OR 1.05, respectively).

- The stage of renal function, eGFR trends and the availability of other options with comparable efficacy are all part of individualized decisions regarding commencing lithium or continuing treatment.

- A baseline eGFR < 60 ml/min should not reflexively prevent starting lithium, although it will require more frequent monitoring. A longitudinal study noted that half of a sample of mean age 55.5 ± 16.8 years and mean eGFR 54 ± 15 ml/min when beginning lithium did not have significant eGFR changes over 7 years.

- Divalproex lacks any impact on dementia risk, and is not more effective than lithium or associated with lower rates of medical service use in older BD-1 patients.

- Unlike many antipsychotics, lithium has no adverse cardiometabolic effects, with emerging literature suggesting cardioprotective properties.

- Some individuals experience higher brain-to-serum ratios with aging, and thus may complain of central nervous system related adverse effects at serum levels that were previously tolerable. These complaints should prompt a discussion about modest reduction in serum levels.

Use of the term "older" is at times based on the speaker's frame of reference, but advancing age is a proxy for the accumulation of factors that influence the relative safety of lithium prescribing, including medical comorbidities which increase CKD risk, medications that interact with lithium, and age-dependent decreases in eGFR [24, 25]. As shown in Figures 7.1 and 7.2, a substantial proportion of BD spectrum patients (25% or more) will be diagnosed after age 51, though many may have been symptomatic for extended periods prior to the initial diagnosis [4]. Patients with BD and SAD-BT continue to experience higher mortality rates from natural causes [52–54]; however, despite this mortality gap vs. age-matched peers, individuals with serious mental illnesses do live longer than in prior decades, so clinicians will routinely encounter older patients who are either long-term lithium users or who are newly diagnosed. While declining eGFR reduces the safety margin for lithium, recent studies indicate that clinicians have become more attentive to the need for increased monitoring in lithium treated patients when eGFR falls below 60 ml/min, to the extent that the biggest source of lithium toxicity risk is not advanced age but concomitant medications [30]. A US hospital system (Kaiser Permanente, Colorado) analyzed data from 3115 lithium treated individuals to identify contributors to lithium toxicity of sufficient severity to require acute care services [30]. After matching patients with an episode of lithium toxicity 1:5 with other lithium treated patients, the most important risk factor for toxicity was adding a potentially interacting medication (odds ratio [OR] 30.30, 95% CI 2.32–394.95)

[30]. Having a higher number of treated chronic diseases (OR 1.28, 95% CI 1.12–1.45), older age (OR 1.05, 95% CI 1.02–1.09) and higher total daily lithium dose (OR 1.00, CI 1.00–1.00) had very modest effects [30]. These findings reinforce the concept that monitoring is but one element in managing older patients on lithium, while collaboration with other health-care providers is also crucial so that use of kinetically interacting medications can be minimized, and that appropriate lithium dosage adjustments and level monitoring can be implemented when those medications are necessary [55].

While monitoring and attention to use of concurrent medications can mitigate lithium toxicity risk, there are legitimate concerns about the overall safety of commencing lithium in patients with low baseline eGFR, and specifically the impact of adding lithium on eGFR progression. In 2021, a Swedish group performed an analysis of CKD progression among new lithium starts with comorbidities and subnormal eGFR. Using a cohort design, the study compared eGFR trajectories in 83 patients with high serum creatinine prior to lithium therapy with 83 individuals with normal creatinine when starting lithium, matched by gender, age when initiating lithium, and duration of lithium treatment [25]. Prior to commencing lithium, the low eGFR group had mean age of 61.2 ± 15.1 years and mean eGFR of 48 ± 14 ml/min. After a duration of 7.9 years on lithium, the annual eGFR decline in the low eGFR group was 1.1 ml/min, a rate that was not significantly different than the 1.5 ml/min annual decline in the reference cohort; however, by the end of the observation period, 48% of the low eGFR group progressed to stage G4–G5 CKD (eGFR < 30 ml/min), compared with only 10% of the reference group. A secondary analysis of the low baseline eGFR cohort sought to identify those factors that differed between the 48% who progressed to stage G4–G5 CKD (progressors, $n = 40$) and the 52% ($n = 43$) who were nonprogressors. It was found that the progressors were significantly older (67.4 ± 9.9 years vs. 55.5 ± 16.8 years), disproportionately female (72.5% vs. 51%) and had lower eGFR (42 ± 11 ml/min vs. 54 ± 15 ml/min) prior to starting lithium ($p < 0.001$ for each comparison) [25]. Progressors also had a greater burden of somatic illness ($p < 0.012$), and higher rates of diabetes mellitus (23% vs. 12%) and cardiovascular disorders (63% vs. 42%), but the difference for those specific causes, lithium dosing or serum levels did not reach statistical significance. Although many mental health providers will not be confronted by the prospect of starting lithium in patients with eGFR < 45 ml/min, there will be reasons that lithium should be used, and reasons why lithium must be continued in those individuals. When indications exist to use lithium, the considerations presented in Info Boxes 7.1 and 7.2 should be part of a treatment plan designed to mitigate further eGFR declines and episodes of lithium toxicity.

(As will be discussed below, there may be rare patients who continue lithium even with end-stage renal disease and the need for dialysis. The process of deciding when and whether to discontinue lithium in the face of declining eGFR is reviewed in Section A3 on safety.)

1 *Efficacy*

While both lithium and divalproex are mood stabilizing agents commonly used for BD-1 mania, the first randomized controlled trial for treatment of late-life mania was not published until 2017 [19]. The GERI-BD study was a double-blind, randomized 9-week trial performed in six academic centers, which examined the comparative efficacy and safety of lithium (10–14 h target level 0.80–0.99 mEq/l) or divalproex (10–14 h target level 80–99 μg/ml) among individuals age ≥ 60 years with BD-1 experiencing a current manic, hypomanic or mixed episode [19]. Response in acute mania trials is defined as ≥ 50% reduction in Young Mania Rating Scale (YMRS) scores, and the week 9 responder analysis revealed no significant difference between the two groups: lithium 79%, divalproex 73%; moreover, the need for adjunctive risperidone was also not significantly different between the two cohorts: lithium 17%, divalproex 14%. Nor were there any significant differences in rates of sedation, nausea or vomiting, but the lithium group tended to have more tremor. The large sample size and prospective, double-blind nature of the trial provides the best evidence that lithium is indeed effective and well tolerated among acute mania patients > 65 years of age [19].

In-Depth 7.1 Methods and Detailed Results of the GERI-BD Study

Treating clinicians were blinded to medication choice by having levels reported as units of both medications without specifying the actual treatment arm (e.g. the laboratory report read: 0.58 mEq/l and 58 μg/l). Levels could be reduced below the target range for safety or tolerability concerns. Exclusions to study participation included a diagnosis of dementia or delirium, a history of rapid cycling, or any contraindication to use of either of the study medications. If individuals demonstrated an inadequate response to mood stabilizer monotherapy after 3 weeks, adjunctive open-label risperidone could be used up to 4 mg/d. The study enrolled 224 subjects with mean age 68.0 ± 6.4 years, of whom 49% were female, 87% were white, and 50% were treated as inpatients. The mood states were classified as follows: 64% mania, 13% hypomania and 23% mixed, with 34% of the study sample exhibiting psychotic features. At the week 9 study endpoint, similar proportions of the lithium (57%) and divalproex (56%) groups achieved target serum levels. Subject attrition rates over the course of the study were also comparable for the two medication arms. At week 3, the attrition rates for lithium and divalproex were 14% and 18% respectively, while at week 9, they were 51% and 44% respectively. The primary outcome measure was change in YMRS score from baseline, and the mixed model analysis significantly favored lithium by 3.90 points (97.5% CI 1.71–6.09; p < 0.0002) (Figure 7.4) [19].

Figure 7.4 Changes in YMRS scores from baseline in a randomized, double-blind trial of lithium vs. divalproex in 226 older bipolar I disorder patients of mean age 68 years with a manic/hypomanic/mixed episode [19]

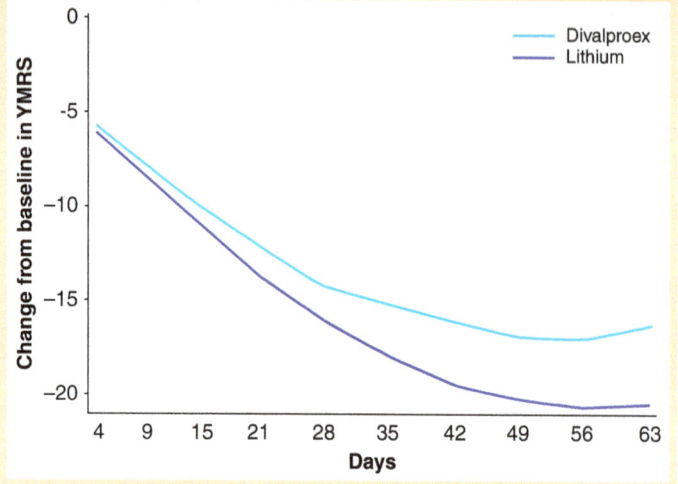

(Adapted from: R. C. Young, B. H. Mulsant, M. Sajatovic, et al. [2017]. GERI-BD: A randomized double-blind controlled trial of lithium and divalproex in the treatment of mania in older patients with bipolar disorder. *Am J Psychiatry*, 174, 1086–1093.)

The efficacy advantage in the GERI-BD study slightly favored lithium over divalproex in older BD individuals, but there are other reasons to consider lithium preferentially in this age group, particularly its neuroprotective effects [15, 16]. The evidence for this is covered extensively in Chapter 1, and consists of both preclinical and clinical data supporting lithium's unique properties in this area [56]. The evidence is so abundant that lithium has been investigated in stroke recovery models and in models of neurodegenerative disorders [57, 58]. For the older BD patient, the most clinically applicable finding relates to reduction of dementia risk [15]. Whether due to inherent mood episode related effects, or the higher prevalence of cardiometabolic disorders and related lifestyle factors (e.g. smoking, diet, sedentary habits), having a BD diagnosis increases dementia risk nearly 3-fold compared with demographically matched peers (OR 2.96, 95% CI 2.09–4.18, p < 0.001); however, long-term use of lithium decreases dementia rates by nearly 50% compared with non-lithium therapies (OR 0.51, 95% CI 0.36–0.72, p < 0.0001). This conclusion comes from a 2020 meta-analysis of cohort and other studies comprising a lithium treated population of 6859 patients on treatment for 3–17 years, and represents a reason to preferentially start or continue lithium in older BD spectrum patients.

In-Depth 7.2 Evidence for Lithium's Protective Effects on Atherosclerosis and Cardiac Function

There are interesting health related effects from lithium noted in recent papers that might also increase the appeal for patients, families and health-care providers. A cross-sectional study of 106 BD-1 outpatients with mean age 44.5 years, 40.6% of whom had concurrent cardiometabolic diseases, used B-mode ultrasound to examine carotid intima-media thickness as a measure of atherosclerotic disease burden [31]. A multivariate regression indicated that higher daily lithium dosage was significantly associated with decreased carotid intima-media thickness in the whole sample, and especially in the younger cohort with age below the sample mean. Another study of 100 BD-1 outpatients used echocardiography and biomarker analyses to examine the cardioprotective effects of lithium in those at higher risk for cardiovascular disease, with higher risk defined as age ≥ 45 years in men or ≥ 55 years in women, or having a diagnosed cardiometabolic disorder [32]. In the high cardiovascular risk group (n = 61), patients on maintenance lithium treatment had significantly lower mean left ventricular internal diameter at end-diastole (Cohen's d = 0.65, p = 0.001) and at end-systole (Cohen's d = 0.60, p = 0.004), and superior performance of global longitudinal strain (Cohen's d = 0.51, p = 0.037) compared with those without lithium treatment.

Although the findings on possible cardioprotective properties warrant further exploration, they complement those from the Global Aging & Geriatric Experiments in Bipolar Disorder trial which showed that lithium treated patients had lower depressive symptom burden, better cognitive performance, less antipsychotic use and fewer cardiovascular comorbidities than non-lithium users [38]. The accumulated findings in the literature should inspire clinicians to advocate for using lithium in older BD patients, and to develop a comfort level with the necessary monitoring in this population.

2 *Lithium Dosing and Kinetics*

It has been known for decades that patients over age 65 have less body water, slower metabolism, and greater burden of comorbid illnesses influencing renal function, and that these differences from younger individuals demand closer monitoring when prescribing lithium [59–61]. While the interplay of age- and disease-related physiological changes and the effects of concurrent medication might seem daunting, the net impact on lithium clearance is readily seen in the 12 h trough lithium level. It thus becomes relatively easy to adjust lithium dosages to maintain a serum level in the range that provides the optimum combination of effectiveness and tolerability for that patient [24]. That the dose-response curve will change in the face of declining renal function is manageable through lithium level monitoring, but what becomes more difficult to track is to what extent age-dependent changes in blood-brain barrier (BBB) permeability might alter the central nervous system (CNS) dose-response curve [33].

In-Depth 7.3 Changes in the Lithium Brain-to-Serum Ratio with Aging

In general, steady state brain lithium levels significantly correlate with serum levels [34, 62], with the brain-to-serum (BTS) ratio averaging 0.50 across multiple studies, meaning that brain levels are 50% lower than serum levels [63]. Yet imaging research uncovered marked interindividual differences in BTS, with older age emerging as one possible factor but not all studies [33–35]. Differences in BTS among age matched patients imply that other biological variables influence lithium CNS transport [64]. Specific concerns about age-related increases in lithium CNS penetration emerged over 20 years ago when a magnetic resonance imaging study in 26 lithium treated BD subjects found that brain lithium levels did not correlate with serum lithium levels for subjects older than age 50 [34]. Moreover, for those older subjects, elevated brain lithium levels were associated with frontal lobe dysfunction on cognitive testing, and higher depression ratings [34].

The clinical implications of studies on BBB changes with aging are 2-fold: (1) For newly started older BD patients, strong consideration should be given to initially managing patients with maintenance lithium levels in the low end of the recommended range (0.6–0.8 mEq/l), and possibly even lower (0.4–0.6 mEq/l), when complaints of CNS related adverse effects (e.g. tremor, new onset cognitive dysfunction) suggest excessive brain exposure [64]. Over time, the level can be adjusted to prevent manic episodes; and, (2) For patients on longer-term lithium treatment, new or increasing complaints of CNS related adverse effects (e.g. tremor, new onset cognitive dysfunction) also indicate alterations in the BTS ratio that might require modest dose and serum level reduction. Perhaps future research might uncover a peripheral marker of CNS lithium exposure, but for the present an increased sensitivity to age-related effects on BBB permeability can help clinicians better understand how peripheral levels that were once ideal for a patient might no longer have the same tolerability profile as the patient ages. As with younger adult patients, lithium is preferentially to be dosed all at bedtime, with dosing decisions based on the 12 h trough serum lithium level.

3 Safety Concerns

The Kaiser Permanente Colorado study previously discussed indicated that the biggest risk for lithium toxicity in older patients relates to introduction of a medication that kinetically interacts with lithium, and not to patient age [30]. Many clinicians are aware of how to manage lithium when using medications associated with significant interactions, to the extent that a 2004 study found use of thiazide diuretics did not result in greater odds of developing lithium toxicity among patients aged 66 and older residing in Ontario, Canada from 1992 to 2001 [22]. Of note, this study also highlighted the fact that furosemide use in an older population might result in a markedly elevated risk of lithium toxicity if not appropriately monitored, somewhat contrary to furosemide's modest effects on lithium clearance in younger adult patients.

Yet the level of sophistication with lithium's kinetic interactions is variable, as is knowledge of the appropriate monitoring frequency for eGFR and lithium levels in older patients. The broader concern thus relates to whether lithium use in an older BD-1 cohort might result in greater need for acute non-psychiatric medical care than an alternative mood stabilizer such as divalproex. The best study to address this issue explored comparative rates of acute nonpsychiatric medical/surgical hospitalization or emergency room (ER) visits during 1-year follow-up in 1388 BD-1 patients age $\geq$ 66 who were discharged from an acute psychiatric hospitalization in Ontario, Canada during the years 2006–2012 (Table 7.1) [23].

As seen in Table 7.1, there were no significant differences between lithium and divalproex treated patients in the proportion with medical admissions, the time to any medical admission after the psychiatric stay, or in the proportion with any nonpsychiatric ER visit. When patients required medical admission, divalproex users had longer lengths of stay than lithium users, but divalproex treated patients also had fewer ER visits than those on lithium. In Cox regression analyses adjusting for age, sex, past medical hospitalization, lithium, divalproex and antipsychotic use (n = 1388), only male gender (HR 1.44, 95% CI 1.15–1.81; p = 0.002) and medical hospitalization in the year prior to the index psychiatric hospitalization (HR 2.22, 95% CI 1.75–2.80; p < 0.001) were significantly associated with a

Table 7.1 Rates of acute nonpsychiatric medical/surgical hospitalization during 1-year follow-up in 1388 bipolar I disorder patients age ≥ 66 years discharged from a psychiatric hospitalization for mania in Ontario, Canada 2006–2012 [23]

	Lithium (n = 279)	Divalproex (n = 452)	Neither lithium nor divalproex (n = 657)	P
Baseline demographic information				
Age	72.4 ± 5.7	71.8 ± 5.4	72.5 ± 5.8	–
Female (%)	61.6%	63.7%	65.0%	–
> 12 years of education (%)	35.8%	30.5%	27.4%	–
Long-term care resident (%)	7.2%	8.8%	5.3%	–
Dementia diagnosis (%)	35.1%	36.7%	35.9%	–
Length of stay during the index psych admission (days)	35.6 ± 47.3	36.7 ± 71.2	33.5 ± 74.2	–
Psychiatric admission in the 1 year prior to the index psych admission (%)	25.1%	32.1%	30.9%	–
Nonpsychiatric hospital admission in the 1 year prior to the index psych admission (%)	21.9%	21.9%	22.7%	–
CKD	11.5%	15.9%	12.0%	–
Outcomes				
Inpatient medical hospitalization	20.8%	21.2%	23.0%	NS
Mean time to medical hospitalization (days)	310.8	317.9	312.7	NS
Length of stay for medical hospitalization (95% CI)	14.8 (7.1, 22.5)	24.5 (10.8, 38.2)	9.6 (7.3, 11.9)	VPA > Li
Any emergency room visit (%)	35.1%	36.9%	41.1%	NS
Number of emergency room visits (95% CI)	2.2 (1.7, 2.8)	1.7 (1.5, 1.9)	2.9 (2.3, 3.4)	VPA < Li

NS = not significant (Adapted from: S. Rej, C. Yu, K. Shulman, et al. [2015]. Medical comorbidity, acute medical care use in late-life bipolar disorder: A comparison of lithium, valproate, and other pharmacotherapies. *Gen Hosp Psychiatry*, 37, 528–532.)

higher incidence of medical hospitalization. No drug group (lithium, divalproex or other) independently contributed to increased risk of medical hospitalization, and mortality rates did not differ significantly between groups, with 3.5% of all patients dying over the year of follow-up. Compared with age-based population data, there were high rates of health service use for all nonpsychiatric medical conditions among older adults with BD-1, but this did not appear to be selectively associated with lithium use. Given the greater extent of medical comorbidity among older BD patients, the authors emphasized a collaborative care approach to prevent acute medical service utilization among late-life BD patients [23], and this recommendation seems prudent to minimize untoward kinetic interactions from new medications, and to manage cooperatively the array of health conditions that are overrepresented among older BD individuals.

The most difficult decision any clinician caring for older BD patients must face is when to consider discontinuing lithium due to the burden of CKD and medical comorbidities. As reviewed in Chapter 5 (Info Box 5.3) and Chapter 8 (Info Box 8.1), this is a difficult decision that should not be made reflexively based on eGFR alone, but which should take into account: a history of psychiatric response, suicide attempts or instability during periods of non-lithium treatments; patient preference; the ability of a patient to manage increasingly stringent monitoring requirements; and the viability of alternative treatment options [50, 65]. In some instances, cognitive testing may be needed to determine patient capacity to assess lithium's risks and benefits. These cases will often necessitate involvement of other treating clinicians, ethicists, family members and stakeholders (e.g. caregivers) to provide input for this complex and individualized decision. That some patients remain on lithium even when receiving hemodialysis speaks to the idea that lithium may be uniquely effective in certain individuals [51], and that innovative solutions can be tailored to support those who cannot remain stable on non-lithium therapies.

 Use of Lithium in Child and Adolescent Bipolar Disorder Patients

 WHAT TO KNOW: USING LITHIUM IN CHILD AND ADOLESCENT BIPOLAR DISORDER PATIENTS

- Pediatric mania is a distinct mood disorder, and one should employ diagnostic criteria based on episodic changes in mood polarity as with adults.
- As with many disorders, earlier onset of BD is often associated with less robust response to treatment. Nonetheless, the core treatment principles are consistent with those employed for adults, especially for

SPECIAL POPULATIONS AND CIRCUMSTANCES

BD-1: mood stabilization, and avoidance of traditional antidepressants for bipolar depression, especially in BD-1. Antipsychotics are very effective for acute mania but can be associated with significant long-term weight gain – unlike lithium, which has limited effects on weight in 28-week studies, and no impact on metabolic parameters.

- An important difference from adult BD-1 treatment is that lithium is the only mood stabilizer indicated for patients under age 18, with US approval for age 7 and higher. Divalproex lacks an indication for pediatric mania, and failed to separate from placebo in a double-blind monotherapy trial. It is used adjunctively at times with lithium nonresponders.

- The relatively high comorbidity with ADHD is one of many issues that face clinicians treating CA-BD patients.

- Pre-adolescent patients have faster renal clearance and often require BID dosing until they reach adult body proportions in their midteens. Use of BID dosing demands adjustment of target serum levels. Failure to do so may result in high rates of GI adverse effects and headache.

- An initial weight based dose of 25 mg/kg/day should be used for preteens and younger adolescents who are not adult sized, with doses adjusted based on levels.

Interest in CA-BD increased significantly 30 years ago as investigators were increasingly able to distinguish childhood mania from the symptoms of attention deficit/hyperactivity disorder (ADHD), while also noting that ADHD comorbidity is not uncommon in CA-BD patients [66–68]. The debate about the characterization of CA-BD and its very existence played out in the literature over the ensuing two decades, but by 2017 the International Society for Bipolar Disorders (ISBD) Task Force felt sufficiently confident to issue its seminal report on CA-BD, whose conclusions are worth quoting verbatim:

> As data have accumulated and controversy has dissipated, the field has moved past existential questions about PBD [pediatric bipolar disorder] toward defining and pursuing pressing clinical and scientific priorities that remain. The overall body of evidence supports the position that perceptions about marked international (US vs elsewhere) and developmental (pediatric vs adult) differences have been overstated, although additional research on these topics is warranted. Traction toward improved outcomes will be supported by continued emphasis on pathophysiology and novel therapeutics [1].

Subsequent literature reinforced that pediatric mania is indeed a distinct mood disorder, and that it should not be inferred solely from a history of severe irritability and aggression [6]. Moreover, as with adults, one should employ diagnostic criteria based on episodic changes in mood polarity over the longitudinal course of the patient's illness to arrive at a BD diagnosis. Indeed, both adolescent and childhood onset BD-1 patients experience a range of symptoms during manic episodes such as euphoria, pressured speech, grandiose ideation, inappropriate laughter and occasionally hypersexuality or psychosis that clearly distinguish this as a mood episode (Figure 7.5) [5].

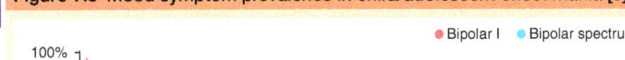

Figure 7.5 Mood symptom prevalence in child/adolescent onset mania [5]

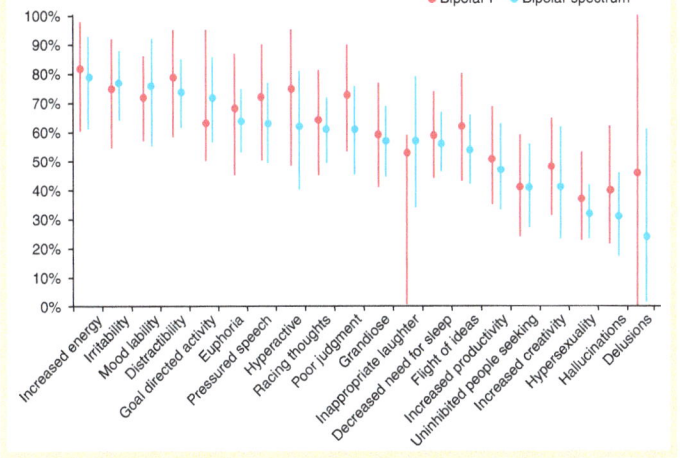

(Adapted from: A. R. Van Meter, C. Burke, R. A. Kowatch, et al. [2016]. Ten-year updated meta-analysis of the clinical characteristics of pediatric mania and hypomania. *Bipolar Disord*, 18, 19–32.)

There is increasing evidence that, prior to the onset of a manic episode, the presentation may be consistent with ADHD [7]; however, while ADHD is typically a stable diagnosis over the patient's lifetime (although the functional impact may change), the prevalence of ADHD in BD patients wanes dramatically, suggesting that the early nonspecific manifestation of BD may have been ADHD, but this is less evident once BD declares itself and patients are treated for the mood disorder [7].

Estimated ADHD prevalence rates from longitudinal and cross-sectional studies range from 73% in childhood to 43% in adolescence, and only 17% in adulthood [69]. That ADHD and BD can coexist should not be minimized, as ADHD is 3 times more common in people with any mood disorder and 1.7 times more common in BD patients compared with those with unipolar major depressive disorder [69]. The relatively high comorbidity with ADHD is one of many issues that face clinicians treating CA-BD patients, but the core treatment principles are largely congruent with adult practices, especially for BD-1: mood stabilization and avoidance of traditional antidepressants for bipolar depression when there is a history of mania [1, 11]. As with other serious mental disorders (e.g. schizophrenia) where onset can occur in patients before the age of 18, medications are the foundation upon which other interventions are added. Effectiveness trials indicate that family psychoeducation plus patient skill-building are well-established treatments, and that these approaches are both acceptable and sustainable in community settings [1].

The ISBD paper highlighted that the presence of mania and the episodic nature of mood symptoms will help clinicians differentiate CA-BD from non-bipolar patients with ADHD or other neuropsychiatric and behavioral disorders [2]. Consistent with a correct diagnosis of the mood disorder, there is significant diagnostic stability among CA-BD, with BD-1 patients displaying high retention of the original subtype (Figure 7.6) [8]. The 2017 ISBD Task Force report reviewed data from 17 studies comprising 31,443 individuals in the age range of 7–21 to generate a weighted average prevalence rate of 2.06% (95% CI 1.44%–2.95%) for CA-BD spectrum disorder [1]. The report noted substantial heterogeneity across study estimates, with differences in the definition of BD explaining the largest portion of variance between studies. Broader definitions had the highest rates, while narrower definitions (i.e. BD-1 or BD-2 only) had lower rates. The weighted average prevalence of BD-1 was 0.49% (95% CI 0.22%–1.09%), with 4 of 12 studies reporting no BD-1 cases [1]. A 2022 meta-analysis examining age of onset across a range of mental disorders indicated that 5.1% will have onset of any BD spectrum diagnosis by age 14, and 13.7% by age 18 [4].

Clinicians who routinely see a younger demographic will inevitably encounter BD patients, and the literature is clear that management of CA-BD can be challenging since early presentation is associated with increased genetic burden and greater disease severity [6]. Childhood onset schizophrenia (COS) is exceedingly rare, but COS patients are largely treatment resistant and only respond robustly to clozapine [70]. Prepubertal onset of BD is not nearly as rare as COS and not necessarily treatment resistant, but long-term follow-up studies show that those with childhood

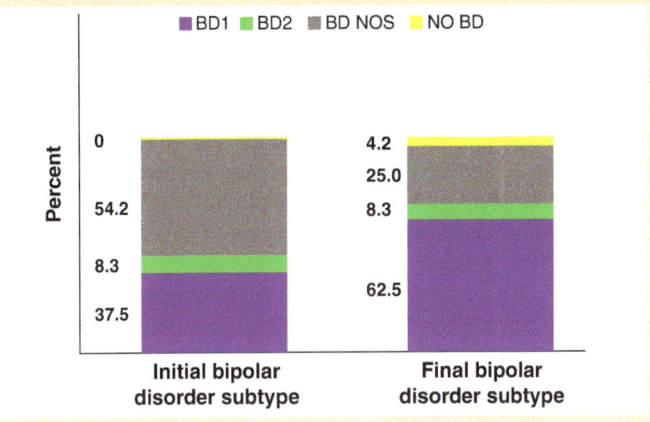

Figure 7.6 Diagnostic stability over 3.86 years of follow-up in a sample of 72 patients with child/adolescent bipolar spectrum disorders, including BD Not Otherwise Specified (BD NOS) (median age of onset 12.6 years) [8]

(Adapted from: M. Ribeiro-Fernández, A. Díez-Suárez and C. Soutullo [2019]. Phenomenology and diagnostic stability of paediatric bipolar disorder in a Spanish sample. *J Affect Disord*, 242, 224–233.)

onset in particular often remain symptomatic with functional impairment into their late teens and early adulthood (Figure 7.3) [9]. These can be complex patients, and all clinicians are advised to acquire one of the comprehensive volumes devoted exclusively to BD in CA-BD patients [71], and, if possible, establish a relationship with a respected clinician who has experience managing these individuals. In this context, it should be recognized that lithium is one of many pharmacological tools to be used in this challenging patient cohort, and that the goal of lithium monotherapy, while laudable, is often not feasible, especially as additional medications may be necessary to achieve mood stability, and to treat depressive or concomitant ADHD symptoms [11]. The 2017 ISBD report and more recent reviews are excellent resources that provide an overview of all the medication options studied in CA-BD, primarily BD-1 [1, 11]. One striking difference from adult BD-1 disorder treatment is that divalproex not only lacks an indication for pediatric mania, it failed to separate from placebo in a 4-week double-blind monotherapy trial in 150 patients aged 10–17 years experiencing an acute manic or mixed episode [72, 73]. Divalproex has been studied adjunctively to lithium, and it does remain an option for residual manic and hypomanic symptoms not addressed by lithium monotherapy [74–76].

For now, lithium is the only mood stabilizing medication with sufficient efficacy data in patients under age 18 to have a child/adolescent US Food and Drug Administration (FDA) indication for acute mania and maintenance treatment of BD-1 disorder [77]. Divalproex lacks this indication, and neither carbamazepine nor lamotrigine have been studied in double-blind CA-BD trials, although adjunctive lamotrigine was explored in a BD-1 long-term maintenance trial where it did not display efficacy [11]. Multiple antipsychotics have US FDA indications in patients aged 10–17 for mixed/manic episodes (aripiprazole, asenapine, olanzapine, quetiapine, risperidone), and two for BD-1 depression (lurasidone, olanzapine/fluoxetine combination), but the established efficacy, safety and kinetics of lithium make it one of the core medications for management of CA-BD-1 patients, especially for maintenance [78]. Despite data supporting lithium's efficacy in this population, there is significant variation in the wording of product labeling throughout the world. Even within the United States, some lithium product labels state that the safety and effectiveness in pediatric patients under 12 years of age have not been determined [79], while others indicate (correctly) that lithium is approved for acute manic or mixed episodes, and for BD-1 maintenance therapy, in patients aged 7 years and older [77]. Outside of the US, labeling in other countries variably suggests that the use in children is not recommended or that lithium should not be used in children [80, 81]. The practice of child psychiatry is largely off label, as many pharmaceutical companies do not pursue indications in this population for commercial reasons. Nonetheless, despite the data indicating that lithium is well tolerated and effective for CA-BD-1, clinicians should abide by their country's practice standards in the use of any medication for patients under 18 years of age. (For a review of the weak evidence supporting lithium's use in the management of conduct disorder or aggressive behavior in children, adolescents or those with intellectual disabilities, please see Chapter 1.)

1 *Efficacy*

The efficacy of lithium for BD-1 in acute manic/mixed episodes, and for BD-1 maintenance, has been established in multiple trials over the past 25 years [10, 18, 82, 83]. One of the earliest and largest clinical trials was a controlled study in which 279 outpatients of mean age 10.1 ± 2.8 years, with no prior exposure to an antimanic agent, and who were experiencing a manic or mixed episode for at least 4 consecutive weeks immediately preceding study entry, were randomized in a 1:1:1 manner to 8 weeks of treatment with risperidone, lithium or divalproex [83]. Symptom raters were blinded, but treatment was open and there was no placebo arm. The mean duration of mania symptoms was 4.9 ± 2.5 years at time of study enrollment, and patients had the following symptom characteristics: elated mood and/or grandiosity: 100%; daily rapid cycling: 99.3%; mixed mania: 97.5%; psychosis: 77.1%. The mean endpoint lithium level was 1.09 ± 0.34 mEq/l, the mean divalproex level was 113.6 ± 23.0 µg/ml, and the mean risperidone dose was 2.57 ± 1.21 mg. Although this study had some methodological limitations, response rates to risperidone (68.5%) were clearly superior to divalproex (24%, $p < 0.001$) and to lithium (35.6%, $p < 0.001$). Unfortunately, risperidone was associated with significantly greater weight gain (risperidone + 3.31 kg, lithium + 1.42 kg, divalproex + 1.67 kg) and prolactin level elevations, compared with either mood stabilizer, raising concerns about its use as maintenance treatment or for any period beyond initial management of acute mania symptoms [11].

Subsequent acute mania trials with antipsychotics possessing more favorable adverse effect profiles (e.g. aripiprazole) provided clinicians an alternative to risperidone, although none were studied vs. lithium. The first randomized, double-blind, placebo-controlled multicenter lithium study enrolled BD-1 subjects aged 7–17 years (median age 11.5 years) with manic or mixed episodes, and compared lithium (n = 53) with placebo (n = 28) for up to 8 weeks [18]. The change in YMRS score was significantly larger in lithium treated participants (–5.51 points, 95% CI –0.51 to –10.50) after adjustment for baseline YMRS score, age, weight, gender, and study site ($p = 0.03$). Of note there was no significant difference between lithium and placebo with respect to weight gain in this trial, although an increase in TSH was seen with lithium (+ 3.0 ± 3.1 mIU/l) but not in the placebo arm (–0.1 $\pm$ 0.9 mIU/l; $p < 0.001$) [18]. As will be discussed in the section on safety below, the increase in TSH appears transient in many patients as maintenance lithium trials do not report clinically significant mean changes from baseline [11, 82, 84, 85]. These and other trials indicate that lithium is effective for pediatric manic/mixed episodes, but that atypical antipsychotics may be particularly helpful in establishing euthymia quickly, a practice pattern very similar to the management of adult mania.

The evidence that initial lithium response portends ongoing stability during maintenance was shown by the results of a double-blind, placebo-controlled, BD-1 maintenance trial published in 2019, examining rates of all cause discontinuation (e.g. mood relapse, adverse effects) [10]. Although the sample size in each arm was small (lithium n = 17; placebo n = 14), those who continued on lithium had a lower hazard ratio for discontinuation compared with those randomized to placebo ($p = 0.015$; Figure 7.7) [10]. The vast majority of discontinuations were due to mood symptom exacerbation, primarily in the placebo treated group. Discontinuation for

Figure 7.7 Lithium vs. placebo in the maintenance treatment of child/adolescent bipolar I disorder (mean age 12.0 years) [10]

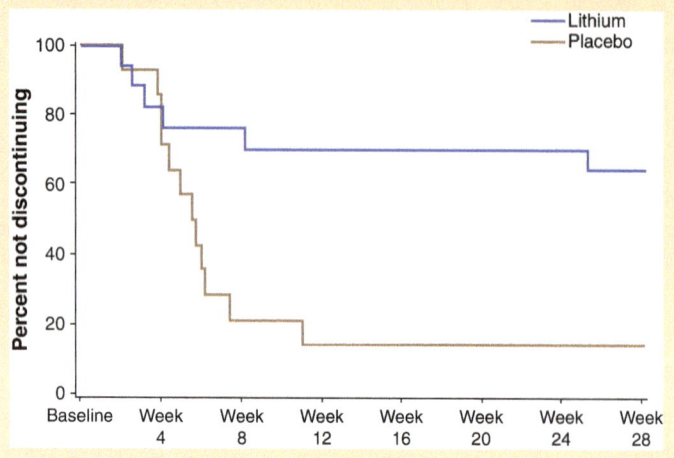

(Adapted from: R. L. Findling, N. K. McNamara, M. Pavuluri, et al. [2019]. Lithium for the maintenance treatment of bipolar I disorder: A double-blind, placebo-controlled discontinuation study. *J Am Acad Child Adolesc Psychiatry*, 58, 287–296.)

other reasons occurred at comparably low rates across both groups. That lithium is effective during maintenance replicates the findings from adult patients; however, as noted previously, earlier onset is often associated with greater disease severity, and many CA-BD patients will require additional medications for mania, depression or other comorbidities (e.g. ADHD, tic disorders) [11–13, 86].

In-Depth 7.4 Lithium Nonresponse and CA-BD-1 Patients

While some CA-BD-1 patients will respond to lithium monotherapy, failure to achieve adequate symptom remission with lithium monotherapy may be relatively common [85]. The best study to exemplify this was a trial of 41 BD-1 outpatients aged 7–17 years experiencing a manic or mixed episode, who demonstrated at least a partial response to 8 weeks of open-label lithium treatment. During the next study phase, subjects were eligible to receive open-label lithium for an additional 16 weeks and up to two adjunctive medications for residual mania symptoms or comorbid psychiatric conditions (e.g. ADHD). Of the 41 subjects who entered the second phase of the study, 60.9% were prescribed adjunctive psychotropics, primarily for resistant mania (31.7%) and for ADHD (36.6%). At the end of this phase, 68.3% of patients met response criteria, and 53.7% were considered to be in remission. The study findings suggest that CA-BD-1 patients who initially respond to lithium for an acute manic or mixed episode will maintain mood stabilization during continuation treatment, but partial responders may be a subgroup with a more difficult-to-treat form of the illness and might not achieve the same extent of symptom reduction even with use of adjunctive medications [85].

There are studies of lithium combined with divalproex for BD-1 patients who exhibit inadequate response to monotherapy demonstrating that the combination is effective despite the lack of positive pediatric mania data for divalproex [74, 75]. Importantly, patients who require combination therapy initially will likely need both medications for ongoing stability, with one trial showing high relapse rates when patients stabilized on combination treatment were placed on mood stabilizer monotherapy, although they could subsequently be restored to euthymia once the combination was resumed [75, 82].

As with adults, the data for lithium use in bipolar II disorder (BD-2) are much more limited, and some of these patients may not need lithium's mood stabilizing properties. Nonetheless, lithium can be considered for bipolar depression or its anti-suicide properties, bearing in mind the limited data supporting lithium's antidepressant effects in BD children [87], and that other medications are specifically approved for BD-1 depression in patients aged 10–17, that are relatively weight neutral and nonsedating (e.g. lurasidone) [1, 11, 88]. The extent to which lithium's putative neuroprotective or anti-suicide properties represent compelling reasons for its use in CA-BD-2 or any CA-BD spectrum patient is an area deserving further study, and one not easily answered from existing data [14].

In-Depth 7.5 Managing Lithium Adherence in CA-BD Patients

Nonadherence with mood stabilizer therapy is common across all ages, and the same is true for CA-BD patients, but conclusions from the existing literature are limited due to significant differences in study methodologies, with a 2021 meta-analysis lamenting that only six studies met inclusion criteria, and only three of these included subjects < 12 years of age [89]. One of the earliest studies tracked pill counts, serum levels and patient/parental self-report as part of a trial examining response to combination lithium and divalproex treatment among 107 patients with CA-BD-1 (mean age 10.5 years at study entry, estimated duration of illness 3.9 years) [90]. Pill counts are one of the most evidence based methods to track oral medication adherence, and are superior to every other method including drug levels, 3rd party report and patient self-report [91, 92]. One working definition of adherence is **taking adherence**, defined as the number of pills taken divided by the number of prescribed doses during the monitoring period [93, 94]. During a mean duration of 11.2 weeks follow-up, pill count adherence was uniformly excellent in this trial: lithium 100%, divalproex 98% [90]. While taking adherence may be outstanding among younger children who might accede to parental directions, this changes over time as teens start to grapple with the illness implications of taking medication daily, and with unpleasant medication related adverse effects. The 2021 meta-analysis noted that no articles reported on interventions to improve adherence in CA-BD, but this will change in the near future.

As reviewed in Chapter 4, Dr. Martha Sajatovic (Willard Brown Chair in Neurological Outcomes at University Hospitals Cleveland Medical Center, and the Rocco L. Motto Professorship in Child & Adolescent Psychiatry) developed Customized Adherence Enhancement (CAE), an evidence based program designed to improve adherence in BD patients [95]. The CAE modules are tailored to each patient's needs and cover four areas: increasing patient knowledge, improving skill at communicating with providers, enhancing motivations for treatment, and identifying issues with medication routines (e.g. unnecessary complexity). Patients are assigned to specific modules based on their individual reasons for nonadherence, and each module is delivered in one-on-one sessions spaced 1 week apart, with a booster session 4 weeks after completion of the last session. The CAE model has proved effective for poorly adherent adults with BD in multiple trials [95, 96], and the delivery of CAE was subsequently modified for the needs of CA-BD patients. The revised treatment is termed CAE for Adolescents and Young Adults (CAE-AYA) and is now being compared with enhanced treatment as usual in a 6-month prospective randomized study [97]. If CAE-AYA is proven effective, it should be offered to CA-BD patients who start to question the need for medication, or who refuse BD medications for a variety of reasons. Bipolar disorder is lifelong, and adherence interventions such as CAE-AYA can provide the knowledge and skills to manage medication adherence among younger individuals who are grappling simultaneously with both illness and developmental issues related to their psychiatric diagnosis.

2 *Lithium Dosing and Kinetics*

Dr. Robert L. Findling (chair of the Virginia Commonwealth University School of Medicine's Department of Psychiatry) has been one of the pioneers in CA-BD lithium research, and his pharmacokinetics studies in CA-BD patients helped establish the dosing regimen used in research and clinical settings [84, 98, 99]. The first dedicated pharmacokinetic trial was a single-dose kinetic study using

20 children of mean age 9.9 ± 1.4 years, and 19 adolescents with mean age 14.0 ± 1.5 years, yielding a mean age for the overall sample of 11.9 ± 2.5 years. As seen in Figure 7.8, there is a biphasic decay curve containing an initial rapid decline with $T_{1/2}$ 2.4 h and a longer terminal phase with $T_{1/2}$ 27 h. Using these data, the estimated multiple dose steady state $T_{1/2}$ arrived at from simulations was 13.1 h with once daily dosing, 14.0 h for BID dosing, and 15.1 h for TID (q8 h) dosing [98]. Although children aged 10–12 had faster lithium clearance than adolescents aged 13–17, the authors did not opt for a weight based algorithm, but instead suggested a dosing strategy loosely based on age, and explored this in an outpatient CA-BD-1 study [84]. This subsequent trial was the first study performed as part of the Collaborative Lithium Trials network, and is referred to in the literature as CoLT 1. That study consisted of two phases: phase I was an 8-week, open-label, randomized, escalating-dose study which contained 3 treatment arms, and phase II a 16-week open-label long-term effectiveness trial [84, 85]. In phase 1, arm I started treatment with lithium 300 mg BID, while the starting dose in arms II and III was 300 mg TID [84]. Patients in arms I and II could have their dose increased by 300 mg/day, depending on clinical response, at weekly visits. Patients in arm III also had mid-week telephone interviews after which they could have the lithium dose increased by 300 mg/day. The investigators found that all 3 treatment arms had similar effectiveness, side effect profiles and tolerability, but detailed pharmacokinetic data were not analyzed in the initial study report [84].

Figure 7.8 Pharmacokinetic single dose modeling of pediatric lithium clearance from a sample of 39 youths with mean age 11.9 years [98]

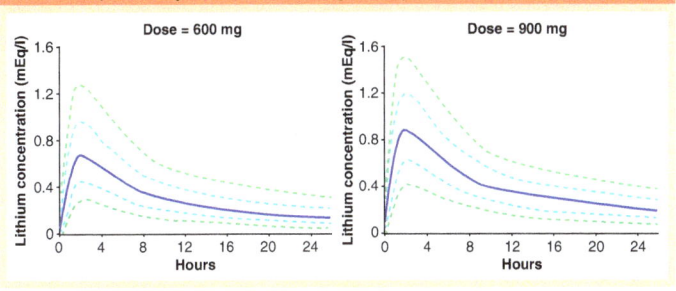

(Adapted from: R. L. Findling, C. B. Landersdorfer, V. Kafantaris, et al. [2010]. First-dose pharmacokinetics of lithium carbonate in children and adolescents. *J Clin Psychopharmacol*, 30, 404–410.)

In 2017, investigators analyzed the entire data set from phases I and II of CoLT 1 to arrive at weight based dosing recommendations [99]. Figure 7.9 shows the kinetic modeling simulation using the dosing recommendation of 25 mg/kg that best fit all of the parameters, while optimizing the balance between efficacy and tolerability [99]. From this dosing strategy of 25 mg/kg/day (administered as divided BID or TID doses) and the response of these CA-BD-1 manic patients to treatment, two important conclusions were reached. The first finding was that the average lithium level required for a 50% reduction in YMRS among manic CA-BD patients was 0.71 mEq/l, but with the caveat that the interindividual variance was 59%. The second finding was that a daily maintenance lithium carbonate dose of 25 mg/kg divided into a BID schedule was predicted to achieve a ≥ 50% reduction in YMRS in 74% of patients, with only 8% of patients expected to have supratherapeutic trough levels > 1.40 mEq/l [99]. While clinicians must acknowledge that significant interindividual variations in lithium clearance demand close level monitoring when starting treatment, the 25 mg/kg dosing recommendation is more evidence based than recommendations in lithium carbonate product labeling, when such recommendations exist at all. For example, a 2020 US package label suggests a lithium carbonate starting dose for pediatric patients weighing 20 to 30 kg of 300 mg twice daily, while any person weighing > 30 kg can initiate therapy at 300 TID [77]. Unlike for adults, clinicians are advised not to use lithium loading

Figure 7.9 Monte Carlo simulations of lithium concentrations for a daily dosage of 25 mg/kg given in two or three divided doses. [NB: The doses administered were rounded to the nearest 300 mg lithium carbonate increment. Where applicable, the higher dose was given in the evening.] [99]

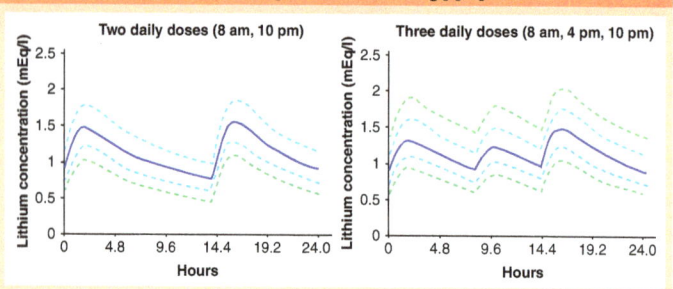

(Adapted from: C. B. Landersdorfer, R. L. Findling, J. A. Frazier, et al. [2017]. Lithium in paediatric patients with bipolar disorder: Implications for selection of dosage regimens via population pharmacokinetics/pharmacodynamics. *Clin Pharmacokinet*, 56, 77–90.)

strategies when managing acute mania in CA-BD, mostly to avoid some of the gastrointestinal (GI) adverse effects that were very prevalent in the CoLT studies [85]. Antipsychotics are effective for CA-BD mania, so their concurrent use lessens concerns that the lithium level achieved with the 25 mg/kg regimen will be subtherapeutic.

Maintenance lithium levels are consistent with those recommended for adult patients, but clinicians should be mindful that the BID dosing commonly used in CA-BD patients will distort the 12 h trough level since half of the dose was administered 24 h prior to the level being drawn (Chapter 3, Table 3.2) [59]. In adults, the morning trough level would be 28% higher were a BID dose converted to a QHS schedule, so consideration should be given to maintaining a morning trough level on BID dosing no higher than 0.78 mEq/l, as this would equate to 1.00 mEq/l if the dose were given QHS only (assuming adult kinetics). As patients enter their midteens, the schedule should slowly be converted to QHS dosing for patient convenience, and to minimize long-term renal effects from divided daily dosing [28]. Some patients may be wedded to BID dosing for a variety of reasons (e.g. historical stability and reluctance to change, prior episodes of gastrointestinal (GI) adverse effects on single QHS doses) but, with patient education, very gradual movement of doses to bedtime, and use of strategies to mitigate GI complaints, most patients can be slowly converted to QHS dosing as they enter their late teens.

3   *Safety Concerns*

During the 16-week second phase of CoLT 1, investigators saw high rates of GI adverse effects and headache, perhaps related to the escalating-dose regimen used in phase I of that protocol [85]. The array of acute adverse effects is very similar to that seen with adults, with the exception of headache as a more prominent complaint, and the absence of significant weight gain on lithium monotherapy, even in 28-week studies [11, 13]. Another difference from adult patients is that increases in TSH levels may be seen in the first 2–3 months of treatment, but in some patients an elevated TSH may decrease over time from these peak levels [11]. Persistently abnormal TSH values will require intervention, but this is one area where collaboration with a specialist (e.g. pediatric endocrinologist) will be helpful to decide on a course of action, including the need for additional thyroid indices to supplement information gleaned from the rising TSH values. As with adults, routine inquiry is the best tool to convey your concern about all adverse effects to the patient, parents and caregivers, and to convey your willingness to manage these issues (see Info Box 7.4). This is especially true for complaints that may be embarrassing (e.g. enuresis) or cause physical discomfort (e.g. abdominal pain, vomiting). While many mental health clinicians will develop a comfort level in using amiloride to manage urine concentration deficits related to lithium use, this is another area where specialist collaboration will be helpful, as few pediatricians will have used amiloride, while a pediatric nephrologist is likely to be aware of its special properties and be able to propose weight based dosing for younger patients. The goal is to address adverse effects as soon as they arise, and to proactively ask about common side effects when not spontaneously offered, to forestall a patient or parent demand to stop lithium.

 Info Box 7.4 Considerations When Using Lithium in Child/Adolescent Bipolar Disorder (CA-BD) Patients

a. **Efficacy:** Lithium remains the only mood stabilizer with a US FDA indication for CA-BD manic/mixed episodes, or for maintenance in CA-BD-1 patients aged 7–17. Divalproex lacks this indication, and neither carbamazepine nor lamotrigine have been studied in double-blind CA-BD trials, although adjunctive lamotrigine was explored in a BD-1 long-term maintenance trial where it did not display efficacy [11]. Divalproex and atypical antipsychotics are used adjunctively with lithium for initial treatment of mania, and at times for maintenance [75]. Multiple antipsychotics have indications for acute mania in CA-BD patients, and two (quetiapine, lurasidone) for BD-1 depression in patients aged 10–17 years. There are limited data on BD-2 in younger patients, but lithium can be considered for those patients who need mood stabilization, or where other properties of lithium are desirable (e.g. anti-suicide effects) [12].

b. **Safety and tolerability:** The adverse effect profile is very similar to adults, but the more aggressive dosing in some trials gave rise to high rates of headache, abdominal pain, nausea and vomiting [85]. Gastrointestinal adverse effects can be addressed in the same manner as with adults: lower lithium doses when possible, use of sustained release preparations or administering lithium with food to slow rapid lithium ion absorption. Long-term studies up to 28 weeks indicate that lithium monotherapy is not associated with significant weight gain [11]. Although TSH monitoring every 6 months is necessary in all lithium treated patients, CA-BD studies note increases over the first 2–3 months, with some improvement over time [11]. Persistent elevations of TSH should be reviewed with a pediatric endocrinologist for the need to examine other thyroid indices and commence treatment. Complaints of thirst or enuresis should be solicited as these represent early signs of polyuria. Once a urine concentration deficit is documented by decreases in the EMUO, consultation with a pediatric nephrologist may be helpful to arrive at a weight based amiloride dose for smaller teens and younger children.

c. **Target levels:** The same as adult levels for acute mania and for maintenance, bearing in mind that, with BID dosing commonly used in

CA-BD patients, the 12 h trough level is distorted since half of the dose was administered 24 h prior to the level being drawn. Adult studies have shown that a morning level obtained with BID dosing should be multiplied by 1.28 to estimate the 12 h trough from QHS dosing. A similar rule of thumb should apply to CA-BD patients to avoid overexposure to lithium. As patients enter their midteens, the schedule should slowly be converted to QHS dosing for patient convenience, and to minimize long-term renal effects of divided daily dosing [28].

d. **Dosing:** For kinetic reasons, an initial weight based recommended dose of 25 mg/kg/day is suggested, with the doses split into BID dosing, especially for children under the age of 13 [98, 99]. As lithium may only be available in certain dosing increments, the larger of the two daily doses is administered at bedtime.

e. **Monitoring frequency:** No differences from adults (see Info Box 7.3), with particular focus on soliciting complaints of polyuria, and measurement of EMUO.

f. **Collaborate:** Develop a collaborative relationship with a pediatrician, and perhaps a pediatric endocrinologist and nephrologist, to assist with management of hypothyroidism and with treatment of lithium-induced nephrogenic diabetes insipidus using amiloride.

g. **Educate:** Family psychoeducation has proven benefits, and patient skill-building is also an evidence based intervention [1]. If the CAE program for adolescents and young adults is also proven to be as effective for this population as for adults, this should be implemented for CA-BD patients with suboptimal adherence [97].

 Lithium Use and Pregnancy

 WHAT TO KNOW: LITHIUM USE AND PREGNANCY

- BD women who discontinue a mood stabilizer during pregnancy have 2-fold higher recurrence risk for any mood episode, and the time spent ill during the pregnancy is 5-fold greater.

- Revised estimates of Ebstein's and other cardiovascular malformation (CVM) risk from 1st trimester lithium exposure were published in a 2020 meta-analysis. The NNH for all CVM was 83 when comparing lithium users and non-users with bipolar disorder [49]. One would need to expose 83 BD individuals to lithium to see 1 additional CVM case compared with lithium non-using peers. For women on doses > 900 mg/d, a rigorous US study provides an NNH of 39. These findings should support the decisions of women whose psychiatric health depends on continuous lithium use to persist with treatment during pregnancy, albeit with appropriate monitoring.

- Lithium prescribers should develop a relationship with an obstetrician familiar with the needs of patients who require lithium, and thereby avoid reflexive demands to discontinue lithium from certain clinicians.
- Lithium levels decrease during pregnancy, and reach their lowest point in the 2nd trimester, 36% below baseline. Monitoring during each trimester can help prevent relapse due to subtherapeutic levels. Trimester-specific ranges exist for TSH to help guide treatment.
- Women with serum lithium levels at the time of delivery under 0.64 mEq/l have more reactive newborns and lower rates of neonatal complications.

1 Intrauterine Exposure and Risk for Ebstein's Anomaly and Other Major Congenital Malformations, and Impact on Development

Women of reproductive age with serious mental disorders are faced with a number of difficult decisions when attempting to strike a balance between their psychiatric stability during pregnancy and breastfeeding and the possible impact of medications on fetal and infant health. Pregnancy itself offers no protective effects on mood stability. In a pooled retrospective analysis of mood recurrence across 2252 pregnancies in 1162 women with BD-1 (479 pregnancies / 283 women), BD-2 (641 pregnancies / 338 women) or recurrent unipolar MDD (1132 pregnancies / 541 women), 23% of those with BD had at least one mood episode during pregnancy, and 52% during the postpartum period (Figure 7.10) [100]. A smaller prospective observational study of 89 pregnant women with BD found that the overall risk of at least one mood episode during pregnancy was 71% [101]. Most mood episodes were depressive or mixed (74%), and 47% occurred during the 1st trimester. Importantly, among those who discontinued their mood stabilizer, the recurrence risk was 2-fold higher, the median time to the 1st mood episode was 4 times shorter, and the time spent ill during the pregnancy was 5-fold greater [101]. The median recurrence latency was also 11 times shorter after abrupt discontinuation of the mood stabilizer compared with a more gradual taper. A subsequent case series of 12 patients confirmed the high risk to BD-1 patients: among the 5 individuals discontinued from lithium, only 1 patient developed mania during the pregnancy, but 4 of 5 became symptomatic in the postpartum period while still off of lithium [102]. In the 7 patients who continued lithium, none were symptomatic during pregnancy, and only 2/7 developed mood symptoms in the postpartum period.

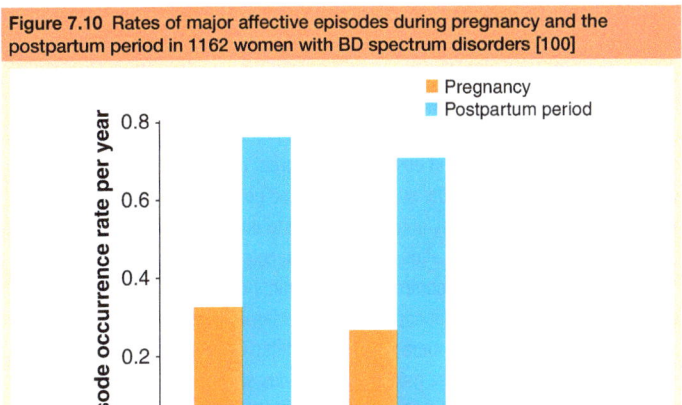

Figure 7.10 Rates of major affective episodes during pregnancy and the postpartum period in 1162 women with BD spectrum disorders [100]

(Adapted from: A. C. Viguera, L. Tondo, A. E. Koukopoulos, et al. [2011]. Episodes of mood disorders in 2,252 pregnancies and postpartum periods. *Am J Psychiatry*, 168, 1179–1185.)

As many BD spectrum women will require lithium treatment for optimum stability, one concern relates to the association of 1st trimester lithium exposure and increased rates of certain major congenital malformations (MCMs), particularly cardiovascular malformations (CVMs) such as Ebstein's anomaly [49]. The early literature relied on spontaneous, nonsystematic reports to various registries and national health-care databases, often generating enormously inflated risk estimates (e.g. 400-fold increased risk) that caused genuine alarm among patients and prescribers alike [103]. While the mechanism by which lithium might induce any MCM from 1st trimester exposure remains unclear, advances in statistical methods have enabled investigators to arrive at empirically sounder conclusions regarding risks for any MCM, and specifically CVM, along with information regarding other pregnancy outcomes (e.g. spontaneous abortion, preterm birth, low birth weight) [49]. The extent of this literature is so vast that a comprehensive 2020 review on lithium exposure during pregnancy and the postpartum period was able to calculate specific estimates, and also to provide guidance on management of lithium levels late in pregnancy to allow for more reactive newborns at the time of delivery [49].

An important aspect of these analyses is that many studies were able to incorporate methods to compare outcomes among lithium exposed women with those among women from diagnostically similar populations [49]. The population of patients receiving lithium has a number of differences from the general population, including health behaviors, access to prenatal care, prevalence of cardiometabolic disorders, and possibly any inherent genetic effects related to the psychiatric disorder itself. Older studies often used general population samples as the comparator group, thereby making it difficult to decide whether the pregnancy outcome related to the medication itself, or to aspects of the patients who received lithium [44]. One method for controlling such confounding bias is to compare outcomes among patients with comparable psychiatric disorders and related risks. For example, the 2020 meta-analysis indicated that 1st trimester lithium exposure appeared to increase risk for spontaneous abortions when compared with any lithium nonuser (OR 3.77, 95% CI 1.15–12.39; NNH 15); however, when the comparison was confined to lithium unexposed patients with affective disorders, the difference was no longer significant [49].

In-Depth 7.6 Ebstein's Anomaly: What It Is and the Association with Psychiatric Disorders Independent of Lithium Use

Ebstein's anomaly occurs when the tricuspid valve between the right atrium and ventricle does not delaminate completely from the underlying myocardium during development. The degree of incomplete delamination is variable and the phenotypes and clinical significance range from a critically ill newborn to an incidental chest X-ray finding of cardiomegaly in an asymptomatic adult [104]. The valve tissue and anatomy are unique to each patient, but they have some underlying commonalities, including displacement of the septal leaflet toward the apex, a billowing anterior leaflet, and areas of tethering restricting leaflet motion. The result is tricuspid regurgitation with differing degrees of right ventricular enlargement and dysfunction [104].

One can appreciate the impact of the psychiatric diagnosis itself when looking at a large European study on Ebstein's anomaly and the association with mental illness, medications or various health conditions [105]. The European registry study was performed using data on 5,644,312 births from 1982–2011 to examine trends in the Ebstein's diagnosis related to improved imaging and detection, and the odds ratios for exposure to maternal illnesses and medications in the 1st trimester. These odds ratios were calculated by comparing Ebstein's cases with cardiac and noncardiac malformed controls, excluding cases with genetic syndromes and adjusting for time period and country [105]. The total prevalence of Ebstein's cases per 10,000 births rose over the 30 years of the analysis from 0.29 (95% CI 0.20–0.41) to 0.48 (95% CI 0.40–0.57) (p < 0.01). Excluding those with genetic syndromes, there were only 250 Ebstein cases, none of which was exposed to lithium; however, mental health conditions associated with use of a variety of psychotropic medications were associated with increased risk for Ebstein's anomaly, but this was not true for those with psychiatric diagnoses who were receiving no medications [105]. As lithium is the only psychotropic known to increase risk for Ebstein's anomaly, the only explanation is that use of other psychotropics is likely a proxy for psychiatric disease severity, and that health behaviors or inherent aspects of the illness itself must be responsible for the risk difference. Studies such as this highlight the need to incorporate women with similar psychiatric and other health risk profiles to best determine medication related effects.

The 2020 meta-analysis of lithium exposure during pregnancy examined 29 papers, of which 20 were good quality, and from these, 13 presented sufficient data for quantitative analysis [49]. The largest of these studies was a 2017 retrospective study that employed US Medicaid data from 2000–2010 that specifically included only those women enrolled from 3 months before their last menstrual period through ≥ 1 month after delivery [44]. From this massive data set, there were 1,325,563 pregnancies, of whom 663 filled at least one prescription for lithium during the 1st trimester. A critical aspect of this analysis was the use of propensity score matching to manage the large number of covariates possibly related to assignment bias (i.e. whether a woman might or might not be given a 1st trimester prescription for lithium). As discussed in Info Box 7.5, propensity score matching is a method to balance the likelihood that the lithium exposed and unexposed groups could have been prescribed lithium, and the propensity score is calculated from a model generated from this specific data set that quantifies a patient's characteristics which influence their likelihood of being prescribed lithium. Comparison groups included those with 1st trimester lamotrigine (LTG) exposure (n = 1945), and those with neither lithium nor lamotrigine use. After propensity score matching, covariates of interest related to the primary outcome (rate of CVM) were then balanced between the groups. Secondary outcomes included the rate of any major MCM, noncardiac congenital malformations (presence of a major malformation in the absence of a cardiac defect), and right ventricular outflow tract obstruction defects (to capture instances where the Ebstein's diagnostic code was not used) [44]. Sensitivity analyses were performed that defined drug exposure as filling ≥ two prescriptions during the 1st trimester, that examined the potential effect of pregnancy termination rates among women treated with lithium, and that examined outcomes only in women who had at least one recorded baseline BD diagnosis.

Info Box 7.5 What Is Propensity Score Matching? [40, 44–46]

a. **The randomized clinical trial (RCT):** A prospective RCT is considered the most rigorous study design to examine the impact of a specific treatment. Because treatments are assigned randomly, this eliminates biases that occur in real world treatment decisions. The random nature of treatment assignment also tends to even out other covariates (e.g. demographic factors, medical and specific illness history, illness severity, etc.) that may influence the outcome. Performing an RCT for certain conditions is not always feasible for a variety of reasons. In the case of evaluating the effects of 1st trimester medication exposure on risk of major congenital malformations (MCMs), such trials would not be deemed ethical.

b. **Real world treatment assignment:** There are numerous reasons why a clinician may choose a particular medication for a patient. When retrospectively examining a large data set exploring new medication prescriptions, one can construct a statistical model based on the pattern of usage in that population that describes the likelihood a particular patient might have been prescribed a medication. For example, one retrospective study used a US Medicaid sample comprising 1,341,715 pregnancies, of whom 9991 received 1st trimester antipsychotic exposure [40]. More than 200 covariates were involved in the model which predicted the likelihood of being prescribed an antipsychotic in the 1st trimester of pregnancy, including geography, the year, psychiatric and nonpsychiatric diagnoses, and prior pregnancy history. From this logistic regression model, one can then take the characteristics of any subject in the entire set of 1,341,715 pregnancies and calculate what their *propensity* would have been to receive the antipsychotic, on a scale of 0 to 1.0. Essentially, this propensity score represents the probability that an individual would be assigned to a treatment based on their demographics and comorbidities present at that time [45].

c. **Propensity score matching:** The idea is that two individuals may have identical propensity scores for receiving a treatment (e.g. 1st trimester antipsychotic exposure), yet one was given the medication and one was not. For example, two women with a bipolar I (BD-1) diagnosis, married, college educated, with similar medical, obstetric and psychiatric histories (and other covariates) might both have a propensity score of 0.45 to be given a prescription for an antipsychotic in the 1st trimester, based on the model generated from the data set of 1,341,715 pregnancies. Despite identical propensity scores, only one of them actually received such a prescription. The fact that both had the same **likelihood or propensity** to get the treatment of interest is the core principle of propensity score matching. In an RCT with 3 treatment arms, each participant has the same propensity of being assigned to any treatment arm: 1/3. By definition, the likelihood is balanced since everyone has the same odds or propensity to be given a certain treatment. With propensity score matching, one can find someone from the group who did receive the treatment of interest (e.g. 1st trimester antipsychotic exposure), and find their propensity score matched peer from the group which did not get the treatment. By propensity score matching everyone from the exposed group to someone in the unexposed group, one can say that mathematically they had the same likelihood of getting the treatment. In general, for patients with the same propensity score, the distribution of measured baseline covariates between the two groups should be very similar.

d. **Covariate balancing:** Propensity score matching means that the two groups had the same likelihood of receiving the treatment. This has nothing to do with the study outcome (e.g. differences in MCM risk from 1st trimester lithium exposure) – it is simply a method for removing the biases from naturalistic treatment assignment in the real world. In most instances, covariates that might influence the outcome (e.g. smoking behavior, substance use) may also be evened out, but the data set is further examined for significant covariate imbalances, and procedures used to even out disparities that might influence the outcome.

The crude unadjusted prevalence of CVM was 2.41 per 100 live births among infants exposed to lithium, 1.15 per 100 among unexposed infants, and 1.39 per 100 among infants exposed to lamotrigine [44]. After adjusting for covariates, the adjusted relative risk (RR) for CVM among infants exposed to lithium was significantly higher than among nonexposed infants (RR 1.65, 95% CI 1.02–2.68), while the adjusted RR for noncardiac defects among infants exposed to lithium compared with nonexposed infants was 1.22 (95% CI 0.81–1.84), a result that was not statistically significant. (Of note, LTG was not significantly different than the unexposed infants for CVM or MCM.) There was a relationship with maternal dose, and those in lithium dosing groups < 600 mg/d or 601–900 mg/d did not have CVM rates that were significantly different from those of their peers. This was not true for those exposed to daily doses > 900 mg (Figure 7.11).

After accounting for potential differences in the probability of pregnancy terminations (spontaneous abortions) in the lithium treated group, the range of plausible adjusted RR for CVM among lithium-exposed infants across all doses was estimated to be 1.67–1.80. To use these data and the dose specific estimates to calculate the number needed to harm (NNH), one must note that the risk for CVM was 1.15 per 100 among unexposed infants. Thus, if the RR across all lithium doses is 1.80, the NNH is 108. If one uses the RR of 3.22 for the high dose group,

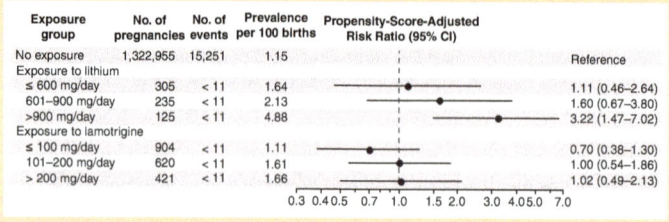

Figure 7.11 Absolute and relative risk of cardiac malformations among lithium-exposed and lamotrigine-exposed infants (vs. unexposed infants) stratified by maternal lithium dose [44]

Exposure group	No. of pregnancies	No. of events	Prevalence per 100 births	Propensity-Score-Adjusted Risk Ratio (95% CI)
No exposure	1,322,955	15,251	1.15	Reference
Exposure to lithium				
≤ 600 mg/day	305	< 11	1.64	1.11 (0.46–2.64)
601–900 mg/day	235	< 11	2.13	1.60 (0.67–3.80)
>900 mg/day	125	< 11	4.88	3.22 (1.47–7.02)
Exposure to lamotrigine				
≤ 100 mg/day	904	< 11	1.11	0.70 (0.38–1.30)
101–200 mg/day	620	< 11	1.61	1.00 (0.54–1.86)
> 200 mg/day	421	< 11	1.66	1.02 (0.49–2.13)

(Adapted from: E. Patorno, K. F. Huybrechts, B. T. Bateman, et al. [2017]. Lithium use in pregnancy and the risk of cardiac malformations. *NEJM*, 376, 2245–2254.)

the NNH is 39. The NNH across all doses is very close to the value of 83 from the 2020 meta-analysis when comparing CVM rates between lithium users and non-users with bipolar disorder [49]. The implication is that, for women who take lithium during the 1st trimester, one would need to expose 83 individuals to see 1 additional CVM case compared with their lithium non-using peers with psychiatric disorders. For women who need daily doses above 900 mg, the NNH of 39 from the US Medicaid data also provides the best evidence for the extent of risk [44].

Although surveillance studies indicate that use of lithium in pregnant women has declined significantly over the past 15 years [106], these revised estimates of MCM risk should support the decisions of women whose psychiatric health depends on lithium (primarily BD-1 and SAD-BT patients) to continue with treatment during pregnancy *at the doses and serum levels that best support psychiatric stability*, albeit with appropriate oversight from their psychiatric provider and obstetrician. When a patient requires > 900 mg/d and her history indicates marked instability at lower daily lithium doses (especially manic relapse with psychosis), it does not seem prudent to risk psychiatric relapse in the interests of lessening 1st trimester exposure and CVM risk by decreasing the lithium dose for 3 months. Even for daily lithium doses > 900 mg, the NNH for CVM is 39 [44], suggesting that the risk–benefit equation for these patients favors continuing lithium in the manner that allows them to remain stable. Conclusions from the 2020 review of lithium exposure during pregnancy provide the most evidence based statement which sums up this literature: "The risk associated with lithium exposure at any time during pregnancy is low, and the risk is higher for first-trimester or higher-dosage exposure" [49].

Info Box 7.6 Considerations in Managing Lithium during Pregnancy

a. Contraception: A 2021 review commented that management of contraception, pregnancy and the psychiatric illness together serve to improve a woman's capacity to function and optimize her mental and reproductive health [107]. Clinical studies and placebo-controlled trials in women with psychiatric disorders generally note comparable or lower rates of depressive mood symptoms in hormonal contraceptive users compared with nonusers. All methods (oral, implants, intrauterine devices) are acceptable, although medical comorbidities may dictate a specific type [107].

b. Education: Patients should receive the latest data on lithium related pregnancy outcomes to decide on the best course of action based on their preferences, history of stability without lithium or when exposed to lower serum lithium levels and doses, and their response to alternative medications.

   i. Spontaneous abortions, preterm birth, low birth weight: Lithium use during the 1st trimester is not associated with increased risk for spontaneous abortions [49]. Lithium use throughout the pregnancy is not associated with increased risk for preterm birth or low birth weight [49]. A Dutch analysis published in 2021 saw an association with increased fetal growth, although the significance is unclear [108].

   ii. Any major congenital malformation (MCM): 1st trimester lithium exposure is associated with an increased risk of MCM compared with any unexposed group (OR 2.03, 95% CI 1.03–3.99; NNH 22), and with a similar risk but numerically lower when the comparison group had an affective disorder (OR 1.75, 95% CI 1.21–2.98; NNH 37) [49].

   iii. Cardiovascular malformation (CVM): 1st trimester lithium exposure is associated with an increased risk of CVM compared with any unexposed group (OR 3.99, 95% CI 1.19–13.43; NNH 37), but the risk was substantially lower when the comparison group had an affective disorder (OR 1.75, 95% CI 1.08–2.84; NNH 83).[49] One study examined dose related effects on CVM risk (Figure 7.11) [44]. After accounting for potential differences in the probability of pregnancy termination, the range of risk ratios (RRs) for CVM among lithium exposed infants across all doses was 1.67–1.80, but only one lithium dosing group differed significantly from unexposed women: those who received > 900 mg/d (RR 3.22; 95% CI 1.47–7.02). The risk for CVM was 1.15 per 100 among unexposed infants, so across all doses (using a RR of 1.80) the NNH was 108. For the high dose exposure group (using the RR of 3.22), the NNH was 39.

c. Monitoring of renal function and lithium levels: Lithium levels decrease on average 24% in the 1st trimester, and reach their lowest point in the 2nd trimester, 36% below the pre-pregnancy baseline [109]. Levels increase modestly in the 3rd trimester, but remain 21% below baseline [109]. For this reason, eGFR and lithium levels should be checked at the end of the 1st trimester (week 12), toward the end of the 2nd trimester (week 24), and once again in the weeks prior to the estimated date of delivery. Lithium levels should always be rechecked 1 week after any dosage change.

d. **Monitoring of thyroid function:** Use trimester-specific reference ranges for TSH [110]. The need to treat subclinical hypothyroidism depends on the TSH and the presence of markers consistent with Hashimoto's thyroiditis [110]. For hypothyroid patients who become pregnant, there is high-quality evidence to recommend an increase in the levothyroxine dose by 20% to 30% when a positive pregnancy test is obtained, and then to contact the treating clinician for follow-up based on trimester-specific TSH ranges.

e. **Time of delivery:** A 2020 review noted that women with serum lithium levels at the time of delivery < 0.64 mEq/l had more reactive newborns and lower rates of neonatal complications [49]. In those whose maintenance levels are ≥ 0.64 mEq/l, consider lowering the lithium dose 1 week before delivery to mitigate some of these issues. The prior lithium dose should be resumed immediately after delivery and continued in the postpartum period. Lithium use was significantly more effective than no lithium use in preventing postpartum relapse (OR 0.16, 95% CI 0.03–0.89; NNH 3) in the two studies which examined this outcome. (See Info Box 7.7 on breastfeeding.)

f. **Balancing risk and lithium exposure:** Maintaining psychiatric stability is the best means to achieve optimal outcomes for the mother and infant. The use of lithium doses/levels in the 1st trimester that are *subtherapeutic for that patient* risks psychiatric relapse. The NNH for CVM on doses > 900 mg/d is 39 [44], arguing that the CVM risk is not inordinately high on that dose, especially when a mother's prior history suggests that lower lithium exposure is associated with rapid relapse.

g. **Collaboration:** Lithium prescribers should develop a relationship with an obstetrician familiar with the needs of patients who require lithium to avoid reflexive demands to discontinue lithium, to arrange for a fetal ultrasound to assess for CVM during the 2nd trimester, and to plan any dose reductions prior to delivery.

As noted in Info Box 7.6, lithium use is not associated with increased risk of preterm delivery or low birth weight, and the short-term effects at time of delivery seem to be lessened when the maternal lithium level is < 0.64 mEq/l [49]. The issue of long-term neurodevelopmental effects from *in utero* psychotropic exposure of any kind are hard to tease out as most studies compare children to peers whose parents did not have a psychiatric diagnosis. The latter is a crucial variable, as periods of maternal illness and the genetic substrate of the psychiatric disorder itself are difficult to quantify but can substantially influence a child's developmental trajectory. There have been extensive studies of longer-term child outcomes from 1st trimester antidepressant exposure; however, despite the enormous sample sizes and multiple publications, a 2022 letter lamented that studying the consequences of *in utero* antidepressant exposure is challenging, particularly because "it is difficult to disentangle the effects of antidepressant use in pregnancy vs. maternal depression and anxiety" [111–113]. With that in mind, only three clinical cohort studies have investigated the consequences of fetal lithium exposure, all of which reported normal development [114]. This is in contrast to clinical studies regarding antipsychotic exposure in which a transient delay in neurodevelopment has been observed in some papers, with a relative risk for neuromotor deficits after *in utero* antipsychotic exposure estimated at 1.63 (95% CI 1.22–2.19) [114].

2 *Changes in Lithium Kinetics during Pregnancy*

Certain types of pregnancy related risks are easily managed, such as adjusting lithium doses to compensate for changes in maternal renal function during pregnancy [109, 115]. Fluid shifts during pregnancy induce a state of hyperfiltration (i.e. increased eGFR), clinically seen as a decrease in serum creatinine values that reach a nadir around week 18, and start to increase in the 3rd trimester (Figure 7.12) [115]. Lithium levels parallel these creatinine trends and this may necessitate dosage adjustment, especially if mood symptoms arise, or if there is a history of instability when levels fall below a certain range. A Dutch group examined 1101 lithium levels in 113 patients throughout the course of their pregnancy and found that levels decreased on average 24% in the 1st trimester, and reached their lowest point in the 2nd trimester, 36% below the pre-pregnancy baseline [109]. Levels increased modestly in the 3rd trimester but remained 21% below baseline, with a slight 9% increase in the postpartum period. A Norwegian study noted a similar effect after examining 25 serum lithium levels from 14 pregnancies in 13 women, and compared these with 63 baseline levels from the same women [116]. Dose-adjusted serum concentrations in the 3rd trimester were significantly lower than baseline (–34%; 95% CI –44% to –23%, p < 0.001) [116]. This state of hyperfiltration is a unique feature of pregnancy, but is easily managed by monitoring eGFR and lithium levels at key intervals during the pregnancy: at the end of the 1st trimester, around week 12; toward the end of the 2nd trimester, at week 24; and in the weeks prior to the estimated date of delivery (Info Box 7.6). Failure to track levels may result in unnecessary mood relapses, relapses that may have been prevented if lithium doses were adjusted in the 2nd trimester to mirror pre-pregnancy levels.

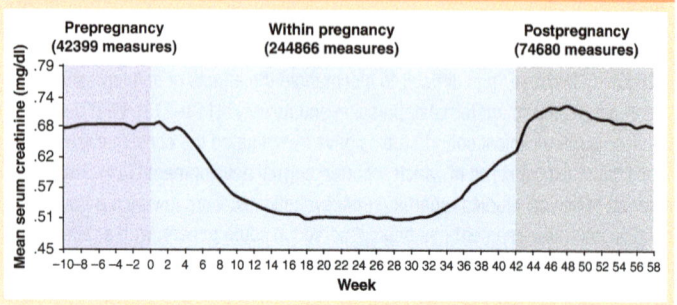

Figure 7.12 Changes in serum creatinine throughout the course of pregnancy [115]

(Adapted from: Z. Harel, E. McArthur, M. Hladunewich, et al. [2019]. Serum creatinine levels before, during, and after pregnancy. *JAMA*, 321, 205–207.)

3   *Managing Lithium at Time of Delivery*

Another reason to monitor lithium levels closely at the end of pregnancy relates to data suggesting that newborns whose maternal lithium level around the time of delivery was under 0.64 mEq/l were more reactive and had fewer neonatal complications [49]. Newborns have relatively immature renal function, and the $T_{1/2}$ of lithium in newborns is estimated at 96 h [43]. Avoiding lithium levels in the upper end of the therapeutic range thus permits the infant sufficient time to gradually clear maternal gestational lithium, especially as the initial exposure from breastfeeding will be relatively modest [43]. Assuming the maternal maintenance lithium level is below 0.64 mEq/l in the latter half of the 3rd trimester, no special action need be taken. For women whose 3rd trimester lithium level is in the range of 0.70–1.00 mEq/l, consider a modest dose reduction 7 days prior to the expected delivery date to achieve a new steady state in the mother and in the infant just prior to birth. When the baseline level is 0.80 mEq/l, this amounts to a 20% dose reduction, while for levels close to 1.00 mEq/l, this corresponds to a 33% dose reduction. Lithium is available in liquid forms (lithium carbonate) and smaller increments than 300 mg (e.g. 150 mg tablets or capsules) to assist with these temporary dosage adjustments. The primary population continuing lithium through pregnancy will be those with BD-1 or SAD-BT, and this patient group is at high risk for postpartum psychiatric complications if a subtherapeutic dose is continued after delivery. The prior baseline stable dose (and level) established during the 3rd trimester should be resumed as soon as possible after delivery. Although only two studies have examined this, lithium was significantly more effective than no lithium use in preventing postpartum relapse (OR 0.16, 95% CI 0.03–0.89; NNH 3) [49]. (Continuation of lithium in the postpartum period while breastfeeding is discussed in Section D.)

4   *Thyroid Issues During Pregnancy*

Renal function is not the only physiological parameter relevant to lithium treatment that changes throughout pregnancy. There are pregnancy related changes in thyroid function to the extent that treatment guidelines from the American Thyroid Association (ATA) on the diagnosis and management of thyroid disease during pregnancy and the postpartum period strongly recommend use of population based trimester-specific reference ranges for TSH to manage pregnant women with a history of thyroid disease [110]. For women who are euthyroid prior to the pregnancy, no additional TSH monitoring is necessary beyond a routine level obtained every 6 months as part of usual lithium related care. However, the ATA guidelines cite high-quality evidence to recommend an increase in the levothyroxine dose by 20% to 30% at the time a positive pregnancy test is obtained in women already receiving thyroid supplementation, with subsequent follow-up by their treating clinician [110]. All women with subclinical hypothyroidism are strongly recommended to begin levothyroxine treatment if the TSH is > 10 mIU/l, although the strength of the evidence is low. There was a weak recommendation to start levothyroxine when the TSH falls between the upper limit of the pregnancy-specific range and 10 mIU/l. Patients with thyroid peroxidase antibodies diagnostic of Hashimoto's thyroiditis should be started on levothyroxine if the TSH is above the pregnancy-specific range, with a weak consideration to starting levothyroxine when TSH is > 2.5 mIU/l, but below the upper limit of the pregnancy-specific range [110].

D   Breastfeeding and the Postpartum Period

WHAT TO KNOW: LITHIUM USE DURING BREASTFEEDING AND THE POSTPARTUM PERIOD

- BD-1 patients are at risk for postpartum psychosis if not adequately mood stabilized. Resumption of pre-pregnancy maintenance doses and levels should be encouraged immediately following delivery to mitigate mood relapse.
- Longitudinal data published in 2022 from 30 breastfeeding dyads found that infant lithium levels were undetectable after the 1st month of age,

but 25% may exhibit inadequate growth in the 1st month. There is no reason to discourage breastfeeding in women on lithium, but the combined use of formula and breastfeeding may help moderate lithium exposure and promote infant growth during the 1st month.

- Develop a relationship with a pediatrician conversant in the latest literature in this area, who is supportive of mothers who wish to continue breastfeeding while on lithium, and who can work cooperatively to implement a rational infant monitoring scheme based on the literature.

- Assistance with nighttime feeding can be an important part of the treatment plan to allow for more uninterrupted sleep.

The decision to continue lithium in breastfeeding mother–infant dyads is as nuanced as those regarding 1st trimester lithium exposure, and reflects the same need to balance patient preferences, potential risks to the infant, and the psychological and health benefits of breastfeeding [42, 43]. An ideal method for examining this issue would involve longitudinal assessment of infant lithium levels, maternal serum levels and their correlation with a range of infant outcomes including growth, TSH and serum creatinine [43]. Due to the paucity of data before 2007 on maternal and infant lithium levels in breastfeeding dyads, the early literature relied on inferences from case reports that were often difficult to interpret for several reasons: (1) some of the clinical observations were obtained shortly after birth and may have reflected peripartum lithium exposure and its short-term impact on infant behavior; (2) cases were reported where maternal lithium levels ranged from 1.00 to 1.50 mEq/l, a maintenance range considered unacceptably high today; and (3) there may have been an impact of concurrent medications [41]. Most cases documented no ill effects of lithium exposure on the infant, but there was one case of lithium toxicity in an infant who became dehydrated, and another of transient lithium toxicity in an infant whose maternal level was 1.50 mEq/l [41].

More cases emerged from 2007 to 2015 that generally indicated no untoward effects of breastfeeding when the mother continued lithium treatment, but with several instances of weight loss, poor feeding or elevated TSH. In one instance, a transiently elevated TSH of 5.14 mIU/l at 1 month postpartum normalized in an infant without the need to stop breastfeeding (6 month value 2.17 mIU/l), while in another case a TSH 7.1 mIU/l resolved after lithium discontinuation [41]. From these case data, multiple sources attempted to arrive at reasonable conclusions, but with widely conflicting opinions [117]. Dr. Thomas W. Hale Ph.D., RPh (Professor of Pediatrics, Associate Dean of Research, Texas Tech University Health Sciences Center) created

Hale's Lactation Risk Category system that places medications on a scale from L1 to L5, with L1 medications considered compatible based on widespread use and presence of controlled trials showing no adverse infant effects, while L5 medications are considered hazardous, with known or potentially serious risk to the breastfeeding infant [117]. In the middle of the last decade, lithium was categorized as L4, indicating that use during lactation is possibly hazardous based on evidence for adverse effects on the infant, but that the benefits from use in the breastfeeding dyad outweigh these concerns when safer drugs cannot be used [117].

In-Depth 7.7 Relative Infant Dose Method to Estimate Medication Exposure During Breastfeeding

The gold standard for assessing infant exposure is direct measurement of infant serum levels and the impact on infant health; however, when these data are not widely available, estimates of infant exposure are created using relative infant dose (RID) calculations that standardize the expected exposure from breast milk by the infant weight. The infant dose in mg/kg/d is calculated by multiplying the drug concentration in breast milk by the daily volume of milk consumed daily (about 150 ml/kg for the average infant) [117]. Mathematically, the RID is simply the ratio of the expected daily ingested infant dose (D_I) divided by the maternal daily ingested dose (D_M): **RID = D_I (mg/kg/d) / D_M (mg/kg/d).** An RID value < 10% is generally considered acceptable in a healthy infant, while RID values > 25% may have an effect on the infant, **if absorbed**, that can potentially be unacceptable. Approximately 90% of medications have an RID < 10%, while only 3% have an RID > 25%. For lithium, RID values are in the range of 12%–30%, a gray area that provides little guidance on expected infant outcomes or serum levels [117].

In-Depth 7.8 Lithium and Breastfeeding: The Literature from 2016–2019

In 2016, a review of mood stabilizer use during breastfeeding found only 26 lithium breastfeeding dyads, but concluded that the incidence of adverse events in infants exposed to mood stabilizers is reported to be very low, and that mood stabilizers can be prescribed without any adverse events in lactating women, albeit with some form of monitoring [118]. The American Academy of Pediatrics and United States National Institutes of Health Drugs and Lactation Database (www.ncbi.nlm.nih.gov/books/NBK501153) arrived at similar conclusions, with the latter providing an extensive review of the literature and suggested methods for monitoring the breastfeeding infant [42]. However, the British Association for Psychopharmacology concluded in their exhaustive 2017 review on the use of psychotropic medications during preconception, pregnancy and the postpartum period that lithium, valproate and carbamazepine should not be prescribed to women with affective disorders who breastfeed [119]. Recommendations posted by the UK Royal College of Psychiatrists in 2018 (www.rcpsych.ac.uk/mental-health/treatments-and-wellbeing/lithium-in-pregnancy-and-breastfeeding) also state that the UK National Institute for Health and Care Excellence, and the British Association of Psychopharmacology, recommend not to breastfeed whilst taking lithium. The accompanying text presents a somewhat mixed message by noting that cases have been reported of women successfully breastfeeding when taking lithium, but also stating that the infant will have to have regular blood tests to monitor the lithium level, thyroid and kidney function, and advising mothers "to check whether your local services can provide the monitoring your baby will need." As no specialized clinical or laboratory monitoring is required, it is unclear what local services might be needed other than a pediatrician to check on the child's overall health periodically, a capable phlebotomist to draw the infant's blood and a standard hospital laboratory to analyze the results.

The literature evolved in 2019 due to the publication of two reviews that described outcomes in 39 dyads. These papers provided a level of clinical detail not seen in prior reviews, and also provided a historical perspective on earlier cases and their limitations [41, 42]. An important point of emphasis is that the vast majority of documented cases showed no ill effects on the infant, especially when maternal lithium levels were < 1.00 mEq/l; that issues during the first postpartum week may relate to effects from peripartum maternal lithium use and exposure to other medications; that infant levels rarely exceed 0.30 mEq/l; and that there is no impact on infant renal or thyroid function in the vast majority of cases [41, 42]. Even with inclusion of peripartum events that might reflect factors other than breastfeeding (e.g. gestational exposure), only 9.4% of cases reported any infant adverse effects, primarily from the literature prior to 2007, and only 9.4% reported any laboratory abnormality (elevated TSH, creatinine or blood urea nitrogen) [42]. The 2019 reviews were reassuring since case reports tend to be heavily skewed toward describing adverse outcomes, yet the absence of longitudinal data was noted as a problem for the field. The ability to recommend any rational monitoring scheme during extended breastfeeding depends heavily on an estimate of infant lithium levels over time, the presence of outliers, and circumscribing the period of greatest infant risk.

Info Box 7.7 Breastfeeding Considerations for Lithium Treated Women [41–43]

a. Educate

    i. Prior to delivery: Consider lowering lithium exposure prior to delivery if the maintenance level is ≥ 0.64 mEq/l [49]. The $T_{1/2}$ of lithium in newborns is 96 h [43], so lessening the carryover from peripartum exposure will be helpful to assure a more reactive newborn, and to minimize the risk of behavioral sequelae from gestational lithium exposure that might interfere with breastfeeding during the first week.

ii. **Safety data:** The 2019 comprehensive review of 39 breastfeeding dyads, combined with 2022 longitudinal data from a case series of 30 breastfeeding dyads, indicate the absence of significant effects from lithium exposure in most infants, although 25% may exhibit inadequate growth in the 1st month [41, 43]. Outliers with respect to lithium levels are rare, but infant lithium levels, TSH and eGFR must be monitored periodically.

iii. **Maternal education:** The mother should be referred to a breastfeeding support group or to an early intervention service if needed. Psychoeducation should be provided for parents or caregivers to monitor infants for signs and symptoms of feeding problems, dehydration, hypotonia or lethargy, or for instances of suspected dehydration, diarrhea or vomiting [41, 43].

b. **Collaborate**

i. **Women continuing lithium from pregnancy into the postpartum period:** The vast majority of mothers who will be breastfeeding were also taking lithium throughout the pregnancy, so there should be an established relationship with an obstetrician and neonatologist. These should be providers who are conversant in the latest literature and recommendations in this area, are supportive of mothers who wish to breastfeed while on lithium, and who can work cooperatively to ensure the health of the mother and baby.

ii. **Women newly initiating lithium while breastfeeding:** Develop a relationship with a pediatrician conversant in the latest literature in this area, who is supportive of mothers who wish to continue breastfeeding while on lithium, and who can work cooperatively to implement a rational infant monitoring scheme based on the literature [41].

c. **Psychiatric considerations**

i. **Sleep:** Despite adequate mood stabilization, sleep deprivation may induce hypomania or mania in certain BD patients. Assistance with nighttime feeding can be an important part of the treatment plan to allow for more uninterrupted sleep.

ii. **Mood stability:** BD-1 patients are at risk for postpartum psychosis if not adequately mood stabilized. Resumption of pre-pregnancy maintenance doses and levels should be encouraged immediately following delivery to mitigate mood relapse [49]. Reinforce with the mother that use of the lithium dose and serum level that ensured stability is the best course of action for all involved, and that the risks from lithium exposure in the infant are now considered modest and manageable with monitoring. Lithium monotherapy may be insufficient to manage depressive symptoms, so options to manage BD depression should be discussed.

A number of questions that persisted in the literature were resolved in October 2022 when a Swedish group published a retrospective study of outcomes in lithium treated women and their breastfed infants born in Stockholm in 2006–2021, using data about infant serum lithium levels and clinical status in the medical records [43]. This study provided information on 30 infants exposed to lithium through breast milk, with a median age at follow-up of 40 days and a range of values extending to day 364. The majority of mothers (26/30) had a BD diagnosis, primarily BD-1, and 90% of the infants had *in utero* lithium exposure. Importantly, 67% of breastfeeding women were also treated with at least one additional psychotropic, including sedatives/anxiolytics (n = 10), antipsychotics (n = 7), antidepressants (n = 6) and psychostimulants (n = 4). From the laboratory data, it was possible to correlate 33 of the infant lithium levels to maternal serum levels. The mean infant–maternal serum level ratio was highest in the first 2 weeks after birth (ratio 0.37) and decreased over time. This trend was reflected in decreasing infant lithium levels after week 2. As noted in Table 7.2, the median infant lithium serum level was 0.10 mEq/l in the 2nd week of life (range < 0.05–0.7 mEq/l), 0.08 mEq/l in weeks 2–4 (range < 0.05–1.2 mEq/l), 0.06 mEq/l in the 2nd month (range < 0.05–0.2 mEq/l) and 0.07 mEq/l after 2 months of age (range < 0.05–0.2 mEq/l). Unexpectedly high lithium concentrations were found in only two infants, both in the 1st month of life. One infant, born at 35 weeks gestation, had a lithium level of 0.70 mEq/l on day 12 of follow-up, 17% higher than the maternal level. The infant was not tired or hypotonic, and the general health was rated as good, but the infant had not gained weight since birth. The infant received formula and was breastfed 75% of the time, so the recommendation was to reduce breastfeeding to 50% and increase use of formula. When checked 4 days later, the infant lithium level was below the limit of detection. The other high infant level was a value of 1.2 mEq/l recorded at 29 days of age, but with no corresponding maternal level obtained at the same time. The infant exhibited normal growth and feeding despite this level, and was thriving despite having experienced a serious postnatal complication at day 2 requiring neonatal ward admission. The infant was partly breastfed, and the mother was told to stop breastfeeding completely. No infant sequelae from the high level were noted in the medical record.

In this sample, the serum creatinine, TSH and electrolytes were normal across all time points, with the exception of one sodium and one potassium level 0.1 mmol/l out of range without clinical significance. While no infants were irritable or displayed hypotonia, 25% did not meet growth expectations during their 1st month; however, aside from the two cases of elevated infant levels noted above,

Table 7.2 Longitudinal data from 30 breastfeeding dyads documenting infant and maternal lithium exposure [43]

Infant age	Infant lithium data				Maternal lithium data			
	Mean level ± SD (mEq/l)	Median level (mEq/l)	Range (mEq/l)	Missing (n)	Mean level ± SD (mEq/l)	Median level (mEq/l)	Range (mEq/l)	Missing (n)
< 2 weeks	0.19 ± 0.20	0.10	< 0.05 – 0.70	0	0.61 ± 0.24	0.70	0.10 – 0.90	1
2 weeks – 1 month	0.16 ± 0.30	0.08	< 0.05 – 1.20	0	0.59 ± 0.14	0.60	0.20 – 0.70	8
1–2 months	0.07 ± 0.0	0.06	< 0.05 – 0.20	1	0.73 ± 0.15	0.70	0.50 – 1.00	15
> 2 months	0.08 ± 0.0	0.07	< 0.05 – 0.20	4	0.62 ± 0.12	0.60	0.50 – 0.90	10

(Adapted from: E. Heinonen, K. Totterman, K. Back, et al. [2022]. Lithium use during breastfeeding was safe in healthy full-term infants under strict monitoring. *Acta Paediatr*, 111, 1891–1898.)

only two other mothers were advised to reduce breastfeeding. The value of this paper is inestimable as it not only increased the data on breastfeeding dyads by 77%, it also provided conclusions not previously available on longitudinal changes in infant lithium levels and clinical outcomes during breastfeeding. The important finding is that serum lithium levels in breastfed infants stabilized at barely measurable levels after the 2nd week of life, and that lithium treatment during breastfeeding can be considered safe with strict follow-up to identify outliers [43]. Even among authors who endorse a low level of risk imposed by maternal lithium use during breastfeeding, there is a decided lack of consensus on necessary monitoring. The proposed scheme in Table 7.3 is but one attempt to assimilate the recent findings from the Swedish study with data from other sources to arrive at a scheme which maximizes early oversight while minimizing unnecessary infant blood draws. The more frequent monitoring during the first weeks is to track the expected carryover from gestational lithium exposure due to the extended $T_{1/2}$ of lithium in the newborn (96 h), the relative immaturity of renal function among newborns, and their greater sensitivity to dehydration [43]. In the end, mothers, pediatricians and psychiatric providers should tailor monitoring schedules to the concerns and needs of each situation, with the goal of providing reassurance and ensuring maternal psychiatric stability and infant safety.

Table 7.3 A proposed monitoring scheme for breastfeeding women who remain on lithium

Infant	Birth	Day 7	4 weeks	8 weeks	3 months	6 months[a]
Lithium level[b]	X	X	X	X[c]	X	X
TSH[d]	X		X	X[c]	X	X
Serum eGFR (creatinine and cystatin C)	X		X	X[c]	X	X
Mother						
Lithium level	X	X[e]			X	X
TSH					X	X
Serum eGFR (creatinine and cystatin C)	X	X[e]			X	X

Comments: Infants are very susceptible to dehydration, and this may precipitate renal dysfunction and lithium toxicity. Any change in clinical status (e.g. irritability, restlessness, poor feeding, hypotonia, lethargy, diarrhea or vomiting) demands clinical evaluation that includes a lithium level, TSH, renal function and electrolytes. Abnormal growth in the first month of life, especially if infant levels are above 0.30 mEq/l, may respond to minimizing other psychotropics, to decreasing the amount of breastfeeding and increasing the use of formula [43]. Cessation of breastfeeding is not typically necessary.

Notes

a. Depending on infant health, consideration can be given to an every 6 month schedule to parallel the adult laboratory requirements, but many pediatricians and mothers may be more comfortable with an every 3 month schedule.

b. The lithium level in the infant at the time of delivery is reflective of peripartum exposure. Clinical decisions about minimizing breastfeeding during the initial 7 days after birth should be driven by the infant's health (e.g. reactivity, hypotonia) and not the lithium level. There is no indication for routine electrolyte monitoring in the infant unless an abnormality is detected at birth.

c. The 8-week monitoring time point can be considered optional for infants with normal growth and good health, as the expected infant lithium level drops after the first 2 weeks of life, and especially after week 4.

d. Elevations in TSH may be transient and may not indicate a clinically significant problem [43].

e. The need for postpartum maternal monitoring is to document the eGFR and lithium level after any fluid shifts following delivery. It is also needed to check the lithium level after resumption of the patient's maintenance lithium dose, since the dose may have been reduced in the week prior to delivery. If the lithium dose must be increased at any time, the lithium level should be rechecked approximately 1 week later. As infant exposure decreases after week 4, one may consider waiting until the next routine time point (e.g. 8 weeks, 3 months, 6 months) to check infant levels if no adverse effects are noted in the infant from the dosage increase.

Dialysis

WHAT TO KNOW: LITHIUM USE DURING HEMODIALYSIS

- A small number of patients may continue lithium while receiving dialysis due to inadequate response to other medications or unique properties of lithium (reduction in suicidality).
- The literature is modest in this area, but indicates that most patients are managed with doses of lithium carbonate ranging from 300 to 600 mg administered following each dialysis session.
- In patients commencing dialysis, obtain a trough serum lithium level prior to each of the three dialysis sessions starting the 2nd week. Adjust the lithium dose to maintain trough levels in the midpoint of the therapeutic range (approximately 0.6–0.8 mEq/l), if tolerated.
- With a short period of frequent monitoring, the trough level and dosing regimen which best suits that patient will become evident.

As eGFR declines significantly, there may be rare patients who have a reason to stay on lithium and who have the cognitive, physical and support resources needed to withstand the demands of dialysis (see Chapter 5, Info Box 5.3) [20, 25]. The greatest challenge in these patients is to solve the pharmacokinetic riddle posed by the intermittent nature of dialysis, and thereby balance efficacy and tolerability. The literature in this area is sparse, comprising 18 total cases, but a 2022 systematic review which covered in detail the treatment course in these 18 patients commented that lithium was clearly effective in all 18 patients, with some demonstrating rapid improvement after initiation, and with 96% able to remain on lithium throughout dialysis treatment that ranged from weeks to 3 years [51]. Since dialysis patients have minimal residual renal function, lithium's elimination $T_{1/2}$ is estimated to exceed 100 hours between dialysis sessions, although the true value is unknown [51]. Maximal serum lithium concentrations are approximately 30% higher than trough levels immediately prior to the next dialysis session, and clinicians will initially make dosing decisions based on predialysis trough levels. The complicating kinetic issues relate to the fact that, during hemodialysis, lithium's elimination $T_{1/2}$ is approximately 1 h, but redistribution following dialysis can make levels less predictable between sessions in certain instances. As an ion, lithium is rapidly distributed via body water into the extracellular fluid following GI absorption, and then slowly into the intracellular compartment over the ensuing 5–10 days

[51]. Dialysis removes 80% of extracellular lithium over a period of hours, but the equilibration process driving lithium across its concentration gradient from intracellular stores back into serum is slow, usually necessitating a lithium dose following each dialysis session. There are, however, interindividual differences in the rate of this postdialysis rebound in serum lithium levels and in the extent of any postdialysis diuresis that promotes further lithium clearance. There are other factors influencing lithium kinetics in dialysis patients, including the type of dialysate itself (e.g. acetate, bicarbonate), dialysis frequency (every 48 h vs. every 72 h), and the type of dialysis (peritoneal vs. hemodialysis) [51]. While multiple factors influence the predialysis serum lithium level, in most patients steady state is achieved within a week following the initiation of dialysis. In the 2022 review, most patients ended up on oral doses of lithium carbonate in the range of 300–600 mg administered following dialysis. Based on the available case data, a practical method for determining an individual patient's lithium requirement is straightforward (Info Box 7.8).

Info Box 7.8 A Method for Determining Lithium Dosing Requirements During Ongoing Dialysis

a. During the first 2 weeks of dialysis, maintain the patient (if possible) on a fixed dose of lithium carbonate (e.g. 300 mg, 450 mg or 600 mg), administered immediately after each dialysis session. If adverse effects arise during the next 1–2 weeks, reduce the dose.

b. Obtain a trough serum lithium level on a stable oral lithium dose prior to each of the three dialysis sessions starting in the 2nd week. Adjust the lithium dose to maintain trough levels in the midpoint of the therapeutic range (approximately 0.6–0.8 mEq/l), if tolerated.

c. If the dose required to place the trough concentration in the maintenance range results in nausea or diarrhea, use the strategies discussed in Chapter 5 (e.g. extended release forms for nausea, food to mitigate nausea or diarrhea). If adverse effects seem related to high peak lithium levels from the single postdialysis dose (e.g. excessive tremor, somnolence, ataxia, myoclonus, etc.), check the serum lithium level on two successive postdialysis days to look for evidence that postdialysis diuresis is causing more rapid lithium clearance in these individuals. In those instances, develop a plan to administer a small lithium dose between dialysis sessions while lowering the postdialysis dose so as to mitigate peak dose (and peak serum level) effects.

d. As many dialysis patients are 60 and above, consideration should be given to using the very low end of the maintenance range (0.4–0.6 mEq/l) due to greater age-related brain penetration of lithium in these individuals, assuming that these levels maintain psychiatric stability.

With a short period of frequent monitoring on a stable oral dose, each patient's kinetic profile will be clear, as will the trough level and dosing regimen which best suits that patient. Among the 18 cases reviewed, 3 patients required daily lithium dosing to better control symptoms and manage the effects of postdialysis diuresis, and 2 patients who were nonadherent with oral therapy had lithium added directly to their dialysate. The 2022 review reported that predialysis lithium levels ranged from 0.3 to 1.3 mEq/l in patients under age 60, and 0.5 to 0.9 mEq/l in patients age ≥ 60 years [51]. Creative and flexible approaches will be necessary in some patients if the standard postdialysis thrice weekly dosing is not ideal, but most patients should be able to tolerate lithium regardless of dosing frequency. Rates of adverse effects among the 18 cases were modest and included thirst (n = 1), elevated serum parathyroid hormone (PTH) and decreased serum calcium (n = 1), somnolence and slurred speech (n = 1), vomiting and myoclonic twitching (n = 1), and ataxia which led to lithium discontinuation (n = 1). Somnolence, slurred speech, myoclonus and ataxia clearly represent symptoms of lithium toxicity that should be manageable by reduction of the postdialysis dose and use of smaller between-dialysis doses to minimize peak dose effects [120, 121]. Elevated PTH and serum calcium may be related to renal dysfunction itself, and also manageable with a calcimimetic agent (e.g. cinacalcet) [122, 123]. Patients who have no other options and for whom lithium has demonstrated unique efficacy need not have lithium withdrawn due to the need for dialysis. Management of such cases requires cooperation from all involved clinicians to obtain levels and communicate about adverse effects, but with diligent and frequent predialysis and postdialysis lithium level monitoring during the early phases of treatment, and the correlation of these levels with response and adverse effects, a clinician can quickly establish the pattern of dosing for each dialysis patient.

 Summary Points

a. Older patients can be maintained on lithium safely, with the laboratory monitoring frequency determined by eGFR, not by age alone. Long-term lithium use decreases dementia rates by 50% in older bipolar disorder patients. The biggest risk for lithium toxicity in this population is the addition of a medication with kinetic interactions, not age itself.

b. Child/adolescent bipolar disorder (CA-BD) is diagnosed based on mood cycling and classic bipolar symptoms, not severe aggression or persistent irritability. Lithium is the only mood stabilizer that is US FDA approved for acute mania and maintenance BD-1 treatment in this population (aged 7–17), with kinetic studies indicating that a daily dose of 25 mg/kg administered on a BID schedule achieves optimal maintenance levels. Lithium monotherapy is not associated with significant weight gain.

c. The latest risk estimates indicate that 1st trimester exposure in lithium treated women is associated with a significantly lower risk for any major congenital malformation (MCM) than previously thought, with a number needed to harm of 37. The risk is dose dependent, but women who need to remain on lithium at a certain dose and serum level for psychiatric stability should not be dissuaded from 1st trimester use, nor encouraged to try lower serum levels in an attempt to minimize MCM risk. eGFR changes throughout pregnancy demand lithium level monitoring and dosage adjustments.

d. Recent additions to the literature on breastfeeding indicate the absence of significant effects in the majority of infants whose maternal levels are < 1.00 mEq/l, with lithium levels barely detectable after the first 2–4 weeks of life. Monitoring of infant lithium levels is important to identify outliers, with the frequency decreasing over time. Inadequate weight gain in the 1st month can occur in 25% of infants, and is manageable by decreasing the amount of breastfeeding and increasing formula supplementation. Clinically significant renal and electrolyte disturbances are not seen in infants, but TSH elevation has been reported. These may be transient, but infant TSH should be monitored periodically along with serum creatinine.

e. Patients who require lithium can be treated while on dialysis once dosing and levels are established utilizing predialysis trough values obtained during the first 1–2 weeks of dialysis treatment. Most of these individuals will receive a modest lithium dosage (e.g. 300–600 mg) administered following each dialysis session (i.e. 3 times per week), but a subset may require more frequent dosing if experiencing significant postdialysis diuresis.

References

1. Goldstein, B. I., Birmaher, B., Carlson, G. A., et al. (2017). The International Society for Bipolar Disorders Task Force report on pediatric bipolar disorder: Knowledge to date and directions for future research. *Bipolar Disord*, 19, 524–543.

2. Singh, M. K., Chang, K. D., Goldstein, B. I., et al. (2020). Isn't the evidence base for pediatric bipolar disorder already sufficient to inform clinical practice? *Bipolar Disord*, 22, 664–665.

3. Baldessarini, R. J., Bolzani, L., Cruz, N., et al. (2010). Onset-age of bipolar disorders at six international sites. *J Affect Disord*, 121, 143–146.

4. Solmi, M., Radua, J., Olivola, M., et al. (2022). Age at onset of mental disorders worldwide: Large-scale meta-analysis of 192 epidemiological studies. *Mol Psychiatry*, 27, 281–295.

5. Van Meter, A. R., Burke, C., Kowatch, R. A., et al. (2016). Ten-year updated meta-analysis of the clinical characteristics of pediatric mania and hypomania. *Bipolar Disord*, 18, 19–32.

6. Findling, R. L., Stepanova, E., Youngstrom, E. A., et al. (2018). Progress in diagnosis and treatment of bipolar disorder among children and adolescents: An international perspective. *Evid Based Ment Health*, 21, 177–181.

7. Comparelli, A., Polidori, L., Sarli, G., et al. (2022). Differentiation and comorbidity of bipolar disorder and attention deficit and hyperactivity disorder in children, adolescents, and adults: A clinical and nosological perspective. *Front Psychiatry*, 13, 949375.

8. Ribeiro-Fernández, M., Díez-Suárez, A. and Soutullo, C. (2019). Phenomenology and diagnostic stability of paediatric bipolar disorder in a Spanish sample. *J Affect Disord*, 242, 224–233.

9. Wozniak, J., DiSalvo, M., Farrell, A., et al. (2022). Long term outcomes of pediatric bipolar-I disorder: A prospective follow-up analysis attending to full syndomatic, subsyndromal and functional types of remission. *J Psychiatr Res*, 151, 667–675.

10. Findling, R. L., McNamara, N. K., Pavuluri, M., et al. (2019). Lithium for the maintenance treatment of bipolar I disorder: A double-blind, placebo-controlled discontinuation study. *J Am Acad Child Adolesc Psychiatry*, 58, 287–296.

11. Sun, A. Y., Woods, S., Findling, R. L., et al. (2019). Safety considerations in the psychopharmacology of pediatric bipolar disorder. *Expert Opin Drug Saf*, 18, 777–794.

12. Stepanova, E. and Findling, R. L. (2017). Psychopharmacology of bipolar disorders in children and adolescents. *Pediatr Clin North Am*, 64, 1209–1222.

13. Duffy, A. and Grof, P. (2018). Lithium treatment in children and adolescents. *Pharmacopsychiatry*, 51, 189–193.

14. Duffy, A., Heffer, N., Goodday, S. M., et al. (2018). Efficacy and tolerability of lithium for the treatment of acute mania in children with bipolar disorder: A systematic review. A report from the ISBD–IGSLi joint task force on lithium treatment. *Bipolar Disord*, 20, 583–593.

15. Velosa, J., Delgado, A., Finger, E., et al. (2020). Risk of dementia in bipolar disorder and the interplay of lithium: A systematic review and meta-analyses. *Acta Psychiatr Scand*, 141, 510–521.

16. Ochoa, E. L. M. (2022). Lithium as a neuroprotective agent for bipolar disorder: An overview. *Cell Mol Neurobiol*, 42, 85–97.

17. De Fazio, P., Gaetano, R., Caroleo, M., et al. (2017). Lithium in late-life mania: A systematic review. *Neuropsychiatr Dis Treat*, 13, 755–766.

18. Findling, R. L., Robb, A., McNamara, N. K., et al. (2015). Lithium in the acute treatment of bipolar I disorder: A double-blind, placebo-controlled discontinuation study. *Pediatrics*, 136, 885–894.

19. Young, R. C., Mulsant, B. H., Sajatovic, M., et al. (2017). GERI-BD: A randomized double-blind controlled trial of lithium and divalproex in the treatment of mania in older patients with bipolar disorder. *Am J Psychiatry*, 174, 1086–1093.

20. Fotso Soh, J., Klil-Drori, S. and Rej, S. (2019). Using lithium in older age bipolar disorder: Special considerations. *Drugs Aging*, 36, 147–154.

21. Lambrichts, S., Detraux, J., Vansteelandt, K., et al. (2021). Does lithium prevent relapse following successful electroconvulsive therapy for major depression? A systematic review and meta-analysis. *Acta Psychiatr Scand*, 143, 294–306.

22. Juurlink, D. N., Mamdani, M. M., Kopp, A., et al. (2004). Drug-induced lithium toxicity in the elderly: A population-based study. *J Am Geriatr Soc*, 52, 794–798.

23. Rej, S., Yu, C., Shulman, K., et al. (2015). Medical comorbidity, acute medical care use in late-life bipolar disorder: A comparison of lithium, valproate, and other pharmacotherapies. *Gen Hosp Psychiatry*, 37, 528–532.

24. Ljubic, N., Ueberberg, B., Grunze, H., et al. (2021). Treatment of bipolar disorders in older adults: A review. *Ann Gen Psychiatry*, 20, 45–55.

25. Golic, M., Aiff, H., Attman, P. O., et al. (2021). Starting lithium in patients with compromised renal function – is it wise? *J Psychopharmacol*, 35, 190–197.

26. Bauer, M. and Gitlin, M. (2016). *The Essential Guide to Lithium Treatment*. Basle: Springer International Publishing AG.

27. Kirkham, E., Skinner, J., Anderson, T., et al. (2014). One lithium level >1.0 mmol/L causes an acute decline in eGFR: Findings from a retrospective analysis of a monitoring database. *BMJ Open*, 4, e006020.

28. Castro, V. M., Roberson, A. M., McCoy, T. H., et al. (2016). Stratifying risk for renal insufficiency among lithium-treated patients: An electronic health record study. *Neuropsychopharmacology*, 41, 1138–1143.

29. Heald, A. H., Holland, D., Stedman, M., et al. (2021). Can we check serum lithium levels less often without compromising patient safety? *BJPsych Open*, 8, e18.

30. Heath, L. J., Billups, S. J., Gaughan, K. M., et al. (2018). Risk factors for utilization of acute care services for lithium toxicity. *Psychiatr Serv*, 69, 671–676.

31. Tsai, S.-Y., Shen, R.-S., Kuo, C.-J., et al. (2020). The association between carotid atherosclerosis and treatment with lithium and antipsychotics in patients with bipolar disorder. *Aust N Z J Psychiatry*, 54, 1125–1134.

32. Chen, P. H., Hsiao, C. Y., Chiang, S. J., et al. (2023). Cardioprotective potential of lithium and role of fractalkine in euthymic patients with bipolar disorder. *Aust N Z J Psychiatry*, 57, 104–114.

33. Moore, C. M., Demopulos, C. M., Henry, M. E., et al. (2002). Brain-to-serum lithium ratio and age: An in vivo magnetic resonance spectroscopy study. *Am J Psychiatry*, 159, 1240–1242.

34. Forester, B. P., Streeter, C. C., Berlow, Y. A., et al. (2009). Brain lithium levels and effects on cognition and mood in geriatric bipolar disorder: A lithium-7 magnetic resonance spectroscopy study. *Am J Geriatr Psychiatry*, 17, 13–23.

35. Machado-Vieira, R., Otaduy, M. C., Zanetti, M. V., et al. (2016). A selective association between central and peripheral lithium levels in remitters in bipolar depression: A 3 T-(7) Li magnetic resonance spectroscopy study. *Acta Psychiatr Scand*, 133, 214–220.

36. Delgado, C., Baweja, M., Crews, D. C., et al. (2021). A unifying approach for GFR estimation: Recommendations of the NKF–ASN Task Force on Reassessing the Inclusion of Race in Diagnosing Kidney Disease. *Am J Kidney Dis*, 79, 268–288.e261.

37. Inker, L. A., Eneanya, N. D., Coresh, J., et al. (2021). New creatinine- and cystatin C-based equations to estimate GFR without race. *N Engl J Med*, 385, 1737–1749.

38. Forlenza, O. V., Hajek, T., Almeida, O. P., et al. (2022). Demographic and clinical characteristics of lithium-treated older adults with bipolar disorder. *Acta Psychiatr Scand*, 146, 442–455.

39. Malhi, G. S., Gessler, D. and Outhred, T. (2017). The use of lithium for the treatment of bipolar disorder: Recommendations from clinical practice guidelines. *J Affect Disord*, 217, 266–280.

40. Huybrechts, K. F., Hernandez-Diaz, S., Patorno, E., et al. (2016). Antipsychotic use in pregnancy and the risk for congenital malformations. *JAMA Psychiatry*, 73, 938–946.

41. Imaz, M. L., Torra, M., Soy, D., et al. (2019). Clinical lactation studies of lithium: A systematic review. *Front Pharmacol*, 10, 1005.

42. Newmark, R. L., Bogen, D. L., Wisner, K. L., et al. (2019). Risk–benefit assessment of infant exposure to lithium through breast milk: A systematic review of the literature. *Int Rev Psychiatry*, 31, 295–304.

43. Heinonen, E., Totterman, K., Back, K., et al. (2022). Lithium use during breastfeeding was safe in healthy full-term infants under strict monitoring. *Acta Paediatr*, 111, 1891–1898.

44. Patorno, E., Huybrechts, K. F., Bateman, B. T., et al. (2017). Lithium use in pregnancy and the risk of cardiac malformations. *NEJM*, 376, 2245–2254.

45. Deb, S., Austin, P. C., Tu, J. V., et al. (2016). A review of propensity-score methods and their use in cardiovascular research. *Can J Cardiol*, 32, 259–265.

46. Thomas, L., Li, F. and Pencina, M. (2020). Using propensity score methods to create target populations in observational clinical research. *JAMA*, 323, 466–467.

47. Kessing, L. V., Gerds, T. A., Feldt-Rasmussen, B., et al. (2015). Use of lithium and anticonvulsants and the rate of chronic kidney disease: A nationwide population-based study. *JAMA Psychiatry*, 72, 1182–1191.

48. Nolen, W. A., Licht, R. W., Young, A. H., et al. (2019). What is the optimal serum level for lithium in the maintenance treatment of bipolar disorder? A systematic review and recommendations from the ISBD/IGSLI Task Force on treatment with lithium. *Bipolar Disord*, 21, 394–409.

49. Fornaro, M., Maritan, E., Ferranti, R., et al. (2020). Lithium exposure during pregnancy and the postpartum period: A systematic review and meta-analysis of safety and efficacy outcomes. *Am J Psychiatry*, 177, 76–92.

50. Werneke, U., Ott, M., Renberg, E. S., et al. (2012). A decision analysis of long-term lithium treatment and the risk of renal failure. *Acta Psychiatr Scand*, 126, 186–197.

51. McGrane, I. R., Omar, F. A., Morgan, N. F., et al. (2022). Lithium therapy in patients on dialysis: A systematic review. *Int J Psychiatry Med*, 57, 187–201.

52. Suetani, S., Whiteford, H. A. and McGrath, J. J. (2015). An urgent call to address the deadly consequences of serious mental disorders. *JAMA Psychiatry*, 72, 1166–1167.

53. Hayes, J. F., Marston, L., Walters, K., et al. (2017). Mortality gap for people with bipolar disorder and schizophrenia: UK-based cohort study 2000–2014. *Br J Psychiatry*, 211, 175–181.

54. Chesney, E., Robson, D., Patel, R., et al. (2021). The impact of cigarette smoking on life expectancy in schizophrenia, schizoaffective disorder and bipolar affective disorder: An electronic case register cohort study. *Schizophr Res*, 238, 29–35.

55. Oakley, P. W., Whyte, I. M. and Carter, G. L. (2001). Lithium toxicity: An iatrogenic problem in susceptible individuals. *Aust N Z J Psychiatry*, 35, 833–840.

56. Puglisi-Allegra, S., Ruggieri, S. and Fornai, F. (2021). Translational evidence for lithium-induced brain plasticity and neuroprotection in the treatment of neuropsychiatric disorders. *Transl Psychiatry*, 11, 366.

57. Haupt, M., Bahr, M. and Doeppner, T. R. (2021). Lithium beyond psychiatric indications: The reincarnation of a new old drug. *Neural Regen Res*, 16, 2383–2387.

58. Almeida, O. P., Singulani, M. P., Ford, A. H., et al. (2022). Lithium and stroke recovery: A systematic review and meta-analysis of stroke models in rodents and human data. *Stroke*, 53, 2935–2944.

59. Amdisen, A. (1977). Serum level monitoring and clinical pharmacokinetics of lithium. *Clin Pharmacokinet*, 2, 73–92.

60. Finley, P. R., Warner, M. D. and Peabody, C. A. (1995). Clinical relevance of drug interactions with lithium. *Clin Pharmacokinet*, 29, 172–191.

61. Tueth, M. J., Murphy, T. K. and Evans, D. L. (1998). Special considerations: Use of lithium in children, adolescents, and elderly populations. *J Clin Psychiatry*, 59, 66–73.

62. Lee, J. H., Adler, C., Norris, M., et al. (2012). 4-T 7Li 3D MR spectroscopy imaging in the brains of bipolar disorder subjects. *Magn Reson Med*, 68, 363–368.

63. Soares, J. C., Boada, F. and Keshavan, M. S. (2000). Brain lithium measurements with (7) Li magnetic resonance spectroscopy (MRS): A literature review. *Eur Neuropsychopharmacol*, 10, 151–158.

64. Luo, H., Chevillard, L., Bellivier, F., et al. (2021). The role of brain barriers in the neurokinetics and pharmacodynamics of lithium. *Pharmacol Res*, 166, 105480.

65. Baldessarini, R. J., Tondo, L., Davis, P., et al. (2006). Decreased risk of suicides and attempts during long-term lithium treatment: A meta-analytic review. *Bipolar Disord*, 8, 625–639.

66. Biederman, J., Wozniak, J., Kiely, K., et al. (1995). CBCL clinical scales discriminate prepubertal children with structured interview-derived diagnosis of mania from those with ADHD. *J Am Acad Child Adolesc Psychiatry*, 34, 464–471.

67. Faedda, G. L., Baldessarini, R. J., Suppes, T., et al. (1995). Pediatric-onset bipolar disorder: A neglected clinical and public health problem. *Harv Rev Psychiatry*, 3, 171–195.

68. Wozniak, J., Biederman, J., Kiely, K., et al. (1995). Mania-like symptoms suggestive of childhood-onset bipolar disorder in clinically referred children. *J Am Acad Child Adolesc Psychiatry*, 34, 867–876.

69. Sandstrom, A., Perroud, N., Alda, M., et al. (2021). Prevalence of attention-deficit/ hyperactivity disorder in people with mood disorders: A systematic review and meta-analysis. *Acta Psychiatr Scand*, 143, 380–391.

70. Kasoff, L. I., Ahn, K., Gochman, P., et al. (2016). Strong treatment response and high maintenance rates of clozapine in childhood-onset schizophrenia. *J Child Adolesc Psychopharmacol*, 26, 428–435.

71. Strakowski, S. M., DelBello, M. P. and Adler, C. M., eds. (2014). *Bipolar Disorder in Youth: Presentation, Treatment and Neurobiology* (1st edn.). New York: Oxford University Press.

72. Redden, L., DelBello, M., Wagner, K. D., et al. (2009). Long-term safety of divalproex sodium extended-release in children and adolescents with bipolar I disorder. *J Child Adolesc Psychopharmacol*, 19, 83–89.

73. Wagner, K. D., Redden, L., Kowatch, R. A., et al. (2009). A double-blind, randomized, placebo-controlled trial of divalproex extended-release in the treatment of bipolar disorder in children and adolescents. *J Am Acad Child Adolesc Psychiatry*, 48, 519–532.

74. Findling, R. L., McNamara, N. K., Gracious, B. L., et al. (2003). Combination lithium and divalproex sodium in pediatric bipolarity. *J Am Acad Child Adolesc Psychiatry*, 42, 895–901.

75. Findling, R. L., McNamara, N. K., Stansbrey, R., et al. (2006). Combination lithium and divalproex sodium in pediatric bipolar symptom re-stabilization. *J Am Acad Child Adolesc Psychiatry*, 45, 142–148.

76. Amerio, A., Russo, D., Miletto, N., et al. (2021). Polypharmacy as maintenance treatment in bipolar illness: A systematic review. *Acta Psychiatr Scand*, 144, 259–276.

77. Glenmark Pharmaceuticals Inc. (2020). *Lithium Carbonate Capsule package insert*. Mahwah, NJ.

78. Amerio, A., Ossola, P., Scagnelli, F., et al. (2018). Safety and efficacy of lithium in children and adolescents: A systematic review in bipolar illness. *Eur Psychiatry*, 54, 85–97.

79. ANI Pharmaceuticals Inc. (2020). *LithoBID package insert*. Baudette, MN.

80. Essential Pharma (2022). *Camcolit Controlled Release product labeling*. Egham, Surrey, UK.

81. **Essential Pharma Limited (2022).** *Priadel Prolonged Release Tablets product labeling.* Birkirkara, Malta.

82. **Findling, R. L., McNamara, N. K., Youngstrom, E. A., et al. (2005).** Double-blind 18-month trial of lithium versus divalproex maintenance treatment in pediatric bipolar disorder. *J Am Acad Child Adolesc Psychiatry*, 44, 409–417.

83. **Geller, B., Luby, J. L., Joshi, P., et al. (2012).** A randomized controlled trial of risperidone, lithium, or divalproex sodium for initial treatment of bipolar I disorder, manic or mixed phase, in children and adolescents. *Arch Gen Psychiatry*, 69, 515–528.

84. **Findling, R. L., Kafantaris, V., Pavuluri, M., et al. (2011).** Dosing strategies for lithium monotherapy in children and adolescents with bipolar I disorder. *J Child Adolesc Psychopharmacol*, 21, 195–205.

85. **Findling, R. L., Kafantaris, V., Pavuluri, M., et al. (2013).** Post-acute effectiveness of lithium in pediatric bipolar disorder. *J Child Adolesc Psychopharmacol*, 23, 80–90.

86. **Shim, S. H. and Kwon, Y. J. (2014).** Adolescent with Tourette syndrome and bipolar disorder: A case report. *Clin Psychopharmacol Neurosci*, 12, 235–239.

87. **Pisano, S., Pozzi, M., Catone, G., et al. (2019).** Putative mechanisms of action and clinical use of lithium in children and adolescents: A critical review. *Curr Neuropharmacol*, 17, 318–341.

88. **Kowatch, R. A., Suppes, T., Carmody, T. J., et al. (2000).** Effect size of lithium, divalproex sodium, and carbamazepine in children and adolescents with bipolar disorder. *J Am Acad Child Adolesc Psychiatry*, 39, 713–720.

89. **Sanchez, M., Lytle, S., Neudecker, M., et al. (2021).** Medication adherence in pediatric patients with bipolar disorder: A systematic review. *J Child Adolesc Psychopharmacol*, 31, 86–94.

90. **Drotar, D., Greenley, R. N., Demeter, C. A., et al. (2007).** Adherence to pharmacological treatment for juvenile bipolar disorder. *J Am Acad Child Adolesc Psychiatry*, 46, 831–839.

91. **Velligan, D. I., Wang, M., Diamond, P., et al. (2007).** Relationships among subjective and objective measures of adherence to oral antipsychotic medications. *Psychiatric Services*, 58, 1187–1192.

92. **Velligan, D. I., Weiden, P. J., Sajatovic, M., et al. (2009).** The expert consensus guideline series: Adherence problems in patients with serious and persistent mental illness. *J Clin Psychiatry*, 70, 1–46.

93. **Yaegashi, H., Kirino, S., Remington, G., et al. (2020).** Adherence to oral antipsychotics measured by electronic adherence monitoring in schizophrenia: A systematic review and meta-analysis. *CNS Drugs*, 34, 579–598.

94. **Meyer, J. M. and Stahl, S. M. (2021).** *The Clinical Use of Antipsychotic Plasma Levels (Stahl's Handbooks).* New York: Cambridge University Press.

95. **Sajatovic, M., Tatsuoka, C., Cassidy, K. A., et al. (2018).** A 6-month, prospective, randomized controlled trial of Customized Adherence Enhancement versus bipolar-specific educational control in poorly adherent individuals with bipolar disorder. *J Clin Psychiatry*, 79, 17m12036 e12031–e12010.

96. **Canales, T., Rodman, S., Conklin, D., et al. (2022).** Combining medication adherence support plus long-acting injectable antipsychotic medication: A post-hoc analysis of 3 pilot studies. *Psychopharmacol Bull*, 52, 41–57.

97. **McVoy, M., Delbello, M., Levin, J., et al. (2022).** A customized adherence enhancement program for adolescents and young adults with suboptimal adherence and bipolar disorder: Trial design and methodological report. *Contemp Clin Trials*, 115, 106729.

98. **Findling, R. L., Landersdorfer, C. B., Kafantaris, V., et al. (2010).** First-dose pharmacokinetics of lithium carbonate in children and adolescents. *J Clin Psychopharmacol*, 30, 404–410.

99. Landersdorfer, C. B., Findling, R. L., Frazier, J. A., et al. (2017). Lithium in paediatric patients with bipolar disorder: Implications for selection of dosage regimens via population pharmacokinetics/pharmacodynamics. *Clin Pharmacokinet*, 56, 77–90.

100. Viguera, A. C., Tondo, L., Koukopoulos, A. E., et al. (2011). Episodes of mood disorders in 2,252 pregnancies and postpartum periods. *Am J Psychiatry*, 168, 1179–1185.

101. Viguera, A. C., Whitfield, T., Baldessarini, R. J., et al. (2007). Risk of recurrence in women with bipolar disorder during pregnancy: Prospective study of mood stabilizer discontinuation. *Am J Psychiatry*, 164, 1817–1824.

102. Deiana, V., Chillotti, C., Manchia, M., et al. (2014). Continuation versus discontinuation of lithium during pregnancy: A retrospective case series. *J Clin Psychopharmacol*, 34, 407–410.

103. Diav-Citrin, O., Shechtman, S., Tahover, E., et al. (2014). Pregnancy outcome following in utero exposure to lithium: A prospective, comparative, observational study. *Am J Psychiatry*, 171, 785–794.

104. Stephens, E. H. and Dearani, J. A. (2022). Ebstein Anomaly – of veils and visions. *JAMA*, 327, 2173–2174.

105. Boyle, B., Garne, E., Loane, M., et al. (2017). The changing epidemiology of Ebstein's anomaly and its relationship with maternal mental health conditions: A European registry-based study. *Cardiology in the Young*, 27, 677–685.

106. Kan, A. C. O., Chan, J. K. N., Wong, C. S. M., et al. (2022). Psychotropic drug utilization patterns in pregnant women with bipolar disorder: A 16-year population-based cohort study. *Eur Neuropsychopharmacol*, 57, 75–85.

107. McCloskey, L. R., Wisner, K. L., Cattan, M. K., et al. (2021). Contraception for women with psychiatric disorders. *Am J Psychiatry*, 178, 247–255.

108. Poels, E. M., Sterrenburg, K., Wierdsma, A. I., et al. (2021). Lithium exposure during pregnancy increases fetal growth. *J Psychopharmacol*, 35, 178–183.

109. Wesseloo, R., Wierdsma, A. I., van Kamp, I. L., et al. (2017). Lithium dosing strategies during pregnancy and the postpartum period. *Br J Psychiatry*, 211, 31–36.

110. Dickens, L. T., Cifu, A. S. and Cohen, R. N. (2019). Diagnosis and management of thyroid disease during pregnancy and the postpartum period. *JAMA*, 321, 1928–1929.

111. Huybrechts, K. F., Palmsten, K., Avorn, J., et al. (2014). Antidepressant use in pregnancy and the risk of cardiac defects. *N Engl J Med*, 370, 2397–2407.

112. Swanson, S. A., Hernandez-Diaz, S., Palmsten, K., et al. (2015). Methodological considerations in assessing the effectiveness of antidepressant medication continuation during pregnancy using administrative data. *Pharmacoepidemiol Drug Saf*, 24, 934–942.

113. Sujan, A. C. (2022). What do we know about in-utero antidepressant exposure, and are these medications safe to use during pregnancy? *Acta Psychiatr Scand*, 145, 541–543.

114. Poels, E. M. P., Schrijver, L., Kamperman, A. M., et al. (2018). Long-term neurodevelopmental consequences of intrauterine exposure to lithium and antipsychotics: A systematic review and meta-analysis. *Eur Child Adolesc Psychiatry*, 27, 1209–1230.

115. Harel, Z., McArthur, E., Hladunewich, M., et al. (2019). Serum creatinine levels before, during, and after pregnancy. *JAMA*, 321, 205–207.

116. Westin, A. A., Brekke, M., Molden, E., et al. (2017). Changes in drug disposition of lithium during pregnancy: A retrospective observational study of patient data from two routine therapeutic drug monitoring services in Norway. *BMJ Open*, 7, e015738.

117. Newton, E. R. and Hale, T. W. (2015). Drugs in breast milk. *Clin Obstet Gynecol*, 58, 868–884.

118. Uguz, F. and Sharma, V. (2016). Mood stabilizers during breastfeeding: A systematic review of the recent literature. *Bipolar Disord*, 18, 325–333.

119. McAllister-Williams, R. H., Baldwin, D. S., Cantwell, R., et al. (2017). British Association for Psychopharmacology consensus guidance on the use of psychotropic medication preconception, in pregnancy and postpartum 2017. *J Psychopharmacol*, 31, 519–552.

120. Caviness, J. N. and Evidente, V. G. (2003). Cortical myoclonus during lithium exposure. *Arch Neurol*, 60, 401–404.

121. Friedman, J. H. (2020). Movement disorders induced by psychiatric drugs that do not block dopamine receptors. *Parkinsonism Relat Disord*, 79, 60–64.

122. Mifsud, S., Cilia, K., Mifsud, E. L., et al. (2020). Lithium-associated hyperparathyroidism. *Br J Hosp Med (Lond)*, 81, 1–9.

123. Pattan, V., Singh, B., Abdelmoneim, S. S., et al. (2021). Lithium-induced hyperparathyroidism: An ill-defined territory. *Psychopharmacol Bull*, 51, 65–71.

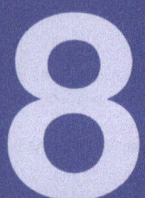

8 Lithium Discontinuation

Advantages of Gradual Tapering; Suicide Risk Following Discontinuation; Efficacy Upon Resumption

PRINCIPLES

- Regardless of bipolar disorder subtype (BD-1, BD-2), gradual discontinuation of lithium (over a minimum of 15–30 days) lengthens the median time to mood episode recurrence approximately 4-fold compared with rapid discontinuation (e.g. over 1–14 days).

- Detailed analyses indicate that rapid discontinuation, stopping for medical reasons, and a BD-1 diagnosis are all significantly and independently associated with early illness recurrence after lithium discontinuation. Longer treatment duration with lithium is not protective.

- Rates of attempted or completed suicides may rise up to 20-fold in the first year after lithium discontinuation. Rapid lithium discontinuation increases this 12-month risk 2-fold compared with a more gradual taper over 15–30 days.

- Lithium appears comparably effective upon resumption after periods of discontinuation, although the time to euthymia may be protracted due to recent mood instability.

INTRODUCTION

WHAT TO KNOW: INTRODUCTION

- Abrupt discontinuation should be avoided and is rarely necessary. Circumstances may arise when there will be strong consideration of lithium discontinuation (e.g. stage G4 chronic kidney disease [CKD]), or when a patient insists on stopping treatment. Gradually tapering lithium over 15–30 days significantly increases the time to mood recurrence.
- Lithium can be reintroduced following discontinuation without loss of efficacy, although patients may suffer from a period of instability until lithium's effects are fully realized.

There are numerous reasons for lithium discontinuation, some patient driven and others motivated by clinician concerns [1]. Focused and early attention to common adverse effects may forestall a certain proportion of somatic complaints leading to lithium refusal, but patients may also stop lithium due to the inconvenience of daily medication; diminished perceived need for lithium during periods of euthymia; a desire to remain in a hypomanic or even manic state (e.g. because they feel more creative or productive, or miss the elevated mood); comparative lack of efficacy for depressive episodes compared with the significant impact on mania; a wish not to be reminded of the illness itself; and not wanting their mood to be regulated by medication [2–4]. While prescribers may employ all of their psychotherapeutic and shared decision-making tools to encourage lithium persistence, oral medication nonadherence is common across all chronic disorders. Despite one's best efforts, there may be little one can do to prevent a patient from self-discontinuing lithium [1]. What remains in the clinician's control is their level of sophistication with use of lithium in patients with medical comorbidity, armed with knowledge of the latest findings indicating that the primary factor in declining estimated glomerular filtration rate (eGFR) in lithium treated patients is the presence of CKD risk factors, assuming that lithium is prescribed using modern precepts (i.e. once daily dosing, 12 h trough maintenance levels ≤ 1.00 mEq/l, and ideally in the range of 0.60–0.80 mEq/l) [5–7].

The idea that older BD patients must be removed from lithium for "safety reasons" is an outdated notion that fails to account for the fact that lithium reduces rates of dementia by 50% in BD spectrum patients [8], that lithium is well tolerated among older patients, and that current clinical practice is to assess renal function and CKD risk based on eGFR and not age, bearing in mind that age is one of two demographic factors used for calculating eGFR [9]. The lack of neuroprotective properties from anticonvulsant mood stabilizers, combined with lithium's robust neuroprotective effects, are compelling reasons to maintain older BD patients on lithium (see Chapter 1) [10]; moreover, recent tolerability and safety data should assuage clinician anxiety about lithium use in this population (also see Chapter 7). Among many papers in this area is a 2021 Dutch study of 135 patients with median age 69 years, of whom only 8.1% had lithium discontinued solely due to adverse effects over a median follow-up of 18 months, with most lithium discontinuations (18.5%) related to psychiatric reasons (lack of efficacy, nonadherence) [11]. Importantly, age, medical comorbidity burden, polypharmacy, renal function and neurological history were not significant predictors of discontinuation due to adverse effects. The authors noted that the overall frequency of lithium discontinuation in their cohort was in line with frequencies reported for younger patients, and stated that older age itself should not be a reason to withhold lithium treatment [11]. Moreover, a study of 1388 older BD-1 patients (age $\geq$ 66 years) documented that, following an inpatient psychiatric hospitalization for mania, the 12-month rates of acute medical care utilization and medical comorbidity were comparable between lithium and valproic acid (VPA) [12]. Even among older patients newly starting lithium (n = 83) with an eGFR at stage G3a or G3b CKD (45–59 ml/min, 30–44 ml/min, respectively), a Swedish study found that a substantial proportion (52%) had limited changes in eGFR over the ensuing 7 years of treatment [9]. Those individuals whose CKD failed to progress after starting lithium had mean baseline eGFR of 54 $\pm$ 15 ml/min and a mean age of 55.5 $\pm$ 16.8 years [9]. As 95% of any sample will be located within 2 standard deviations on either side of the mean, this implies that 47.5% of this cohort had ages in the range of 55.5–89.1 years. Those who experienced further eGFR changes were older (mean age 67.4 $\pm$ 9.9 years) when starting lithium, but also had significantly lower baseline eGFR (42 $\pm$ 11 ml/min) and greater medical comorbidity [9]. Mean lithium level did not distinguish those whose renal function remained stable compared with those whose eGFR declined further. The conclusion from this study is that age is not the sole determinant of further renal risk, and neither is lithium exposure – it is the presence of CKD comorbidities and very low baseline eGFR.

The lithium literature over the past decades has also provided insights into evidence based methods for managing hypothyroidism, hyperparathyroidism and polyuria, thereby obviating reflexive decisions to discontinue lithium if patients develop those adverse effects [13–17]. Moreover, increasing sophistication with the uncommon but potentially serious Brugada syndrome allows many asymptomatic patients diagnosed solely from a screening ECG to remain on lithium. Despite the diagnostic

ECG pattern, provocative electrophysiology with intravenous doses of sodium channel blockers (e.g. ajmaline) often shows limited genetic penetrance for Brugada syndrome, thus permitting use of lithium [18, 19]. As clinicians become more adept at identifying and managing lithium's array of adverse effects, especially those patients who can or should remain on lithium despite low eGFR, there will be a decreasing need to stop lithium for medical conditions or age alone, but discontinuation may be necessary in certain circumstances. What the past three decades of research has shown is that the method of deprescribing lithium can have a tremendous impact on short-term mood stability, regardless of the reason why lithium is being stopped.

Irrespective of BD subtype, studies over the past 30 years have reproducibly found that stopping lithium over 1–14 days accelerates the time to the first mood episode compared with a more gradual taper over 15–30 days [20]. A 1993 study in 64 BD spectrum patients previously stable on lithium monotherapy for an average of 3.6 years found that the hazard ratio (HR) of a new manic episode during the next 12 months was 2.8-fold greater after rapid (< 2 weeks) discontinuation, and rapid discontinuation increased the risk of a depressive episode 5.4-fold [20]. By 1999, there was sufficient literature for a review to examine 28 studies across the mood disorder spectrum (BD, unipolar major depressive disorder [MDD]) and conclude that discontinuing lithium was followed by a sharp increase in morbidity and suicidality in the first year, but that gradual discontinuation markedly reduced, and not merely delayed, recurrences of mania or depression [21]. Although studies dating back to the 1950s demonstrated a 90% reduction in mood episodes during lithium treatment of BD-1 patients, the 1999 review confirmed this finding, noting that during lithium treatment the mood recurrence rate averaged $1.5 \pm 2.4\%$ per month, compared with $26 \pm 34\%$ per month during periods off lithium ($p < 0.001$) [21]. Moreover, in the first year off lithium, rates of serious suicide attempts or completed suicides increased 20-fold, and the rate of suicide related fatalities increased by a factor of 12.6 [22]. Not surprisingly, rapid lithium discontinuation increased the rate of suicidal acts nearly 2-fold compared with a more gradual taper.

The good news for patients who resume lithium is that reintroduction following discontinuation is not associated with significant loss of efficacy [21]. There had been some debate in the literature based on results of two studies published in 1995 [23, 24], but a 2013 review found three trials that disputed this contention [25], and studies as recent as 2022 provide further support for the notion that lithium is equally effective upon resumption [26]. What is clear from naturalistic outcomes in BD-1 patients and from results of lithium discontinuation studies is that many patients may experience significant morbidity after lithium discontinuation even when placed on second generation antipsychotics (SGAs) or other effective mood stabilizers (e.g. VPA, carbamazepine) [26, 27]. That alternative therapies may not be comparably effective for BD spectrum patients, and may not possess lithium's anti-suicidal and neuroprotective properties, are important considerations for any clinician-motivated decision to stop lithium, and should also be conveyed to patients considering lithium discontinuation. While patients typically resume their prior baseline upon recommencing lithium, they may experience further morbidity until euthymia is recaptured, a process that may not occur instantaneously upon restarting lithium [28].

A · Rapid Lithium Discontinuation Increases the Risk for Mood Recurrence

WHAT TO KNOW: THE CONSEQUENCES OF RAPID LITHIUM DISCONTINUATION

- There are three important variables associated with early mood recurrence in the 12 months following lithium discontinuation: rapid lithium withdrawal ($\leq$ 14 days) (odds ratio [OR] 4.27), BD-1 subtype (OR 5.19) and having lithium stopped for medical reasons (OR 4.98).
- In the first 12 months after lithium is discontinued, 67% of BD patients experience a mood recurrence, and rates of suicidal behavior increase markedly, up to 20-fold, but diminish significantly after the first year.

The initial finding of the 1993 study that rapid lithium discontinuation over 1–14 days significantly influenced the time to mood recurrence and frequency of subsequent mood episodes in BD was an unexpected outcome that demanded replication, especially as the sample size was modest (n = 64) [20]. That gradually stopping lithium over 15–28 days would have such a marked differential effect was not easily explained, and to some extent remains incompletely understood aside from general explanations that a more gradual loss of lithium's homeostatic properties might permit more time for development of adaptive cellular processes [21]. A 1996 study of 161 BD patients on lithium 4.2 ± 3.1 years was the next publication to examine the differential effects of discontinuing treatment abruptly (1–14 days) or gradually (15–30 days), and the investigators also found that gradual discontinuation reduced the median time to mood recurrence 5-fold (gradual 20.0 ± 5.8 months vs. rapid 4.0 ± 0.7 months; $p < 0.0001$) [29]. In addition, the median time in remission for the rapidly discontinued cohort was 2.3 times shorter than their mean cycling interval before lithium (6.3 vs. 14.6 months; $p < 0.0001$). Patients also remained stable over the next 3 years off lithium 20 times more frequently after gradual than rapid discontinuation (37% vs. 1.8%; $p < 0.0001$) [29].

A 1997 study in 78 BD spectrum patients came to the same conclusions. When lithium treatment was discontinued rapidly over 1–14 days the median time to any mood recurrence was 2.5 months, but was 5.6 times longer (14.0 months) following gradual discontinuation over 15–30 days [30]. Lastly, a much larger study examined symptom trajectory over the first year after lithium discontinuation in 300 clinically stable BD spectrum patients. The principal reason for lithium discontinuation (51%) was patient decision to stop treatment based on clinical stability. In the first 12 months after lithium was removed, 67% experienced a mood recurrence, and rates of suicidal behavior increased 20-fold, although the extent of suicidal behavior diminished significantly after month 12 [22]. Suicide related fatalities were also 14 times more frequent after discontinuation of lithium. Replicating a finding from prior studies, early mood recurrence was 2.5-fold lower, and suicidal risk was 2.0-fold lower, after slow ($\geq$ 15 days) vs. rapid (1–14 days) discontinuation of lithium [22].

Table 8.1 Multivariable logistic regression model of time to first mood episode among 200 BD patients following discontinuation of lithium carbonate [31]

Factor	Odds ratio [95% CI]	p value
Rapid (1–14 days) vs. gradual ($\geq$ 2 weeks) lithium discontinuation	4.27 [2.26–8.08]	< 0.0001
Medical reason for stopping lithium	4.98 [2.36–10.5]	< 0.0001
BD-1 (vs. BD-2) subtype	2.04 [1.10–3.76]	0.02
Years of lithium treatment	1.00 [0.99–1.01]	0.70

(Adapted from: R. J. Baldessarini, M. Pinna, M. Contu, et al. [2022]. Risk factors for early recurrence after discontinuing lithium in bipolar disorder. *Bipolar Disord*, 24, 720–725.)

In an attempt to quantify factors that increase risk for mood recurrence during the first 12 months after stopping lithium, a 2022 publication analyzed data from 227 BD spectrum patients [31]. Consistent with other studies, the mean latency to any new mood episode was 11.7 months. In a multivariable logistic regression model that looked at numerous variables including patient demographics, duration of lithium use and mood stability on lithium (as measured by mood episodes per year), BD subtype (BD-1 vs. BD-2), rapid vs. gradual discontinuation, and reason for discontinuing lithium, only three factors were significantly and independently associated with early mood recurrence during the next 12 months: rapid lithium withdrawal (odds ratio [OR] 4.27), BD-1 subtype (OR 5.19) and, importantly, having lithium stopped for medical reasons (OR 4.98) (Table 8.1) [31]. The median time to a first new episode was 4.0 months after rapid vs. 13.0 months after gradual discontinuation (p < 0.0001) (Figure 8.1). Duration of prior lithium treatment did not modify this effect in the final logistic regression model. This study reinforces that stopping lithium for medical reasons should be a deliberate, well-informed decision that might require consultation with a psychopharmacologist who can help determine the feasibility of managing the patient on lithium (Info Box 8.1). In instances where lithium is to be discontinued due to patient or clinician decision, this should proceed gradually over a minimum of 15–30 days to lessen the risk of abrupt destabilization due to the independent effect of rapid lithium withdrawal, even if other mood stabilizing therapies have already been added.

Figure 8.1 Kaplan–Meier survival analysis of time to first mood episode among 200 BD patients following gradual discontinuation of lithium carbonate (over ≥ 2 weeks; n = 95) vs. rapid discontinuation (1–14 days; n = 105) [31]

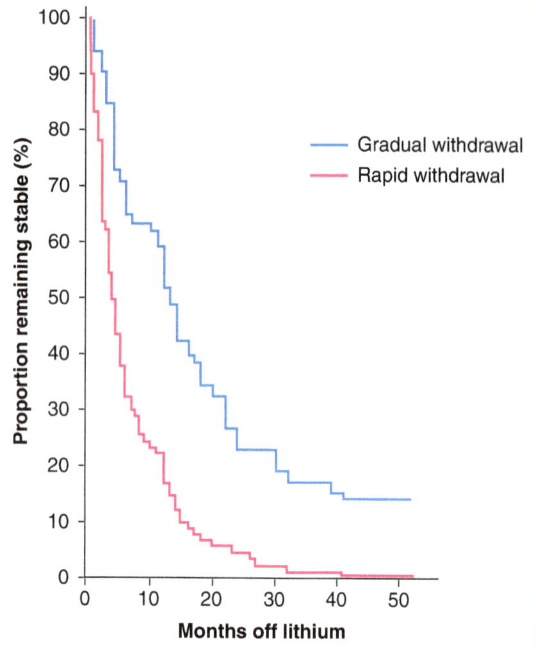

(Adapted from: R. J. Baldessarini, M. Pinna, M. Contu, et al. [2022]. Risk factors for early recurrence after discontinuing lithium in bipolar disorder. *Bipolar Disord*, 24, 720–725.)

Info Box 8.1 Concerns When Considering Discontinuing Lithium for Medical Reasons

a. Does the patient have a compelling reason to remain on lithium?

i. Is there evidence of therapeutic failure on non-lithium therapies? Alternative treatments may not be equally efficacious for many BD patients [27, 32, 33]. Lack of adequate effectiveness during prior trials of non-lithium therapies, particularly suicide attempts during periods when receiving other treatments, when the patient was nonadherent with lithium or when lithium was held, all present compelling reasons why remaining on lithium is a prudent course of action. (If lithium is stopped due to renal dysfunction, see Chapter 5, Info Box 5.3, for thoughts specific to management of CKD, and the feasibility of lithium use with low eGFR or during dialysis.)

ii. Is the patient a capable decision maker? In instances where there is doubt about the patient's cognitive abilities, a formal cognitive assessment may be necessary to decide whether a conservator must be appointed to assist with decisions. This is especially true when there is concern that the patient does not fully appreciate the medical consequences or burdens of stopping or continuing lithium treatment.

b. Does the patient have a strong preference for remaining on lithium? Despite the availability of feasible alternative treatments for certain individuals, some patients may be unwilling to consider other options due to the longstanding nature of their stability on lithium, negative experiences with non-lithium treatments, cognitive impairment, or significant underestimation of the burdens imposed by dialysis. As noted above, a competency assessment may be necessary in certain circumstances.

c. Does the patient's medical status preclude use of other evidence based options? Although no one medication may be equivalent to lithium as BD monotherapy, BD-1 patients have better outcomes when on a mood stabilizer compared with antipsychotic monotherapy, with divalproex and carbamazepine having ample data for BD maintenance [27, 33]. Even if the patient's medical condition permits anticonvulsant mood stabilizers, use of lithium may still be appealing in certain circumstances, and possibly offers greater efficacy.

 Psychiatric Course after Lithium Discontinuation and a Switch to Other Medications

 WHAT TO KNOW: PSYCHIATRIC COURSE AFTER LITHIUM DISCONTINUATION AND A SWITCH TO OTHER MEDICATIONS

- Following a switch from lithium to other agents, naturalistic data sets show that restarting lithium was associated with better outcomes than remaining on VPA or any other mood stabilizer monotherapy. Moreover, patients on quetiapine and olanzapine monotherapy had higher hospitalization risk compared with those not on antipsychotics.

Regardless of the reason for discontinuation, the fate of a patient who stops lithium presents three areas of concern: (a) that patients will experience short-term morbidity and possible mortality since non-lithium options may not be therapeutically equivalent; (b) that, even among eventual responders, there may be significant difficulty in restoring a patient to their clinical baseline; and (c) that patients may no longer respond after reinitiating lithium [28]. Until we have robust biomarkers of future treatment response for the complete array of BD related medications, the first issue will never disappear, but a 2022 study of BD outcomes following lithium discontinuation emphasizes that other treatments may not be equally effective [26]. Using three Finnish national health-care registers (1987–2018), the authors identified all individuals with a BD spectrum diagnosis who had used lithium for at least 1 year and for whom lithium use ended due to reasons other than death or hospitalization. After excluding those with a concurrent schizophrenia spectrum diagnosis, the sample totaled 4052 individuals with a median 2.7 years of lithium use before discontinuation [26]. Medication options were compared within class (e.g. mood stabilizers to nonuse of mood stabilizers), and the outcome measures included psychiatric hospitalization or all cause treatment failure (psychiatric hospitalization, death or change in medication). The mean length of follow-up was 8.9 ± 6.2 years from lithium discontinuation to hospitalization, death or study end. Although the results were not analyzed by BD subtype, the use of mood stabilizers, especially lithium, VPA and carbamazepine, is typically heavily weighted toward BD-1 patients. For the primary outcome of psychiatric hospitalization while on mood stabilizer monotherapy, VPA had lower risk than nonuse of mood stabilizers (HR 0.83, 95% CI 0.71–0.97); however, resumption of lithium was associated with lower risk of all cause treatment failure (HR 0.82, 95% CI 0.76–0.88) than remaining on VPA or any other mood stabilizer monotherapy (Figure 8.2) [26]. Moreover, quetiapine and olanzapine monotherapy were associated with increased hospitalization risk compared with antipsychotic nonuse, echoing naturalistic studies in BD-1 patients demonstrating greater treatment failure on antipsychotic monotherapy [27]. It is worth noting that the use of a long-acting injectable (LAI) antipsychotic or one specific oral antipsychotic (chlorprothixene) was associated with lower hospitalization rates than antipsychotic nonuse in the Finnish study, indicating that certain antipsychotics can keep BD patients out of the hospital, although they may not completely address the full mood spectrum of the bipolar illness. This study and others emphasize the need to avoid anticonvulsant agents with no proven benefit for acute mania or BD maintenance when lithium is withdrawn (e.g. gabapentin, oxcarbazepine, topiramate) [32–37]. Gabapentin is of particular concern as ongoing use in BD patients is associated with a 2-fold increased risk of completed suicide [38–40].

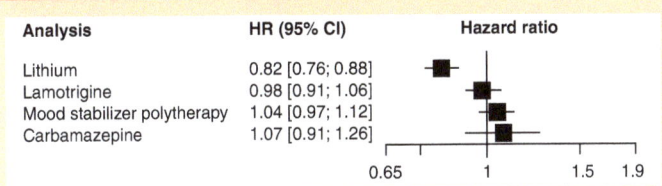

Figure 8.2 Using valproate as the reference, a within-individual Cox regression analysis of treatment failure with mood stabilizer monotherapy following lithium discontinuation shows that resumption of lithium is superior to trying other options [26]

Analysis	HR (95% CI)	Hazard ratio
Lithium	0.82 [0.76; 0.88]	
Lamotrigine	0.98 [0.91; 1.06]	
Mood stabilizer polytherapy	1.04 [0.97; 1.12]	
Carbamazepine	1.07 [0.91; 1.26]	

(Adapted from: M. Holm, A. Tanskanen, M. Lahteenvuo, et al. [2022]. Comparative effectiveness of mood stabilizers and antipsychotics in the prevention of hospitalization after lithium discontinuation in bipolar disorder. *Eur Neuropsychopharmacol*, 61, 36–42.)

C Lithium Response after Resumption

WHAT TO KNOW: LITHIUM RESPONSE AFTER RESUMPTION

- Tolerance to lithium's mood stabilizing properties does not occur, and stability of response extends at least to 20 years in long-term follow-up studies.
- Recent studies indicate lithium is equally effective upon resumption in the majority of patients; however, stability may not be instantaneously regained upon restarting lithium, and this fact must be communicated to patients who wish to discontinue lithium.

The question of nonresponse to lithium after resumption is one that has percolated in the literature after two papers appeared in 1995 which noted that certain individuals who were prior responders did not do as well when lithium was restarted [23, 24]. The quality and breadth of the data on this subject are not great, and a 2013 meta-analysis focusing on this issue found only five relevant publications (n = 212), with two studies indicating lithium was less effective after discontinuation and reintroduction, but three studies seeing no decreased effectiveness [25]. Moreover, the pooled odds ratio (OR) for relapse after interruption of lithium treatment compared with continuous treatment was 1.40 (95% CI 0.85–2.31), a result that was not statistically significant (p = 0.19) [25]. This finding is reassuring, and parallels conclusions from other papers indicating that tolerance to lithium's mood stabilizing properties does not appear, and that stability of response extends at least to 20 years in long-term follow-up studies [41]. Although lithium will be effective upon resumption in the vast majority of patients, the price to pay can be a period of prolonged instability. Using a data set of 873 lithium treated subjects in Norrbotten, Sweden, the investigators performed a mirror image outcomes analysis for the cohort of 194 individuals who had clinical data 2 years before and 2 years after lithium discontinuation [28]. In the 2 years after lithium discontinuation, 51% of patients with BD-I/SAD-BT (n = 100) and 46% with BD-2/ other BD (n = 94) were on an alternate mood stabilizer. Despite the use of other medications, the BD-1/SAD-BT subgroup experienced a significant increase in the proportion who required psychiatric admission: 18% in the 2 years prior to lithium discontinuation vs. 56% after discontinuation (p < 0.001); moreover, there was also a significant increase in the total number of admissions in this subgroup: 33 while on lithium vs. 130 after stopping lithium (p < 0.001) [28]. In the subgroup with a prior mania history, the overall increase in admissions was for mania and depression, and this occurred irrespective of lithium reinitiation, reflecting the reality that destabilization due to lithium discontinuation is not always quickly rectified in some patients [28]. It is worth noting that the effect on psychiatric hospitalization was not seen for the BD-2/other BD group. Nonetheless, these recent Swedish and Finnish studies reinforce the importance of addressing adverse effects to decrease the odds of lithium discontinuation, and of managing lithium in patients with CKD or medical comorbidities. These studies also highlight the risk posed by ineffective non-lithium options and the possibility that lithium reinitiation may not immediately restore euthymia and stability [25, 42].

 Summary Points

a. Clinicians can forestall lithium discontinuation by becoming adept at managing adverse effects, and in using lithium among those with medical comorbidities, including CKD.

b. Rapid lithium discontinuation over 1–14 days should be avoided as it increases the risk of early mood recurrence 4-fold compared with a more gradual taper of at least 15–30 days. Rapid lithium discontinuation also doubles the risk for serious suicide attempts and fatalities.

c. Patient decision is a primary reason for lithium discontinuation. Nonetheless, clinicians should communicate that other therapies may not provide equivalent efficacy, especially in areas of suicidality or neuroprotection.

d. Lithium appears equally effective upon resumption, but this effect might not be instantaneous, and that should also be conveyed to patients. The loss of stability is often relatively quick, but achieving euthymia may be more difficult.

References

1. Öhlund, L., Ott, M., Oja, S., et al. (2018). Reasons for lithium discontinuation in men and women with bipolar disorder: A retrospective cohort study. *BMC Psychiatry*, 18, 37–46.

2. Van Putten, T. (1975). Why do patients with manic-depressive illness stop their lithium? *Compr Psychiatry*, 16, 179–183.

3. Jamison, K. R., Gerner, R. H. and Goodwin, F. K. (1979). Patient and physician attitudes toward lithium: Relationship to compliance. *Arch Gen Psychiatry*, 36, 866–869.

4. Vestergaard, P. and Amdisen, A. (1983). Patient attitudes towards lithium. *Acta Psychiatr Scand*, 67, 8–12.

5. Kirkham, E., Skinner, J., Anderson, T., et al. (2014). One lithium level > 1.0 mmol/L causes an acute decline in eGFR: Findings from a retrospective analysis of a monitoring database. *BMJ Open*, 4, e006020.

6. Clos, S., Rauchhaus, P., Severn, A., et al. (2015). Long-term effect of lithium maintenance therapy on estimated glomerular filtration rate in patients with affective disorders: A population-based cohort study. *Lancet Psychiatry*, 2, 1075–1083.

7. Castro, V. M., Roberson, A. M., McCoy, T. H., et al. (2016). Stratifying risk for renal insufficiency among lithium-treated patients: An electronic health record study. *Neuropsychopharmacology*, 41, 1138–1143.

8. Velosa, J., Delgado, A., Finger, E., et al. (2020). Risk of dementia in bipolar disorder and the interplay of lithium: A systematic review and meta-analyses. *Acta Psychiatr Scand*, 141, 510–521.

9. Golic, M., Aiff, H., Attman, P. O., et al. (2021). Starting lithium in patients with compromised renal function – is it wise? *J Psychopharmacol*, 35, 190–197.

10. Gerhard, T., Devanand, D. P., Huang, C., et al. (2015). Lithium treatment and risk for dementia in adults with bipolar disorder: Population-based cohort study. *Br J Psychiatry*, 207, 46–51.

11. Flapper, M., van Melick, E., van Campen, J., et al. (2021). Tolerability of lithium: A naturalistic discontinuation study in older inpatients (≥ 60 years). *Int J Geriatr Psychiatry*, 36, 1231–1240.

12. Rej, S., Yu, C., Shulman, K., et al. (2015). Medical comorbidity, acute medical care use in late-life bipolar disorder: A comparison of lithium, valproate, and other pharmacotherapies. *Gen Hosp Psychiatry*, 37, 528–532.

13. Kinahan, J. C., NiChorcorain, A., Cunningham, S., et al. (2015). Diagnostic accuracy of tests for polyuria in lithium-treated patients. *J Clin Psychopharmacol*, 35, 434–441.

14. Schoot, T. S., Molmans, T. H. J., Grootens, K. P., et al. (2020). Systematic review and practical guideline for the prevention and management of the renal side effects of lithium therapy. *Eur Neuropsychopharmacol*, 31, 16–32.

15. Pattan, V., Singh, B., Abdelmoneim, S. S., et al. (2021). Lithium-induced hyperparathyroidism: An ill-defined territory. *Psychopharmacol Bull*, 51, 65–71.

16. Ketteler, M., Bover, J. and Mazzaferro, S. (2022). Treatment of secondary hyperparathyroidism in non-dialysis CKD: An appraisal 2022s. *Nephrol Dial Transplant*. https://doi.org/10.1093/ndt/gfac236.

17. Lerena, V. S., León, N. S., Sosa, S., et al. (2022). Lithium and endocrine dysfunction. *Medicina (B Aires)*, 82, 130–137.

18. Brugada, J., Campuzano, O., Arbelo, E., et al. (2018). Present status of Brugada Syndrome: JACC state-of-the-art review. *J Am Coll Cardiol*, 72, 1046–1059.

19. Ravi, V., Serafini, N. J., Pulipati, P., et al. (2020). Lithium-induced Brugada pattern: A case report and review of literature. *Cureus*, 12, e9351–e9537.

20. Faedda, G. L., Tondo, L., Baldessarini, R. J., et al. (1993). Outcome after rapid vs gradual discontinuation of lithium treatment in bipolar disorders. *Arch Gen Psychiatry*, 50, 448–455.

21. Baldessarini, R. J., Tondo, L. and Viguera, A. C. (1999). Discontinuing lithium maintenance treatment in bipolar disorders: Risks and implications. *Bipolar Disord*, 1, 17–24.

22. Baldessarini, R. J., Tondo, L. and Hennen, J. (1999). Effects of lithium treatment and its discontinuation on suicidal behavior in bipolar manic-depressive disorders. *J Clin Psychiatry*, 60, 77–84.

23. Koukopoulos, A., Reginaldi, D., Minnai, G., et al. (1995). The long term prophylaxis of affective disorders. *Adv Biochem Psychopharmacol*, 49, 127–147.

24. Maj, M., Pirozzi, R. and Magliano, L. (1995). Nonresponse to reinstituted lithium prophylaxis in previously responsive bipolar patients: Prevalence and predictors. *Am J Psychiatry*, 152, 1810–1811.

25. de Vries, C., van Bergen, A., Regeer, E. J., et al. (2013). The effectiveness of restarted lithium treatment after discontinuation: Reviewing the evidence for discontinuation-induced refractoriness. *Bipolar Disord*, 15, 645–649.

26. Holm, M., Tanskanen, A., Lahteenvuo, M., et al. (2022). Comparative effectiveness of mood stabilizers and antipsychotics in the prevention of hospitalization after lithium discontinuation in bipolar disorder. *Eur Neuropsychopharmacol*, 61, 36–42.

27. Wingård, L., Brandt, L., Bodén, R., et al. (2019). Monotherapy vs. combination therapy for post mania maintenance treatment: A population based cohort study. *Eur Neuropsychopharmacol*, 29, 691–700.

28. Öhlund, L., Ott, M., Bergqvist, M., et al. (2019). Clinical course and need for hospital admission after lithium discontinuation in patients with bipolar disorder type I or II: Mirror-image study based on the LiSIE retrospective cohort. *BJPsych Open*, 5, e101–112.

29. Baldessarini, R. J., Tondo, L., Faedda, G. L., et al. (1996). Effects of the rate of discontinuing lithium maintenance treatment in bipolar disorders. *J Clin Psychiatry*, 57, 441–448.

30. Baldessarini, R. J., Tondo, L., Floris, G., et al. (1997). Reduced morbidity after gradual discontinuation of lithium treatment for bipolar I and II disorders: A replication study. *Am J Psychiatry*, 154, 551–553.

31. Baldessarini, R. J., Pinna, M., Contu, M., et al. (2022). Risk factors for early recurrence after discontinuing lithium in bipolar disorder. *Bipolar Disord*, 24, 720–725.

32. Lahteenvuo, M., Tanskanen, A., Taipale, H., et al. (2018). Real-world effectiveness of pharmacologic treatments for the prevention of rehospitalization in a Finnish nationwide cohort of patients with bipolar disorder. *JAMA Psychiatry*, 75, 347–355.

33. Kishi, T., Ikuta, T., Matsuda, Y., et al. (2021). Mood stabilizers and/or antipsychotics for bipolar disorder in the maintenance phase: A systematic review and network meta-analysis of randomized controlled trials. *Mol Psychiatry*, 26, 4146–4157.

34. Chengappa, K. N. R., Schwarzman, L. K., Hulihan, J. F., et al. (2006). Adjunctive topiramate therapy in patients receiving a mood stabilizer for bipolar I disorder: A randomized, placebo-controlled trial. *J Clin Psychiatry*, 67, 1698–1706.

35. Kushner, S. F., Khan, A., Lane, R., et al. (2006). Topiramate monotherapy in the management of acute mania: Results of four double-blind placebo-controlled trials. *Bipolar Disord*, 8, 15–27.

36. Vasudev, A., Macritchie, K., Watson, S., et al. (2008). Oxcarbazepine in the maintenance treatment of bipolar disorder. *Cochrane Database Syst Rev*, CD005171.

37. Kishi, T., Ikuta, T., Matsuda, Y., et al. (2022). Pharmacological treatment for bipolar mania: A systematic review and network meta-analysis of double-blind randomized controlled trials. *Mol Psychiatry*, 27, 1136–1144.

38. Pande, A. C., Crockatt, J. G., Janney, C. A., et al. (2000). Gabapentin in bipolar disorder: A placebo-controlled trial of adjunctive therapy. Gabapentin Bipolar Disorder Study Group. *Bipolar Disord*, 2, 249–255.

39. Fullerton, C. A., Busch, A. B. and Frank, R. G. (2010). The rise and fall of gabapentin for bipolar disorder: A case study on off-label pharmaceutical diffusion. *Medical Care*, 48, 372–379.

40. Leith, W. M., Lambert, W. E., Boehnlein, J. K., et al. (2019). The association between gabapentin and suicidality in bipolar patients. *Int Clin Psychopharmacol*, 34, 27–32.

41. Berghöfer, A., Alda, M., Adli, M., et al. (2013). Stability of lithium treatment in bipolar disorder – long-term follow-up of 346 patients. *Int J Bipolar Disord*, 1, 11–18.

42. Orsolini, L., Pompili, S. and Volpe, U. (2020). The "collateral side" of mood stabilizers: Safety and evidence-based strategies for managing side effects. *Expert Opin Drug Saf*, 19, 1461–1495.

Index

For EU product safety concerns, contact us at Calle de José Abascal, 56–1°, 28003 Madrid, Spain or eugpsr@cambridge.org.

www.ingramcontent.com/pod-product-compliance
Ingram Content Group UK Ltd.
Pitfield, Milton Keynes, MK11 3LW, UK
UKHW020432181225
466164UK00003B/187